Contents

KU-677-539

Foreword from our partners

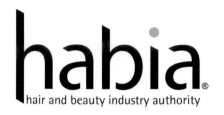

Nothing stands still; and this is certainly true in the world of professional beauty. The ongoing advances in technology in this exciting and dynamic industry lead to new products, equipment and treatment techniques which mean new therapists need a book that reflects these changes to prepare them to meet the standards required by industry, their future employers and clients.

As one would expect from the number one beauty author, Lorraine Nordmann has taken all the advances and incorporated them in this superb book that reflects industry expectations, best practice with a strong focus on client care and professional attitudes.

Lorraine is never one for holding back, and her sense of understanding the complexity of the industry shows by the way she has the ability to write in an engaging style; keeping the content simple yet making you feel that her considerable knowledge and experience are at your fingertips and you're fired up ready to go. Lorraine has excelled herself again, making sure that this edition will be well read and will leave a lasting impression on what the industry requirements are.

Jo Goodman
Habia

About VTCT

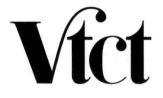

VTCT is a government approved specialist awarding organisation responsible for qualifications in the beauty therapy, complementary therapy, hairdressing, sports, fitness, hospitality and catering sectors.

VTCT has been in existence for over 50 years, and in fact it was VTCT who originally coined the phrase *Beauty Therapy*. VTCT has remained at the forefront of developing the vocational system of qualifications in the UK and internationally.

VTCT invests in many charitable projects which support education and training in the beauty therapy industry. VTCT is the main sponsor and organiser of Worldskills UK (Beauty Therapy competitions) and VTCT also fund the development of the European and British Standard for Beauty Salon Services. In addition, VTCT donates charitable funds to disfigurement charities, prison education and other worthwhile causes linked to the beauty therapy sector.

VTCT has the widest and most diverse range of qualifications in the beauty industry and is leading on many new initiatives in technical and professional education, including qualification and apprenticeship reforms, online assessment and innovative teaching and learning programmes.

VTCT develops innovative, fit for purpose qualifications via beauty therapy technical expert panels made up of employers, industry experts and educationalists from all over the UK.

HABIA SERIES LIST

Beauty therapy

Beauty Basics: The Official Guide to Level 1 Revised 3e *Lorraine Nordmann*

Beauty Therapy – The Foundations: 7e *Lorraine Nordmann*

Professional Beauty Therapy – Level 3 5e *Lorraine Nordmann*

The Complete Make-up Artist, 3e: *Penny Delamar*

The Pocket Guide to Key Terms for Beauty Therapy *Lorraine Nordmann and Marian Newman*

The Complete Guide to Make-up 1e *Suzanne Le Quesne*

The Encyclopedia of Nails 2e *Jacqui Jefford and Anne Swain*

The Art of Nails: A Comprehensive Style Guide to Nail Treatments and Nail Art 1e *Jacqui Jefford*

The Complete Nail Technician 3e *Marian Newman*

Manicure, Pedicure and Advanced Nail Techniques 1e *Elaine Almond*

An Holistic Guide to Reflexology 1e *Tina Parsons*

SPA: The Official Guide to Spa Therapy at Levels 2 and 3 *Joan Scott and Andrea Harrison*

Nutrition: A Practical Approach 1e *Suzanne Le Quesne*

Hands on Sports Therapy 1e *Keith Ward*

The Anatomy and Physiology Workbook: For Beauty and Holistic Therapies Levels 1–3 *Tina Parsons*

The Anatomy and Physiology CD-Rom

The Official Guide to the Diploma in Hair and Beauty Studies at Foundation Level 1e *Jane Goldsbro and Elaine White*

The Official Guide to the Diploma in Hair and Beauty Studies at Higher Level 1e *Jane Goldsbro and Elaine White*

Hairdressing

Begin Hairdressing: The Official Guide to Level 1 3e *Martin Green*

Hairdressing – The Foundations: The Official Guide to Level 2 Revised 7e *Leo Palladino and Martin Green*

Professional Hairdressing: The Official Guide to Level 3 7e *Martin Green and Leo Palladino*

The Pocket Guide to Key Terms for Hairdressing *Martin Green*

eXtensions: The Official Guide to Hair Extensions 1e *Theresa Bullock*

Salon Management *Martin Green*

Men's Hairdressing: Traditional and Modern Barbering 3e *Maurice Lister*

Hairdressing for African & Curly Hair Types From a Cross-Cultural Perspective 3e *Sandra Gittens*

The World of Hair Colour 1e *John Gray*

Hair Extensions: Additions and Integrations *Dawn Reilly, author on behalf of Balmain Hair*

Patrick Cameron: Dressing Long Hair 1e *Patrick Cameron and Jacki Wadeson*

Patrick Cameron: Dressing Long Hair 2 1e *Patrick Cameron and Jacki Wadeson*

Professional Men's Hairdressing: The Art of Cutting and Styling 1e *Guy Kremer and Jacki Wadeson*

The Official Guide to Foundation Learning in Hair and Beauty 1e *Jane Goldsbro and Elaine White*

About the author

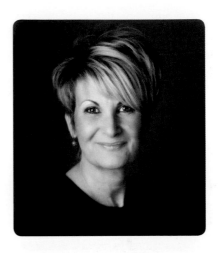

Lorraine Nordmann has over 30 years of experience in the beauty therapy industry and is as enthusiastic today as when she first entered it. This seventh edition of Beauty Therapy: The Foundations aims to share Lorraine's on-going passion and commitment to raising the profile of the industry, now a major employer and significant contributor to the UK economy, with spending on beauty worth an estimated £17 billion.

A note from the author

Providing an inclusive and personalised service that not only meets but exceeds every client's expectation should be the goal for every treatment you deliver. Readers of this book will learn the specific requirements, essential skills, values and behaviours required to meet the latest National Occupational Standards and provide a service to be proud of.

Industry role models share their insight and expertise in each chapter and confirm the importance of the professional standards underpinning everything you do.

I hope this text supports your training in order to qualify and enter this industry as a confident professional beauty therapist.

I wish you every success in your future career.

Lorraine Nordmann

About the book

Throughout this textbook you will find many colourful text boxes designed to aid your learning and understanding as well as highlight key points. Here are examples and descriptions of each:

ROLE MODEL

Lorraine Nordmann, Beauty Therapy Author

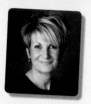

Role model boxes give you an inspirational glance into the knowledge and experience of a trusted industry expert, helping to motivate, guide and support you in your studies.

Products, tools and equipment

◆ Help you prepare for each practical treatment and show you the tools, equipment and products required.

TOP TIP

Shares the author's experience and provides positive suggestions to improve knowledge and skills in each subject.

HEALTH & SAFETY

Draws your attention to related health and safety information essential for each technical skill.

Quotations from role models feature throughout most chapters and provide you with practical and helpful advice.

Lorraine Nordmann

Directional arrows point you to other parts of the book that explore similar or related topics, so you can expand your learning.

Revision aid

Questions to help test your knowledge and understanding as you progress through the book.

ALWAYS REMEMBER

Helpful author insight, advising you on useful points not to forget.

ACTIVITY

Featured in the book to provide additional tasks for you to further your understanding.

ASSESSMENT OF KNOWLEDGE AND UNDERSTANDING

At the end of each chapter there is a useful revision section which has been specially devised to help you check your learning and prepare for your oral and written assessments.

Use these revision sections to test your knowledge as you progress through the course and seek guidance from your supervisor or assessor if you come across any areas that you're unsure of.

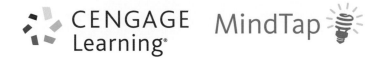
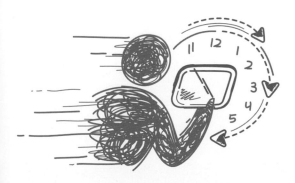

Acknowledgements

The author and publishers would like to thank the following

Elizabeth Rose Whiteside for her ongoing love and support.

Virginia Thorp, for her meticulous professional dedication in the conception and production of this seventh edition of Beauty Therapy: The Foundations.

Pamela Linforth, Human Resources Director at Ellisons, leading supplier of hairdressing and beauty resources, including training.

Marion Main, Tanya Ahmed, Karen Muircroft and Aysha Ahmed for the Asian bridal make-up work and step by step guide.

Marian Newman for her kind permission to use the nail art content.

Laura Holdstock, Centre Training Manager, VTCT.

Tracey James, Development Officer, Habia.

For their contribution as industry role models

Janice Brown	Daniella Norman
Annette Close	Lorraine Onorato
Laura Dicken	Tina Rook
Maureen Evans-Olsen	Andy Rouillard
Marion Main	Shavatah Singh
Marian Newman	Sam Sweet

Credit list

Chapter 1

© Milady, a part of Cengage Learning 11b, 16t; Babtac 19; Cengage Learning 7.1, 7.3, 8.3, 27b, 31m, 53.1, 53.2, 53.3, 53.4, 53.5, 53.6, 53.7, 53.8, 53.9, 53.10, 53.11, 53.12, 56tl, 56tr, 58t, 61b, 70, 75t, 80, 82, 94, 108, 114t, 114b, 115; Cengage Learning /V.Thorp 24; Chubb Fire & Security 41b, 42tl, 42tl2, 42mm, 42ml, 42bm; Collin UK 109b; Courtesy of Dermalogica 96t; Depilex 47 br; Ellisons 10, 28b, 46, 47tl, 47tm, 48, 101m,112; Habia 28t, 98t; HMSO 35tl; HSE 21b, 26b, 28m, 29t, 29b, 30, 31b, 32t, 32b, 34t, 35tr, 37, 38, 45, 51ml, 51mm, 51mr, 56br; Janice Brown 20t; Jessica 98b; Lash Perfect 98m, 99b; Maureen Evans-Olsen 11t; Mii 100, 102, 103; Nathan Portlock Allan Photography/Media Select International for Cengage Learning 7.4, 21t, 27t, 67b, 96b; Phorest Salon Systems 75b; Recycle Now 39t.1, 39t.2, 39t.3, 39m, 39b; Sam Sweet 93t; Shutterstock 7.2, 8.1, 9.1, 9.2, 15, 35b, 58m, 59b, 60, 71, 74r, 76, 79, 81t, 93b, 109t; Simon Jersey 6.1, 52t, 52b; Thalgo 99t; Thinkstock 2, 4, 6.2, 7.5, 8.2, 9.3, 9.4, 16b, 20b, 26t, 34b, 36t, 36b, 40t, 40b, 41t, 47b, 49, 54t, 54b, 57, 58b, 61t, 62, 66, 67t, 69, 72, 74l, 81b, 84, 85, 87, 91, 95l, 95r, 97, 106, 101t, 101b, 106; Tina Rook 59t; VTCT 5; World skills 55

Chapter 2

© Dallas Events Inc., 2008; used under license from Shutterstock.com 195t; © Milady, a part of Cengage Learning 122bm, 123b, 124t, 133, 134, 167b, 172b, 185b, 208t; © Milady, a part of Cengage Learning, photography by Larry Hamill 142; Carlton Beauty and Spa Group 211; Cengage Learning 122br, 123t, 124bl, 124br, 125, 127, 135.1, 135.2, 136.2, 139, 140m, 141, 143t, 144, 145b, 148b, 149t, 150t, 150m, 153t, 153b, 154t, 154b, 155b, 156t, 157, 159b, 160.1, 160.2, 160.3, 160.4, 160.5, 161.1, 161.2, 161.3, 161.4, 161.5, 162, 165t, 165b, 166t, 166b, 167t, 168, 170, 171l, 171r, 172t, 172m, 173, 174, 175t, 175b, 176t, 176m, 176b, 177t, 179, 180t, 180b, 181tr, 181mr, 181bl, 183l1, 183l2, 183l3, 183l4, 183l5, 183l6, 183r1, 183r2, 183r3, 183r4, 183r5, 183r6, 184l1, 184l2, 184l3, 184l4, 184l5, 184l6, 184r1, 184r2, 184r3, 184r4, 184r5, 184r6, 185tl, 185tr, 185ml, 185mr, 187, 188, 189l, 189m, 189r, 191t, 191m, 191b, 192t, 192b, 193t, 193b, 194b, 197l, 198t, 200, 201, 202tl, 202tr, 202m, 202b, 203, 204b, 205, 206m, 206b, 208m, 208b, 210l, 210r, 212, 213, 215, 216l, 216r, 216t, 217m, 218t, 218mr, 218br, 218bl, 219l, 219r; Courtesy of Dermalogica 149b; Dr A L Wright 140b; Dr John Gray, The World of Skin Care 128, 146t, 150b; Dr M H Beck 146b; Hugh Rushton 145t; Nathan Portlock Allan Photography/Media Select International for Cengage Learning 152; Shutterstock 140t, 143b, 169; Shutterstock (MMUTLU) 163l; Thinkstock 120, 122t, 122m, 126, 131t, 131b, 136.1, 137, 147t, 147b, 148m, 149m, 151t, 151b, 155t, 156b, 158, 159t, 163r, 175m, 177b, 178, 182tl, 182bl, 182br, 190, 194t, 195b, 196t, 196b, 197r, 198b, 204t, 206t; Unilever 148t;

Chapter 3

© Milady, a part of Cengage Learning 244.7, 244.8, 245.1, 245.2, 245.3, 245.4, 245.5, 245.6; Cengage Learning 217b, 235, 239, 240; Delmar Cengage Learning 253.3, 259t; DermNet NZ 252.3, 257.3; Dr A L Wright 246.4, 248.2, 249.1, 250.1, 250.2, 252.1, 259m; Dr John Gray, The World of Skin Care 233, 234l, 254b, 257.2, 258t, 260.1, 260.2, 260.3, 260.4; Dr M H Beck 246.1, 254t, 255t, 255m, 255b, 256.2, 257.1, 258b, 259b; Ellisons 232t; Nathan Portlock Allan Photography/Media Select International for Cengage Learning 223t, 226t, 231, 232b, 234m, 234r, 251t, 251b; Permission of The National Cancer Institute 256.3, 256.4; Shutterstock (CLS Design) 248.1; Shutterstock (Eric Fleming Photography) 247.2; Shutterstock (Faiz Zaki) 247.1; Shutterstock (Guentermanaus) 256.1; Shutterstock (Heiko Barth) 246.3;

470.4, 470.5, 470.6, 471t, 473.2, 473.3, 473.4, 473.5, 473.6, 474l.1, 474l.2, 474l.3, 477t, 477b, 483tl, 483tm, 483tr, 483bl, 483bm, 483br, 484tl, 484tm, 484tr, 484bl, 484bm, 484br, 485tl, 485tm, 485tr, 485bl, 485bm, 485br; Korres Natural products 429b; Make-up by www.julianfrancis.co.uk and photography by Thomas Sergeant 478; Marion Main 426, 486tl, 486tm, 486tr, 486bl, 486bm, 486br, 487tl, 487tm, 487tr, 487bl, 487bm, 487br, 488tl, 488tm, 488tr, 488ml, 488mm, 488mr, 488br; Mii 441t, 448t, 448b, 449t, 449m, 457mr, 472m, 472b, 476l.2; Nathan Portlock Allan Photography/ Media Select International for Cengage Learning 427b, 429t, 430t, 433tl, 433tr, 438, 439b, 440t, 440m, 440b, 441m, 441b, 443, 444m, 444b, 446tl, 446tr, 452t, 452b, 455tl, 455tr, 457bl, 458, 461b, 463r.3, 463r.4, 463r.5, 464tm, 464tr, 465tl, 466tr, 467m, 467b, 469t, 472tr, 474b, 475t, 475b, 476tl.1, 476tr, 482t, 482b; Photo used by permission of Iredale Mineral Cosmetics Ltd. 467t, 472tm; Shavata 466tl; Shutterstock 427tl, 427tr, 427m, 456t, 479tl, 479r.1, 479r.2, 479r.3, 479r.4; Thinkstock 424, 428t, 428b, 430b, 432br, 434, 439t, 439m, 442, 463tl, 464bm, 464br, 465tr, 468t, 473.1, 480

Chapter 7

© Habia 498l; © Milady, a part of Cengage Learning 501tl, 501tm, 501ml, 501mm, 501bl, 501bm, 505t, 540t, 548, 575t, 575ml, 575mr, 575b; Beauty Express 500t, 500b, 501mr, 501br, 502br, 523.1, 544t, 544b, 545, 546t, 559r.1, 559r.2, 559r.3, 569l.3, 569l.4, 569l.5, 570, 578m, 579.1, 580l.1, 580l.2, 580l.3, 580b, 581mr, 582tr, 585, 586tm, 586tr, 586b, 587l, 587r, 591l, 591m, 593; Cengage Learning 503t, 504b, 518tl, 518tm, 518tr, 518bl, 518bm, 518br, 519tl, 519tm, 519tr, 519ml, 519mm, 519mr, 519bl, 519bm, 519br, 520tl, 520tm, 520tr, 520ml, 520mm, 520mr, 520bl, 521t, 522t.1, 522t.2, 522t.3, 522t.4, 522t.5, 522m.1, 522m.2, 522m.3, 522bl.1, 522bl.2, 530tl, 530tm, 530tr, 530ml, 530mm, 530mr, 530bl, 530br, 531tl, 531tm, 531tr, 531ml, 531mr, 531bl, 531br, 540b, 553bl, 553bm, 553br, 554tl, 554tm, 554tr, 554ml, 554mm, 554mr, 554bl, 554bm, 554br, 555tl, 555tm, 555tr, 555ml, 555mm, 555mr, 555bl, 555bm, 555br, 556tl, 556tr, 556ml, 556mr, 556b, 557tl, 557tm, 557tr, 557b, 558t, 558m, 562tl, 562tm, 562tr, 562ml, 562mm, 562mr, 562bl, 562bm, 562br, 563tl, 563tm, 563tr, 563bl, 563bm, 563br, 564br, 566, 572, 582m; Courtesy of Mavala 535l, 535r; DermNet NZ 508.1, 509.2, 512.3, 514.3, 550.2, 551.1; Dr A L Wright 507.4, 508.4, 509.3, 510.1, 510.2, 510.3, 511.1, 511.2, 511.3, 512.1, 512.2, 549.2, 549.3, 551.2; Dr John Gray, The World of Skin Care 515; Dr M H Beck 507.3, 509.1; Ellisons 523.2, 524b, 526b, 539, 544mr, 546b, 559r.4, 569l.1, 569l.2, 569r.5, 573t, 577l.1, 577l.2, 578b, 579.2, 579.3, 579.4, 580m, 582tl, 586tl, 586m, 589, 592b; Habia 546m; Jessica 501tr, 565m; Ken Franklin/Video4 Ltd 504m, 538tl, 538bl, 544ml; Laura Dicken 494b; Margaret Dabbs 541b; Marian Newman 494t, 521b, 534, 583l, 583r, 584l, 584m, 584r; Mavala 565b; Nail Delights 569r.1, 569r.2, 569r.4, 569l.6; Nataliya 567b; Nathan Portlock Allan Photography/Media Select International for Cengage Learning 498r, 499, 502mr, 502br, 504t, 505b, 517t, 517b, 523.3, 523.4, 523.5, 524t, 525t, 525m, 525b, 526t, 527, 528tl, 528tm, 528tr, 528ml, 528mm, 528mr, 528bl, 528bm, 528br, 536l, 536m, 536r, 537tl, 537tm, 537tr, 537bl, 537br, 538tm, 538tr, 538br, 542b, 553t, 558b, 559l, 560tl, 560tm, 560tr, 560bl, 560bm, 560br, 564tl, 564tr, 564bl; Salon Systems 565t, 569r.3; Shutterstock 495t, 495b, 497, 506.1, 506.2, 507.1, 507.2, 508.2, 508.3, 508.5, 514.1, 514.2, 532t, 541t, 542t, 543, 549.1, 550.1, 529; Thinkstock 492, 502tr, 503b, 524mr, 524ml, 526m, 532b, 533l, 533r, 550.3, 567t, 567m, 568t, 568b, 571b, 573b, 574, 576b, 577r.1, 577r.2, 581ml, 581bm, 582b, 591r, 592t; Tracey Stephenson 571t, 576tl, 576tm, 576tr, 576ml, 576mr, 577r.3, 577r.4, 578tl, 578tr, 581tl, 581tr, 581mm, 581bl, 581br

Chapter 8

Andy Rouillard 600b; Annette Close 600t; Beauty Express 608t, 608mr, 608b, 609ml, 609mm, 609mr, 609b, 615, 626t, 635b.1, 635b.2; Cengage Learning 603b, 619; DermNet NZ 617t; Ellisons 608ml, 609t, 628t, 630t, 631t, 632b, 634m, 634bl, 634bm, 634br, 635tl, 635tm, 635tr, 635ml, 635mm, 635mr, 636b; Encyclopedia of Hair Removal, Gill Morris and Janice Brown 606m; Habia 610; Ken Franklin/Video4 Ltd 630m.1, 630m.2, 630m.3, 630m.4, 630b.1, 630b.2, 630b.3, 630b.4; Milady 606t, 611b, 618m.2, 618b; Milady Standard Esthetics 633tm; Nathan Portlock Allan Photography/Media Select International for Cengage Learning 602t, 602b, 603t, 604t, 611t, 617m, 620, 621, 622t, 622m, 622b, 623t, 623b, 624l, 624m, 624r, 625tl, 625tr, 625ml, 625mr, 625b, 626b, 627tl, 627tr, 627m, 628ml, 628mr, 628bl, 628br, 629t, 629ml, 629mm, 629mr, 629b, 631bl, 631bm, 631br, 632tl, 632tr, 632ml, 632mr, 633tl, 633tr, 633bl, 633br, 634t, 638bl, 638bm, 638br, 636t; Shutterstock 601l, 601r, 604b, 605t, 605b, 616.1, 616.2, 616.3, 617b, 618t, 618m.1; Sterex Electrolysis 614t; Thinkstock 598, 605m, 606b, 614b, 627b

1 The Business of Beauty Therapy

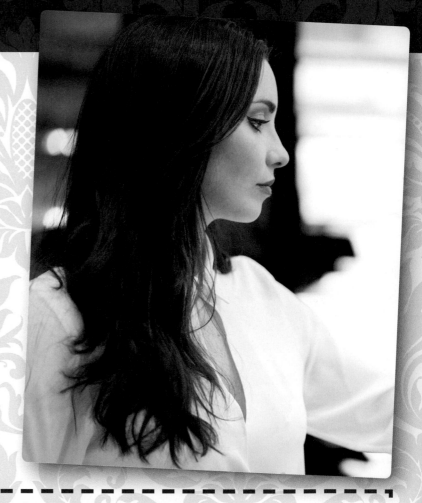

LEARNING OBJECTIVES

This chapter covers the business of beauty therapy and provides an overview of the essential knowledge, understanding and skills required to be a successful professional beauty therapist and effective within your work role. You have an important role in making the workplace a successful and pleasant environment to work in.

Which chapters provide coverage for your training route?

Core chapters

Chapter1: The Business of Beauty Therapy

Chapter 2: The Science of Beauty Therapy

Chapter 3: Consultation Practice and Techniques

Core chapters plus the following for Beauty therapy route

Chapter 4: Facials

Chapter 5: Eyelash and Eyebrow Treatments

Chapter 6: Make-up

Chapter 7: Hand and Foot Services

Chapter 8: Wax Depilation (including threading)

Core chapters plus the following for Make-up route

Chapter 5: Eyelash and Eyebrow Treatments

Chapter 6: Make-up

Core chapters plus the following for Nails route

Chapter 7: Hand and Foot Services (including nail art and gel polish)

Core chapters plus the following for the Beauty Consultancy route:

Chapter 4: Facials

Chapter 6: Make-up

You will learn more about the following:

◆ The beauty sector, market and industry.

◆ Career opportunities and progression.

◆ The importance of professional image and reputation, and the part you play.

◆ Client care and communication at all stages of the customer journey.

◆ The essential work ethics, skills, values and behaviours that are required to competently carry out your work role.

◆ The importance of keeping yourself professionally updated and aware of current developments within the beauty industry and related technologies.

◆ Law, legislation and industry codes of practice and compliance requirements that are related to different workplace activities.

◆ Selling techniques.

◆ Promotional and marketing techniques and activities, which raise publicity for the business, its brand image, products and treatments in order to support sales and growth.

◆ The resources used to manage business information on sales, stock, clients, staff and appointment bookings.

◆ The duties of a receptionist, which include maintaining the reception environment, attending to clients, handling enquiries and payments and making appointments.

◆ Identifying appropriate additional treatments and products for your clients that meet their requirements and expectations.

KEY TERMS

Accident	Continuing professional	HSE (Health and Safety	PPE (Personal
Allergic reaction	development (CPD)	Executive)	Protective
Apprenticeships	Contract of employment	Human resources	Equipment)
Appointment (making	Credit card	Hygiene	Receptionist
and scheduling)	Demonstration	Job description	Risk
Behaviours	Debit card	Legal requirements	Salon services
Body language	Disciplinary	Liability insurance	Self-management
Cheques	Discrepancies	Marketing	Skills
Client care	Enquiries	Message taking	Skin sensitivity
Client record	Ethics	Method of payment	tests
Code of practice	Gift voucher	Posture	Values
Communication	Hazard	Promotion	Vouchers
Complaints procedure	Health and safety policy	Promotional activities	Workplace

The business of beauty

The beauty industry covers spending on cosmetics, personal care and professional treatments. It is a major contributor to the UK economy and is reported to be worth over £17 billion*.

The professional beauty sector in the UK covers a wide variety of treatments. The UK treatment market was worth £1.91 billion** in the year to the end of October 2014. The largest proportion of this spend was through beauty salons.

Qualifying in beauty therapy at Level 2 provides you with the opportunity to work across a range of diverse skill areas, offering treatments that improve or enhance the appearance of your clients' skin, nails or eyes. Each treatment received or product purchased should make your client feel more confident in their appearance and overall wellbeing.

To be a competent, successful beauty therapist, the practical **skills** and knowledge learned should be applied consistently in order to match the treatment, service or product needs of every client. The result will be a satisfied client who will return to you. They may become your best advert for the business, sharing their positive experience.

Employment opportunities

When you have successfully qualified at Level 2 you can enter employment or progress your training, gaining a further or higher qualification. Some examples of the different opportunities you may consider are:

◆ junior therapist in the workplace

◆ retail in cosmetics and skincare, referred to as a make-up consultant

◆ on-line beauty retail distributor

◆ franchise, renting your own treatment room or space

◆ business owner

◆ specialist in an occupational area, for example providing eye treatments in a lash and brow bar (there is an increasing trend for employers to look for staff specialising in certain skills)

◆ freelance, working for yourself, visiting clients' homes or workplaces

◆ freelance, working in the media including 'blogging' and 'vlogging'

◆ spa environment within a fitness club or hotel

◆ spa and beauty therapy general treatments in a day spa

◆ luxury wellbeing services in a health spa resort

◆ premium brand skincare therapist at an 'in-store' salon

◆ cruise liner, as part of a beauty and spa team

◆ holiday resort, as part of a beauty and spa team

◆ airport lounge pre-flight beauty treatments

◆ sales representative promoting a particular product, treatment or company brand.

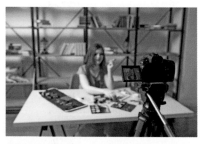

A female vlogger presenting make-up tutorial

*Source: Mintel 2015;   **Kantar World Panel Beauty.

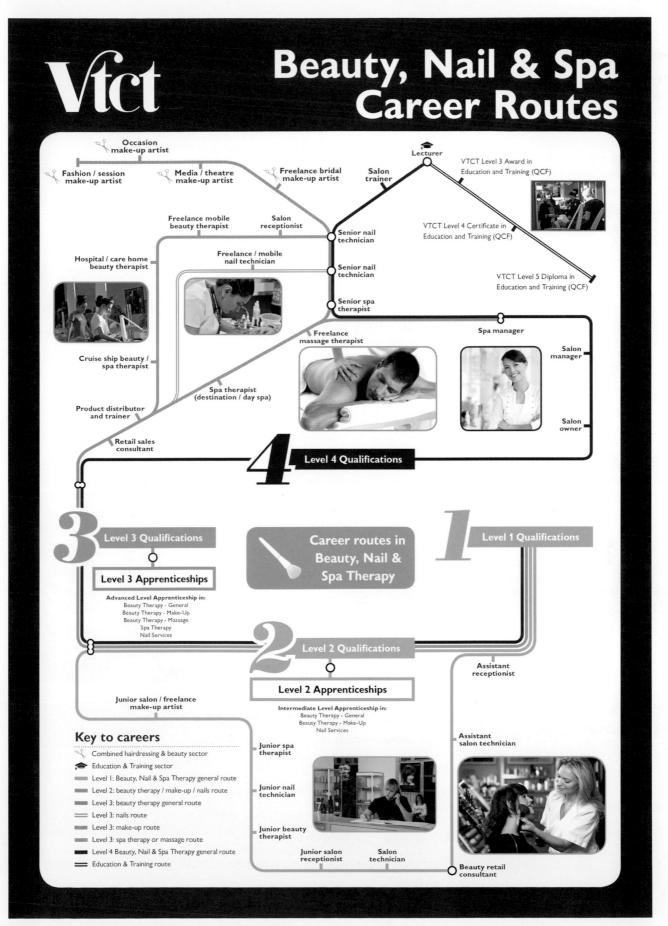

Beauty, Nail & Spa Career Routes

VTCT

Occasion make-up artist

Fashion / session make-up artist

Media / theatre make-up artist

Freelance bridal make-up artist

Salon trainer

Lecturer

VTCT Level 3 Award in Education and Training (QCF)

VTCT Level 4 Certificate in Education and Training (QCF)

VTCT Level 5 Diploma in Education and Training (QCF)

Freelance mobile beauty therapist

Salon receptionist

Senior nail technician

Senior nail technician

Senior spa therapist

Hospital / care home beauty therapist

Freelance / mobile nail technician

Freelance massage therapist

Spa manager

Salon manager

Cruise ship beauty / spa therapist

Spa therapist (destination / day spa)

Salon owner

Product distributor and trainer

Retail sales consultant

4 Level 4 Qualifications

3 Level 3 Qualifications

Level 3 Apprenticeships

Advanced Level Apprenticeship in:
Beauty Therapy - General
Beauty Therapy - Make-Up
Beauty Therapy - Massage
Spa Therapy
Nail Services

Career routes in Beauty, Nail & Spa Therapy

1 Level 1 Qualifications

Assistant receptionist

Assistant salon technician

2 Level 2 Qualifications

Junior salon / freelance make-up artist

Level 2 Apprenticeships

Intermediate Level Apprenticeship in:
Beauty Therapy - General
Beauty Therapy - Make-Up
Nail Services

Key to careers

- Combined hairdressing & beauty sector
- Education & Training sector
- Level 1: Beauty, Nail & Spa Therapy general route
- Level 2: beauty therapy / make-up / nails route
- Level 3: beauty therapy general route
- Level 3: nails route
- Level 3: make-up route
- Level 3: spa therapy or massage route
- Level 4 Beauty, Nail & Spa Therapy general route
- Education & Training route

Junior spa therapist

Junior nail technician

Junior beauty therapist

Junior salon receptionist

Salon technician

Beauty retail consultant

A guide to beauty industry careers from awarding body VTCT

TOP TIP

Real work experience

Whilst you are training, it is important to gain experience in the beauty work environment. You will gain experience of work, skills, values and behaviours required, client interaction and care, the importance of retail sales and reception, and when competent you will be able to offer those treatments.

Career progression opportunities

You may wish to continue your training and there are a number of routes you could follow to progress further. Some examples you may consider include:

◆ Business owner

◆ Level 3 beauty therapist

◆ Other associated occupational qualifications in spa, make-up and media, and nail services

◆ Further training to gain advanced practical techniques and maintain your Continuing Professional Development (CPD). It is important to keep yourself up-to-date and capable of meeting emerging industry trends.

When you achieve your level 2 qualification in beauty therapy, you can continue to update and advance your skills through further study where relevant to your career path/goals or employment appraisal targets relating to your employer's business objectives.

Beauty related work roles

The wide range of different job opportunities available in the beauty related industries with a brief explanation of these various occupational work roles are described below. Some of these may require further training.

Occupational work role	Description of activities	
Beauty therapist	Beauty therapists provide beauty treatments and treatments which, if qualified to Level 3, may include those listed in this table. They also provide advice to clients and promote related beauty products to support the treatments they offer. Beauty therapists may be salon based, work from their own home or travel to a location such as the client's home.	
Make-up artist	Make-up artists apply preparatory skincare, make-up and provide services which enhance the eyes such as eyelash enhancement systems. They will often also style the hair of performers and presenters for TV, film, theatre, fashion shows, live performances and photo shoots. They may be employed in a department store where their primary role is to retail products for a particular company or brand. Increasingly, this may include the delivery of express make-up services that allow the customer to receive personalised, professional advice on their application.	

(Continued)

Occupational work role	Description of activities	
Electrologist	A specialist in hair removal who uses electrical epilation to permanently destroy the hair follicle to stop hair growth. A sterile needle is used to apply an electric current with short wave diathermy technique which may include galvanic current electrical equipment.	
Nail technician	A specialist in nail services and treatments including care of the natural nail with manicures and pedicures, nail finishes including gel polish and nail art application and artificial nail enhancement techniques.	
Manicurist/pedicurist	A manicurist/pedicurist, usually a beauty therapist or nail technician, specialises in applying treatments for the hands (manicure) and feet (pedicure) with the aim of improving or maintaining their health and appearance through the provision of specialised treatments and retail promotion of related products.	
Massage therapist	The massage therapist provides massage treatments and techniques to the face, head and body. This may be performed *manually*, where the massage therapist's hands manipulate the client's skin, tissue and underlying muscles, or *mechanically* using a machine. Massage techniques can achieve a relaxing or stimulating effect and create a feeling of well-being.	
Aromatherapist	Aromatherapists treat a variety of physical conditions and psychological disorders using essential aromatic oils that are extracted from flowers, trees, fruit and herbs, selected for their therapeutic properties.	

(Continued)

Occupational work role	Description of activities	
Reflexologist	In reflexology every part of the body is reflected in a precise area, or reflex point, on the feet and hands. The reflexologist works on the foot or the hand as appropriate, using a precise technique based upon the application of finger point pressure on the reflex zones of the feet and hands to restore the flow of energy through the body.	
Complementary therapist	A practitioner providing treatment alongside or in addition to conventional medicine. This is referred to as 'complementary medicine' as the two practices *complement* each other. The practitioner treats the client's body and mind as a whole and this is often referred to as an 'holistic approach'.	
Cosmetic beauty consultant	Usually employed by a cosmetic company in a retail environment or freelance, cosmetic beauty consultants sell cosmetics and advise customers on the right products to meet their requirements.	

(Continued)

Occupational work role	Description of activities	
Sales representative	Promotes a particular product, treatment or company 'brand'. They are often experts in their field and can offer technical support and training within the beauty related industries through continuing professional development (CPD). CPD maintains an individual's expertise and awareness of current beauty related industry practice.	
Receptionist	The receptionist receives clients entering the beauty work area, handles enquiries, makes appointments, deals with client payments and maintains the appearance of the reception area. The receptionist should always take care of clients in a polite, efficient manner, particularly while questioning them to find out what they require.	
Salon manager	The salon manager, supervisor or team leader supervises and supports other colleagues with additional responsibilities which may include the day-to-day running of the business, complying with all workplace legislation, maintaining resource levels and monitoring staff performance and attainment towards any specific targets.	
Teacher	Teachers are qualified and trained to teach their occupational skills and assess their learners' competence or capability across a variety of courses and levels. Evidence is required of significant related occupational experience and further education in teacher training is required.	

(Continued)

Occupational work role	Description of activities	
Trainer	Trainers are qualified to train learners in a variety of courses, often in specific CPD courses. Evidence is required of significant related occupational experience and further education in training delivery is required.	

Industry role models

In the beauty industry there are many role models who, through their broad experience and passion for their work, are ambassadors for the industry. They can provide inspiration to those entering the industry. These may include the people you work with on a day to day basis.

Our industry role models have shared their valued 'tips of the trade' in each chapter of this book. The industry role models featured are detailed below.

Role model	Find out more
Maureen Evans-Olsen, World Skills UK	Chapter 1 The Business of Beauty Therapy
Janice Brown, Director, HOF Beauty	
Tina Rook, Head of Saks Education	
Sam Sweet, Sweet Squared LLP	
Daniella Norman, Education Operations Manager, Dermalogica UK	Chapter 3 Consultation Practice and Techniques; Chapter 4 Facial Treatments
Shavatah Singh, Shavatah Brow Studios	Chapter 5 Eyelash and brow services
Lorraine Onorato, Founder and Principal, The National School of Threading	
Marion Main, Glasgow Clyde College	Chapter 6 Make-up
Laura Dicken, Managing Director, Podology	Chapter 7 Hand and foot services
Marian Newman, Freelance session nail technician, author and industry consultant	
Andy Rouillard, Owner, Axiom Bodyworks and Axiom Wax Academy	Chapter 8 Wax depilation and threading hair removal
Annette Close, General Manager, Australian Bodycare UK	

ALWAYS REMEMBER

Create a positive work environment

An important factor in the success of any business is the commitment of the staff to provide a consistently high standard of service and client care. In order to be effective, all staff must be confident in their job role. The aim is to perform treatments to the highest standard, whilst maintaining positive, professional working relationships and creating a happy, productive atmosphere, which is obvious to the client.

INDUSTRY ROLE MODEL

MAUREEN EVANS-OLSEN Head of Education and Development, Worldskills UK

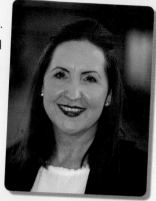

Do what you love to do To be successful in industry whether you are employed or freelance, you have to be great at what you do and therefore it is important that you love your job role and the skills you are developing.

Every day and situation will bring with it new challenges, and so in order to be successful, a positive problem solving approach to your technical skills development will assist you to succeed. As a beauty therapist, every client will present you with a different challenge and each should be treated as an individual. Your ability to manage yourself and be proactive, along with daily, weekly and monthly planning will support you in your approach to your skill development and will enable you to reach your goals.

Your goals will include excelling in your technical skills development but that is not enough. Communication and genuinely caring for others is paramount to success in this industry as well as a confident approach to treating clients, planning your time well, selling on products to reinforce treatments, and increasing the number of clients you treat.

Don't be afraid to fail and foster a willingness to learn In a supportive framework failures can lead you to your greatest success and enable you to learn and grow. During the safety of the training environment practice and confront all of those weak areas until they become your strengths.

Ask for, and follow the advice of your lecturers, employers and trainers. You may get conflicting advice, but that will come from a rich tapestry of experience. Remember what works for one will not work for another so try each piece of advice and see if it works for you.

Competition is a great way to support your development and a really good method of gaining feedback. During competition you are faced with a particular challenge and are expected to fulfill the requirements in a short time span, the competition will seek out excellence. For more information take a look at the WorldSkills website www.worldskillsuk.org

What are employers looking for? In the beauty industry employers are looking for a range of skills depending on the size and style of the organisation:

1. Great communication skills with beautiful manners and a positive attitude.
2. Excellent technical skills with the willingness and capacity to take on new learning.
3. Confidence, a strong presence and the ability to build rapport with co-workers and clients.
4. Commitment and dedication to your skill with a flexible approach to working hours.
5. Professionalism with strong ethics, attention to detail and a commitment to high standards.

Getting started

Your education and studies will equip you with the practical skills, knowledge and understanding to work competently. In order to gain employment and be successful these must be supported by good employability skills. These are the necessary workplace skills, **values** and **behaviours** required by employers. See later in this chapter for more details on skills, values and behaviours.

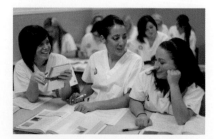

Continuously develop your treatment skills and knowledge

The workplace

People are the most important resource in a business that makes profits from the delivery of treatments and retail sales. To maximise business performance, every employee should complete their allocated duties and responsibilities to the best of their ability and staff should work together as a team. An employer would regard these attributes as being as important as qualifications.

Personal performance at work As an employee, you should be aware of the goals of the business so that you understand what is expected of you in helping achieve them. A job induction provides you with general and essential information when you first start work. It may include:

◆ a description of the work environment

◆ facilities

◆ health and safety

◆ security

◆ the staffing structure

◆ roles and responsibilities of colleagues and how they relate to your welfare.

It will also tell you who to report to if you require support or advice in any area outside of your responsibility, or if you have any concern or receive a complaint. The induction should leave you feeling more confident about the expectations required from you and how you will be supported in achieving them. Your responsibilities are outlined in a **job description**.

The job description can also be used when reviewing your own performance in your role. This is called self-appraisal or evaluation. It is important to ensure that you are meeting all requirements of the job role and, if not, identify why this is so that it can be resolved.

ALWAYS REMEMBER

Human Resources (HR)

Employees in the business are known as 'human resources' or 'HR'. This term is used to refer to their qualifications, skills and abilities.

ALWAYS REMEMBER

Job description

The job description informs employees what is expected of them. It details to whom they are responsible and for what they are responsible.

A sample job description is provided below.

Sample job description for a beauty therapist

Job title:	Beauty therapist
Reporting to:	Salon manager
Location:	Based at salon as advised
Overall purpose:	To ensure the highest standards of customer care and treatments at all times.
	To maintain a competent standard of technical knowledge and practical skill, ensuring that current methods and techniques are used and that the salon training, practices and procedures are followed.
Key responsibilities:	◆ Achieve individual, team and company Key Performance Indicators (KPIs).
	◆ Maintain the company's service standards set for all beauty treatments.
	◆ Present professional standards and a well-groomed appearance at all times.
	◆ Provide clients with up-to-date information on the range of products and beauty treatments available to them.
	◆ Carry out client consultations in accordance with company guidelines.
	◆ Evaluate the needs of the client and recommend the relevant beauty treatment.
	◆ Actively promote the products and market the service of the beauty salon.
	◆ Assist with promotion and marketing activities as required.
	◆ Assist with the professional development of others where necessary.
	◆ Ensure your own and the customers' health and safety requirements are met at all times.
	◆ Assist your manager in ensuring the maintenance of salon resources.
	◆ Maintain 'good housekeeping' standards, ensuring tidiness, safety and good working practices are adhered to, in order to meet statutory health and safety requirements.
	◆ Maintain company security practices and procedures.
	◆ Undertake any additional tasks and duties as defined by your manager.
Personal indicators:	◆ Keep up-to-date with beauty products and equipment at all times.
	◆ Achieve all sales and activity targets as agreed.
	◆ Maximise the business on all new sales opportunities.
	◆ Keep your Continuing Provisional Development (CPD) record up to date.

For reasons of safety and effectiveness it is important that you work only within your job role at all times. Perform the skills that you are qualified to undertake. Non-compliance can result in harm to yourself or others and you could be liable for any incorrect working practice.

A written statement of the terms of employment or **contract of employment** (which includes all terms and conditions listed below) should be given to an employee within two months of them becoming employed.

The statement or contract includes the names of the employer and employee, the date that employment commenced, and when the period of continuous employment began. It will also include details of the job description.

Terms and conditions should be listed, including the following:

◆ scale or rate of pay

◆ payment interval, e.g. weekly, monthly

REVISION AID

What is the purpose of a job description?

ACTIVITY

Staff roles and responsibilities

List the different roles and responsibilities of employees in your workplace.

This will be useful because you will know who to refer to in different situations. In addition, clients and visitors to the workplace may also request this information.

HEALTH & SAFETY

Only ever work within your job role in any activity carried out in the workplace.

◆ hours of work

◆ holiday entitlement, including bank holidays and how holiday pay is calculated

◆ length of notice requirements

◆ work location

◆ job title, roles and responsibilities

◆ **disciplinary** rules and disciplinary procedure (or it should state where this can be found)

◆ other policies and procedures to be complied with, e.g. environmental policy; social media policy (or it should state where these can be found).

Information should also be provided on reporting absence, eligibility for sickness pay, pension schemes, etc. (or it should state where these can be found).

As well as the rights of clients, the business has a legal obligation to protect the rights of the employee.

ALWAYS REMEMBER

Payment

◆ A statutory national minimum wage was introduced in 1999 and is updated each year. The national living wage was introduced in April 2016 for those aged 25 and over. For further information, see the website: www.gov.uk/national-minimum-wage-rates

◆ As part of an employee's contract of employment, bonuses and commission are identified, if applicable.

◆ A detailed written pay statement should be provided before or when an employee is paid. This should identify any deductions and what they are for.

◆ Sick pay may be provided by the employer identified in the employment contract, or if this has not been agreed, an employee may be entitled to statutory sick pay (SSP). For more information on SSP see www.gov.uk/statutory-sick-pay.

ALWAYS REMEMBER

Workplace pensions

Under the **Pensions Act 2008** every employer in the UK must enrol certain employees into a pension scheme and contribute towards it. This is called automatic enrolment. If you employ at least one person you are an employer and have certain legal duties.

The rules that are associated with workplace pensions are quite complex and include who is eligible, when you have to start a scheme and how much the employer/employee has to contribute.

You must enrol all workers who are:

◆ aged between 22 and the State Pension age

◆ earn at least £10,000 a year

◆ work in the UK.

To find out if and when employees should be enrolled into a workplace pension scheme you can check the government website www.thepensionsregulator.gov.uk for further details.

Employment and the Equality Act (2010)

The government has set in law certain legislative requirements to protect employees from discrimination and harm. The Equality Act 2010 was set up to protect people from being discriminated against in the **workplace** and in society. This single Act replaced a number of different laws that previously covered discrimination, such as the Sex Discrimination Act, Race Relations Act and Disability Discrimination Act. The Equality Act (2010) also covers a variety of laws, including equal pay and working conditions. It is unlawful within the Act to discriminate against anyone with 'protected characteristics'.

Under the Equality Act 2010 the nine protected characteristics are as follows:

◆ age

◆ disability

◆ gender reassignment

◆ marriage and civil partnership

◆ pregnancy and maternity

◆ race

◆ religion or belief

◆ gender

◆ sexual orientation.

For more detailed information on equality and rights, including Codes of Practice, you can visit the Equality and Human Rights Commission website: www.equalityhumanrights.com

Working Time Regulations (1998)
The Working Time Regulations implement the European Working Time Directive into British law and aim to ensure that employees are protected against adverse conditions with regard to their health and safety caused by working excessively long hours with inadequate rest or disrupted work patterns.

The Working Time Directive provides for the following:

◆ Working hours must be limited to an average of no more than 48 hours per week. An employee can agree to work more but it must be in writing.

◆ Employees are entitled to one uninterrupted rest day in every seven.

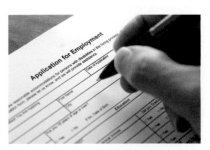

Discrimination is against the law

◆ A working day should be no longer than 13 hours, although this will depend upon the agreed break between each shift.

◆ Night workers are entitled to a break of 11 consecutive hours in each 24-hour period.

◆ If working more than 6 hours per day, employees are entitled to a minimum 20-minute break.

◆ After 3 months employment, employees are entitled to 4 weeks paid holiday a year. Holiday pay is pro rata for part-time employees.

Employability skills

These are the skills that make you employable. They will help you gain employment, be successful and contribute to your career progression. All these skills can be learnt.

Examples of the skills a professional beauty therapist is required to have are shown below.

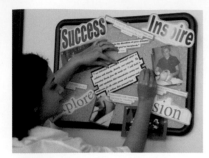

Keep focused on your goals. Identify the skills, values and behaviours that are going to get you there.

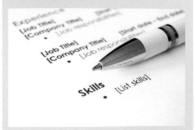
◆ **Professional:** presenting a consistent, positive image of yourself and the business.

◆ **Courteous:** you should treat everyone with respect through verbal and non-verbal communication. This should be applied in the use of social media too.

◆ **Discreet:** you must be tactful and cautious in all communication and self expression. Certain topics may be unsuitable for discussion, including the expression of personal opinions that may cause offence or embarrassment to the other person. Always think before you speak.

Remember, never pass on information related to clients or colleagues without formal agreement to do so. This is in compliance with the Data Protection Act (1998) discussed later in this chapter.

◆ **Personable:** a successful business requires staff who are personable or pleasant. This is described as having 'people skills'. These staff will moderate their behaviour as appropriate to the situation.

◆ **Enthusiastic:** employers want employees who are self-motivated, proactive, have high aspirations and are willing to work hard to achieve them.

◆ **Responsible:** your employer will expect you to think carefully when performing any activity to avoid unnecessary error. Self-management is a positive attribute to ensure all necessary activities are completed competently and timely.

Skills, values and behaviours

The following section reviews the occupational standards and employability skills that underpin the delivery of professional beauty therapy treatments. These are classified under the headings: skills, values and behaviours.

Skills

These are competencies you need to carry out your work role.

◆ The ability to be able to self-manage, termed **self-management**. This will include the skills of using initiative and decision making. This should always be within the limits of your authority.

◆ To use effective verbal and non-verbal **communication** skills, selecting the most appropriate method to communicate with others.

◆ To respond efficiently to others seeking assistance/information, providing information that will be relevant and helpful in relation to business services.

Values

Most values relate to personal attitude and standards of behaviour and include:

◆ **A willingness to learn:** including learning about new treatments, products and changes to workplace practices – and on personal reflection, learning from experience!

◆ **A flexible attitude:** you need to be able to adapt to new situations or working conditions (as long as these are fair and realistic). In the day-to-day operation of the business things cannot always be planned for.

◆ **A team player ethos:** you should know your role and what you contribute to the purpose of the team. People need to feel comfortable and supported to work well together, achieving a team spirit!

◆ **A positive attitude:** it is important to be personable with good people skills. This means having a positive attitude, being able to work co-operatively and communicate well with others.

◆ **Personal and professional ethics:** these uphold the industry standards and beliefs. Professional ethics are about being responsible, having integrity and doing what is moral and just. These ethics should be evident in the way you personally conduct yourself.

Behaviours

Behaviour relates to your conduct and requires that you do the following:

◆ Ensure that your organisation's and industry standards of appearance and behaviour are met.

◆ Greet clients in a respectful yet friendly manner at all times.

◆ Communicate with clients in a way that makes them feel valued and respected.

◆ Treat clients courteously, offering assistance willingly at all times.

◆ Ensure that your behaviour is adapted in consideration of client diversity and in respect of different circumstances.

◆ Use appropriate assessment and questioning techniques, in order that you fully understand client expectations and that they will feel confident with the information you have provided.

◆ Respond promptly and positively to client's questions and responses made.

Every beauty treatment and work-related activity may include and combine any or all of the above. Check your employer's workplace policy to help you understand how to fulfil these important employability skills in your workplace.

Workplace policy

The workplace policy communicates standardised workplace operational procedures and protocols or rules, which includes the skills, values and behaviours expected from its employees. These may be written, but not all workplace procedures require this. What is essential is that employees understand the reasons for the workplace policy, their responsibility in policy implementation and the standard operating procedures and comply with them. The workplace policy may include the following:

◆ job descriptions and responsibilities, policies and procedures

◆ treatment operational procedures including reception

◆ **ethics**

◆ health, safety and **hygiene** procedures

◆ personal presentation and standards of appearance

◆ working hours and time keeping

◆ absence procedure

> **REVISION AID**
>
> What do you understand by the terms: 'skill', 'values' and 'behaviours', in relation to the workplace?

ACTIVITY

Great customer care experience

Think of an occasion when you received what you considered to be a great customer care experience.

a What was the context?

b What features of this experience made it both memorable and special?

c Did you tell others about it?

This demonstrates the importance of great customer care. You have remembered it. The same activity could be completed for poor customer care.

ACTIVITY

Personal ethics

What would you say are your personal work ethics? (e.g. always be honest, respect colleagues.)

ALWAYS REMEMBER

Qualified to practise as a Level 2 beauty therapist

Even when you have qualified you will continue to be judged on your performance every day, by your clients and others. You will find that your skills may need to be developed further, even though you have just qualified. There will be standards of treatment delivery that are unique to each beauty workplace and business targets to be met. Be prepared to retrain and update your skills whenever necessary.

REVISION AID

How would you describe workplace ethics?

- behaviour, disciplinary and grievance procedures
- drugs and alcohol use
- eating and drinking protocol (health and safety)
- **client care**, defining the service expectations of the customer journey
- communication skills
- relationships with clients
- relationships with other professionals (including colleagues)
- social media (personal use)
- salon environment, environmental and sustainability procedures.

Overall, if the policy is consistently implemented the client will know they can expect to experience a great service whenever they visit.

We will now look further into how policy implementation may be applied in the workplace; these are also discussed within each chapter.

We are going to start with ethics.

Ethics

Working ethically means behaving in ways that are morally correct, being both fair and honest. It means considering the impact of all actions taken in relation to the operation of the business. Ethical businesses always consider that the outcomes of decisions made in the workplace are morally correct. As a provider of skincare treatments, it is important that you are competent, advise the clients on products that will meet their needs and treat all clients equally. These are examples of implementing work ethics.

Business ethical decisions may consider the impact of decisions made on others, for example staff, clients, local community and the environment.

If you use a skincare brand that is ethical in its source of ingredients, you could tell your clients that you use a brand that considers the environment in its production. This can be used in **marketing** as additional good publicity for the salon's business image.

In business, someone's personal ethics may not be totally in line with their professional workplace ethics. However, it is essential that in the workplace professional ethics are demonstrated by staff who consistently provide a great service. This ensures the requirements of the workplace policy are adhered to. When this is not the case there should be a procedure for reporting this.

TOP TIP

Fairtrade brand: an example of business ethics

The Fairtrade Foundation has ethics associated with its brand. Consumers understand the ethical principles behind the brand and choose to pay more for products that consider the environment and pay a reasonable wage to those involved in the production of the merchandise.

ALWAYS REMEMBER

Personal and professional ethics defined

"**Personal ethics** refers to the ethics that a person identifies with in respect to people and situations that they deal with in everyday life."

"**Professional ethics** refers to the ethics that a person must adhere to in respect of their interactions and business dealings in their professional life."

Definitions according to a Government of New Zealand website.

Beauty therapy has a code of ethics. This is a code of behaviours and expected standards for the professional beauty therapist to follow. These will uphold the reputation of the industry and ensure best working practice for the safety of the industry and members of the public. Professional bodies produce Industry Codes of Practice for their members. A business may have its own **code of practice**. Although not a legal requirement, this code may be used in criminal proceedings as evidence of improper practice.

Code of Ethics

1 **Towards BABTAC**
   a) By not bringing the profession as a whole into disrepute.
   b) By protecting collective morality. Members should not professionally associate themselves with any person or premises which may be deemed to be unprofessional or disreputable, as such an Association which may put the good name of the therapist and of BABTAC at risk.

2 **Towards clients** (concerned with the individual therapist/client relationship)
   a) Appointments must be kept. If unforeseen circumstances arise every effort must be made to make the client aware of the treatment cancellation.
   b) Client confidentiality – personal information should be kept private and only used for the specific purpose for which it is given, namely, to enable the therapist to carry out a safe and effective treatment.
   c) Information concerning the client and views formed must be kept confidential. The member should make every effort to ensure that this same level of confidence is upheld by receptionists and assistants where applicable.
   d) Client treatment details should remain confidential. Possible exceptions are the following;
      i) The client's knowledge and written consent are obtained.
      ii) There is a necessity for the information to be given, for example if the client is being referred onto another professional.

The exceptions are:
      iii) If the therapist is required by law to disclose the information.
      iv) If the therapist considers it their duty for the protection of the public.

If a therapist has information of a criminal nature the member is advised to take legal advice.

An excerpt from *The BABTAC Handbook*, code of ethics, www.babtac.com/www.babtac.com
BABTAC, The British Association of Beauty Therapy and Cosmetology

ALWAYS REMEMBER

Code of Ethics

As a professional beauty therapist it is important that you adhere to a code of ethical practice. As a student member you may wish to join a professional body, which will issue you with a copy of its agreed minimum standards.

INDUSTRY ROLE MODEL

JANICE BROWN Director, HOF Beauty (House of Famuir Ltd)

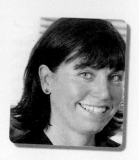

"My career journey has taken me from working in (and later managing) a group of salons, through sales, teaching, training, research and development. I am currently Director of HOF Beauty Ltd. Along the way I have specialised in electrolysis and hair removal. I am the co-author of the *Encyclopaedia of Hair Removal*, along with Gill Morris. I am proud to say that I have been able to make a real difference to people's lives by helping to correct skin, body and hair growth issues. I hope I have also been able to inspire and encourage fellow beauty therapists through the training I have provided. In the course of my career I have been fortunate enough to travel the world and work with wonderful people. Beauty therapy for me is not only a career but a true passion."

Health and safety in the workplace

Health and safety should be considered at all times. This is to guarantee the safety of yourself, all staff, clients and also any visitors to the workplace. *Health* is a state of wellbeing. *Safety* is the absence of risks.

There is a large body of legislation relating to health and safety at work. You need to understand how health and safety law, duties and responsibilities apply to you and others, and how to implement it, check for compliance and take appropriate action when necessary, which will safeguard you too.

Taking care of all in the workplace

When working in a service industry, you are legally obliged to provide a **safe and hygienic work place environment.** The workplace is an area or building where people work. This applies whether you are working in a hotel, retail environment such as a department store, a spa, a leisure centre or a private beauty salon, or operating a freelance beauty therapy service where you may be working in clients' homes. You must pay careful attention to health and safety to control and minimise any risk from something that can cause harm.

Your employer is responsible for:

◆ providing a safe working environment

◆ carrying out risk assessments to identify potential hazards

◆ taking relevant action, and

◆ adopting procedures that eliminate risk

◆ providing health and safety training

◆ On-going training which will ensure staff are confident and consistently apply the appropriate health and safety policies and procedures in compliance with the law.

Your role in implementing health and safety practice as a Level 2 beauty therapist is that you are responsible for checking that all statutory and workplace practices are being

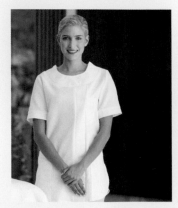

complied with and carried out correctly on a daily basis in every undertaking within your area of responsibility. Workplace practices are all activities, procedures and use of resources that are carried out by staff in the workplace.

You have responsibility for yourself, your clients and colleagues and will be required to:

◆ meet the required standards for personal presentation and wear appropriate PPE

◆ have a current knowledge of all relevant health and safety legislation and any updates

◆ have an understanding of the identification and elimination of risks in the workplace

◆ attend health and safety training provided

◆ ensure that all health and safety legislative documentation is recorded as required

◆ inform the relevant person if there is a shortage of any resources to ensure these are available at all times to comply with required practice and procedures as outlined in the workplace policy

◆ ensure equipment is checked every time before it is used to ensure it is in good working condition

◆ participate in all health and safety training updates to ensure compliance requirements are met

◆ inform colleagues of potential health and safety problems and report non-compliance issues if observed – legislative compliance is not optional!

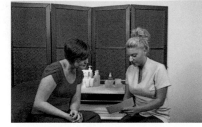

Performing a client consultation is health and safety practice and in compliance with the Health and Safety at Work Act as you check the client's suitability for the treatment, acting responsibly and not endangering yourself or others.

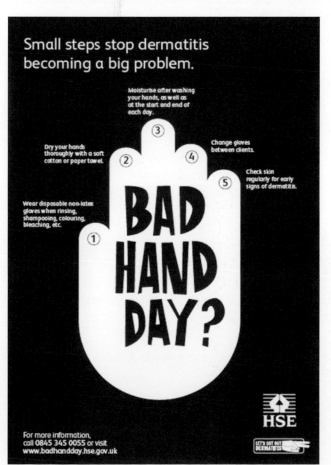

Health and safety poster informing the reader how to avoid the occupational disease, dermatitis. An HSE campaign pioneered by Habia.

ALWAYS REMEMBER

Safely controlling hazards and risks

Employees must work together to provide a safe and healthy workplace. As soon as a **hazard** is observed (anything that has potential to cause harm), this must be dealt with dependent upon the level of responsibility or reported to the designated authority so that the problem can be put right, preventing a risk. A **risk** is the likelihood of potential harm from that hazard happening.

Legal responsibilities

Failure to comply with legislation can have serious consequences for employers, employees and the business. If you cause harm to your client, or put them at risk, you will be held responsible. The result of this will cause loss of client trust and reputation; this may have a financial impact on the business, and you may be liable to **prosecution**, with the possibility of being fined or at worst, imprisoned.

There is a good deal of legislation relating to health and safety to inform you of and guide you in carrying out your responsibilities. You will need to know and understand which laws relate to beauty therapy. Health and safety issues specific to a job role or working methods are identified in the knowledge and understanding for each National Occupational Standard (NOS) and are referred to in each technical chapter.

It is important that you obtain and read all relevant publications. The **Health and Safety Executive (HSE)** is the body that provides guidance and information on all aspects of health and safety legislation. It also regulates and enforces health and safety. Your Local Authority can also be contacted for advice. For certain treatments the business premises are inspected, including the work area, and working practices reviewed to ensure they meet minimum standards. In addition, manufacturers provide instructions on equipment and products, which must always be checked. Even if you are familiar with the content, you should check just in case for any update so this can be followed. There may also be local bye-laws that are enforced through your local authority regulations. These will differ from one authority to another.

ACTIVITY

Know your responsibilities – keep up-to-date

Health and safety information is continually updated. For the latest information, you can find out more at **www.hse.gov.uk.**

Visit Habia.org to research current beauty therapy health and safety legislation and minimum compliance standards.

Legislation relevant to workplace operation can also be found in the Habia Health and Safety pack for beauty and nails.

TOP TIP

Guidance

As the standards setting body for beauty therapy, health and safety resource packs are available from Habia. These provide guidance in implementing health and safety policy and legislation in the beauty therapy workplace.

Codes of practice are also available from Habia, sharing best and mandatory working practice approved by both industry experts and health and safety advisors. Approved codes of practice are recognised by the HSE.

Professional beauty related membership organisations will also provide guidance on current industry advice and best practice.

The Health and Safety at Work Act (1974) The Health and Safety at Work Act (1974) (HASAWA 1974) is the main piece of legislation and covers many other health and safety regulations which are also discussed. This is continually reviewed with the introduction of new legislation as necessary. It lays down the minimum standards of health, safety and welfare required in each area of the workplace – Approved Codes of Practice (ACOP) are provided that detail the expected standards for compliance. It is the employer's legal responsibility to implement the Act and to ensure that, so far as is reasonably practicable, they manage the health and safety at work of the people for whom they are responsible and of those who may be affected by the work they do. Your role is an employee to implement these requirements within your job responsibilities.

This will include the following.

◆ Always act responsibly, ensuring your actions will not endanger yourself or others.

◆ Work with your employer or relevant person to fulfil all necessary duties.

◆ Never use anything other than for its intended purpose, in the interests of health and safety.

◆ Pass on all incidents, accidents and unsafe practices to your employer or relevant person.

The HASAWA also affects those who operate freelance and do not have a specific workplace base.

Officers from the Health and Safety Executive (HSE) or your Local Authority (LA) enforce health and safety law by visiting the workplace to regulate or check compliance with all relevant health and safety legislation.

For some treatments the local council requires a registration for licence to practice, which must be applied for and approved before you can begin to practice. This includes treatments such as massage and ear piercing. The purpose of this is to confirm the workplace premises meets the regulatory requirements and the beauty therapist is qualified to undertake the treatments offered.

If non-compliance or any area of dangerous work practice is identified, an improvement notice is issued and it is the responsibility of the employer to remove this danger within a designated period of time. Failure to comply with the notice will lead to prosecution. A business can be forced to stop providing a particular product or service or closed completely until all danger to employees or clients has been removed. Such workplace closure involves the issuing of a prohibition notice.

Your job description will include expected workplace standards, including health and safety operations. Good health and safety knowledge and understanding will help you meet the required responsibilities of health and safety legislation to be adhered to and workplace practices to be adopted.

HEALTH & SAFETY

The Health and Safety Information for Employees Regulations (1989) (HSIER 1989): Health and safety notice

Every employer is obliged by law to display the health and safety law poster in the workplace. This explains the responsibilities of employees, what actions to take if a health and safety problem arises and employment rights. A leaflet is available called *Your health and safety – a guide for workers*. Both poster and leaflet are available from the HSE on the website: http://www.hse.gov.uk/pubns/.

TOP TIP

It is good practice to have health and safety information filed centrally storing all current guidance including any updates to legislation. This may be in your workplace policy. This may be paper based or electronic, as long as it is up to date and readily accessible.

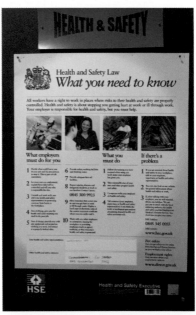

HSIER poster

At induction, staff should be made aware of relevant health and safety information. This includes hygiene procedures as identified in the workplace policy. Examples of topics you will cover will require that you:

◆ have read and understand the workplace health and safety policy

◆ know who to inform if there is any health and safety risk they cannot resolve within their level of authority

◆ have received a copy of the Health and Safety Law leaflet or are referred to the location of the Health and Safety Law poster

◆ are aware of where health and safety guidance publications, procedures and documentation are stored

◆ participate in emergency procedure training, e.g. action to take in the event of a fire or other emergency

◆ know first aid and accident procedures, including who to inform

◆ know manual handling best practice techniques and correct use of display screen equipment

◆ understand Control of Substances Hazardous to Health (COSHH) guidance

◆ understand personal protective equipment requirements.

If an employee is required to work on their own, there is a requirement for training, monitoring of any identified risks and supervision of this work requirement to ensure the employee's wellbeing.

Health and Safety Information for Employees Regulations (HSIER) (1989)

Amended in 2009 to reflect legislation updates, the purpose of the HSIER is to ensure all employees understand both their right to a safe and healthy workplace and their part in providing a good standard of health and safety.

The regulations require the employer to provide employees with the approved health and safety law information in the form of a standardised poster or leaflets. HSIER information is available from the HSE and is provided in different formats to suit the business and aid understanding, considering the diverse needs of the employee.

Each employer of more than five employees must formulate a written **Health and Safety Policy** for their business. For those employers with less than five employees this policy does not have to be written. The policy content states who should do what, when and how. The HSE and Habia have resources and examples providing guidance on how to create a written policy.

The policy is generally in three parts:

◆ objectives of the workplace health and safety policy

◆ responsibilities for duties and actions

◆ implementation of the policy, operational systems and procedures.

The policy must be issued and discussed with each employee at induction to ensure they understand the responsibilities that affect them. In addition the Health and Safety Policy may be displayed, for example on a noticeboard.

The health and safety policy should be dated and reviewed regularly to ensure it meets all relevant legislation guidelines, including updates.

Regular health and safety checks should be made and procedures reviewed to ensure that safety is being satisfactorily maintained. Health and safety training should also be carried out regularly and recorded.

In addition to the HSIER poster and Health and Safety Policy, further health and safety rules and regulations and examples of compliance to be displayed for all employees to access include:

◆ the fire evacuation procedures

◆ Employer Public Liability Insurance certificate

◆ first-aid guidance and arrangements.

Hazards and risks

Employees must always work together with their employer to provide a safe, secure and healthy workplace. A **hazard** is anything that has the potential to cause harm. As soon as an employee observes a hazard in the workplace, this must be dealt with or reported to the relevant person so that the problem can be put right. A **risk** is the likelihood of the potential hazard happening, and therefore causing harm.

The employer or responsible person should carry out a risk assessment to identify the potential hazards in the workplace.

All processes, activities and substances used in the workplace should be considered for their potential to cause injury or harm. Any hazards that have the potential to cause harm should be recorded with actions to be taken to reduce or prevent the risk. This is a legal requirement.

For employers with fewer than five employees, it is not necessary to write these down, although it is good practice to refer to the procedures for compliance and amendment as necessary.

General workplace hazards include:

◆ obstructions to routes including corridors, stairways and fire exits

◆ spillages on the floor and breakages.

◆ trailing leads from equipment

◆ overloaded plug sockets

◆ water placed near electrical equipment

◆ poor manual lifting and working techniques

◆ cross-contamination through poor hygiene practices.

Obstructions An obstruction is anything that blocks the traffic route in the work environment. In an emergency, such as a fire, an obstruction could delay people leaving the building, cause injury or prevent the emergency services entering the premises. All staff should be trained in the importance of keeping walkways and doorways clear at all times.

Spillages and breakages Any breakage or spillage should be dealt with immediately and in the correct way. For example, breakage of glass can cause cuts, while spillages may cause somebody to slip and fall.

ACTIVITY

Workplace health and safety rules

The health and safety policy identifies the employer's commitment to health and safety and how it is managed, who does what, when and why. Identify the rules, practices and procedures that apply to you in your workplace's health and safety policy.

HEALTH & SAFETY

Hazard example: stock delivery

When receiving a delivery, never leave it in a place it where it may be an obstruction. Do not leave it near high temperatures either, because if the products are flammable, it may ignite.

ALWAYS REMEMBER

Health and safety staff training

Employees are required to understand the difference between a hazard and a risk. They must also know how to deal with low-risk hazards within their responsibility, following the workplace health and safety policy and other legal requirements. Health and safety training is an important part of your CPD and a requirement to fulfill your job role.

ACTIVITY

Identifying hazards and risks

What is a hazard?

What is a risk?

a Give an example that can demonstrate this for a beauty therapy treatment.

b What measures should be taken to prevent the potential hazard becoming a risk?

ALWAYS REMEMBER

Use your initiative

You should use your initiative and deal with hazards within your responsibility. Follow workplace policy and requirements.

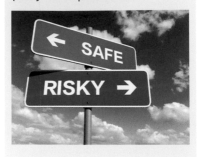

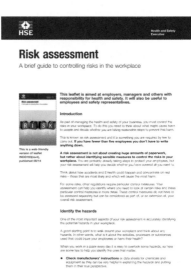

Risk assessment: A brief guide to controlling risks in the workplace

Trailing leads from equipment These should not be in an area where someone could trip. Tuck or secure them out of the way. When not in use, equipment may be unplugged.

Overloaded plug sockets This may cause the total current to exceed the power rating of the socket supply. Sufficient power sockets should be provided for each work station on the basis of the equipment required to be used.

Water placed near equipment This is highly dangerous. Water is an excellent conductor of electricity which can travel through you and to the ground leading to electric shock. Therefore, water near mains electricity is a serious hazard. Remember to keep your hands dry when touching anything electrical.

Poor lifting and working techniques Incorrect techniques and posture when lifting and working can lead to injury and repetitive strain injury (RSI). This is discussed later in this chapter. Correct techniques and assistance should be used whenever possible e.g. use of trolleys.

Cross-contamination Careless hygiene will lead to transmission of harmful micro-organisms, leading to infection. Appropriate hygiene procedures should be followed at all times.

Employers must:

◆ evaluate the possible risks associated with the identified hazard

◆ identify who may be at risk from the hazard and how

◆ identify the action or procedure that should be put in place to reduce or remove the risk.

A hazard should be dealt with immediately to prevent incident or injury. However, some hazards cannot be fixed immediately and in this case a solution should be put in place to control the risk. An example would be a flood.

Staff should know who to report hazards to if it is outside the limit of their responsibility or authority.

As workplace practices can change, activities should be reviewed regularly by the person responsible.

Some hazards require specific control measures, which are regulated through the Control of Substances Hazardous to Health (COSHH) Regulations 2002 (as amended).

Control of Substances Hazardous to Health (COSHH) Regulations (2002) (as amended) The Control of Substances Hazardous to Health (COSHH) Regulations (2002) requires employers to identify the substances used in their workplace that are hazardous to health. Many substances that seem quite harmless can prove to be hazardous if used or stored incorrectly. A hazardous substance is anything that can harm your health. These can come in many forms and include:

◆ chemicals, including those contained in products

◆ fumes

◆ dusts

◆ vapours

◆ mists

◆ gases

◆ germs.

Employers are responsible for assessing the risks from all materials used, identifying any hazardous substances and controlling exposure to them to prevent ill health. Any hazardous substances identified must be formally recorded in writing and given a hazard risk rating. Safety precaution procedures should then be put in place and training given to employees to ensure that the procedures are understood and will be followed correctly to store, handle, use and dispose of all substances hazardous to health. Examples of this include wearing protective equipment such as gloves, protective eye wear, aprons and masks.

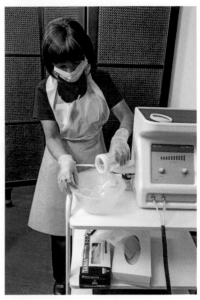

Beauty therapist wearing personal protective equipment: gloves, mask and apron, while safely disposing of potentially hazardous waste

ACTIVITY

COSHH risk assessment

The HSE website provides guidance and example COSHH risk assessments for different industries. Hairdressing is provided as an example.

Using the headings of the COSHH risk assessment provided below, think of further hazards in the workplace and identify who could be at risk, the level of the risk and what action should be taken to reduce the risk.

TOP TIP

Visit the HSE website on COSHH and beauty for key messages and industry related guidance: http://www.hse.gov.uk/coshh/industry/beauty.htm.

Step 1	Assess the risks.	Assess the risks to health from hazardous substances used in or created by your workplace activities.
Step 2	Decide what precautions are needed.	You must not carry out work which could expose your employees to hazardous substances without first considering the risks and the necessary precautions, and what else you need to do to comply with COSHH.
Step 3	Prevent or adequately control exposure.	You must prevent your employees being exposed to hazardous substances. Where preventing exposure is not reasonably practicable, then you must adequately control it (e.g. shampooing – wear non-latex gloves).
Step 4	Ensure that control measures are used and maintained.	Ensure that control measures are maintained properly and that safety procedures are followed.
Step 5	Monitor the exposure.	Monitor the exposure of employees to hazardous substances, if necessary.
Step 6	Carry out appropriate health surveillance.	Carry out appropriate health surveillance where your assessment has shown this is necessary or where COSHH sets specific requirements.
Step 7	Prepare plans and procedures to deal with accidents, incidents and emergencies.	Prepare plans and procedures to deal with accidents, incidents and emergencies involving hazardous substances, where necessary.
Step 8	Ensure employees are properly informed, trained and supervised.	You should provide your employees with suitable and sufficient information, instruction and training.

Process for undertaking COSHH risk assessment

COSHH Risk assessment - EXAMPLE ONLY						
Company name		Staff member responsible		Review date		
What are the hazards?	Who might be harmed and how?	What are you already doing?	What further action is necessary?	Action by whom?	Action by when?	Done
Aerosols (list the ones used in your workplace)	Everyone in the workplace but in particular the user of the aerosol and the client. Risk of fire, explosion and intoxication from flammable gases and irritant chemicals.	Ensuring aerosols are stored below temperature of 50°C and are not pierced or burnt. Avoiding inhalation of contents.	Look for aerosols with non-flammable gases if possible.	Name of staff member	Date	Date
Nail polish remover (list the ones used in your workplace)	Beauty therapists, trainees and clients. Irritant to the skin and eyes. Moderately toxic if swallowed or inhaled.	Always resealing after use. Not using on damaged or sensitive skin. Avoid breathing in.	Ensure that products are stored in a cool place and never place in unlabelled containers.	Name of staff member	Date	Date

An example COSHH risk assessment

Toxic   Gas under pressure   Harmful irritant

Flammable   Explosive   Harmful to the environment

Oxidising   Serious long term health hazard   Corrosive

International hazard symbols

Hazardous substances are usually identified through the use of known symbols, examples of which are shown here. Any substance in the workplace that is hazardous to health must be identified on the packaging, which will also explain how to store and handle the substance correctly, as well as how to dispose of it.

Hazardous substances may enter the body via:

◆ the eyes

◆ the skin

◆ the nose, by **inhalation** – breathing in

◆ the mouth, by **ingestion** – swallowing.

Each beauty product supplier is legally required to make available guidelines called material safety data sheets (MSDSs) on how materials should be used and stored; these will be supplied on request. When a product is 'dangerous for supply', i.e. with a hazard symbol, by law a safety data sheet must be provided.

It is important to use the safest products that are available and comply with the Cosmetic Product Enforcement regulations.

ALWAYS REMEMBER

You need COSHH control measures that prevent risk and do so every day. Everybody must be familiar with the COSHH assessment risk control measures and safety precautions must be followed by employees in order that any risk is actively reduced.

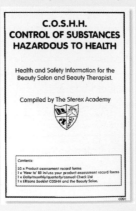

C.O.S.H.H.
CONTROL OF SUBSTANCES
HAZARDOUS TO HEALTH

Health and Safety Information for the
Beauty Salon and Beauty Therapist.

Compiled by The Sterex Academy

Contents:
50 x Product assessment record forms
1 x 'How to' fill in/use your product assessment record forms
1 x Daily/monthly/quarterly/annual Check List
1 x Ellisons Booklet COSHH and the Beauty Salon.

ACTIVITY

Hazard checklist

◆ Does any product that you use have a hazard symbol?

◆ Does any procedure you provide produce a hazardous substance, i.e. dust or fumes?

◆ Can the substance enter the body in any way?

◆ What procedure or practice is in place for the use of this product to prevent potential injury or harm?

REACH 2007 is a European Union Regulation concerning the:

Registration, **E**valuation, **A**uthorisation and restriction of, **CH**emicals.

REACH was introduced to provide a high level of protection to human health and the environment from the use of chemicals. It is known that chemicals can be irritant, toxic and corrosive. It is important that such hazardous chemicals are identified and controlled accordingly. It operates alongside COSHH and is designed to improve the information provided by chemical manufacturers through the provision of adequate safety data sheets.

Cosmetic Products Enforcement Regulations (2013) This piece of legislation consolidates earlier regulations and incorporates current European Market Directives. Part of consumer protection legislation, it requires that cosmetics and toiletries are safe in their formulation and for use for their intended purpose before being placed on the market, as well as that they comply with labelling requirements, instructions for use and disposal.

It is an offence to supply cosmetic products that are likely to cause damage to human health.

Certain substances are prohibited, e.g. certain fragrances, preservatives and colourings. Specific labelling is required.

The Trading Standards Service will provide advice on the manufacture and supply of cosmetic products.

TOP TIP

Reach

Further guidance can be found on the HSE website: www.hse.gov.uk/reach.

REVISION AID

What is a hazard? What is a risk?

TOP TIP

Cosmetic Products (Safety) Regulations labelling information requirement includes

◆ Function of product.

◆ The name and address of the supplier.

◆ A list of the ingredients in descending order of weight or volume, located on the packaging.

◆ Durability information and symbols to ensure it is used whilst in a satisfactory condition.

◆ Ingredients: precautions must be identified to avoid any unwanted reaction, e.g. allergic reaction.

◆ The preservatives and UV filters used should be identified.

◆ The batch code must be shown.

HEALTH & SAFETY

HSE COSHH guidance

A COSHH essentials information document is available at www.coshh-essentials.org.uk. It covers a broad range of activities and provides advice for products that have data sheets. Where not available specifically for your industry it is recommended that you look for that which is most similar. Supplement this with manufacturer safety data sheets.

The HSE publication *A step by step guide to COSHH assessment* (ISBN 9780717627851) gives advice and guidance on assessing workplace activities under the Control of Substances Hazardous to Health Regulations 2002. There is also a publication entitled *The Control of Substances Hazardous to Health Regulations 2002*, which covers approved code of practice and guidance by HSE Books (ISBN 9780717665822).

HEALTH & SAFETY

COSHH assessment

All hazardous substances must be identified when completing the risk assessment and implementing control measures. This includes cleaning agents such as a wax equipment cleaner. Where possible, high-risk hazardous products should be replaced with lower-risk, environmentally friendly products. The COSHH assessment should be reviewed on a regular basis and updated to include any new products.

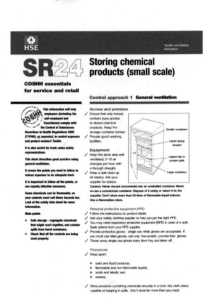

COSHH essential guidance for the service industry

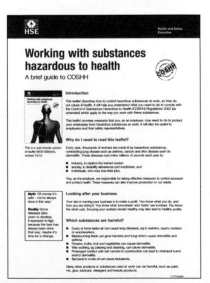

Guide to working with hazardous substances

Reporting of Injuries, Diseases and Dangerous Occurrences Regulations (RIDDOR) (2013 regulation 4)

RIDDOR requires the reporting and recording by the employer or responsible person of employee work-related deaths and specified injuries, cases of reportable work-related occupational diseases and certain 'dangerous occurrences' (near miss accidents) to the HSE. In addition, accidents involving others should be reported; for example clients. Guidance on what constitutes a RIDDOR incident and how this should be reported is located in the HSE RIDDOR guide and on the HSE website, www.hse.gov.uk/riddor/.

Cases where employees suffer personal injury resulting in seven consecutive days absence from work (including non-working days) requires notification. When this occurrence results in death or specified injuries, it must be reported by telephone immediately, followed by a written report on the appropriate HSE documentation. In all cases where personal injury occurs, an entry must be made in the workplace **accident book**. It is a legal requirement to keep an accident book. This will form part of your risk assessment procedures to ensure health and safety is managed to avoid potential harm. Where visitors to the work premises, such as clients, are injured and taken to hospital for treatment, this must also be reported. RIDDOR is a legal requirement and assists enforcing authorities, such as the HSE and local authorities, to assess if there is a need for further investigation and action to avoid further occurrences.

As an employee it is a requirement to inform your employer of a dangerous occurrence, death or major injury at work and work-related illnesses such as occupational dermatitis. This will allow the responsible person such as your employer to fulfill their obligations in relation to RIDDOR.

A record of any specified reportable injury, occupational disease or dangerous occurrence (incidents with potential to cause harm) must be retained after it happened in accordance with the HSE requirement. Information should include:

- the date, time and place
- how it was reported
- personal details of persons involved
- a brief description of the injury, disease or dangerous occurrence.

The Management of Health and Safety at Work Regulations (1999)

These regulations require employers to make formal arrangements for maintaining and improving working conditions and practices to meet the requirements of the Health and Safety at Work Act. This includes training for required employees to ensure their competency and to monitor risk in the workplace, referred to as 'risk assessment'. Employers are required to:

- identify and record any potential hazards
- assess the potential risks associated with the hazard
- identify who is at risk from the hazard
- identify how the risk is to be reduced or removed
- train staff to recognise and control risks
- put in place emergency procedures
- systematically review the risk assessment process regularly.

ALWAYS REMEMBER

Occupational related diseases

Where a disease has occurred or become worse due to the type of work undertaken, this must be reported as a RIDDOR case as a reportable occupational disease. Examples include occupational dermatitis, occupational asthma, carpal tunnel syndrome and tendonitis of the hand and forearm.

TOP TIP

When to report a RIDDOR incident

The HSE website provides guidance of what constitutes a reportable major injury, occupational disease and dangerous occurrence.

Reporting accidents and incidents at work

A brief guide to the Reporting of Injuries, Diseases and Dangerous Occurrences Regulations 2013 (RIDDOR)

RIDDOR guide

When employee circumstances change, such as when an employee becomes pregnant, the potential risks should be reviewed and appropriate action taken.

Where there are five or more people employed, the Act includes a requirement to:

◆ introduce a health monitoring system, making the change if the risk assessment monitoring system identifies a need

◆ record the risk assessment details.

Compliance with this Act will help to ensure that risks are controlled safely and effectively.

ACTIVITY

During the working week identify any hazards. For each one, identify the risk that could occur and what action needs to be taken to control this risk. If this is within your job role responsibility you could action this immediately, or if not you may need to pass it onto your employer.

Follow up this task by discussing your findings with your employer.

This is a compliance measure for the **Management of Health and Safety at Work Regulations (1999).**

Date	Hazard	Risk	Control action required/taken

Personal Protective Equipment (PPE) at Work Regulations (2002)

The **Personal Protective Equipment (PPE) at Work Regulations (2002 as amended)** require employers to identify – through a risk assessment – those activities or processes which require special protective clothing or equipment. When identified as necessary, PPE must be available, effective and in sufficient supply. PPE includes aprons, gloves and particle masks. Wax depilation is an example where PPE is a necessary requirement in the form of disposable gloves and apron because of the high risk of contamination with blood or body tissue fluid. PPE should also be available for clients to protect them adequately whilst receiving a treatment in your workplace. The PPE must be fit for purpose. An example is protecting their upper clothing whilst receiving an eye lash tinting treatment. Failure to do this could form the grounds for a possible claim, through treatment negligence.

Employees are required to wear protective clothing and use protective equipment provided for their own safety and welfare, and make employers aware of any shortage so that supplies are maintained.

PPE for handling chemicals

ACTIVITY

PPE risk assessment

Carry out your own risk assessment in the workplace. List the potentially hazardous substances that you may be required to handle. What are the risks and how may these be reduced or removed? What protective clothing and equipment should be available to reduce the risk?

Staff training should be provided on the correct use, application, removal and disposal of PPE. Employee compliance with the use of PPE should be monitored. If not used the reasons why should be investigated as this can then become a risk. For example, the development of the skin disease *primary dermatitis* may be caused by regular contact with a substance for which PPE is recommended. Therefore, by not using the appropriate PPE, the skin becomes irritated and inflamed.

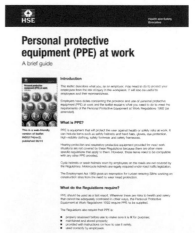

PPE Guidance

HEALTH & SAFETY

PPE Gloves

If there is a chance you may come into contact with body tissue fluids or chemicals, wear single use disposable non-latex (synthetic) nitrile or PVC formulation gloves that are powder-free. These must be the correct size for your hands. Latex gloves are known to cause allergic reactions (and in some cases the development of asthma) and are not recommended. PPE should be 'CE' marked; this indicates that it complies with the Personal Protective Equipment Regulations (2002) and satisfies basic safety requirements. Another useful source of information is the British Safety Industry Federation (www.bsif.co.uk).

To avoid the potential for contamination when removing single use disposable gloves, follow the steps shown on this website and below: http://www.hse.gov.uk/skin/posters/glovesingleuse.pdf.

Health and Safety Executive

Correct removal of gloves
Single use gloves (splash resistant)

Follow the steps shown

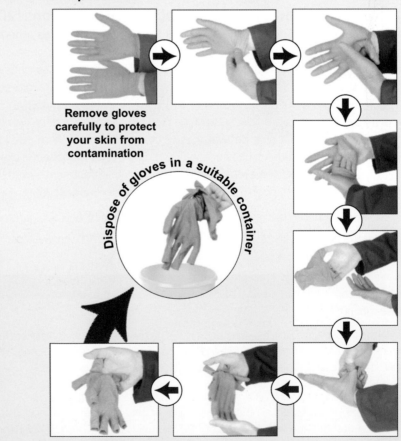

Remove gloves carefully to protect your skin from contamination

Dispose of gloves in a suitable container

www.hse.gov.uk

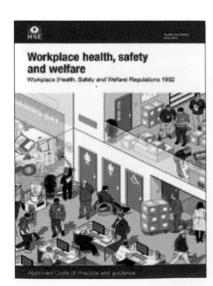

Workplace health, safety and welfare
Workplace (Health, Safety and Welfare) Regulations 1992

Workplace (Health, Safety and Welfare) Regulations (1992)

The Workplace (Health, Safety and Welfare) Regulations (1992) cover a broad range of basic health, safety and welfare issues to maintain a safe, healthy and secure working environment. Employers and employees need to be aware of and comply with their responsibilities as required in these regulations. The regulations aim to ensure the workplace meets the health, safety and welfare needs of all in the workplace.

The Equality Act 2010 also requires the access and facilities provided at the business premises must be equal for all, regardless of age, disability, gender reassignment, marriage and civil partnerships, pregnancy and maternity, race, religion or belief, sex or sexual orientation. The Workplace Regulations include **legal requirements** in relation to the following aspects of the working environment.

◆ The maintenance of the workplace and equipment in efficient working order.

◆ Adequate ventilation to ensure the air is changed regularly and hazardous vapours and materials are removed. Fresh air should be drawn from outside the workplace.

◆ The working temperature should be regulated by how physically demanding the work being carried out is. For work that is not severely physical, the temperature should be a minimum of 16°C for employees to be comfortable without requiring additional clothing. If the temperature becomes too high or too low, temperature stress can be suffered.

◆ Lighting should be adequate to enable people to move safely and perform tasks competently; local lighting is required to assist effective, safe service delivery of treatments such as electrical epilation and intimate waxing.

◆ The cleanliness of furniture, equipment, furnishing and fittings.

◆ The correct handling and disposal of waste materials.

◆ Floors and traffic routes should be of an even, safe surface to prevent trips and falls and strong enough for any weight they are required to support. Traffic routes should enable people to move easily. Dimension of doors and stairways are an important consideration, especially for disabled access.

◆ Safe workplace premises layout, and dimensions adequate for people to move about and for services being carried out.

◆ Windows, doors, gates and walls should be safe and fit for purpose.

◆ Workstations should be suitable for the people using them and the work being carried out. Adequate postural support should be provided.

◆ Safety protections against falling objects and safe storage of objects.

◆ Washing facilities of hot and cold running water should be available with hand detergent and a hygienic means of drying hands.

◆ Facilities for staff to rest and eat meals should be suitable.

◆ Drinking water with adequate high quality supply.

◆ Facilities for changing and storage of clothing should be adequate and secure.

◆ Sanitary conveniences for all staff and clients should be suitable and sufficient. Males and females should have a separate room unless it can be used by only one person at a time and can be locked.

◆ Fire exits are clearly located and accessible and firefighting equipment is available and maintained.

ALWAYS REMEMBER

Workplace temperature and ventilation

The workplace temperature should be a minimum of 16°C within 1 hour of employees arriving for work. The environment should be well ventilated or carbon dioxide levels will increase, which can cause nausea. Many substances used can become hazardous without adequate ventilation. If the working environment is too warm, this can cause heat stress, a condition recognised by the HSE.

REVISION AID

What is PPE used for in the workplace?

"Always have a tidy and safe work area and consider storage of clients' bags and clothes."

Janice Brown

ECO TIP

Environmentally friendly water on tap

Mains supplied water cooling systems are considered to be more environmentally friendly than bottled water by avoiding plastic waste and removing transport costs.

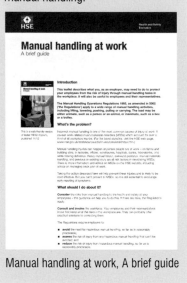
Manual Handling Operations Regulations (1992) The Manual Handling Operations Regulations (1992) apply in all occupations where manual handling occurs. The Regulations define manual handling as 'any transporting or supporting of a load (including the lifting, putting down, pushing, pulling, carrying or moving thereof) by hand or bodily force'. The aim is to prevent skeletal and muscular (muscles that attach to bone) disorders and repetitive strain disorders (as a result of performing repeated actions) due to poor working practice, which accounts for 50 per cent of workplace absence. The employer is required to carry out a risk assessment of all activities undertaken that involve manual lifting.

Manual handling should be risk assessed as a requirement to provide safe working conditions in the Management of Health and Safety at Work Regulations 1999.

The risk assessment should provide evidence that the following have been considered:

◆ risk of injury

◆ the manual movement involved in performing the activity

◆ the physical constraint the load incurs

◆ the environmental constraints imposed by the workplace

◆ workers' individual capabilities

◆ action taken in to minimise potential risks.

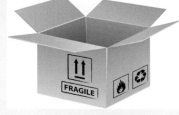
Manual lifting and handling Wherever possible manual handling should be avoided if there is a risk of injury. Use the appropriate equipment provided to move heavy loads and steps to access shelving. The HSE provides guidance of workplace measures to be implemented to reduce risk. Following training it is advisable to take care of yourself when moving goods around the workplace. Assess the risk. Do not struggle or be impatient: get someone else to help.

Ensure others will not be affected by your actions. For example, make sure you can see where you are going when moving objects.

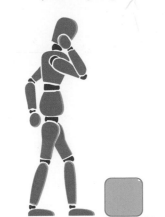

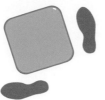

Ensure you feel stable before you lift and move the object.

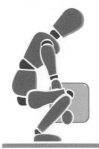

Bend the knees, keep the back straight. Lean slightly forward over the load and ensure you have a good grip of the object. You should be able to move the object smoothly with minimum effort and without twisting.

Consider where you are going to move the load to. If too large / heavy can it be made smaller?

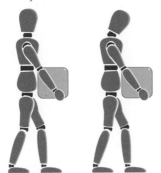

Carry the heaviest part nearest to your body.

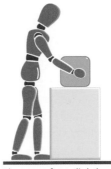

Place one foot slightly forward to support balance.

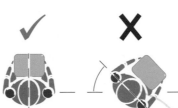

Lifting and carrying

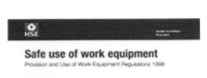

Safe use of work equipment
Provision and Use of Work Equipment Regulations 1998

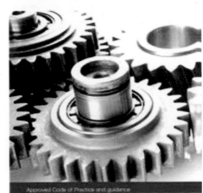

Approved Code of Practice and guidance

Provision and Use of Work Equipment Regulations (PUWER) (1998)

The **Provision and Use of Work Equipment Regulations (PUWER) (1998)** lay down the important health and safety controls on the provision and use of work equipment both new and second hand. These regulations include the use of mobile equipment, which is transported by freelance beauty therapists. They state the duties for employers and for employees, including the self-employed. The regulations apply to both old and new equipment. They identify the requirements in selecting suitable equipment and in maintaining it so that it is fit for purpose. They also discuss the information provided by equipment manufacturers and instruction and training requirements in the safe use of equipment. Specific regulations address the dangers and potential risks of injury that could occur during operation of the equipment and not using it for its intended purpose.

Suitable safety measures should be in place including protective devices available and warning signage as appropriate. Equipment should only be used by those who are adequately trained in its use.

Health and Safety (Display Screen Equipment) Regulations (1992)

The **Health and Safety (Display Screen Equipment) Regulations (1992)** cover the use of display screen equipment including computer screens. If your workplace employs a receptionist or has an online order operation, these regulations will probably be relevant to them. They specify acceptable levels of radiation emissions from the screen and identify correct **posture**, seating position, permitted working heights and rest

Receptionists in the workplace often use a computer throughout the working day, the Display Screen Equipment Regulations are relevant to their work.

TOP TIP

Work equipment

Health and safety consultant, Wendy Nixon, gives this important advice:

"How many of us try to multitask and use more than one piece of work equipment at the same time? This is a common problem among beauty therapists who are required to answer the telephone and make appointments. Trying to balance the telephone on your shoulder whilst writing or typing can cause musculoskeletal problems such as neck and back pain but can be solved easily by providing a headset for the telephone, allowing free movement of both hands and encouraging a good posture."

ACTIVITY

Identifying electrical hazards

Make a list of electrical equipment you use in the workplace and potential electrical hazards that may occur with them e.g. damaged cables.

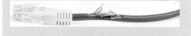

HEALTH & SAFETY

Electrical equipment safety

Take appropriate care when using electrical equipment.

For example, check that depilatory wax is at the correct recommended working temperature before use and that the equipment is not faulty when carrying out wax depilation treatment.

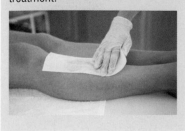

periods. Employers have a responsibility to comply with this regulation to ensure the welfare of their employees, avoiding the potential risks of eyestrain, mental stress and muscle fatigue.

TOP TIP

Display Screen Equipment Regulations 1992

As an employee it is your responsibility to work in a healthy way. Examples of good practice include the following.

◆ Hold the lower arm horizontally to the keyboard and adjust screen height so that the eyes are the same height as the top of the DSE screen.

◆ Make sure there is sufficient space around the DSE to avoid restricting physical movements, which could lead to problems with vision and posture.

◆ Avoid unnecessary glare; the screen should not face the windows or bright light.

◆ Take short regular breaks and change activities to avoid fatigue.

Electricity at Work Regulations (1989)
If unsafe or used carelessly, electricity can harm or even kill. The Electricity at Work Regulations (1989) state that every piece of equipment is to be maintained to prevent danger.

These regulations state that every piece of electrical equipment in the workplace should be maintained in good working order to prevent danger. Items of beauty equipment are often used regularly each day, e.g. wax depilation equipment. Therefore, they should be systematically checked to ensure they are in good working order. Equipment should be tested by a competent person. The necessity for testing will depend upon its use. The regulations require that equipment is safe for use. This is called portable appliance testing or PAT. A written record of testing should be kept, which can be made available for inspection if required.

In addition to PAT testing, a trained member of staff should regularly check all electrical equipment for safety; every three months is recommended. It is good practice to keep records of the check, including:

◆ competent person's name/contact details

◆ itemised list of electrical equipment complete with each piece's unique serial number for identification purposes

◆ date of purchase/disposal

◆ date of inspection.

However, electrical equipment should be safety checked every time it is used.

Report it, remove from use and make safe as immediately as practicable if any of these potential hazards are observed:

◆ exposed wires in flexes and plugs

◆ burn marks indicating overheating

◆ loose screws and wiring

◆ temperature setting thermostat does not seem to be working

◆ cracked plugs or broken sockets

◆ worn cables

◆ overloaded sockets.

Although it is the responsibility of the employer to ensure all equipment is safe to use, it is also the responsibility of the employee to always check that equipment is safe before use and to never use it if it is faulty. This complies with the requirements of public **liability insurance**. Failure to do so could lead to an accident, which could be considered careless or negligent.

Any pieces of equipment that appear faulty must be immediately reported, checked and repaired before use. They should ideally be labelled to ensure that they are not used by accident.

Remember Electrical equipment should always be used according to the manufacturer's instructions and its intended use. As it is for professional use it should be fit for purpose.

First aid Employers must manage the provision of first aid in the workplace to ensure they have appropriate and adequate first-aid arrangements in the event of an accident or illness occurring. This regulation also applies to the self-employed.

What is adequate first aid will depend upon each workplace and requires an assessment of the potential first-aid needs.

Detailed information can be found in the **Health and Safety (First Aid) Regulations 1981**, Guidance on Regulation.

It is recommended that at least one person holds a basic first-aid qualification. An amendment to the regulations in 2013, removed the previous requirement for the HSE to approve first aid training and qualifications.

All employees should be informed of the first-aid procedures including:

◆ where to locate the first-aid box

◆ who is responsible for the maintenance of the first-aid box

◆ which staff member to inform in the event of an accident or illness occurring

◆ the staff member to inform in the event of an accident or emergency

◆ calling the ambulance service in an emergency situation.

The Health and Safety (First Aid) Regulations (1981) state that workplaces are required to manage first-aid provision. An adequately stocked first-aid box should be available that complies with health and safety first aid regulations. This should contain a minimum level of first aid equipment.

ALWAYS REMEMBER

Your first-aid kit should include the following items.

No. of employees	1–5	6–10	11–50
First-aid guidance notes	1	1	1
Individual sterile adhesive dressings	20	20	40
Sterile eye pads	1	2	4
Sterile triangular bandages	1	2	4
Safety pins	6	6	12
Medium size sterile unmedicated dressings	3	6	8
Large size sterile unmedicated dressings	1	2	4
Extra-large size sterile unmedicated dressings	1	2	4

HEALTH & SAFETY

Electricity at Work Regulations 1989

For more information on these regulations, visit www.hse.gov.uk /electricity.

TOP TIP

First-aid booklet

HSE Guidance publication

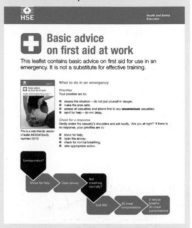

Basic advice on first aid at work; you can download a free copy at www.hse.gov.uk/pubns/indg347.pdf. This can be stored in the first-aid box.

HEALTH & SAFETY

First aid

◆ This should only be given by a qualified first aider.

◆ A first-aid certificate is only valid for 3 years and must be renewed after this period. This may mean additional first-aid training.

◆ Know what action you can take *within your responsibility* in the event of an accident occurring. The appointed person should take action if someone is injured, becomes ill, an ambulance is required or the quality and content of the fist aid box requires checking.

◆ An accident book should be available to record details of any accident that has occurred. This information should be reviewed when looking at risks in the workplace.

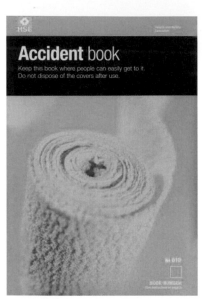

HSE accident book

Accidents An accident is an unplanned and uncontrolled event with potential to cause injury. Accidents in the workplace usually occur through negligence by employees or unsafe working conditions. Details of accidents involving clients should also be recorded, as they may be required in the instance of legal action being taken.

Employers are required to provide an accident book to record any accidents that occur in the workplace.

Any accidents occurring in the workplace must be dealt with following the workplace policy and details recorded on a **report form** and entered into an **accident book**. Incidents in the accident book should be reviewed regularly to see where improvements to working practice can be made. Details of injuries from accidents at work that must be reported under the Reporting of Injuries, Diseases and Dangerous Occurrences Regulations (RIDDOR) should be recorded also. The report form requires more details than the accident book – you must note:

◆ the date and time of accident
◆ the date of entry into the accident book
◆ the name of the person or people involved
◆ details of how the accident occurred
◆ the injuries received
◆ the action taken
◆ what happened to the person immediately afterwards (e.g. went home or to hospital)
◆ name and address of the person who provided service
◆ the signature of the person making the entry.

In the instance of an accident, first aid should only be carried out by employees qualified to do so.

Disposal of waste Waste is generated as part of the day-to-day operation of the business and as a result of treatments delivered. Waste should be sorted and disposed of according to its risk in an environmentally-friendly way. Failure to do so can result in legal action.

TOP TIP

Recognising recycling symbols

OPRL – On-Pack Recycling Label

A variety of recycling labels appear on packaging. The label will indicate if the packaging is recyclable, how widely it is recycled and where.

Some examples are shown below.

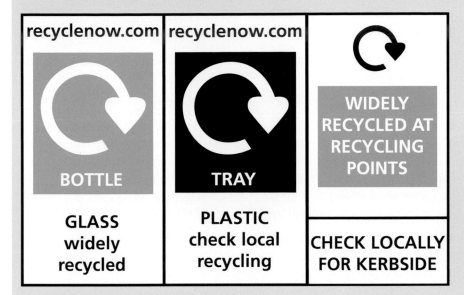

Mobius loop

This symbol means that the item is capable of being recycled. It does not necessarily mean that the item will be accepted in all recycling collection systems.

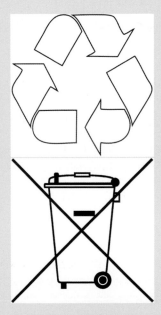

Waste electrical

If an electrical item has this symbol, it means it can be recycled.

Visit the website for further information: https://www.recyclenow.com/recycle/packaging -symbols-explained.

Remember to recycle your waste wherever possible. Recycling means that your waste is processed into new materials and conserve other natural resources that would have been used otherwise. This protects the environment as the alternative is landfill or incineration, creating pollution.

Waste you may consider recycling includes:

◆ *Paper waste* such as magazines and cardboard boxes. Every tonne of paper recycled saves 17 trees.

◆ *Glass waste* from bottles, glass accessories related to equipment such as steamer glass water jars.

Energy saved from recycling one glass bottle will power a light bulb for four hours.

◆ *Plastic waste* from packaging, plastic containers and bottles that contain cosmetics. Recycling one plastic bottle can can save enough energy to power a light bulb for six hours.

◆ *Aluminium waste* from drink cans. The energy saved by recycling one can will run a television for three hours.

◆ *Organic compostable waste* from sources such as flowers or fruit.

General waste that is not hazardous should be disposed of in an enclosed waste bin fitted with a polythene bin liner that is durable enough not to tear. The bin should be regularly cleaned and disinfected in a well-ventilated area. Protective gloves should be worn whilst doing this. When the bin is full, the liner should be sealed using a wire tie and placed ready for refuse collection. If the bin liner punctures, the damaged liner and waste should be placed inside a second bin liner.

Some waste is hazardous and is a risk to health as well as the environment. This may have the potential to be inflammable, explosive, corrosive or poisonous, referred to as toxic. Batteries and fluorescent tubes are examples of hazardous waste.

ALWAYS REMEMBER

Waste Electronic and Electrical Equipment Regulations (WEEE) (2013)

These regulations place responsibilities on manufacturers, importers, retailers and salons to ensure the safe disposal of electrical products when you are sold a replacement product. Retailers must make available the facility for unwanted items to be disposed of. These regulations apply however the item was purchased: direct, internet, mail order or telephone. Examples include portable microcurrent equipment that you may retail. Every year an estimated 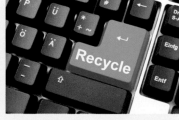 two million tonnes of WEEE items are disposed of in the UK. Nearly 25% of electrical waste and electronic equipment that is taken to household waste recycling centres can be reused.

Clinical waste is waste that is contaminated with human body tissue or bodily fluids and is classed as high risk hazardous waste. This includes waste that has come into contact with blood or urine. Hazardous waste must be handled following the COSHH procedures and training by the employer. This should be disposed of as recommended by the Local Authority environment agency in accordance with the Controlled Waste (Amendment) Regulations (1993). Items that have been used in the skin, such as ear studs or facial micro lances, should be safely discarded in a disposable sharps container. Contact your environmental health department to check on waste disposal arrangements for different hazardous items.

Any items that could cause injury to others, such as broken glass, should be placed in a secure container.

Remember to handle chemicals correctly, referring to your COSHH data sheets. Always dispose of chemicals in an environmentally-friendly way.

ALWAYS REMEMBER

Waste classification

1 Before waste is moved or disposed of, it should be classified. This will ensure that hazardous waste is disposed of appropriately. It is a good idea to have recycling containers that separate your waste, making later waste disposal easier and safer.

2 Apply your knowledge of categories of waste when recycling and disposing of waste. This will prevent harm to people and the environment by reducing waste.

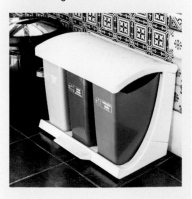

Certain treatments carried out in beauty therapy, such as ear piercing and depilatory waxing have an additional risk because of the possibility of contamination between blood or body tissue fluids. Good infection control systems are essential. An Environmental Health Inspector can visit your premises to ensure the guidelines listed in the local Government Miscellaneous Provisions Act (1982) relating to the treatment area are being met in terms of levels of hygiene and competence.

Fire

The **Regulatory Reform (Fire Safety) Order (2005)** replaces all previous legislation relating to fire, including fire certificates that no longer have any validity. This law is applicable to England and Wales only. Northern Ireland and Scotland have their own similar legislation. Local fire and rescue authorities have responsibility for enforcing this legislation.

The Regulatory Reform (Fire Safety) Order (2005) places responsibility for fire safety onto the 'responsible person', which is usually the employer. The 'responsible person' will have a duty to ensure the safety of everyone who uses their premises and those in the immediate vicinity who may be at risk if there is a fire. The 'responsible person' must carry out a fire safety risk assessment. This must be kept updated, and may be completed as part of the regular risk assessment responsibilities. If there are more than five employees, this must be in writing.

The aim is to ensure there are adequate and appropriate safety measures in place when the risk is identified so that a fire can be avoided but, in the event of a fire, it can be controlled without harm or loss of life.

Fire risk assessments will include:

◆ identifying and removing any obstacles that may hinder fire evacuation

◆ ensuring that suitable fire detection equipment is in place, such as a **smoke alarm**

◆ making sure that all fire exits and escape routes are clearly marked and free from obstructions

◆ testing fire alarm systems regularly to ensure they are in full operational condition.

All staff must be trained in fire and emergency evacuation procedures for their workplace. The **emergency exit route** will be the easiest route by which staff and clients can leave the building safely. Fire action plans should be prominently displayed to show the emergency exit route. Fire fighting equipment should be available and maintained, to be used only by those trained to use it.

A 'smash glass' type alarm may be activated to instigate evacuation and alert the fire brigade to attend. Check and ensure the building is safe before re-entering.

Fire training and improvement

◆ Training must be given to new staff during their induction.

◆ Training must be regularly updated for all staff.

◆ Fire drills must be held at regular intervals.

◆ Following a fire drill, feedback should be given on any risks that need to be actioned.

Firefighting equipment
Firefighting equipment must be available, located in a specified area. The equipment includes fire extinguishers, blankets, sand buckets and water hoses. Firefighting equipment should be used only when the cause of the fire

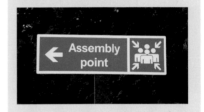
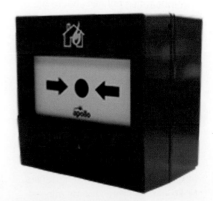

Fire alarm-smash glass type

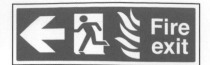
Fire exit sign

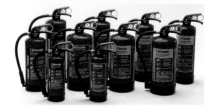
Fire extinguishers showing colour denoted for use

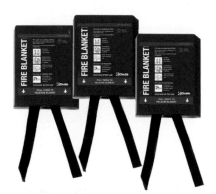
Fire blankets

has been identified – using the wrong extinguisher could make the fire worse. Using the incorrect fire fighting equipment may:

◆ cause the fire to spread or reignite
◆ cause injury including electrocution.

There are six classifications of fire of which the most relevant for the salon are A, B and C. Symbols used to identify these classifications and the relevant choice of fire extinguisher are shown in the diagram *Fire extinguisher symbols* (below). Never use firefighting equipment unless you are trained in its use.

Fire extinguishers Fire extinguishers are available to tackle different types of fire. These should be located in a set place known to all employees. It is important that these are checked and maintained as required.

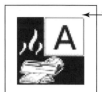
Class A Fire – Carbonaceous materials such as paper and wood.

Class B Fire – Flammable liquids such as petrol and paints.

Class C Fire – Flammable gases such as methane and acetylene.

Electrical hazard symbol – For extinguisher products safe on electrical fires.

Fire extinguisher symbols

This chart illustrates the type of fire extinguisher medium suitable for specific risks and classification of fires.

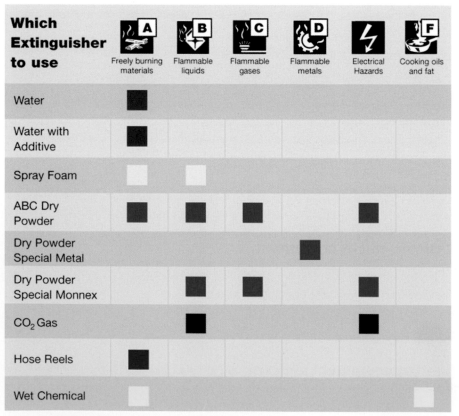

Which Extinguisher to use	A Freely burning materials	B Flammable liquids	C Flammable gases	D Flammable metals	Electrical Hazards	F Cooking oils and fat
Water	■					
Water with Additive	■					
Spray Foam	□	□				
ABC Dry Powder	■	■	■		■	
Dry Powder Special Metal				■		
Dry Powder Special Monnex		■	■		■	
CO₂ Gas		■			■	
Hose Reels	■					
Wet Chemical	□					□

Causes of fire and choice of fire extinguishers

Fire blankets are used to smother and extinguish the flames of a burning liquid or if a person's clothing is on fire. **Sand** is used to soak up liquids if these are the source of the fire, and to smother the fire. **Water hoses** are used to extinguish large fires caused by paper materials and the like – buckets of water may be used to extinguish a small fire. *Turn off the electricity first!*

Never put yourself at risk – fires can spread quickly. Leave the building at once if in danger and raise the alarm by telephoning the emergency services on the fire and rescue service emergency telephone number **999**.

Other emergencies

In addition to accidents, medical or health emergencies and fire, other possible emergencies that could occur relate to fumes and flooding. Learn where the water stopcock and gas mains supply are located. In the event of a gas leak or a flood, switch off the mains gas supply and shut off the water stopcocks. Open the window to increase ventilation. Evacuate the building following the fire drill procedure and contact the appropriate emergency service.

It is a good idea to get a gas detector, which sounds when it detects a gas leak. Never switch on an electric switch as this could cause a spark and ignite the gas. By law gas appliances and fittings must not be used if thought to be unsafe.

In the event of a bomb alert, staff must be trained in the appropriate emergency procedures. This will involve recognition of a suspect package, how to deal with a bomb threat, evacuation of staff and clients and contacting the emergency services. Your local counter-terrorism security adviser will advise on bomb security.

Inspection and registration of premises Inspectors from the HSE of your Local Authority enforce the Health and Safety law including relevant bye-laws. For certain Local Authorities there is a requirement to register the business and beauty therapist(s) performing treatments. They visit the workplace to ensure compliance with government legislation.

If the inspector identifies any area of danger, it is the responsibility of the employer to remove this danger within a designated period of time. The inspector issues an **improvement notice**. Failure to comply with the notice will lead to prosecution. The inspector also has the authority to close a business until they are satisfied that all danger to employees and the public has been removed. Such closure involves the issuing of a **prohibition notice**.

Certain services carried out in beauty therapy, such as ear piercing, pose additional risk as they may produce blood and body tissue fluid. Inspection of the premises is necessary before such services can be offered to the public. Such services are included in the local bye-laws guidelines and it is important that those guidelines in the **Local Government (Miscellaneous Provisions) Act (1982)** relating to this area are being complied with as well as other relevant health and safety laws. When the inspector is satisfied, a **certificate of registration** will be awarded. This usually lasts for as long as the individual registered remains in the district.

Insurance

Insurance must cover all activities in the workplace. The insurance should be appropriate to your employment circumstances and associated considerations. Optional cover should be considered including property damage, equipment and product loss.

ACTIVITY

Causes of fires

Can you think of several potential causes of fire in the salon? How could each of these be prevented?

HEALTH & SAFETY

Carbon monoxide fumes

When gas does not burn properly it creates poisonous carbon monoxide, which may not be apparent to you, but can kill.

It is important that gas appliances are regularly safety checked by a competent person.

Gas detection alarms are available to detect gas leaks.

ACTIVITY

Skin piercing and the Miscellaneous Provisions Act

Obtain a copy of your local authority bye-laws for skin piercing. Note the recommendations and check your compliance.

ALWAYS REMEMBER

Bye-laws

A bye-law is a law set by a statutory body such as the Local Authority. Each local authority is able to introduce its own bye-laws under the Miscellaneous Provisions Act.

Always check the bye-laws of your local authority and how they may affect you.

Public liability insurance protects employers and employees against the consequences of death or injury claim to a third party while on the premises. This also covers damage to client possessions. This does not relate to claims by employees.

Professional indemnity insurance extends the public liability insurance to cover named employees against claims. This is an important consideration when performing high-risk services such as electrical epilation.

Product and **treatment liability insurance** is usually included with your public liability insurance, but you should check this with the insurance company. Product liability insurance covers you for risks that might occur as a result of the products you are using and/or selling. Treatment risk cover may provide client compensation where there is a claim for injury as a result of treatment.

It is a legal requirement under the **Employers' Liability (Compulsory Insurance) Act 1969** that every employer must have employer liability insurance. This provides financial compensation to employees should they be injured as a result of an accident in the workplace. A current employers' liability insurance certificate must be displayed in a prominent place indicating that the policy has been obtained.

Security

Security concerns should be the responsibility of all staff to minimise theft and to keep the workplace and its goods secure. Procedures should be in place stating responsibility and the actions to be taken for different activities and circumstances. Usually the police are the contact service when dealing with an incident or security threat. Insurance companies will assess the effectiveness of security measures before providing insurance cover. Workplace policy and procedures should be identified and may refer to the following:

◆ people and possessions, including client records

◆ premises

◆ products and equipment

◆ stock

◆ cash and cash equivalents.

Internal theft by employees may result in disciplinary action, dismissal, fines and criminal prosecution.

Suspicious behaviour should be dealt with as appropriate.

There may be occasions when client behavior is inappropriate. You may need to tactfully ask a client or other visitor to leave your work premises if you feel there is a security risk or their conduct is inappropriate (e.g. a client is being abusive). Guidance for client etiquette may be provided on expectations and consequences to ensure a safe, secure and relaxing environment for all users.

Your demeanour must remain calm and positive, and you must keep to the facts of why you are taking action. All actions should be taken in line with your workplace policy.

ACTIVITY

Health and safety staff awareness training

Where are the following found in your workplace, explain the number, types and format as applicable e.g. dry powder, blue label fire extinguisher in the salon reception.

Item	Workplace location
Fire extinguisher(s)	
Information sheets stating how products should be stored/used (MSDS – Material Safety Data Sheets)	
Health and safety workplace information	
First-aid kit	
Sterilisation/disinfection equipment	
PPE	
Fire exit(s)	
Accident book	

Hygiene and infection control in the workplace

When performing treatments on different clients there is a risk of cross-infection. Infection control is the method used to remove or reduce the spread of potentially harmful microorganisms that can inhabit the work environment. Carrying out infection control procedures is a legal requirement and will also promote your professional image.

Infections

Effective hygiene and infection control is necessary to prevent cross-infection and secondary infection. Infection can occur through poor practice, such as the use of tools that are not sterile. Reusable (as opposed to disposable) tools and equipment become contaminated – infected with skin debris, known as cross-contamination. An infection can be recognised by red and inflamed skin, or the presence of pus. All staff must be trained in and carry out effective workplace decontamination procedures to remove or destroy the contamination. These procedures can be detailed in the workplace policy on health, safety and hygiene.

Cross-infection occurs because some microorganisms are contagious and they may be transferred through personal contact or by contact with an infected tool that has not been disinfected or sterilised. Cross-infection can occur through blood contamination and skin or nail infections.

HEALTH & SAFETY

Work related violence

The HSE defines this as 'any incident in which a person is abused, threatened or assaulted in circumstances relating to their work'.

This should be dealt with in the same way as any other risk assessment in the workplace, identifying the hazards and procedures for staff to implement.

REVISION AID

Which set of regulations determines fire safety in the workplace?

ACTIVITY

Avoiding cross-infection

List the different ways in which infection can be transferred in the salon.

How can you avoid cross-infection in the workplace?

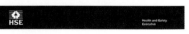

Blood-borne viruses in the workplace

Guidance for employers and employees

Is this guidance useful to me?

If you are an employee or employee, self-employed or a safety representative, and involved in work where exposure to blood or other body fluids may occur, you should read this guidance. It will help you to understand:

- what blood-borne viruses (BBVs) are;
- the types of work where exposure to BBVs may occur and how BBVs are spread;
- the legal duties of employers and employees;
- the action to be taken after possible infection with a BBV;
- special considerations for first aiders.

Detailed guidance on BBVs is already available for those in certain industries, for example health care (see 'Further reading'). This simple leaflet will be of particular use to those in occupations where such detailed guidance is not available.

What are blood-borne viruses (BBVs)?

BBVs are viruses that some people carry in their blood and which may cause severe disease in certain people and little or no symptoms in others. The virus can spread to another person, whether the carrier of the virus is ill or not.

The main BBVs of concern are:

- hepatitis B virus (HBV), hepatitis C virus and hepatitis D virus, which all cause hepatitis, a disease of the liver;
- human immunodeficiency virus (HIV) which causes acquired immune deficiency syndrome (AIDS), affecting the immune system of the body.

These viruses can also be found in body fluids other than blood, for example, semen, vaginal secretions and breast milk. Other body fluids or materials such as urine, faeces, saliva, sputum, sweat, tears and vomit carry a minimal risk of BBV infection, unless they are contaminated with blood. Care should still be taken as the presence of blood is not always obvious.

Blood-borne viruses in the workplace information

ALWAYS REMEMBER

Sterilisation

Sterilisation is the killing of organisms, such as bacteria, fungi and parasites.

Disinfection

Disinfection is the elimination of the most harmful microorganisms (but not including their spores, which are single-celled reproductive units) from surfaces or objects.

HEALTH & SAFETY

UV lamp usage

UV light is dangerous, especially to the eyes. The UV lamp must be switched off before opening the cabinet.

A record must be kept of usage because the effectiveness of the lamp decreases with use.

ECO TIP

Electricity consumption

Switch off all electrical equipment at the end of business where its use is not necessary. This includes the UV cabinet.

Glass-bead steriliser

Secondary infection can occur as a result of injury to the client during the treatment, or if the client already has an open wound. Bacteria can penetrate the skin and cause infection.

Sterilisation and **disinfection** procedures are used to minimise or destroy the harmful microorganisms that could cause infection: bacteria, viruses and fungi.

Infectious diseases that are contagious **contra-indicate** beauty treatment: they require medical attention. People with certain other skin disorders, even though these are not contagious, should not be treated by the beauty therapist, as treatment might lead to secondary infection.

Sometimes people may have a contra-indication they are not aware of, such as a blood-borne virus. If hygiene practice is not followed there is a risk of contamination from blood-borne virus transmission, including hepatitis B and C and HIV/Aids. Hepatitis B can be transmitted in small volumes of blood too small to be visible, so effective sterilisation methods and hygiene practice are essential.

HEALTH & SAFETY

Blood borne viruses: Hepatitis B immunisation

It is recommended that if you are performing treatments, such as wax depilation, where you may come into contact with blood, you should be immunised against hepatitis B to protect both yourself and clients.

For more information refer to the HSE guidance *Blood-borne viruses in the workplace* available at www.hse.gov.uk/pubns/indg342.pdf.

Sterilisation and disinfection Sterilisation is the total destruction of all living microorganisms. Disinfection is the destruction of most, but not all, microorganisms and aims to reduce the number of microorganisms (not including spores, which are their single-celled reproductive units) to a level that will not lead to infection. Sterilisation and disinfection techniques practised in the beauty work environment involve the use of physical agents, such as radiation and heat; and chemical agents, such as antiseptics and disinfectants.

All objects should be thoroughly cleaned before sterilisation or disinfection to remove surface dirt and debris.

Radiation A quartz mercury-vapour lamp can be used as the source for **UV light**, which minimises the level of harmful microorganisms. UV light has limited effectiveness and cannot be relied upon for complete sterilisation. Radiation only destroys microorganisms on the surface that the UV rays strike, requiring the object to be turned. For each surface of the object, follow the manufacturer's recommended exposure time.

HEALTH & SAFETY

If you have any cuts or abrasions on your hands, cover them with a clean dressing to minimise the risk of secondary infection. Disposable gloves may be worn for additional protection.

Certain skin disorders are contagious. If you are suffering from any such disorder you must not work, but seek medical advice immediately.

Face masks may be worn when working in close proximity to the client.

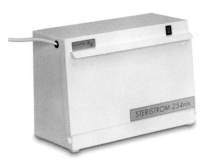

UV light cabinet

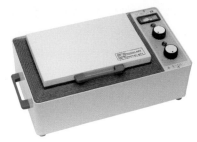

Dry-heat sterilising cabinet

Heat Dry and moist heat may both be used in sterilisation.

Dry heat One method is to use a dry hot-air oven. This is similar to a small oven, and heats to 150–180°C. It is seldom used in the salon. Also available is a glass bead steriliser where tiny glass beads are heated in an insulated container to between 190–300°C. This is suitable only for small, clean metal objects.

Moist heat The autoclave (similar to a pressure cooker) is a moist heat method of sterilisation where, because of the increased pressure, the water reaches a temperature of 121–134°C. Autoclaving is the most effective method and highly recommended for sterilising objects in the beauty workplace.

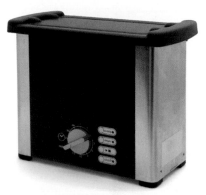

Ultrasonic cleaner

"Alcohols, such as surgical spirit, should not be used to clean equipment and furniture in the salon, particularly those with laminated or painted surfaces, as they have a stripping effect over time. Alcohol is also flammable and so should never be used to clean wax heaters that are switched on or not cool."

Janice Brown

Disinfectants and antiseptics If an object cannot be sterilised, it should be placed in a chemical disinfectant solution. A disinfectant destroys most microorganisms, but not all. **Hypochlorite** is a disinfectant; bleach is an example of a hypochlorite. It is particularly corrosive and therefore unsuitable for use with metals. Use on hard surfaces, such as work surfaces, and non-corrosive materials such as plastic tools. Always use as directed by the manufacturer.

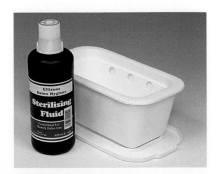

Disinfection tray with liquid

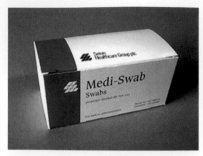

Medi-Swabs (sterile isopropyl tissues)

Ammonium compound disinfectants such as 'Barbicide' can be used with metal and plastic items. Alcohol impregnated wipes are a popular way to clean the skin using an ingredient such as isopropyl alcohol.

An **antiseptic** prevents the multiplication of microorganisms. It has a limited action, and does not kill all microorganisms.

All sterilisation and disinfection techniques must be carried out safely and effectively following the manufacturer's instructions for correct use.

1   Select the appropriate method of sterilisation or disinfection for the object. Always follow the manufacturer's guidelines on the use of the sterilising unit or agent. Wear PPE gloves as required to avoid skin irritation, which could lead to a skin disorder.

2   Clean the object in clean water and detergent, such as liquid soap, to remove dirt, debris and grease. (This is often referred to as cleansing in the salon). Dirt left on the object may prevent effective disinfection or sterilisation.

3   Dry it thoroughly with a clean, disposable paper towel.

4   Sterilise or disinfect the object, allowing sufficient time for the process to be completed. Contact with all surfaces of the object must be made.

5   Following disinfection/sterilisation, handle the object with clean tongs or protective gloves. Place objects that have been sterilised or disinfected in a clean, covered container, ideally labelled with the date. After 24 hours the object will be clean but not disinfected. This length of time is extended where a procedure is used that places the object in a vacuum sealed bag.

6   Keep several sets of the tools used regularly; this will allow you to carry out effective sterilisation following each use.

Workplace policy   It is important that you support others in maintaining a healthy, safe salon environment. Your workplace policy regarding hygiene rules and procedures may include the following requirements:

◆ **Health and safety.** Follow the health and safety policies and procedures for the workplace.

◆ **Personal hygiene.** Maintain a high standard of personal presentation and hygiene. Wash your hands before and after every treatment, and in addition to this as necessary, with a detergent containing chlorhexidine gluconate, which protects against a wide range of bacteria. The addition of isopropyl alcohol provides a stronger hand disinfectant, removing surface bacteria and fungi, and is widely used for skin cleansing.

◆ **Cuts on the hands.** Always cover any minor cuts on your hands with a protective waterproof dressing.

◆ **Cleaning rotas.** It is a good idea to have a cleaning rota that details what should be cleaned, when, how and by whom. If staff are off sick, jobs require reallocation.

If you have contract cleaners, the telephone number should be available in the event they do not arrive.

◆ **Cross-infection.** Take great care to avoid cross-infection in the workplace. This is prevented by professional, effective consultation and treatment procedures. Never treat a client who has a contagious skin disease or disorder, or any other contra-indication. Refer the client tactfully to their GP.

◆ **Use hygienic tools.** Never use an implement unless it has been effectively sterilised or disinfected, as appropriate.

◆ **Disposable applicators.** Wherever possible, use disposable products to minimise contamination.

◆ **Working surfaces.** Clean all working surfaces (such as trolleys and couches) with a chlorine preparation, diluted to the manufacturer's instructions. Cover all working surfaces with clean, disposable paper tissue. Remember to wear PPE when using cleaning materials.

◆ **Equipment.** Clean equipment, concentrating on areas such as knobs and digital pads. Cotton buds are great for cleaning hard to access areas.

◆ **Product containers.** Regularly clean pump tops and necks of tubes.

◆ **Gowns and towels.** Clean gowns and towels must be provided for each client. Towels should be laundered at a temperature of 60°C.

◆ **Laundry.** Dirty laundry should be placed in a covered container and dealt with according to the laundry procedure.

◆ **Waste, including clinical waste and non-contaminated waste.** Waste must be disposed of following the COSHH procedures and guidelines provided by the environmental health department and training by the employer. For contaminated waste, comply with the Controlled Waste Regulations (1992). Put waste in a suitable container lined with a disposable waste bag. A yellow 'sharps' container and heavy duty yellow bag should be available for clinical waste contaminated with blood or tissue fluid, e.g. contaminated wax depilation waste. Protective gloves should be worn to avoid risk of contamination.

◆ **Eating and drinking.** Never eat or drink in the treatment area of the salon. It is unprofessional and harmful chemicals may be ingested.

In the day-to-day running of the business you have a responsibility to implement working practice that is both efficient and environmentally friendly.

Environmental and sustainable working practices

Compliance with requirements for environmental and sustainable working practices is monitored through **The Environmental Protection Act**. This Act of Parliament brings in a system of unified pollution control for the disposal of waste to land, water and air. Enforcing authorities such as the Local Authority monitor compliance.

Having environmental and sustainable working practices in your workplace is cost effective and shows good citizenship.

Environmental top tips are provided throughout this book.

A busy beauty business can use a lot of resources and create a great deal of environmental waste. Both employers and employees can contribute to reducing this waste. The aim of sustainability is to use minimal resources whilst achieving maximum efficiency.

REVISION AID

What is the difference between the hygiene control methods 'disinfection' and 'sterilisation'?

ALWAYS REMEMBER

Appropriate hygiene procedures

Always follow manufacturers' guidelines on the use and suitability of chemical agents and equipment used. If you don't, this may be ineffective but also damage tools and equipment.

"Remember: smoking, eating and drinking during the course of a treatment allows close contact with the mouth, transferring microorganisms to the hand, which can then spread from or to the client."

Janice Brown

ECO TIP

Disposable towels will reduce the quantity of towels that require laundering.

TOP TIP

Cleaning schedule

For general hygiene procedures and to maintain the cleanliness of the work area, a schedule can be created identifying what should be done when and by whom.

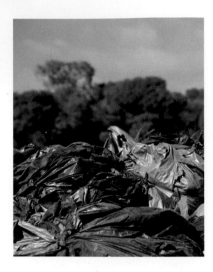

ALWAYS REMEMBER

Sustainability is about doing more with less.

ECO TIP

Team commitment

Your business's environmental and sustainability policy should be reviewed regularly to see how practice can be improved. There are environmental business awards in recognition of best practice.

ALWAYS REMEMBER

Environmentally friendly terminology

Commitment to being environmentally friendly is also known as being 'eco-friendly' or 'green', meaning that you endeavour to minimise harm to the environment and put this into your working practice.

The environmental effect of all workplace operations should be assessed. Performance should be regularly reviewed for improvement.

A starting point is to have a business environmental policy. This shows the commitment by the business and provides instruction on what actions are to be taken, the benefits and who does what and when. *Environmental and sustainable practices* can be an agenda item into which all staff can contribute their ideas.

The following working practice can be considered.

◆ Use available technology rather than paper wherever possible.

◆ Recycle whenever possible; many items can be recycled, including light bulbs.

◆ Minimise waste and use only the required amount of product within a treatment.

◆ Use and dispose of products safely as recommended by the workplace instructions and manufacturer or legislative guidelines.

◆ Use renewable resources, those that can be easily replenished.

◆ Use biodegradable packaging for disposal of waste. Recycle your waste where possible, use colour-coded waste bags that are, of course, made from recycled materials.

◆ Some beauty companies will provide incentives such as refill facilities and a free product on the return of used packaging.

◆ Dispose of chemicals safely, not down the sink.

◆ With the increase in use of electronic and digital technology, consider the safe disposal of e-waste such as discarded electronic devices.

◆ For hospitality drinks, rather than disposable plastic cups revert back to cups and glasses that can be washed.

◆ Choose ethical and responsible suppliers wherever possible, such as 'Fair Trade' products, e.g. tea and coffee.

◆ If using wooden spatulas, purchase from sustainable wood sources (managed forests).

◆ Buy in bulk, reducing trips to the wholesaler and buy locally, supporting other local businesses.

◆ Use recyclable consumable materials where possible, e.g. couchroll tissues and cleaning products.

◆ Switch off equipment at night.

◆ Use light bulbs that minimise energy use. Although initially more expensive they use less energy, saving money in the long term!

◆ Switch off lights and equipment when not in use (for lighting only if safe to do so)!

◆ Sensor light switches reduce the amount of time a light is on for. They respond to movement; inactivity will result in the lights going into hibernation mode, preventing unnecessary energy usage.

◆ Only fill the kettle with the amount of water required to be heated.

◆ Turn down the heating thermostat rather than opening the windows, this will save money too! Switch it off or lower it when the business is closed.

◆ Choose energy-efficient appliances wherever possible, e.g. washing machine; look for an 'A' rating.

◆ If using air conditioning (which uses a significant amount of energy) only use it when necessary and keep the windows closed when in use.

◆ Insulation should be installed where possible to reduce energy used.

◆ Choose recycled, eco-friendly furniture and low-chemical paints.

◆ Staff can be encouraged to reduce their journey 'carbon footprint'; examples include using public transport, cycling to work and car sharing.

ACTIVITY

Sustainable practice

In what ways can you further improve sustainable practice in your workplace?

Create a checklist that you can monitor to check for improvement.

REVISION AID

Why is environmental practice an important consideration for all in the workplace?

ACTIVITY

Look to see if there are any hazard pictograms which state care that should be taken in a product's use, storage or disposal.

Some examples are shown below. Identify their meaning and how this will affect your safe handling of the product.

  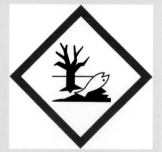

TOP TIP

Always aim to reduce waste and reuse or recycle. This will save money, which could be invested in staff training.

Personal appearance, hygiene and health

Personal appearance

Your personal appearance enables the client to make an initial judgement about the professional standards of the salon, so all staff need to make the correct impression. Employees in the workplace should always reflect the desired professional image and look the part.

Due to the nature of many of the treatments offered, beauty therapists are required to wear protective, hygienic workwear, referred to as PPE. An overall may comprise

TOP TIP

Professional image

A professional image instills confidence in clients, who trust that they will be treated in a certain way, professionally and with respect.

HEALTH & SAFETY

Workplace Policy

Your workplace policy will advise you of the standards for personal presentation and any additional requirements in relation to your appearance.

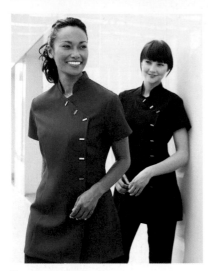

Female workwear

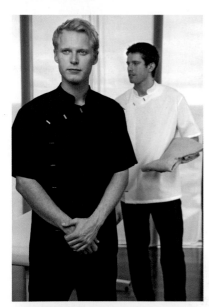

Male workwear

HEALTH & SAFETY

Tattoos and piercings

Your workplace policy may state a preference in terms of whether piercings and tattoos can be physically displayed.

a dress, a jumpsuit or a tunic top, with co-ordinating trousers, with choice and length suited to the work role. The use of a colour such as white, immediately shows the client that you are clean and professional. However, a fresh, clean overall should be worn each day.

If the business employs a receptionist, they may wear different clothing but it should be smart, functional and appropriate to their role and the image of the business.

Skincare Make-up, if worn, should be appropriate to your work role and the skincare suited to your skin type. A healthy facial appearance will be a positive advertisement for your work. First impressions count!

Jewellery Keep jewellery to a minimum, such as a wedding ring, a watch (which requires removal during treatment application therefore a popular alternative is a fob watch) and small stud earrings. Facial piercings are increasingly popular but their acceptability may be covered or discussed as part of your workplace policy on appearance and dress code in maintaining a professional appearance.

Nails A beauty therapist's work requires nails on the hand to be short, neatly manicured and free of nail polish. Nail length can interfere with the application of the treatment, such as massage and electrical epilation and some clients may be allergic to nail polish. Artificial nails, (including gel polish) should not be worn. This rule has an exception, however. If you are specialising in nail services, it is important to promote nail finish.

Shoes Ideally you should wear flat, well-fitting, comfortable shoes that enclose your feet fully, offering protection but allowing the toes to spread. Remember you may be on your feet most of the day and this action will prevent future foot and postural disorders caused by ill-fitting shoes!

Personal hygiene

It is vital that you have a high standard of personal hygiene. You are going to be working in close contact with people. Guidance should be provided when necessary to reinforce the need.

Cross-contamination can be avoided if you exercise a high level of compliance with personal hygiene practice. Bodily cleanliness is achieved through daily showering or bathing. This removes stale sweat, dirt and bacteria, which cause body odour. An antiperspirant or deodorant may be applied to the underarm area to reduce perspiration (sweat) and therefore the smell of body odour. Clean underwear, socks or tights should be worn each day.

Hands Your hands and everything they touch are covered with microorganisms (or 'germs'). Although most are harmless, some can cause ill-health or disease. Hands should be washed regularly with a hand detergent, particularly after using the toilet and especially before eating food. Hands must always be washed before and after treating each client, and during a treatment if necessary. Washing your hands before treating a client minimises the risk of cross-infection, and presents to the client a hygienic, professional, caring image. The hand detergent may contain chlorhexidine gluconate, which protects against a wide range of bacteria.

RECOMMENDED HAND-WASHING ROUTINE

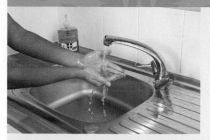

1 Wet your hands, wrists and forearms thoroughly using running water.

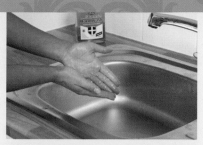

2 Apply around 3–5 ml of liquid soap.

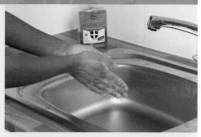

3 Start the lathering process, rubbing palm to palm.

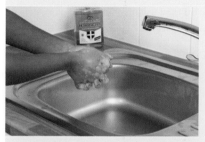

4 Interlock fingers and rub, ensuring a good lather.

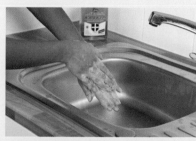

5 Rub right hand over back of left, then left over right hand.

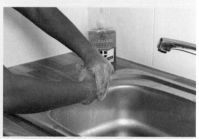

6 Rub with fingers locked in palm of hand, ensuring fingertips are cleaned.

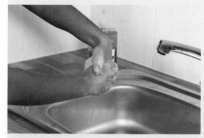

7 Lock thumbs and rotate hands.

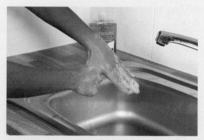

8 Grasp thumb with hand and rotate, repeat with opposite thumb.

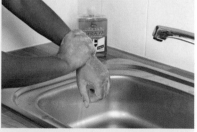

9 Rotate hand around wrist, repeat on opposite wrist.

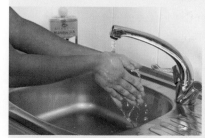

10 Rinse hands and wrists thoroughly using running water.

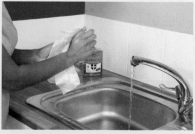

11 Dry the hands and wrists thoroughly using a clean, disposable paper towel or warm-air hand dryer.

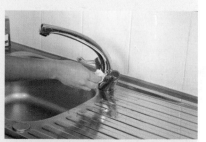

12 Turn off the tap using a clean paper towel to avoid contaminating the hands. Dispose of the paper towel without coming into contact with any part of the waste bin.

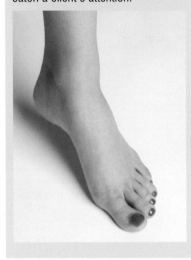

The addition of isopropyl or ethyl alcohol provides a stronger hand disinfectant, removing surface bacteria and fungi and is widely used for skin cleansing.

After washing your hands it is important to dry them thoroughly and apply a moisturiser or barrier cream to replace the skin's natural oils.

Disinfectant hand gel may also be applied to clean hands before treatments are delivered.

Skin on the hands should be regularly checked for dryness or soreness. If this occurs, hand maintenance systems should be reviewed, including PPE.

HEALTH & SAFETY

Hand cleanliness

Wash your hands with liquid soap from a sealed dispenser. This should take 10–20 seconds. Don't refill disposable soap dispensers when empty: if you do they will become a breeding ground for bacteria and the chemical interactions may reduce the cleaning property.

Disposable paper towels ideally from recycled paper or eco-friendly, low energy warm-air hand dryers should be used to thoroughly dry your hands.

ECO TIP

Water Use

When washing hands, reduce water use by:

◆ using the correct amount of soap

◆ avoiding leaving the tap running unnecessarily whilst washing hands

◆ using hot water only when necessary as this will reduce energy consumption to heat the water.

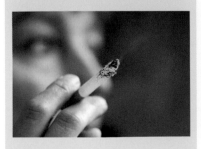

Feet Keep feet fresh and healthy by washing them daily and then drying thoroughly, especially between the toes, to avoid foot infections such as athlete's foot. Deodorising foot powder may then be applied. Foot lotions are recommended to maintain skin moisture, preventing dry skin conditions.

Oral hygiene Avoid bad breath by brushing teeth at least twice daily and flossing the teeth frequently. Remember, some foods such as garlic can be present on the breath the following day.

Use of breath fresheners and disinfectant mouthwashes can help to freshen the breath. Visiting the dentist regularly will maintain healthy teeth and gums. Avoid smoking, eating strong flavoured foods that could cause offence when in close contact with clients.

Hair Your hair should be clean and tidy. It should be cut regularly to maintain its appearance, and shampooed and conditioned as often as needed. If long, your hair should be worn off the face, and taken to the crown of the head. Medium-length hair should be clipped back, away from the face, to prevent it falling forwards and restricting your vision.

Diet, exercise and sleep A beauty therapist requires lots of energy. To achieve this you need to eat a healthy, well-balanced diet, take regular exercise and have regular sufficient sleep – between seven and eight hours per night is recommended.

Staff training is important to raise awareness of problems that can arise from poor work-related posture, or health complaints when providing services. Client comfort is important but it is equally important that the beauty therapist is comfortable too when delivering each service.

Posture

Posture is the way you hold yourself when standing, sitting, walking and in day-to-day movements. Recognising good posture is important to avoid developing postural faults. Correct posture enables you to work longer without becoming tired; it prevents muscle fatigue, repetitive strain injury (RSI) and stiff joints; and it also improves your appearance.

Good standing posture If you are standing with good posture, this is how you will look:

- head up, centrally balanced
- shoulders slightly back and relaxed
- chest up and out
- abdomen flat
- hips level
- fingertips level
- bottom in
- knees level
- feet slightly apart, and weight evenly distributed.

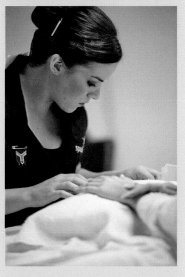

HEALTH & SAFETY

Working Time Regulations

A 20 minute break is required when working for 6 hours or more. This is important when carrying out repetitive tasks, where further breaks may be required or the inclusion of other treatment activities using different postural movements.

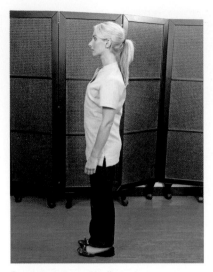

Good posture – standing

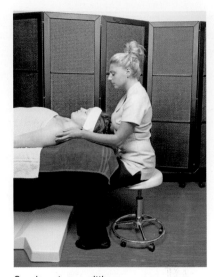

Good posture – sitting

TOP TIP

When performing treatments in a standing position:

◆ Position yourself so that you do not have to unnecessarily overstretch or stoop.

◆ Ensure you have sufficient room around you to avoid unnatural restriction of body movement.

TOP TIP

When performing treatments in a sitting position:

◆ Position yourself so that you do not have to overreach.

◆ Ensure you have sufficient room around you to avoid unnatural restriction of body movement.

◆ Ensure that you keep your feet on the floor for stability.

HEALTH & SAFETY

Repetitive strain injury (RSI)

If you do not follow correct postural positional requirements when performing treatments, and take recommended breaks between delivery of the same treatment such as single lash extensions, your muscles and ligaments may become overstretched and overused, resulting in repetitive strain injury (RSI). This may lead to you being unable to work in the short term – and potentially – long term in the occupation!

HSE provide guidance on managing upper limb disorders in the workplace. Management of avoidance of RSI is the employer's responsibility as part of the general duties under the Health and Safety at Work Act 1974 and the Management of Health and Safety at Work Regulations 1999.

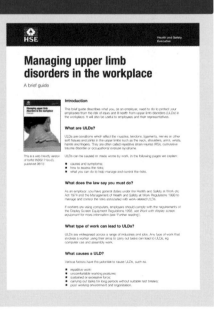

REVISION AID

Why is a therapist's posture an important consideration when carrying out treatments?

Good sitting posture Sit on a suitable chair or stool with a good back support and follow these tips:

◆ Sit with your lower back pressed against the chair back.

◆ Keep your chest up and your shoulders back.

◆ Distribute your body weight evenly along your thighs.

◆ Keep your feet together and flat on the floor.

◆ Do not slouch or sit on the edge of your seat.

HEALTH & SAFETY

Seating to be for purpose and individual's needs

Employers are required to provide seating for their employees that is both suitable and safe for the needs of the individual and the requirements of the job role. This may require the purchase of ergonomic equipment such as back and foot rests, seating and treatments couches which are height adjustable. Where required, training should be provided to ensure compliance with safety seating.

Regular risk assessments should be made in compliance with the Management of Health and Safety Regulations 1999. Special need requirements for staff should be covered under the Workplace (Health, Safety and Welfare) Regulations 1992 and the Equality Act 2010.

ACTIVITY

The importance of posture and position when working

1 Which treatments will be performed sitting and which standing?

2 In what way will your treatments be affected if you are not sitting or standing correctly?

3 How can incorrect sitting and standing affect you physically?

4 How can you take responsibility to avoid postural related injury in your day-to-day work?

Working hours and time keeping

Absence from work

If you are unexpectedly absent from work, you need to let others know as soon as practicable. Contact must be made as early as possible, in order that the client treatment schedule can be reviewed and rescheduled to minimise disruption and avoid client disappointment.

Following an absence you may be required to provide a Medical Statement (or a doctor's note) and complete sickness forms in relation to your absence.

Punctuality

To ensure the efficient workflow throughout the working day, all staff must be punctual to fulfill their work obligations. If you are late, clients' treatments will be delayed. This will have a knock-on effect throughout the working day and may result in loss of clients. Changes to working hours, breaks and treatment delivery can arise in order to accommodate different situations, e.g. staff sickness, changes to appointment bookings, or as a result of poor staff punctuality at the start of the day, which is unacceptable. There should be an effective system to communicate any change to those staff affected.

Time management – every minute counts!

Management of working time is important to ensure that all responsibilities and duties are completed. This also requires self-management skills. Managing your time effectively makes you more productive.

Working in an efficient, tidy manner will save time, as your work area will need minimal preparation for each client. It will also prevent tools and products being mislaid if they are kept in the correct designated place.

It is also important to carry out treatments in a commercially viable time to avoid overrunning. This will avoid disruption to delivery of treatments and avoid delay of subsequent client appointments. Where a delay does occur, clients may be contacted to suggest a revised time.

ALWAYS REMEMBER

Financial effectiveness

As well as people, remember that time is another resource that contributes to the financial effectiveness of the business.

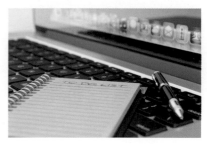

To do list

ALWAYS REMEMBER

Efficiency

Being tidy, putting things back where they should be after use, will mean the next person may use them straight away with no disruption to treatment delivery. One of the most annoying losses of time is caused by careless use of equipment and resources.

ACTIVITY

Investigate the commercial timings for treatments in salons in your location.

Reception requires the application of excellent organisational skills and systems to ensure it operates efficiently, manages and maximises the potential clientele and leaves a positive, lasting, professional impression on each client.

Reception essentials

When booking clients for a treatment it is essential that sufficient time is allocated for the treatment, including consultation and aftercare advice. In a salon, if you have a receptionist, their role is important to ensure that clients are booked correctly for their treatment. They are also responsible for arranging and confirming relevant pre-treatment tests have been received.

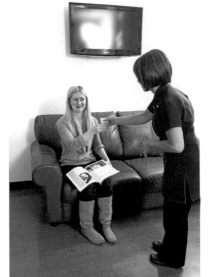

Ensuring your client's wait is enjoyable

TOP TIP

Managing work flow

In the case of treatments overrunning their allocated time, use your initiative and where applicable, follow your supervisor's advice on the appropriate action to take. If the client cannot wait, the solution may be to offer an alternative beauty therapist or an alternative treatment time. If the client is able to wait, make the wait as enjoyable as possible, for example offer refreshments or magazines. Another beauty therapist may be able to prepare the client for you.

ALWAYS REMEMBER

Working under pressure

On occasions you will be extremely busy, and may feel tired and irritable. This is not your client's or colleague's problem. Remain cheerful, courteous and helpful at all times. Use your initiative in helping others at busy times.

You must be able to cope with the unexpected:

◆ clients arriving late for appointments

◆ clients' treatments overrunning their allocated treatment time

◆ double bookings, where two clients require treatment at the same time

◆ clients who have a contra-indication to the treatment

◆ faulty equipment requiring you to offer an alternative treatment if possible, or rearrange the booking

◆ the arrival of unscheduled clients

◆ changes to the bookings.

With effective teamwork such situations can usually be overcome.

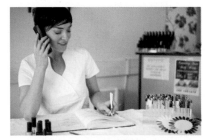

Booking client appointments

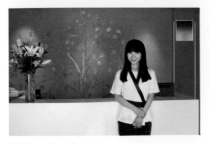

Welcoming clients

The reception area should feel welcoming and well organised to clients.

Important reception skills include welcoming and receiving clients and visitors to the business on arrival, handling enquiries, making appointments, dealing with client payments and generally maintaining the appearance and organisation of the reception area. Dealing with people in a polite, efficient manner and using good communication and questioning skills to find out exactly what they require is an important part of this role.

INDUSTRY ROLE MODEL

TINA ROOK Head of Saks Education

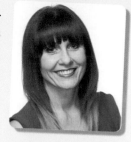

At the age of 14 I had an interview with the careers teacher at school. I knew exactly what I wanted to do – I always had – to be a beauty therapist! But I didn't really know what it entailed; all I knew was that I was going to make a living out of it.

I was lucky as I managed to get a job straight out of college in a local beauty salon. It was a small salon with just two beauty rooms at the back of the hairdressers, and while it was a fantastic experience, I knew I wanted to work in a larger salon that offered more advanced beauty services.

So my next step took me to a larger beauty salon, with 10 treatment rooms, fitted with toning tables and tanning facilities. The salon offered more modern, advanced techniques and treatments in beauty therapy. It was really exciting to learn new skills and develop a better insight into the beauty trade.

From salon to sea: cruise ships were my next adventure. I think this is not only where I got my sea legs, but I also got a real taste of what being a beauty therapist was all about. The job was very demanding but not as glamorous as you might imagine. It was also extremely rewarding, not to mention the crew parties and travelling to some of the most beautiful places in the world. I had the time of my life!

When I finally returned home, I wanted to share my knowledge and experience with others so teaching felt like the natural path to take. I started working for a small training provider delivering beauty therapy qualifications. Subsequently, I applied for a job at HABIA where I worked as the Qualifications Development Manager. My role was instrumental in developing one of the first apprenticeships in beauty therapy. During this time I also set up my own beauty salon, offering a full range of services including nail enhancements. Thereafter, I joined Saks Education. And as they say – the rest is history!

First impressions

Reception is usually a client's first and also final impression of the business, whether this is on the telephone or in person when they visit. Clients observe and remember the quality of this service. It is important that the appearance of the receptionist is impeccable, and their attitude and response to any query are knowledgeable and extremely helpful. Remember, first impressions count, so ensure that clients consistently get the *right* impression!

ALWAYS REMEMBER

Transferable skills

If providing a reception service it is important to apply the following knowledge and skills:

◆ Health and safety legislation
◆ Consumer protection legislation
◆ Selling skills
◆ Continuing Professional Development (CPD): keeping up-to-date with current products and services
◆ Stock control
◆ Communication: written and verbal.

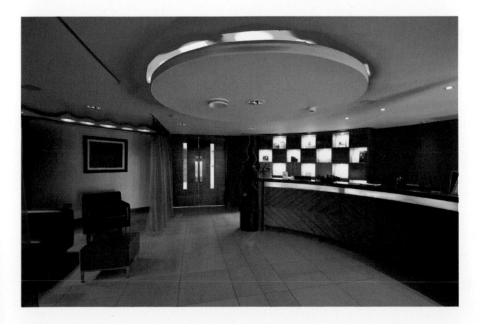

"Remember, first impressions count. You only get one chance to make a good first impression and it only takes a few seconds for a client to form a judgement whether they like you or not."

Tina Rook

ALWAYS REMEMBER

Seek the guidance of others

If you are unable to answer any query or are unsure of the best way to handle a situation, know to whom you can refer and when to do so.

Clients need to feel valued. Excellent **interpersonal skills** are essential in a receptionist. These skills are the way in which you communicate and interact with other people, and require you to adapt and moderate your behaviour depending upon the circumstances. Your interpersonal skills are judged with everything you say and do. Clients will reach conclusions based upon your behaviour. Considering this you should always:

◆ act positively and confidently whatever the circumstance

◆ speak clearly

◆ be friendly, appear approachable and smile; show empathy depending on the situation

◆ when face-to-face look at the client to acknowledge them, show interest and read their facial expressions

◆ use good listening skills, actively hear what they are saying to you and how they are saying it, noting their tone

◆ be interested in everything that is going on around the reception area

◆ give each client your full attention and respect.

TOP TIP

Cleanliness

An attractive heavy-duty foot mat at the entrance to reception will protect the main floor covering from becoming marked. This may be embossed with the business logo.

Keep the entrance clean and smart at all times to reduce the hazard of accidents occurring from slipping on wet flooring.

"Remember, as the front of house receptionist you are the first person that a client will see when they walk through the door. You are an advert for your salon and as such your hair, make-up and dress should reflect this."

Tina Rook

ACTIVITY

Planning a reception area including access considerations for all users

Design a reception area, to scale, appropriate to a small or large beauty business. Discuss your choice of wall and floor coverings, furnishings and equipment, giving the reasons for their selection. Consider clients' comfort, and health and safety, and disability adjustments, e.g. easy to reach door handles for wheelchair users.

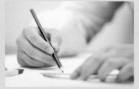

To help you plan this you may refer to a specialist beauty equipment suppliers' brochure or online information.

Reception area

Location Reception is usually situated at the front of the business premises; in a large department store, reception may be a cosmetic counter. It should be clean, tidy and inviting.

If the business has a window this can be used to attract and capture the attention and interest of potential clients passing by. Clients who are waiting in reception, however, may seek privacy, so if there is a window this should be attractively screened and the seating should be situated away from the view of the main window if possible.

Size The entrance to reception should wherever possible accommodate wheelchair access. There should be adequate seating, and an area in which to hang clients' coats and wet umbrellas. If the entrance floor becomes wet for any reason, all necessary action should be taken immediately to avoid slippage.

HEALTH & SAFETY

Equality Act 2010 – access to the business premises

The Equality Act 2010 was set up to protect people from being discriminated against in the workplace and in society. It replaced a number of different laws including the Disability Discrimination Act. Your business provides an everyday service that those with disabilities have a right to access and you are required to make reasonable adjustments to enable this. It is important every effort is made to comply with this legislation. The location of the reception and access design should take this into account. Failure to make reasonable adjustments can result in legal action being taken.

As a receptionist, if a client informs you of a disability, you should always ask what you can do to assist them.

For more information on this or accessibility issues visit **www.gov.uk/browse/disabilities**.

Hospitality is important and shows the salon's commitment to client care. If the client arrives early or their treatment is likely to be delayed, offer magazines or refreshments such as coffee, herbal teas or water. Clients may also like refreshments following their treatment, for example while waiting for their nail polish to dry, or between treatments. Seasonal refreshments may be provided, for example mulled wine and mince pies during the festive period.

If your salon has a relaxation area, ensure this area is kept tidy and refreshments are available, if provided. This is also used as a type of reception area where clients can relax as they wait for their treatment.

Magazines should be stored in an area of the reception. They should be collected as necessary and returned to this area. Magazines should be renewed regularly and if in poor condition, put in the recycling bin. Some clients may wish to access their electronic devices. If available, you can offer guest wireless access. This is especially helpful if you are in an area with limited wi-fi connectivity.

Smoking (tobacco and e-cigarettes) It is illegal to smoke on enclosed or partially enclosed business premises and you are required by law to display a mandatory sign stating this. Out of courtesy if you have an area where clients are able to smoke outside you may inform them of this. Clearly signpost where clients can and cannot smoke. Battery operated e-cigarettes, personal vaporisers (PVs) and electronic nicotine delivery systems (ENDS) which are an alternative to smoking tobacco are increasingly popular. The long term effects of their use are unknown and they fall outside tobacco smoking legislation. It is wise for their use to be included in the workplace policy for both employees and visitors. It may be required to have a separate area for e-cigarette smokers to tobacco smokers as they may be trying to stop smoking.

TOP TIP

Window displays

Windows provide great opportunities to show eye-catching displays that help market your business and products. You can change the theme according to the time of year and special calendar events.

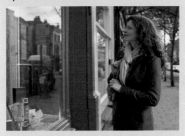

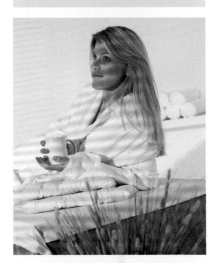

Client relaxing between treatments

ALWAYS REMEMBER

The definition of a person with disabilities

The Equality Act (2010) defines a person with disabilities as someone who has a physical or mental impairment that has a substantial and long-term negative effect on their ability to do normal daily activities.

HEALTH & SAFETY

Eating and drinking

The receptionist and other employees should not eat or drink at reception for reasons of hygiene and to maintain a professional appearance.

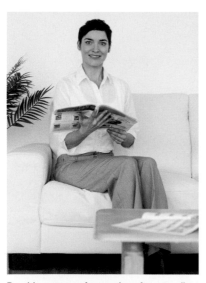

Provide a range of magazines for your client

Decoration The reception area should be decorated tastefully in keeping with the décor in the rest of the salon. Attractive posters promoting proprietary cosmetic ranges, products and treatments may be displayed on the walls. These should be renewed regularly to keep a fresh feel. Framed certificates of the staff's professional qualifications can be displayed, as well as local authority byelaws, registration with the local authority and insurance certificates.

Decorative plants or fresh flowers displayed on reception are attractive. Avoid heavily fragranced flowers which could cause respiratory problems to some people.

A television is often sited in reception. This may also be used to promote **salon services**. Promotional DVDs or web links are available from beauty manufacturers and suppliers or you can upload your own materials. These can capture your clients' interest and awareness about further products and treatments.

Reception resources The reception area should be uncluttered. The main equipment and furnishings required for an efficient reception include the following:

◆ *A reception desk* The size of the reception desk will depend on the size of the business; some businesses such as health spas employ several receptionists. The desk should include shelves and drawers; some have an in-built lockable cash or security drawer. The desk should be at a convenient height for the client to make a payment, note down the appointment time etc. It should also be large enough to house the **appointment** book or computer (or both). Consider clients who may be in a wheelchair – the desk must be accessible to them so you can communicate effectively with them and handle their payments.

◆ *A comfortable receptionist chair* The receptionist's chair should provide adequate back support and be the correct height for working at a computer screen.

◆ *A computer* Computers are used to store and analyse data about clients, for example picking up appointment trends for services and product sales. They are also used to book appointment schedules, to carry out automatic stock control, handle electronic communication (e.g. email), send text appointment reminders and also as a follow up communication informing clients about offers and promotions or using social media to post useful information, photographs or videos. They are frequently used to record business details such as accounts and marketing information. They can also be programmed to recommend specific services on the basis of personal data about the client! Space should be provided for a printer if required. A shredder is useful to dispose of confidential information when necessary.

◆ *A calculator* This is used for simple financial calculations, especially if the salon does not have a computer.

◆ *Stationery* This should include price lists, paper-based gift **vouchers**, appointment cards and a receipt pad. Keep a supply available in line with your salon policy.

◆ *A notepad* This is for taking notes and recording **messages**.

◆ *Address business cards and telephone contact details* All frequently used telephone numbers should be available in an electronic or non-electronic format.

◆ *Sales-related equipment* Items such as till rolls, credit card related equipment and resources and a cash book if used.

◆ *A telephone with answer phone/voicemail facility* Voicemail allows clients to notify you, even when the salon is closed, of an appointment request, or an unavoidable change or cancellation. You can then re-schedule appointments as quickly as possible. If you are working on your own, this voicemail facility avoids interruptions during a service, yet without losing custom.

◆ *A fax machine* This is becoming less popular as a communication system but may be available at reception. The fax is capable of transmitting text and images via a telephone line to another fax machine. This is useful when information needs to be passed on quickly.

◆ *Client records* **Client records** hold confidential data and record the personal details of each client registered at the salon. They should be kept in alphabetical order in an electronic format or a filing cabinet or a card-index box, and should be ready for collection by the beauty therapist when treating new or existing clients.

Each card records:

◆ the client's name, address (home and email) and telephone numbers

◆ age and gender

◆ medical information including medication taken

◆ any known health contra-indications (such as allergies) and contra-actions

◆ treatment aims and outcomes

◆ consultation outcomes related to the client, which will assist in planning future treatments

◆ treatments received, products used and purchased

◆ person to contact in the event of an emergency

◆ personal notes, including likes and dislikes; these help maximise the enjoyment of each visit.

These details may be updated by the receptionist at a later stage following the client's treatment. An electronic database may be used to maintain client records, which makes updating client data easier and more accessible. It can also be used in conjunction with other business software packages.

◆ *Salon policies (also on the website if available)* These can be displayed at the reception area. This may include information about smoking, pre-treatment skin tests, client etiquette, cancellation of appointments time lines etc.

◆ *Pens, pencils and a rubber* Make sure these stay at the desk and are in good condition!

◆ *A display cabinet* This may be used to store retail products and items sold by the salon.

◆ *Retail displays* These should be inspiring in their presentation and available for the client to try and purchase products.

◆ *Waste bin* A covered, lined waste bin may be provided at the reception area. Ensure this is emptied regularly following salon policy, with consideration to waste recycling.

Data Protection Act (DPA) (1998)

The **Data Protection Act (1998)** This legislation is designed to protect the client's privacy and confidentiality, control the way information is handled and to give legal rights to people who have information stored about them. With more businesses using computers to store and process personal data, access to confidential information is becoming increasingly possible. It is necessary to ask the client personal questions before the treatment plan can be finalised. As a receptionist it is important that access to confidential client information is stored in a secure area following the client service, whether on a computer or organised paper filing system. Inform the client that their personal details are being stored and will only be accessed by those individuals who are authorised to do so. Remember also: do not provide confidential information over the telephone or in email correspondence.

ALWAYS REMEMBER

Data Protection Act (DPA) (1998)

This legislation requires employees to:

◆ comply with the use and storage requirements of client records

◆ only use data for its intended purpose

◆ keep data accurate and up to date

◆ retain data for the specified time limit

◆ securely password protect electronic information

◆ allow client access to data on request.

To be aware of the full legislation requirements for the DPA visit **www.legislation.gov.uk**.

ACTIVITY

Designing a client record/salon treatment menu

Design a client record be used to record the client's personal details, treatment details and treatment plan. Alternatively, you could design a salon treatment information menu explaining the different treatments available, timing and cost. Be creative, and include a business name you may wish to use in the future. Relate the design of each to the training route you are studying towards.

TOP TIP

Electronic mail (email)

Email is a more popular method of communication today. If your salon has an email address this should be provided to your clients. Also, collect your clients' email addresses as an alternative method of communicating if preferred.

The receptionist duties

The receptionist's duties include:

◆ providing outstanding customer care

◆ maintaining a clean and hygienic the reception area and resources including product displays

◆ recognising and dealing with risks and hazards within the work environment

◆ looking after clients and visitors on their arrival; sometimes during their time in the salon; and on departure

◆ providing hospitality and making clients feel valued and comfortable, for example providing refreshments, especially if their appointment is delayed or they are early. Friendly 'small talk' is important as is provision of magazines for the client to read. How far your hospitality will go depends on how busy you are and their requirements. For example, if they have several bags you may offer to carry these to the treatment area for them, opening the door when the client leaves, thanking them for their service and wishing them a great day is a nice gesture.

HEALTH & SAFETY

Cleanliness of the reception area

In a large salon a professional cleaner may be employed to maintain the hygiene of the reception area. In a smaller salon this may be the responsibility of the receptionist, identified as a duty on your job description. Reception must be maintained to a high standard at all times. Use quieter periods for this purpose and to check retail stock levels etc.

TOP TIP

Useful contact numbers

It is useful to have the contact details of other service providers that a client may ask for that you could personally recommend. Examples include local taxi companies, hairdressers and florists. You may work collaboratively with these businesses displaying their business cards.

◆ answering telephone calls, listening to voicemails and other electronic communication systems within your responsibility

◆ taking and passing on messages

◆ dealing with **enquiries** face-to-face, by telephone, fax, email, social media and possibly text

◆ scheduling and cancelling appointments

◆ dealing with complaints and compliments

◆ telling the appropriate beauty therapist that a client or visitor has arrived

◆ dealing with deliveries

HEALTH & SAFETY

Deliveries to reception

You may have to receive and sign for deliveries at reception, confirming their arrival.

These should be dealt with at the earliest possibility to avoid them causing an obstruction, for security and for checking accuracy against the delivery note.

◆ assisting with retail sales and marketing

◆ operating the payment point and handling different types of payments

◆ filing client records (increasingly this is performed electronically)

◆ handling client records in relation to sales and marketing activities.

The receptionist should know:

◆ the name of each member of staff, their role and their area of responsibility

◆ who to refer different enquiries to that they are unable to deal with themselves

◆ the business hours of opening, and the days and times when each beauty therapist is available

◆ the range of treatments or products offered by the salon, their duration and their cost

◆ any booking service restrictions such as skin testing requirements

◆ who to refer different types of enquiries to

◆ the person in the salon to whom you should refer reception problems

◆ any current discounts and special offers that the business is promoting

◆ the benefits of each treatment and each retail product

◆ the approximate time taken to complete each treatment

◆ how to schedule follow-up treatments.

TOP TIP

Name badges

It is a good idea for the receptionist to wear a badge indicating their name and position.

HEALTH & SAFETY

Client wellbeing on the business premises

Just in case a client should become ill whilst on the premises, a contact number should be recorded on the client's contact details. The receptionist should also know the qualified first aider and emergency service numbers.

ALWAYS REMEMBER

Receptionist duties

Follow your procedural guidelines for the receptionist role to ensure that the best quality of service and client experience is provided.

TOP TIP

Opportunities for promoting products and treatments

Within your area of training and responsibility, bring to the attention of clients waiting in the reception area any new products, treatments or promotions.

Skin sensitivity patch tests   Before clients receive certain treatments it may be necessary to carry out pre-treatment **skin sensitivity patch tests** to determine if a client is suitable for the treatment. The skin sensitivity test is often carried out at reception, and the receptionist will be able to perform such tests once they have been trained. Every client should undergo a skin test before a chemical treatment such as a permanent tinting service to the eyelashes or eyebrows. Further tests may be necessary, depending on manufacturer's guidelines and the client sensitivity, as well as their previous treatment history, before services such as semi-permanent eyelashes or wax depilation. Further details on skin tests can be found in the section entitled Pre-treatment tests in Chapter 3.

As a receptionist it may be your responsibility to check that necessary tests have been received on client arrival. Ensure you follow your salon's policy for this.

TOP TIP

Client/visitor attention at reception

It is important to give the right amount of attention to all clients according to their specific requirements, to ensure client satisfaction. This must always be considered in a busy situation where a client may be kept waiting. Always acknowledge their arrival.

It may be necessary for visitors to sign in dependent upon the workplace policy. For health and safety you need to be aware who is on the premises. Have a sign-in book available for this purpose.

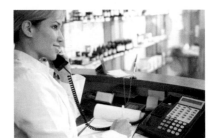

A receptionist should cheerfully welcome the client, even if engaged on another task.

The importance of good communication

Clients make quality judgements based on their experience. Good communication skills are essential to business success. For the receptionist, this includes **verbal communication**, that is face-to-face, over the telephone or written communication including email, and **non-verbal communication**, that is communicating through our facial expressions, body movements and gestures, referred to as body language. Conclusions about how we see other people are based on their behaviour both spoken and unspoken.

Always remember the **diversity** or range of people you will come into contact with and adapt your communication accordingly.

"Remember there are different ways in which you can communicate with clients. Always be aware of your body language and how this can be interpreted by others. Be cautious when sending written communications and how this can be translated."

Tina Rook

TOP TIP

Eye contact

In some cultures eye contact is considered to be disturbing or inappropriate. Always consider client diversity.

REVISION AID

What are the main duties of the salon receptionist?

Communication should always suit the situation. In all situations speak clearly and concisely, avoid rushing the conversation even in busy trading situations. Avoid slang words and informal phrases such as 'hang on a minute'. Your tone of voice is important; you should always aim to appear calm, cheerful, helpful, knowledgeable and professional. Your voice and manner should inspire confidence and trust.

Adopting good posture will also positively affect your speech and professional appearance. You will also sound and look more energised.

Non-verbal communication Sometimes unconsciously our body language may contradict what we are actually saying. It is an important receptionist skill to be able to interpret the body language and mood of clients. Observing client behaviour will assist you in understanding their expectations and how they wish to be treated.

Your body language should be open and attentive. For example, you can nod your head and smile in agreement to demonstrate you are listening to what the client is saying but remember not to fold your arms across your body as this can appear negative.

"The way you say things can be interpreted differently, depending on the tone of your voice, eye contact and your facial expressions."

Tina Rook

ACTIVITY

Non-verbal communication

In conversation you give signals through your behaviour that informs others what you may be thinking, feeling and whether you are really listening or not.

1 What do you think the following facial and body signals indicate?

◆ a smile
◆ eyes semi-closed
◆ head tilted, and resting on one hand
◆ head nodding
◆ frowning
◆ fidgeting.

2 Can you think of further facial or body signals and what they may communicate?

Asking questions It is important to ask verbal questions to ensure, for example, that you are confident and understand what the client is asking, or telling you. Do not be embarrassed to do this. You may ask 'open', 'probing' or 'closed' questions as appropriate. Always ask open questions if you need more information. Open questions cannot be answered with a 'yes' or 'no'. They start with words like 'what', 'when', 'who' or 'why'.

Ask probing questions to gain more information: these are usually follow-up questions. For example, use them if you do not fully understand a client's response to a question.

Closed questions are used when you need to confirm something quickly or specifically. These are answered 'yes' or 'no'. Listen carefully to correctly identify the client's service requirements.

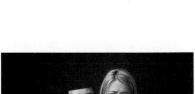

Always project a positive facial expression

Telephone communication technique

A good **telephone technique** can gain clients; a poor technique can lose them. Here are some guidelines for good technique:

◆ **Answer quickly** On average, a person may be willing to wait up to nine rings: try to respond to the call within six rings. If you are unavailable, make use of an answer phone voicemail facility which provides a short message explaining what the caller should do. Set aside time to follow up messages that have been left. In the case of text messages, ensure they are followed up promptly.

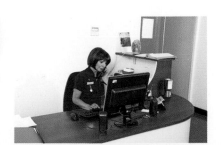

Telephone communication technique; always sound calm, cheerful, helpful, knowledgeable and professional

◆ *Build a rapport* by introducing yourself when you answer the telephone.

◆ *Be prepared* Have information and writing materials available in the event you need to write down a message or record an instruction. It should not normally be necessary to leave the caller waiting while you find something.

◆ *Be welcoming and attentive* Speak clearly without mumbling, at the right speed. Pronounce your words clearly, and vary your tone. Sound interested, and never abrupt.

Remember: the caller may be a new client ringing several salons, and their decision whether to visit your salon may depend on your attitude and the way you respond to their call.

Here are some more ideas about good telephone technique:

◆ *Smile* – this will help you put across a warm, friendly response to the caller.

"Smile when you answer the telephone! A smile can be heard in your voice and speaks a thousand words."

Tina Rook

◆ *Alter the pitch of your voice* as you speak, this will create interest

◆ *As you answer give the standard greeting for the salon* – for example: 'Good morning, Visage Beauty Salon, Susan speaking. How may I help you?'

◆ *Listen attentively* to the caller's questions or requests. You will be speaking to a variety of clients: you must respond appropriately and helpfully to each caller.

◆ *Evaluate the information* given by the caller, and be sure to respond to what they have said or asked.

◆ *Use the client's name* if you know it; this personalises the call.

◆ *In your mind summarise the main requests from the call.* Ask for further information if you need it.

◆ *If you have an enquiry that you cannot deal with yourself* refer to the relevant person promptly for assistance. Inform the client what you are doing.

◆ *At the end of the conversation* repeat the main points clearly to check that you and the client have understood each other.

◆ *If the client is new* check that they know where the business is located and where to park – is there a parking fee? Ask if they have any further requests or questions that you can assist with. Be helpful and informative.

◆ ***Close the call pleasantly*** – for example, 'Thank you for calling, Mrs Smith. We look forward to seeing you. Goodbye.'

If you receive a business call, or a call from a person seeking employment, always take the caller's name and telephone number. The relevant staff can then deal with the call as soon as they are free to do so.

> "As a receptionist you cannot have a bad day as you are always in view of your customers, either face-to-face or on the telephone. The person on the end of the telephone cannot see how busy or harassed you are, so always speak clearly and politely."
>
> *Tina Rook*

ALWAYS REMEMBER

Personal calls

Check the salon's policy on personal calls. Usually they are permitted only in emergencies and at agreed times of the working day. This is so that staff are not distracted from clients, the workplace operations and to keep the telephone land line free for clients to make appointments. Also, using your personal mobile phone is unprofessional, inattentive and inappropriate at reception. Your attention should stay focused on the responsibility of managing the reception area and ensuring your clients' satisfaction and welfare.

Transferring telephone calls

If you transfer a telephone call to another extension, explain to the caller what you are doing and thank them for waiting. If the extension to which you have transferred the call is not answered within nine rings, apologise and explain to the caller that you will ask the person concerned to ring back as soon as possible. Take the caller's name and telephone number and offer to take a message. Always make sure the person gets the message.

Taking messages

Messages taken by telephone should be recorded neatly usually on a message or 'memo' pad or sent electronically via email or text. Each message should record:

◆ who the message is for

◆ who the message was from

◆ the date and the time the message was received

◆ accurate details of the message, including the reason for the communication, details of information requested or to be passed on

◆ the telephone number or e-mail address of the caller

◆ the name of the person who took the message.

When taking a message listen attentively. Repeat the details you have recorded so that the caller can check that you've got it right. Pass the message directly to the correct

TOP TIP

Cordless phones

If your business uses a cordless phone or a mobile phone, keep it in a central location where it can easily be found when it rings. After each call, be sure to return the phone to its normal location.

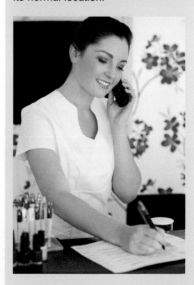

person as soon as possible. This may be via memo note, telephone, in person or electronically via text or email as appropriate. The important thing is that the message should be received in time to be acted upon.

An example memo

TELEPHONE MESSAGE RECEIVED			
To	Angela	Date	15.11.17
From	Jenny Heron	Time	9.30 am
Number	01632 960496	Taken by	Sandra

Please ring Jenny Heron regarding her appointment this Saturday

TOP TIP

Poor service

A client who has received a poor response to their telephone call may tell others about it.

Social media can quickly create a negative image of the business.

As part of the review of the quality of service provided, some businesses will perform an independent assessment of the quality of calls and their handling. This means that some calls will be recorded and may lead to further training where required to improve customer service.

ACTIVITY

Positive verbal communication with clients

Listen to experienced receptionists and notice the positive features of their communication with clients.

ACTIVITY

What do you need to know?

Think of different questions that you might be asked as a receptionist. Then ask an experienced receptionist what the most common requests are.

TOP TIP

Using your initiative when taking messages

It is important to interpret the mood of a client leaving a message. If they are making a complaint listen to their complaint, ensure you have the key facts and where possible provide a time that somebody will get back to them. Never become angry or defensive yourself.
If skilled, you should be able to calm and provide reassurance to the complainant.

Listening skills

It is important to listen closely to what people are saying to you in your receptionist role, whether face to face or not, to ensure you correctly identify the purpose of any enquiry in order to choose the correct response when dealing with it.

Listening skills include:

◆ being focused on the other person, giving them your full attention

◆ ensuring that your facial expressions communicate your interest

◆ not interrupting the other person when they are speaking

◆ using positive body language to communicate your interest; examples include maintaining eye contact, nodding your head and leaning forward

◆ observing the other person's body language, interpreting what it is telling you while you listen

◆ summarising what the other person has said to confirm understanding

◆ asking further questions as necessary if unsure in order to give the right response

◆ asking a client to rephrase what you have said in their own words if they appear confused.

Dealing with a dissatisfied client or complaint

The receptionist is usually the first contact with the client (either face-to-face or through telephone contact) and may have to deal with an awkward or difficult situation. Considerable skill is needed if you are to deal constructively with such a situation, which could be a potentially damaging to the reputation of the business.

Follow your business procedure for handling **complaints**. Procedures are useful as they provide direction and can be regularly audited to identify emerging problems or trends in the service provided that may require correction and can be targeted through relevant staff training. If ignored these problems could be harmful to the business.

In such situations, never become angry, defensive or awkward yourself. Always remain calm, courteous and diplomatic, listen without interrupting and communicate confidently and politely.

1   Listen to your client as they describe their problem, without making judgments. Do not make excuses for yourself or for colleagues. Do not interrupt.

2   Ask questions to check that you have the full background details. Summarise the client's concerns to confirm this.

3   If possible, agree on a course of action, offering a solution if you can. Check that the client has agreed to the proposed course of action. It may be necessary to consult the relevant person before proposing a solution to the client. If you are not sure, always check first.

4   Log the complaint: the date, time, client's name, context of the complaint and the course of action agreed.

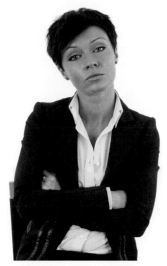

Dealing with a dissatisfied client

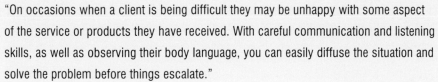

"On occasions when a client is being difficult they may be unhappy with some aspect of the service or products they have received. With careful communication and listening skills, as well as observing their body language, you can easily diffuse the situation and solve the problem before things escalate."

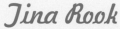

Tina Rook

Compliments

There should also be a system for handling compliments. It is good to identify those aspects of the business that are successful. Communicating this information is also rewarding and motivational for staff and can be used in marketing activities.

ALWAYS REMEMBER

Behaviour breeds behaviour

If you behave calmly, the client will become less angry. If you become angry, the client will become even angrier!

Your behaviour can affect the other person for the worse or the better.

Appointments

Making correct entries in the **appointment book** or salon **computer** is one of the most important duties of the receptionist. The way you handle client records and the information held on them must conform to the Data Protection Act. Always handle confidential information in line with salon policies and legal requirements.

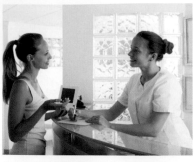

Appointment booking

As a receptionist you must be confident with the application of the salon's appointment system, treatment times and any abbreviations used.

Each beauty therapist will usually have their name at the head of a column. Entries in columns must not be reallocated without the consent of the beauty therapist or responsible person, unless they are absent.

Appointment bookings

When a client calls to make an appointment, record the client's name, confirm the accurate spelling of their name and the service they require. Allow adequate time to carry out the treatment. Inform the client how long their treatment will take.

Take the client's telephone number or other contact details in case the beauty therapist falls ill or is unable to keep the appointment for some other reason. If the client requests a particular beauty therapist, be sure to enter the client's name in the correct column.

TOP TIP

Gaining client satisfaction

Occasionally you will have to disappoint a client such as when cancelling their appointment or explaining they cannot proceed with a treatment for reasons of health and safety, e.g. contra-indication or contra-action. You should be able to do this without offending or upsetting the client. Consider your tone of voice, how you are going to present the information and what alternative options there may be. Through your words and tone you should be able to demonstrate genuine empathy and resolve to recover the situation.

In addition, software enabling online appointment booking and scheduling is becoming more popular. This is accessed through the business website and clients can book appointments and view the business's information (treatments offered, promotions, etc.) at any time. The business can make the final decision to accept or reject the appointment. As receptionist this may be your responsibility. Always spellcheck any electronic communication forwarded to clients – it is important that salon correspondence is of a professional standard.

ACTIVITY

Reception role play

With colleagues, act out the following situations, which may occur when working as a receptionist. You may wish to video the role plays for review and discussion later.

1   A client arrives very late for an appointment but insists that she be treated.
2   A client questions the accuracy of the bill.
3   A client comes in to complain about a service received previously. (Choose a particular service.)

Alternatively you may choose to do this as a written activity with a discussion of your answers.

Finally, the hours of the day are recorded along the left-hand side of the appointment page, usually divided into 15-minute intervals. You must know how long each treatment takes so that you can allow sufficient time for the beauty therapist to carry out the treatment in a safe, competent, professional manner. If you don't allow sufficient time, the therapist will run late, and this will affect all later appointments. On the other hand, if you allow too much time, the beauty therapist's time will be wasted and the salon's income will be reduced. Suggested times to be allowed for each treatment are listed below and provided in each technical treatment chapter.

Ensure that you regularly check scheduled appointments and plan ahead where you can see any potential problem – put a strategy in place to rectify it. This may involve asking others to help you.

Confirm the name of the beauty therapist who will be carrying out the treatment, the date and the time.

Finally, confirm or estimate the cost of the treatment to the client.

Treatments are usually recorded in an abbreviated form as shown below. All those who use the appointment page must be familiar with these abbreviations. Some examples that may be used are shown below.

Treatment	Abbreviation	Treatment time allowed*
Make-up lesson		75 mins
Cleanse and make-up: day	C/M/up day	30 mins
special occasion	C/M/up special	45 mins
Eyebrow shaping	E/B reshape or trim	15 mins
Eyebrow tint	EBT	10 mins
Eyelash tint	ELT	20 mins
Manicure	Man	45 mins
Pedicure	Ped	50 mins
Leg wax: half	½ leg wax	30 mins
three-quarter	¾ leg wax	30–40 mins
full	F/leg wax	45 mins
Bikini wax	B/wax	15 mins
Underarm wax	U/arm wax	15 mins
Arm wax	F/arm wax	30 mins
Facial wax: includes upper lip and chin	F/wax	10–15 mins
upper lip	U/lip	10 mins
chin wax	C/wax	10 mins
Eyebrow wax	E/B wax	15 mins
Threading	EB/Thread re-shape	20 mins
	F/Thread:	10–15 mins
	U/lip	10 mins
	C	10 mins
Ear pierce	E/P	15 mins
Facial	F	60 mins

(Continued)

Treatment	Abbreviation	Treatment time allowed*
Artificial eyelash extension systems strips/individual flare/single lash	F/Lash:	10–20 mins
	F/flare ext	20 mins
	Part/flare ext	10 mins
	F/strip ext strip	10 mins
	F/SL Ext	60–120 mins (depending on effect required)
	Part/SL Ext	30/45/60 mins (depending on maintenance or effect required)

*Treatment time does not include preparation for service and consultation.

If an appointment book is used, write each entry neatly and accurately. It is preferable to write in pencil: appointments can be amended by erasing and rewriting, keeping the book clean and clear.

Electronic appointment booking systems, if used, allow you to read the appointment schedule and add or edit appointments immediately. These can be printed and passed to the relevant staff member for information.

Appointment cards may be offered to the client, to confirm the client's appointment. The card should record the treatment, the date, the day and the time. The beauty therapist's name may also be recorded. Or if used a text appointment may be electronically forwarded.

When the client arrives for their treatment, draw a line or checkmark through their name to indicate that they have arrived.

If the client cancels, indicate this on the appointment page *immediately*, usually with a large C, placed through the booking. This enables another client to take the appointment.

If a client fails to arrive, the abbreviation DNA ('did not arrive') is usually written over the booking. The client's telephone number should then be used to see if a re-booking is required. To reduce the possibility of missed appointments, the receptionist should confirm appointments with clients 48 hours in advance or use a texting reminder service, if available.

Use the relevant recording icon if using an online appointment booking system.

Some businesses will have a policy to charge for a missed appointment. To discourage clients from missing appointments, it may be a policy to take a deposit when booking appointments.

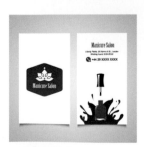

An appointment card can also provide the business contact details

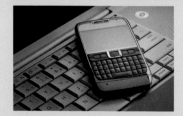

THERAPIST	JAYNE	SUE	LIZ
9.00	Mrs Young		
9.15	1/2 leg wax	Jenny Newley	
9.30	Carol Kreen	EL T/EBT	
9.45	Full leg wax	EB trim	
10.00	B / Wax		
10.15		Sandra Smith	Sue Lowe
10.30	Ms Lord E/B wax	C / M / up	C / M / up
10.45			Strip / lash
11.00		Mrs Jones	
11.15		U/arm wax	
11.30		F/arm wax	Carol Brown
11.45			E/P
12.00			
12.15			
12.30	Nina Farrel		
12.45	Man		
1.00	Ped		
1.15		Sue Yip E/P	
1.30	1/2 leg wax	T Scott	
1.45		3/4 leg wax	
2.00	Karen Davies	U/arm wax	
2.15	Facial		
2.30			
2.45			Pat king
3.00			C / M / up
3.15	Anne Wood		Man
3.30	Man		
3.45	E/B Reshape		
4.00			

DAY   SATURDAY   DATE   15th JANUARY

DNA

Appointments page

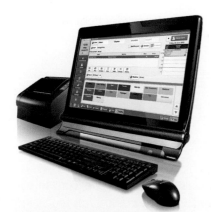

Salon software system

TOP TIP

Treatment time allowed

Dependent upon the manufacturer's guidelines and the treatment needs of the client, including any procedure modifications required, the treatment times may take less or more time.

Dealing with appointment problems

You are often required to use your initiative in helping colleagues and clients and be able to cope with the unexpected such as:

◆ Clients arriving late for appointments. Discuss the options, reassure the client that you will always try to accommodate them. It may not be their fault and if arriving for a relaxation treatment the receptionist will have an important role in supporting the client to relax. A client can always have the option to re-book the treatment if necessary. If a client's treatment cannot be completed to the correct standard due to lack of time it is preferable to explain this to the client and re-book.

◆ Where a client is always late. You will need to discuss this with a supervisor and appropriate action taken to deal with this. Perhaps offering a later appointment. Tact is essential in all situations.

◆ Double-bookings, with two clients requiring treatment at the same time. The important outcome is that the client is not disappointed and will return. Be honest about the mistake, why it has occurred and try to resolve the situation in order that the client receives the treatment wherever possible. An alternative therapist may be able to offer the service or a goodwill complimentary gesture may be offered.

◆ The arrival of unscheduled clients. Always try to find out why they have chosen to arrive for the treatment. It may be that you ran a promotion and they have responded to it; it could be word of mouth, another client may have recommended the salon or treatment. Ensure the client has a positive experience and capture any marketing intelligence for future planning.

◆ Staff absence with a column of appointments! Inform the client as early as possible if the appointment has to be cancelled. That is why it is important to always have contact details for your clients. Wherever possible consider how the treatment can be accommodated. Another beauty therapist may be able to carry out the treatment but it is important to confirm with the client if this will be acceptable – some clients may be unhappy to have an alternative beauty therapist allocated.

Effective teamwork can usually overcome any of the above situations. Inform your colleague/supervisor of the problem immediately and, dependent upon your experience, state what action needs to be taken or ask them to support you in identifying a solution. You must always:

◆ aim to accommodate clients

◆ not disadvantage or compromise any clients in terms of quality of treatment

◆ keep the client informed of what action is being taken

◆ state how long any delay to treatment will be and if this is unsuitable offer an alternative future appointment

◆ ensure the client is happy with the treatment they have received

◆ use your excellent communication skills!

Thanking the client for their visit As well as welcoming clients to the business, receptionists also have a role to play in ensuring they receive appreciation for their visit.

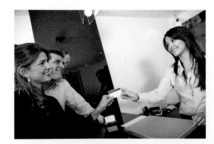

Receptionist returning a card used for payment to the client

Check to see if they have enjoyed their treatment. If not, make a note and then this important feedback can be given to the relevant person.

There may be a satisfaction questionnaire available to gather feedback.

Check if they would like to rebook their next appointment.

You should also make clients aware of any retail or product promotions that can provide the opportunity for up-selling.

Following their departure you may have an electronic automated facility whereby you can thank new clients for their visit. You may be required to generate birthday or festive cards, so taking the client's details correctly is essential.

Handling payments Every business will have a policy for handling cash and for handling the payment. Clients can choose from a wide range of payment methods. It's important that you handle each payment efficiently and correctly. Not all businesses accept every **method of payment** so this should be checked in your training.

It is important that you have received training and are confident to take payment in the client's preferred method, which may be cash or cash equivalent (i.e. **gift voucher**), cheque or payment card.

Before processing payment confirm what it is the client is paying for, i.e. the treatments received and/or the products to be purchased. Confirm the price; ask how they would like to pay. Gaining client confirmation will reduce **discrepancies** later. Always check for any defects in products as you process a sale, i.e. breakage or leakage. If you are responsible for **stock control** when a product is found to be defective a replacement product is required.

> **TOP TIP**
>
> **Advertisement vouchers**
>
> Sometimes the salon may publish other offers, such as a discount on producing a newspaper advertisement for the salon or a website voucher. The advertisement voucher is a form of payment, and must be collected following your workplace procedure.

The payment point

Types of payment points

Manual tills With **manual tills** a lockable drawer or box is used to store cash: this may form part of the reception desk. Each transaction must be recorded by hand.

At the end of the working day, record the total cash register in a book, to ensure that accurate accounts are kept. Records of petty cash, small amounts of monies used for expenditures, e.g. milk for clients' coffee, must also be kept so that the final totals will balance.

Automatic tills Electrical **automatic tills** use codes, one for each kind of service or retail sale. These are identified by keys on the till. Using these with each transaction makes it possible to analyse the salon's business each day or each week.

With each sale during the day a receipt is given to the client; the total is also recorded on the till's **audit roll**.

Automatic tills also provide **subtotals** of the amounts taken: these can be cross-checked against the amount in the till, to determine the daily takings:

◆ The X reading provides subtotals throughout the day, as required.

◆ The Z reading provides the overall figures at the end of each day. This includes a breakdown of payment types and the time they occurred.

Computerised tills Computerised tills provide the same facilities as automatic tills, with additional features to help with the business, including trading patterns, record-keeping, including client service cards, service history, stock records, calculate staff takings and commission (payment paid to the therapist as a percentage of their takings) if paid.

Both electronic and computerised tills help calculate the client's bill for you, including change to be given.

Electronic scanning facilities are also available. These use infrared light to read barcodes. Inbuilt electronic circuitry detects the price and sends it to the point of sale equipment, such as a computer or cash register till.

Equipment and materials required

◆ *Calculator* This is useful in totalling large amounts of money or when using a manual till.

◆ *Card processing equipment* Where an electronic payment system is used a special till roll which provides a printout for yourself and a copy for the client is required.

◆ *Cash float* At the start of each day you need a small sum of money comprising coins and perhaps a few notes, to provide change: this is called the **float**. (At the end of the day there will be money surplus to the float: if no mistakes have been made, this should match the takings.) At the start of the working day the float amount should be checked.

◆ *Till roll* This records the sales and provides a receipt. Keep a spare to hand. If you're using a manual cash drawer, you'll need a **receipt book**.

◆ *Audit roll* The retailer's copy of the till roll.

◆ *Cash book* This is a record of income and expenditure, for a manual till.

◆ *Other stationery* A date stamp and a salon name stamp (for cheques), pens, pencils and an eraser, and a container to hold these.

Security at the payment point

Be aware that the reception is usually entered from the street outside, so security should be foremost at all times. Always close the cash drawer firmly following a cash transaction – never leave it open. Do not leave the key in the cash drawer, or lying about reception unattended. Large amounts of money should never be left in the till. Regularly remove money from the till and store in a secure area, often a safe, before it is banked in line with your workplace policy. Times should be varied when banking monies to ensure personal safety and security from possible theft.

Some members of staff will be appointed to authorise cheques and credit card payments.

Errors may occur when handling cheques or when operating an electronic or computerised payment point. Don't panic! If you can't correct the error yourself, seek assistance – but don't leave the cash drawer unattended and open.

Be aware of stolen cards and forged notes and coins. Check for this at every payment transaction and follow the workplace policy if presented. Remember that this must be handled sensitively as the client may not know they are in receipt of a cash forgery.

TOP TIP

Cash float

Businesses that take credit and debit card payments, or cheques rather than cash, will not usually require much cash in the float. It is always sensible to have a little more than you think you will need. A typical float will be £50 made up of denominations of £10/£5 notes, £2/£1 coins and silver coins.

ALWAYS REMEMBER

Maintaining cash in the till

If there is too little change in the till, inform the relevant person. Running out of change would disrupt service and spoil the impression clients receive.

You may periodically be informed of cards that are invalid, on a credit card warning list from the service provider. If you receive a card that is on a credit card warning list, politely detain the customer, hold onto the card, and contact your supervisor, who will implement the workplace procedure. If the card is unsigned, do not allow the cardholder to sign the card unless you first get authorisation from the credit card company's service provider. (The service provider's telephone number should be kept near the telephone.)

ACTIVITY

Fraud

Find out about your salon's policy in the case of fraudulent monetary transactions, using either cash or cards. What actions should you take if you find yourself in this situation?

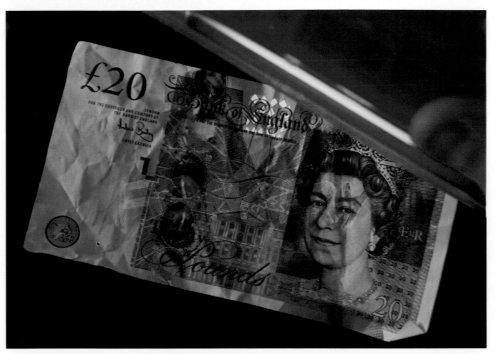

Forged note detector

TOP TIP

Forgeries

Hold notes to the light to check for forgeries. You should be able to see the watermark (picture of the Queen's head), the continuous metal strip that runs through the note and a hologram decal in the mid-left section of the note.

An UV detector machine may also be used to check for forgeries.

A special pen can be used which detects if the note is a forgery.

The police will often provide a list of forged bank note numbers to businesses to be aware of.

Suspected forged notes should be returned to the bank where they will be investigated.

REVISION AID

How can security be maintained at the payment point?

Discrepancies In the event of a **cash discrepancy** (difference) where the sales and takings do not balance, an investigation will be required. This will be completed by a supervisor. Where the discrepancy cannot be traced this must be logged and may be required to be reported externally. If theft has occurred, this should be reported to the police. Staff will usually be dismissed, but may also be prosecuted, when they have committed theft.

REVISION AID

How would you handle an error made at the payment point?

Methods of payment

Cash   When receiving payment by **cash**, follow this sequence:

1   Accurately enter or 'ring up' the items into the till and press 'subtotal' to calculate the charge for the services/products received. Inform the client of the amount to be paid.

2   Check that the money offered is **legal tender** – that is, money you will be able to pay into your bank. (Your salon will probably not accept foreign currency, for example.) Also be aware of counterfeit (fake) money, checking the validity of bank notes.

3   Place the customer's money on the till ledge until you have given change, or at least state to the customer verbally the sum of money that they have given you.

4   If using a till, press the total button, equal to the sum of cash you have been given.

5   When providing change verbally count the change as you give it to the client. This will help avoid payment disputes.

6   Thank the client and give them a receipt.

7   If a client disputes the change given as too little, ask how much money they are missing. Inform the client that when the takings are cashed at the end of the day if there is a surplus and it matches that amount they will be reimbursed. Ensure that you have the client's details so that you can inform them of the outcome the next day. Always follow your salon policy.

A cheque

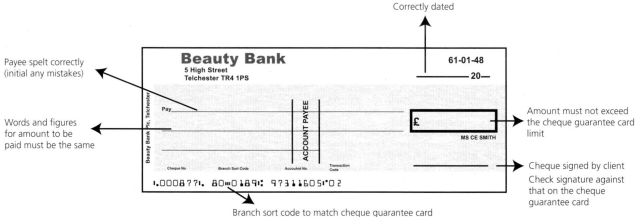

Correctly dated

Payee spelt correctly (initial any mistakes)

Words and figures for amount to be paid must be the same

Amount must not exceed the cheque guarantee card limit

Cheque signed by client
Check signature against that on the cheque guarantee card

Branch sort code to match cheque guarantee card

Beauty Bank
5 High Street
Telchester TR4 1PS

61-01-48

20—

Pay

£

MS CE SMITH

ACCOUNT PAYEE

Cheque No   Branch Sort Code   Account No.   Transaction Code

Cheques   Cheques are an alternative form of payment to cash.

Some businesses are no longer accepting cheques as it is becoming more costly to accept as a form of payment and less popular.

When receiving payment by cheque, follow this sequence of checks:

1   The cheque must be correctly completed.

2   The cheque must be made payable to the business, the spelling must be correct (you may have a salon stamp for this).

3   The day, date and month should be correct.

4   The words and figures written on the cheque must match those in the box.

5   Any errors or alterations must have been initialled by the client.

6   The cheque must be signed by the client.

If your workplace accepts debit or credit cards it is important to know this. Usually there will be signage displayed stating which will be accepted.

Debit cards Debit cards authorise the immediate debit of the cash amount from the client's account and are an alternative to writing a cheque. You cannot perform this kind of transaction unless your salon has an electronic terminal. This processes payment automatically through a telephone connection (chip and PIN). The card processing company applies a fixed fee for each transaction made.

Credit cards Credit cards can be used only if your business has an arrangement with the relevant credit card company. A fixed percentage of the total bill is charged by the card processing company for this arrangement.

As the business is required to pay for every transaction with credit and debit cards there may be a minimum spend applied.

Credit cards allow the client to 'buy goods now and pay later' with interest paid each month on the outstanding balance if not paid off in full.

Electronic payment systems An electronic computerised terminal may be used for payment by both credit and debit cards. A portable wireless option enables payment from your clients anywhere in the business premises.

Increasingly credit card terminals also provide an option for processing mail order and telephone order payments from your clients.

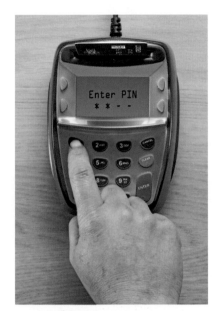

1 The card is placed into the chip and PIN machine at the point of sale. The card is verified as genuine.

2 When prompted, the 'AMOUNT' should be input of the total sale. If a mistake is made you can clear the figures using the CLEAR button.

3 The client then checks the amount is correct and enters their unique 4 digit personal identity number (PIN). Look away whilst the PIN is entered. The transaction will be declined if the PIN is incorrect. Electronic payment authorisation is immediately provided by the bank and transferred electronically.

For security purposes if the PIN number is entered three times incorrectly, the card is declined and is deactivated. The client will be required to contact their bank in this instance.

Some clients with mobility issues may be unable to use the digital pad and use a chip and signature card system instead. PIN key pads have been designed with raised areas for visually impaired people.

A receipt is provided and should be given to the client. A duplicate copy is retained by the business which is used when calculating takings.

Mobile card readers are now available which work with mobile phones to process payments. These are convenient for beauty therapists working at different locations.

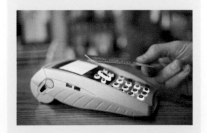

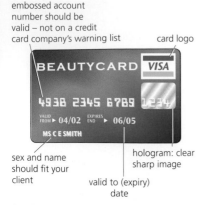

embossed account number should be valid – not on a credit card company's warning list

card logo

BEAUTYCARD VISA

4938 2345 6789 1234

VALID FROM ▶ 04/02   EXPIRES END ▶ 06/05

MS C E SMITH

sex and name should fit your client

hologram: clear sharp image

valid to (expiry) date

Credit card checks

A debit or credit card will show the following:

1   The card logo for a debit or credit card is at the lower right-hand corner on the front of the card.

2   The hologram should have a clear, sharp image and be in the centre right of the card.

3   The date on the card must be valid: if it is out-of-date ask for another form of payment.

4   The sex (Ms, Miss, Mrs, Mr) and the name of the customer must fit your client.

5   The cardholder's signature on the reverse of the card must match the name on the front of the card.

6   The cardholder's card number should be embossed and across the width on the front of the card.

7   The cardholder's card number must not be one of those on the credit card company's warning list.

Charge cards   Some businesses accept charge cards such as American Express. These differ from credit cards in that the account holder must repay to the card company the complete amount spent each month. They are considered a more convenient alternative to cash.

Gift vouchers   Gift vouchers are purchased from the salon as pre-payments for beauty therapy services or retail sales. Check the following:

◆   There is usually a specific time period in which gift vouchers must be used. Check to see if this is the case and if they are still valid.

◆   For security purposes some vouchers will have a reference number to reduce the risk of fraudulent copies. The voucher reference number can then be tracked back to the date of purchase and its value, which can be validated.

◆   Cards are also available registered on a database. The value on the card can be read and the credit value debited accordingly.

◆   Vouchers are processed as cash against the treatment. Check the value of the voucher, and remember to request another form of payment if the cost of the service is higher than the voucher. You must be able to process part payments accurately and confidently.

Loyalty cards

Increasingly clients may receive an incentive reward for their customer loyalty and spend with the business. The card records progress towards an agreed target, which may be redeemed against treatments/products as agreed as part of the loyalty scheme. It can be used for further marketing activities that may increase the numbers of new clients to the business, such as 'recommend a friend' to gain loyalty rewards.

It is important that all financial transactions are handled competently. However busy you are, always follow the guidelines for handling each method of payment.

If you are ever unsure when handling a financial transaction or make a mistake, inform your supervisor immediately. It may be that you have to be discreet when doing this, for example if a client has handed you a forged bank note!

Behaviour

In the beauty business it is your knowledge, skills and overall professionalism that are your greatest strengths. Your professional reputation is important to your success, and the opinions of professional colleagues and your clients will influence this.

It is essential that your behaviour and how you conduct yourself are considered professional at all times. Outside the workplace be mindful of your actions and how these may be perceived. Your workplace policy may state that you do not socialise with clients outside work; this includes communication through social media.

Inappropriate behaviour may lead to the application of the **disciplinary** procedure. Employers can take disciplinary action for their employees' actions outside work hours. In such cases, these would be actions that might harm the reputation of the business. This can include inappropriate postings on social media.

Drugs and alcohol

Treatments must never be carried out if you are under the influence of drugs or alcohol. Your competence will be affected, putting yourself, clients and possibly colleagues at risk. Any accident as a result will be termed negligent and you would be liable. Your behaviour at work should be in accordance with your workplace policies and must not endanger yourself or others.

Recognising professional practice

Within the beauty industry, there is now a professional register set up to recognise adherence to best professional practice and qualified therapists which is supported by other professional bodies in the industry. This Register of Beauty Professionals was established by the government approved standard setting body, Habia (the Hair and Beauty Industry Authority) in partnership with the sector skills council, SkillsActive. Membership on this public register aims to provide assurance for clients and employers where the professional criteria and eligibility for registration have been met.

Registration criteria require that you:

◆ are qualified to practice

◆ have skills and knowledge that reflect current practice, achieved through continuing professional development (CPD)

◆ uphold the Professional Register Industry 'Code of Ethical Conduct', which defines good practice and is governed by four principles:

1 Professional Standards

2 Rights

3 Relationships

4 Personal and Business Responsibilities and Safe Working Practices.

Continuing professional development (CPD)

The most successful beauty therapists are educated, up-to-date and aware of what is new in the beauty industry. This means that they are able to deliver the best possible treatment and advice to meet their clients' needs.

ALWAYS REMEMBER

Disciplinary policy

It is important that there is a disciplinary policy that is understood. This usually has several stages but dismissal may be a sanction where there is evidence of 'Gross Misconduct'. There should also be an 'appeal' process, to reconsider the outcome.

ALWAYS REMEMBER

Social Media policy

It is good practice for a business to have a policy for social media use. on what is acceptable and what is not.

Social media is the use of internet-based tools on PCs, laptops, tablets and smart phones for communication and interaction.

ALWAYS REMEMBER

Professional body membership

As a member of a professional body such as BABTAC, your professional status and ethical commitment to standards is promoted to those users of beauty therapy services.

TOP TIP

Register of Beauty Professionals

To find out more about the personal benefits of the Register of Beauty Professionals visit www.registerofbeautyprofessionals .co.uk.

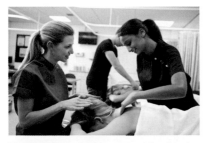

Staff training supports your professional development

CPD is the term used by professionals to provide evidence of activities undertaken to maintain their knowledge and skills related to their profession. It is recommended that CPD is updated annually. Examples of activities include visits to trade exhibitions, subscriptions to journals, attendance at seminars and further training.

For some beauty therapists there is a requirement to record CPD hours undertaken related to their job role, for example those involved in training and assessment. This will ensure that up-to-date technical information informs their training.

Staff training

Staff training is important and should be on-going from induction to inform you about new treatment techniques or salon policy updates.

Product knowledge, both technical and retail, is important. Good product knowledge will increase retail and treatment sales and increase client confidence. As a member of staff you have a responsibility to be aware of current legal requirements relating to the sale and retail of goods.

Communication skills and client care

Communication can be described as the exchange of information between two people or groups of people, that is effectively understood. It has been discussed as an important skill for the receptionist.

Positive communication, therefore, is the effective sharing of information between two or more people, which is clearly understood. Conclusions about how we see other people are based upon both spoken and unspoken communication. Clients make quality judgments based upon their contact with the business.

Communication is often referred to as an employment soft skill. Such soft skills can be described as an individual's personal qualities. This also includes their attitudes and ethics (principles, behaviour, morals and beliefs).

Good or positive communication skills will help you to:

◆ gain the confidence of your clients and others in the workplace

◆ develop a professional rapport with your clients and others in the workplace

◆ correctly identify your clients' needs

◆ confidently promote products and services

◆ resolve quickly any misunderstandings, complaints or disputes.

Always consider the diverse needs of your clients and other people in the workplace. Diversity means differences and people's differences are many including:

◆ personality

◆ beliefs and attitudes

- ◆ age
- ◆ religion and spirituality
- ◆ background and culture
- ◆ physical disabilities including hearing and visual impairment.

Adjust your method of communication accordingly to achieve positive communication with everyone you come into contact with. This may be face to face or not.

Communication can be verbal or non-verbal.

> **TOP TIP**
>
> When talking on the telephone, always smile! It can be heard in your voice.

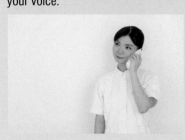

> **TOP TIP**
>
> **Non face-to face communication**
>
> When communicating over the telephone, your face cannot be seen, therefore it is important to consider your tone of voice, volume and clarity.

> "Clients have a vast choice of salons, so by creating the right atmosphere, giving excellent service and paying attention to detail, you will encourage the client to return to YOU."
>
> *Janice Brown*

> Communication and beautiful manners are a necessity in the beauty industry and this starts with your care and understanding of each client's needs. The use of both spoken communication and body language will enable you to build up trust, respect and above all the rapport you need to exceed your clients' needs. Your client is your free advertising campaign.
>
> *Maureen Evans-Olsen*

Verbal communication

Verbal information may be provided via the telephone, other electronic media or given to a client at consultation or during the treatment.

Verbal communication occurs when you talk directly to another person, either face to face or over the telephone. To assist effective communication, always speak clearly, slowly and precisely. Your tone of voice is important, sound calm, cheerful and helpful. This will help gain client confidence. Avoid chattering constantly and allow others the opportunity to speak. Avoid interrupting the client while they are speaking; this can appear rude and you may miss important information. Always listen carefully and be patient.

Having developed a rapport with your client, centre the conversation on them, they should be made to feel important. Consider the client's needs; a nervous client may need to be reassured.

Non-verbal communication

Clients can be made to feel intimidated, uncomfortable or ignored – without even saying anything! This is because you also communicate with your eyes, face and body,

> **REVISION AID**
>
> How would you explain non-verbal communication?

transmitting your feelings. This is called 'body language' or **non-verbal communication**. Therefore, how you look and how you behave in front of your clients is very important too. Interpreting your client's body language is an important skill to develop. Learn to notice your client's behaviour; observe their eyes, body, arm and hand movements. An instinctive 'feel' for a client's behaviour can be developed with experience.

Listening skills When listening to your client, give them your undivided attention; this lets them know you are listening. If you are face to face with the client, make eye contact. You must ensure that you *hear* and *understand* what the other person is saying. Then you will be able to *respond* appropriately to what they have said or asked. Do not be afraid of silence, allow the other person to think and consider when listening.

Become a good listener: this will help you identify your client's treatment requirements, expectations and consider if these are realistic. You can then guide the conversation appropriately.

Questioning skills Asking your client a question allows you to find out the information you need to know and learn more to help you make decisions. When asking questions, never interrogate your client or talk down to them, and avoid technical jargon, which can be off-putting – instead use commonly understood words.

Ask open questions; those that encourage the client to talk and cannot be answered with just *'yes'* or *'no'* (these are called closed questions). Closed questions are used when you need to confirm something. Probing questions can be used and are necessary when you need to gain further information. You may need to use these when specific information is required to assist you in making a decision, e.g. 'How long exactly do you want to wear your eyelashe extensions for?' when deciding which type to apply.

Professional work relationships

Clients

A professional relationship should be maintained, which is quite different from that enjoyed with close friends. To maintain this professional rapport, people who were met initially as clients, should not be seen socially outside of the workplace and should not be accepted as a social media friend.

A significant part of your job role is to provide excellent client or customer care. Many businesses have a customer care statement that outlines the standards of treatment and service they may expect. These standards can then be used to measure client satisfaction, monitoring if the treatment standard is being met and if not, allowing you to investigate why, and taking the appropriate action to address the problem.

Clients want to enjoy their experience when they visit your workplace. Remember, they are paying for your service. It is important that at every visit they are made to feel satisfied and comfortable, with their needs met. Always treat your client as a guest in your workplace.

This experience is often referred to as the 'customer journey'. The customer service expectations should start from the moment they enter the salon until they leave.

ACTIVITY

Do you have a client care statement?

How well do you provide client care? Monitor yourself against the statement and ask colleagues for feedback too.

ACTIVITY

How good are we?

Client feedback

A questionnaire is useful to monitor client satisfaction.

Questionnaires can be anonymous and collected at a central point. Reception is ideal. This can be in addition to electronic questionnaires.

Identify several questions to ask your clients.

ALWAYS REMEMBER

Create a positive work environment

An important factor for the success of the business is the commitment of each employee to provide a consistently high standard of client care. For this to occur it is important that all staff are confident and effective in their job role. Carrying out treatments to the highest standard, whilst maintaining positive working relationships with colleagues, creates a happy, productive work environment that is obvious to the client.

Gaining client feedback

To check the quality of client care you should capture your clients' views. Client feedback can be gathered in a variety of ways, both formally and informally.

Client questionnaires can be used to measure performance against the service standards. They can be used at random to gather feedback. For example, rating satisfaction with the service received that day or things that they would like to see introduced that would improve their experience.

Occasionally you could incentivise this important quality check by carrying out a random spot check. You can contact clients and gain feedback from those who have recently received salon services and reward them with a gift voucher, for example.

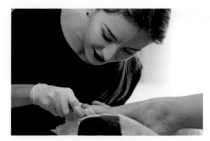

Client care: provide a consistently high standard of service

TOP TIP

What clients want

According to a report from LivingSocial (The Local Beauty Report 2015), which polled 1,114 women from 11 cities across the UK and Ireland, factors that are important include:

◆ price, with 64% saying it was important

◆ location, 37% preferred to visit salons closer to their home

◆ online and face-to-face reviews from friends influenced choice, 39% said recommendations were an important factor when choosing a salon.

Always consider whether you have dealt with each client adequately and responded to their needs appropriately. Sometimes clients are unhappy with an aspect of their service or perhaps a product purchased. Unfortunately, problems in which the client cannot be appeased do sometimes arise. Most complaints are easily resolved but require a procedure to deal with them. A **complaints procedure** is a formal, standardised approach adopted by a business to handle any complaints. It is important all staff are familiar with and trained in the correct implementation of the complaints procedure.

Dealing with client complaint or dissatisfaction
When you are aware of a client complaint, you should play your part in ensuring that it is resolved quickly. If a client is dissatisfied, they may appear angry and complain or they may say nothing. However they react, remember that a dissatisfied client is bad for business.

You may be required to deal with a dissatisfied client:

◆ Stay calm and listen to the client's complaint.

◆ If you are unable to handle it, refer it as quickly as possible to somebody who can. Inform the client of your actions at all times. (It is important that you know the limits of your authority when handling a complaint.)

◆ Inform the relevant person. This may be the manager, receptionist or senior beauty therapist depending upon the nature of the complaint.

◆ Establish the facts and take appropriate action as laid down in your client complaints procedure.

◆ Always aim to repair the relationship, although at times this may not be possible.

◆ Not all clients are genuine in their complaint – establish the facts and tactfully advise the client of the outcome.

◆ Always remain courteous, professional and create a positive impression.

ALWAYS REMEMBER

Social media

Social media may be used by a dissatisfied client to share their experience. This could be potentially damaging for the business. When an issue or complaint arises, always try and resolve the problem by contacting them to arrange to discuss it personally. This action should be completed by the designated person.

Avoiding client dissatisfaction
Some dissatisfied clients will voice their dissatisfaction; others will remain silent and simply not return to the salon. This situation can often be prevented through good client care and effective communication.

◆ Always ensure that the client has a thorough consultation before any new treatment. This should be carried out by an employee with the appropriate technical expertise.

◆ Regularly check the client's satisfaction. If there is any concern that you cannot handle, inform the relevant person of this immediately.

◆ Inform the client of any disruption to treatment. Do not leave them wondering what the problem may be. Politely inform them of the situation, for example 'I'm sorry but we are running 10 minutes late – are you able to wait?' If your salon has the facilities, you may offer them a drink.

◆ Inconvenience caused by disruption to treatment can usually be compensated in some way. It is important to resolve problems and keep clients satisfied.

Clients should be advised of the complaints procedure. If you are not able to deal with it immediately, they should be left with the confidence in knowing how it is to be dealt with and how and when they will be contacted with an update and outcome, and ideally by whom.

Client care is vital. Clients provide the business with income and ultimately pay the staff's wages. The success of the business depends upon client satisfaction.

Colleagues

Good working relationships with managers and colleagues lead to the best employee engagement. This is where employees are committed and enthusiastic about their work and role in the business. Engaged employees make positive colleagues.

Always work to the best of your ability. Request support and guidance from other colleagues, but only when needed. It is important that you use your initiative whenever possible. When seeking support or guidance, always do this courteously at an appropriate time and from the appropriate person.

If you are unsure of how to proceed with any task or duty, always request further support and guidance. If you receive any request for support or guidance always respond to this clearly and courteously.

Use your time effectively. If you are not busy, offer to help your colleagues.

Every member of staff, or the team, plays a different role, each ensuring the success of the business. Poor working relationships create an unpleasant environment for both staff and clients. A great portion of your time is spent in the workplace, working alongside your colleagues. If the environment becomes stressful this will affect your effectiveness.

Professional relationships with colleagues should be maintained at all times.

Professional conduct

◆ Be polite and courteous with colleagues at all times.

◆ Never talk down to colleagues.

◆ Never ridicule or lose your temper with a colleague in front of others.

◆ If personal issues arise between yourself and a colleague, these should not be displayed. Settle grievances (reasons for complaint) as soon as possible, or job satisfaction and productivity can be affected.

If a dispute with a colleague occurs, remember:

◆ Your behaviour can affect others for the worse or better. Remember 'behaviour breeds behaviour'. Stay calm and the other person will become calm; become angry and so will the other person.

◆ Do not be defensive; this is negative behaviour.

◆ Behave appropriately for the workplace, remembering your workplace's policy on code of conduct.

◆ Explain yourself and your issues clearly; avoid repeating yourself.

◆ Listen to the other person's response without interrupting.

◆ Make suggestions that will resolve the dispute. What outcomes are required?

◆ Agree a solution, negotiating this and including the other person's ideas.

◆ Agree together to move forward.

If the dispute cannot be resolved, it must be referred to a responsible member of staff to deal with.

For a team to work effectively, problems should be addressed as soon as they arise and it is important that harmonious relationships are rebuilt. If ignored this can lead to workplace stress, which can negatively affect the health and wellbeing of staff and could result in absence from work.

Grievances

If you feel you are in conflict with other staff or are being treated unfairly, you may wish to submit a grievance using the grievance and appeals procedure. All staff should be made aware of the grievance and appeals procedure and where it can be found at the time of their induction. The procedure aims to address situations as soon as they arise, investigating and wherever possible resolving the problem. In some cases this will mean that disciplinary action against an individual is taken. This is certainly the case where there is evidence of harassment or bullying against individuals.

A disciplinary procedure should be provided to each employee, which will emphasise the importance of staff behaviour. This is essential in the case of complaints, poor performance, staffing issues and misconduct.

Personal performance

Your ability to meet the expected standards is referred to as personal effectiveness. Standards that you will be assessed against include:

◆ the National Occupational Standards (NOS) for Beauty Therapy

◆ workplace operating standards

◆ awarding body performance criteria and essential knowledge and understanding

◆ personal targets.

Targets In order to develop personally and to improve your skills professionally, it is important to have personal targets against which you can measure your achievements.

If these are confidential, the workplace policy regarding confidentiality should be observed.

Targets should follow the **SMART** principle:

◆ **Specific** – clearly defined

◆ **Measurable** – quantifiable in some way

◆ **Agreed** – between both parties

◆ **Realistic** – can the target be met? Is it achievable?

◆ **Time bound** – completed within a fixed time period.

To an employer it is important that you are consistent. You must always perform your skills to the highest standard. You should present and promote a positive image of the industry and the business in which you are employed and which you represent.

> Be successful, keep learning and don't stand still. The industry will continue to develop and you must stay ahead by seeking out new developments and enhancing your skill set.
>
> *Maureen Evans-Olsen*

Productivity

Productivity targets are set for the business through strategic plans, budgets and sales targets. From these, they are broken down to team and individual targets.

For instance, if there is a new treatment that the business has decided to offer, then a decision will be made as to how that new treatment will pay for itself and bring more money into the business. This is a financial target. In order to achieve this, a productivity and development target will be needed for the individual beauty therapist. It is likely that you will require training on the treatment and then you will have sales targets set for the number of treatments to be performed and for the number of product sales to be made alongside treatment. Salon management software or electronic dashboards may be customised for business needs. An example could be a diary for each employee showing their productivity performance against target.

This shows how the productivity targets for technical (the treatment) and product sales go together and also how the individual training sessions all link up.

Personal development plans are necessary to make sure that the individual beauty therapist is always learning and improving, bringing added value to the business and also preventing them from becoming bored, staying motivated and retaining their clients.

Personal targets will include:

◆ *Technical sales:* individual treatments and courses, link-selling of treatments such as encouraging someone who has half leg waxing to have underarm and bikini waxing when they mention a forthcoming holiday. Each beauty therapist will have their own targets, which will be linked to their ability to perform the treatments, their expertise and experience.

◆ *Retail sales:* the products that go with the treatments for aftercare or to continue the maintenance programme at home. If the salon also has a retail sales section for customers who can just walk in without having treatments, this can be an effective way of making extra revenue. Each salon employee should have a retail sales target and view it as a professional way of supporting their treatments and part of their job description.

ALWAYS REMEMBER

Productivity targets

Productivity targets are for: retail sales, technical services, treatments and personal learning.

ALWAYS REMEMBER

Employee incentives

Some companies provide rewards for employees who achieve results and develop ideas for increased productivity, helping the business achieve its goals. Commission is a method of rewarding individuals who achieve and exceed targets.

When making recommendations, clearly show the benefits of implementing your suggestions.

ALWAYS REMEMBER

Productivity targets

Productivity targets can be achieved by cross-selling, advising or recommending the purchase of additional products to enhance the benefit to be achieved from the client's treatment. For example, when a client receives a nail service, you can recommend nail products for use at home to maintain and enhance the finish. An appointment should be made for any treatment, especially where a follow up maintenance service is recommended.

◆ Keep clients informed of any special offers and promotions.
◆ Keep abreast of current and seasonal trends.
◆ Productivity targets need to be kept up-to-date.

◆ *Standards of work:* high standards are essential to be professional and to give exceptional customer service and care.

◆ *General tasks:* tasks that are needed to be done around the salon including stock taking, hygiene maintenance, keeping equipment in good condition.

◆ *Personal development targets:* (personal learning) such as improving confidence, selling skills, customer care skills and communication, and training targets such as learning new treatments and for those that the salon offers but in which you have not been trained. These need to be agreed.

Personal productivity and development time-bound targets should be set and agreed, for which employee performance will be reviewed at regular intervals.

Appraisals

Appraisals or progress reviews are an important method of communication, where one member of staff looks at the way another member of staff is performing in their job role or training. It is usual for an employee to receive an appraisal from their line manager on a regular basis.

Appraisals provide an opportunity to review an individual's performance against set targets. Each member of the team will have their own strengths and weaknesses and it is important to make the most of their strengths and work out an action plan to improve weaknesses with appropriate personal goals.

A performance appraisal will look at:

◆ results achieved against agreed targets

◆ additional accomplishments and contributions.

This may seem daunting, but it is an important and useful process. You can also use it to your advantage.

◆ Identify with your supervisor the tasks you see that need to be accomplished, and how these will be met.

◆ Identify your development training needs: this will provide you with a greater range of skills and expertise. It will ultimately improve your opportunities for promotion, giving you increased responsibilities.

◆ Identify obstructions that are affecting your progress. Look for guidance and support on how these can be overcome.

◆ Identify and amend any changes to your work role.

◆ Identify what additional responsibilities you would like.

◆ Identify and focus on your achievements to date against targets set.

◆ Update your action plan, which will help you achieve your targets.

If personal targets are not being met, it is important to identify the problem. Following this, new performance targets should be put in place to resolve any difficulties and prevent unsatisfactory performance.

If you meet the standards before the target date, inform your appraiser, who will review new targets for completion.

At the next appraisal the agreed objectives and targets set for the previous period will be reviewed.

Believe in yourself and use any small setbacks and failures as new opportunities for growth. Use other successful individuals (trainers, lecturers, bloggers and employers) as mentors, learning from them and their mistakes, this will help you as you perfect your craft. Above all else love what you do.

Maureen Evans-Olsen

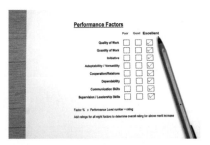

Employee evaluation form

TOP TIP

Developing confidence and experience in the job role

Further opportunities to develop your skills and experience include:

◆ attending trade seminars

◆ subscribing to professional trade magazines

◆ active participation in training and development activities

◆ observing and talking to colleagues with advanced skills and further experience

◆ gaining evidence of your Continuing Professional Development

◆ using time effectively and practising. All skills take time to master; the more you practise the more skilled and efficient you will become.

Performance review for a trainee beauty therapist

Name:	Jeanette Manners
Job title:	Trainee junior beauty therapist
Date of appraisal:	19th February 2018
Objectives:	To obtain competence within: improving and maintaining facial skin condition across the scope.
Notes on achievement:	Competence has been achieved for most facial skin condition scope requirements.
Training requirements:	Further training and practice is needed within the area of facial massage.
Any other comments on performance by appraiser:	Jeanette has achieved most of the objectives set out during the last performance review for carrying out waxing services.
Any comments on the appraisal by the staff member appraised:	I feel that this has been a fair appraisal of my progress although I did not achieve all of my performance targets and need to organise time more productively. *J Manners*
Action plan: Targets to be achieved:	◆ To achieve occupational competence across the scope for facial skin condition. ◆ To undergo further training and practice in hair removal techniques using setting wax. ◆ To take assessment for hair removal using setting wax.
Date of next appraisal:	19th June 2018

Being positive about negative feedback Your appraisal may not always be a positive experience. It is important to be positive about improvements and any recommendations to improve your performance, and to work towards achieving these.

Not meeting targets may ultimately result in a disciplinary procedure, which can lead to dismissal.

Your achievement of the productivity targets set leads to the financial effectiveness of the business.

If you are unhappy about your appraisal there should be a grievance process or appeal where an independent and impartial review can take place to assess if your appeal is valid or not.

Selling and promotion

Each business needs to continually review what products and treatments they offer. Keeping up-to-date with new or improved treatments and products benefits the salon by maintaining client interest and improving overall the results that can be achieved. This will help to keep your client satisfied and loyal.

INDUSTRY ROLE MODEL

SAM SWEET Co-founder, Sweet Squared LLP

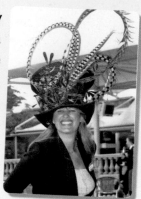

What do you find rewarding about your job? Beauty professionals are smart, artistic individuals, who have raw natural talent and artistic flair. It gives me a tremendous buzz knowing that these professionals have been able to garner self-respect and confidence from doing something that they love!

What do you find challenging about your job? Trying to convince beauty professionals of how important ongoing education is to their careers. Keeping up-to-date with training is vital and ultimately leads to much happier consumers.

What makes a good beauty therapist? Don't have a competitive spirit, have a creative one. If you are always worrying about what your competitors are doing then you lack confidence in what you are doing. Concentrate on your own business as only that will make you truly successful.

Clients expect more and more from the treatments or products they receive, to meet their individual requirements and to be personalised for them. Your professional advice will help inform them of what is new to the market and realistically what is achievable, providing them with a greater choice. Financially this is also an important benefit to the business.

When communicating information about special offers and additional treatments to clients this may be face-to-face, in writing, by telephone or text message, by email or online, via a website or social media such as Facebook or Twitter.

TOP TIP

Be part of a successful thriving industry

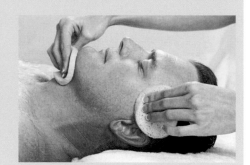

According to a 2015 Mintel research report the UK beauty industry turnover is valued at over £17bn and employs over a million workers, according to Cosmetic Executive Women (CEW) UK. The CEW study noted that there were a number of trends continuing to emerge in the beauty and skincare sector during 2015. These were:

1 an increase in men's skincare;

2 organic skincare rising in popularity; and

3 the over 50s market continuing to grow in importance and spending power.

When clients select a treatment or product they do so for one or a number of reasons. This may be:

◆ to improve appearance, e.g. eye service or manicure

◆ for a special occasion, e.g. make-up application; nail art

◆ for therapeutic reasons, to receive a quality professional service in tranquil surroundings, e.g. a spa de-stress facial massage

◆ for aspirational reasons, to achieve the appeal of an advertising campaign, for example radiant, healthy looking skin

TOP TIP

Client loyalty

Businesses must continuously source and launch new or improved products and services to be able to compete in a competitive market place. However, it is equally important for a business without local competitors to positively promote the industry to encourage their clients to try new services or products to maximise the service benefits that can be gained.

◆ to seek professional guidance on what would best suit their needs, e.g. skincare advice to deal with specific needs i.e. sensitivity

◆ for performance: the product or treatment has guaranteed results, i.e. an eyelash tint to darken the lashes permanently before a holiday

◆ to maintain the benefits of a particular treatment they have received before, e.g. repeat booking for leg waxing service

◆ for social reasons: they enjoy visiting the salon just as much as receiving the treatment

◆ to give a friend a treatment or product as a gift, e.g. a **gift voucher**

◆ value for money: the product or treatment is on promotion at a discounted price.

Whatever the reason, you want the client to feel satisfied that their choice was correct and that they enjoy the experience of using the product or receiving the treatment and tell others – thus promoting the business.

TOP TIP

Professional advice

Your personal professional guidance is a significant asset to the business as a unique selling point (USP). The client can purchase a product that is professionally endorsed, ideal for their needs and they can touch and smell it as well as be educated on the best way to get the most out of it.

"Don't have a competitive spirit, have a creative one. If you are always worrying about what your competitors are doing then you lack confidence in what you are doing. Concentrate on your own business as only that will make you truly successful."

Sam Sweet

The importance of retail sales

Retail sales are of considerable importance to the business: they are a simple way of greatly increasing the income without too much extra time and effort. Beauty therapy treatments are time-consuming and labour-intensive; up-selling a product in addition to providing the treatment will greatly increase the profitability.

Clients need to be regularly informed about what products and treatments the business is promoting. Earlier in this chapter we looked at the importance of creating that first, initial positive impression to the client through personal appearance. Staff knowledge of products and treatments is just as important to ensure personal effectiveness and to gain client confidence and trust in you.

Demonstrate a thorough and expert understanding of your products including:

◆ ingredients

◆ unique properties

◆ the beneficial effects they have

◆ how the products should be used

◆ how they complement each other, and

◆ the overall results that can be achieved.

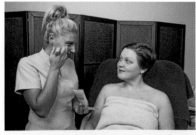

Demonstration of product application technique

If you get this right the client will remain loyal to you and this enables the business to grow. For example, a facial treatment might take 1 hour and cost the client £40.

You might then sell the client a moisturiser costing £40, of which £10 might be clear profit. Supposing that you sold eight products each day each yielding £10 profit. That would be a profit of £80 per day or £400 per week, or £1600 each month and thus, £19 200 profit over the whole year: a significant sum when consistently achieved with different clients.

TOP TIP

Client refreshments

Healthy light refreshments may be promoted as an additional retail opportunity. Clients receiving a treatment at lunchtime may value this service. A client having a range of treatments may have the cost of a lunch built into the service package.

A glass of champagne may be offered whilst receiving a treatment making their retail beauty experience feel extra special!

ACTIVITY

'Express' services or treatments

Increasingly, clients have a fast-paced lifestyle. This requires treatments delivered quickly and efficiently, often referred to as 'express', meaning fast. Examples include express artificial lash enhancements for that unexpected special occasion.

What other treatments may be offered as an 'express' service? Is the treatment adapted in any way to reduce timing in the delivery of the service? If so, how?

TOP TIP

Seasonal sales opportunities

The client's skincare preparations should change according to the different seasons. As such, the client should be advised on products that are most suitable to maintain skin health and appearance. This gives you the opportunity to educate your clients on the need to change skincare routines and promote products maintaining client interest with the product range and their loyalty to its use.

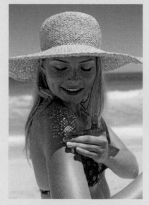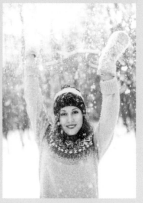

When promoting products or treatments, find out first about your client's needs and expectations. This will help you select the appropriate treatments or products which meet their requirements. Consider the following. What is the client's main concern? What would they like to achieve – their hope from either using a product or receiving a treatment? This information will guide you on selecting and advising them of the most suitable product or treatment:

◆ Is a skin sensitivity patch test necessary before the treatment? Ensure there will be sufficient time to carry out any necessary tests when promoting a treatment, to avoid disappointment.

TOP TIP

Express services

If you offer express services, make sure you explain to the client the difference between the express service and the full treatment. Remember, when the client experiences an express service this provides an opportunity to explain the benefits of receiving the full treatment to the client.

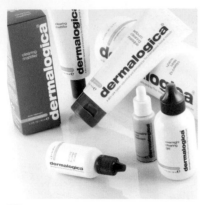

Skincare retail products

TOP TIP

Consumer awareness

According to Consumer Insights research, 90% of UK buyers of natural and organic personal care products said 'avoidance of synthetic chemicals' was important or very important to them and they would be willing to pay more.

As well as ingredients that have a positive effect on their health, consumers want to know that they will work and increasingly they require evidence of this, according to research by Diagonal Reports.

HEALTH & SAFETY

Contra-indications

If the client appears to have a contra-indication to the treatment they wish to receive, advise they seek medical approval first. Comply with your workplace policy and insurance company requirements regarding this.

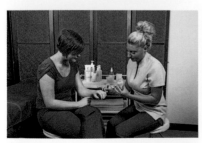

Demonstrating a product and describing its features and benefits

◆ Is the client allergic to any particular substance, contact with which should be avoided? Check the ingredients of any product if a client identifies they have an allergy.

◆ Does the client have a skin, nail disorder or disease which might contra-indicate use of a particular product or receiving a particular treatment? Contra-actions (undesirable or unwanted reactions) must always be noted if they occur, together with the action to take, which must be explained to the client. This information may be required in the future if questioned why the contra-action occurred and what advice was provided.

◆ Is the client planning to use a product over a skin disorder, i.e. cuts and abrasions? If so, is this safe? Always provide professional guidance.

◆ Find out what treatments the client has received before. Were they satisfied or disappointed in any way with them? If so, find out why this was.

◆ How much is the client used to spending on products? You can tactfully find this out by asking about what they are presently using: this will give you an idea of the types of product they have experience with using, and the sort of prices they are used to paying.

◆ Consider your client's values. Does the client have an interest in organic and eco-friendly products and those that have not been tested on animals? Guide them to the relevant choice.

Bearing in mind the client's needs, you can now guide them to the most suitable treatment or product. This is where your expertise and knowledge are so important: you can describe fully and accurately the features and benefits of the services and products you can offer.

Features and benefits

This can be repeated later to help the client make a purchase decision when there are several items to consider.

A **feature** is the uniqueness or individuality of a product or service, e.g. new technology in the ingredient formulation of a product or the design technology of a piece of equipment.

A **benefit** is the gain to be made by the client from using the product or treatment.

The features and benefits help to explain the treatment or product's Unique Selling Points (USP) which make it special.

TOP TIP

Features and benefits

A *feature* is the product's specialist ingredients, or what the treatment includes.

A *benefit* is what the client can expect from buying the product or receiving the treatment. The client will be more interested in the benefits of the products or treatment received – what it can do for them. The benefits will ultimately be the measure of the satisfaction with a product or treatment.

"Find a brand that you love and believe in. Customers will trust your judgement. Stay on trend and bring things into the salon that will sell."

Sam Sweet

Selling products

The products themselves must be presented to the client in such a way that they seem both attractive and desirable: the presentation should encourage the client to purchase them. The packaging and the product should be clean and in good condition, and **testers** should be available wherever possible so that the client can try the product before purchasing it.

You may also display cards with details of products which provide the USP of these products in an engaging and personal way.

The final choice of product is with the client, of course, but often the client will ask for a recommendation, for example if they cannot decide between two possibilities. It is in these circumstances that your ability to answer technical questions fully, from a complete knowledge of the product, will help in closing the sale. Speaking with confidence and authority on the one product that will particularly suit the client's requirements may well persuade them to buy it. You may also mix and match, select and display those products that are your top recommendations for the client. Make it as interactive as possible, allowing the client to touch and smell the products.

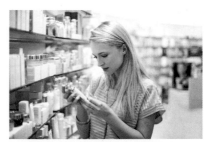

Professionally advise the client on which are the correct products to meet their requirements

Product suitability

If the client has not used the product or received the service before there is always a possibility of an allergic reaction.

Skin sensitivity patch tests If the client has not tried a product or received a service before, or if there is doubt as to how their skin will react, a skin sensitivity patch test must always be carried out. These details and outcomes are updated on the client record.

1 Select either the inner elbow or the area behind the ear. The skin here is thinner and more sensitive.

2 Make sure the skin is clean.

3 Apply a little of the product/s, using a clean applicator.

4 Leave the area alone for 24 hours.

5 If there is no reaction after 24 hours, the client is not allergic to the product: they can go ahead and use it. If there has been any itching, soreness, erythema, or swelling in the area where the product has been applied, the client is allergic to it and should not use it.

If the client does not know what an **allergic reaction** is – or how to recognise an allergy – it is important that you describe it to them (red, itchy, flaking and even swollen skin). If they experience this following a service they should contact you immediately for further advice, or in the case of product intolerance stop applying the product the client suspects is producing it.

Techniques in selling

The first rule of selling is: *know your products*. This applies to all retail products and to all salon services.

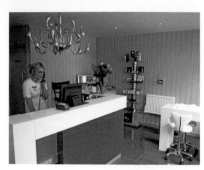

Retail products are usually located in the salon reception for the client to view

Staff training

It is important that everybody is knowledgeable and able to answer the client's questions – this includes the receptionist who is often the first and last person the client comes into contact with in a salon. In conversation, especially during quieter periods, they have opportunities to discuss products and services informally. Receptionists are also closely placed to point-of-sale (where purchases are made) displays and can inform clients of incentive items such as loyalty cards and **promotional activities**.

Often product companies provide training either at the business or at another venue. This is a great opportunity to update your knowledge and skills, which you will be able to share enthusiastically with your clients. Certificates to prove training are usually provided and these should be professionally displayed in the workplace.

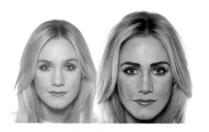

"When giving advice, always ensure you don't give opinions but that your advice can be backed up with facts."

Sam Sweet

It is not always possible for all staff to take part in training unless it is on a day when the business is closed. It is important that new information is passed on to these colleagues to ensure standardisation. Team meetings are a good opportunity to discuss workplace policy and new products and promotions.

Information on products and services must be available for clients to read, and eye-catching **displays** should be set up to gain attention both outside and inside the workplace. Be aware of your **competitors** and their current advertising displays and campaigns.

If your business has a website ensure that it is kept updated. It is a great resource for sharing any product or service promotions. If you have the software facility, clients may be able to purchase products or services online also.

Methods of promoting products and services

When promoting products and services it is good to raise client interest and awareness by considering the following:

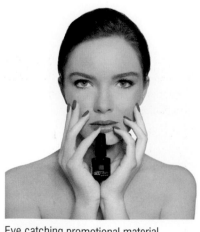

Eye catching promotional material

◆ Provide these at a time when the business is not normally open. This allows you to be more creative in the workspace you have for the promotional activity. **Demonstrations** are an ideal way to introduce potential clients to products and services.

◆ Eye-catching promotional material (usually provided by the product supplier): displays in the window will encourage new clients! Also point of sale are an ideal place to stimulate interest both in counter and floor displays. Promotional material should be changed regularly to maintain interest. Think of all the special dates in the calendar year, there are lots of great marketing occasions that should not be missed.

◆ Updated salon literature discussing benefits and costs of products and services may be provided. These may be available as hard copies and duplicated online, available for download wherever possible.

◆ A promotional launch event, where clients can enjoy a social event and perhaps book services or buy products at discounted prices, may be held.

TOP TIP

Promotional launch events

Promotions are an ideal opportunity to establish your new product line with special offers. Clients may have the opportunity to:

◆ purchase products at a special discounted rate

◆ purchase products with complimentary gifts

◆ receive complimentary samples.

Clearly signpost these offers at different areas of the salon, i.e. reception and service treatment rooms, using professional marketing materials. Provide the opportunity for the client to try the products.

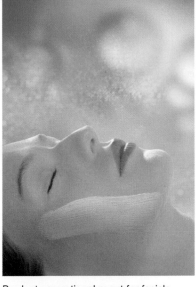

Product promotional event for facials

◆ Promotional packages may be presented at reduced cost or limited edition products can be purchased.

◆ Sample products may be given following a service or given away with the purchase of a service for the client to try at home.

◆ Products to enhance the service may be promoted, e.g. specially formulated mascara to wear with individual false lashes that enhance the overall result, ensuring client satisfaction.

◆ If you have a website you may wish to promote products and services on your home page. Special offers may be featured and you may have the facility for clients to book online.

◆ Special events or occasions: e.g. if the client is going on holiday, recommend travel-size products.

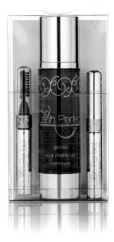

Lash care kit

Finally, remember if promoting a particular service or product such as nails – your nails should look great!

"You know much more than your client and as such must carry the confidence and the courage of your convictions when recommending the correct treatment for them."

Sam Sweet

Know your products   Product usage must be discussed with clients, as necessary, and advice given on which product will best suit each of them. The only way to be able to do this is to memorise the complete range: all your products, including for example, which skin types or service conditions each is for, what the active ingredients are, when and how each should be used, and its cost. Any questions asked must be answered with

ACTIVITY

Learn all about the services and product range offered

Learn about and memorise the services and product range sold in your workplace. Once you have learnt this, memorise the cost of the products. Clients will regularly enquire about such information.

ACTIVITY

Updating your knowledge

Professionally, it is recommended that you update your skills and knowledge annually, referred to as **continuous professional development (CPD)**. This allows you to be aware of current skills and trends. Keep a record or log of the different training activities you have been on.

TOP TIP

Product knowledge and loyalty to the product

Use the products yourself. It is always good to be able to speak from experience and shows your confidence in them. You will also be able to give tips on how best to use and gain the best result from them.

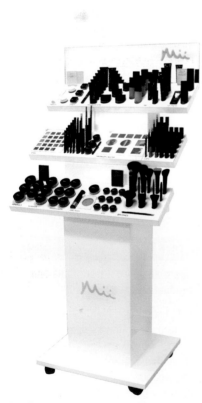

Retail products available for sale

authority and confidence. Clients expect the staff in the beauty salon to be professionals, able to provide expert advice:

◆ speak with confidence and enthusiasm

◆ avoid confusing technical words

◆ explain the benefits and personalise these, matching them to the needs of each client.

If the client requests advice on products or services that are outside of your responsibility refer them to the relevant colleague who has the expertise. You may have information literature you are able to provide to your client that will prevent possible loss of a sale, so pass it on.

> "Attend education updates at least twice a year. Updating your skills and mastering new ones will always keep you ahead of the pack."
>
> *Sam Sweet*

Information to read The **information** available to clients may start from the window display. If available use the **window adverts** if supplied with product ranges, and promote information that advertises the salon's services. Wherever you are situated it is important that potential customers know you are there.

Posters are supplied with good-quality product ranges, and most suppliers provide **information leaflets** for clients. Use the posters and **display cards** in the reception area; clients can then help themselves, and read about the products and their benefits. This will generate questions – and sales.

ACTIVITY

Collecting promotional information

Collect information leaflets from local beauty businesses and skincare/make-up product retailers in department stores. Is this literature attractive? Does the presentation encourage interest which may lead to sales?

Research wholesalers and beauty/make-up product companies for information about the display packs they supply with their products.

Look at websites also. What do you consider are the key features of a good business website?

Product and retail displays Two types of display are usually used in the beauty salon. In the first, the display is there simply to be looked at, and seen as part of the decor. It should be attractive and artistically arranged, and can use dummy containers. It is not meant to be touched or sold from, so it can be behind glass or in a window display.

In the second, products are there to be sold. The display should include testers so that clients can freely smell and touch. Products should be well stocked indicating they are popular. They may also be accessible dependent upon your workplace policy. Each product must be clearly priced, and small signs placed beside the products or on the edge of the shelves to describe the selling points of each product.

This sort of active display must always be in the part of the salon where most people will see and walk past it – the area of 'highest traffic'.

ACTIVITY

Evaluating product displays

Whenever you can, look at product displays through the 'eyes of a client' and judge their neatness, cleanliness, product availability, availability of clear pricing and information to read.

Compare the best with the worst and write a list stating why you have come to these judgements.

ACTIVITY

Importance of location and generating client interest

In your nearest large town, go into the big department stores and note where the cosmetic and perfumery department displays are situated. Is location important? Are some busier than others? If yes, why do you think this is, what are they doing to attract client interest?

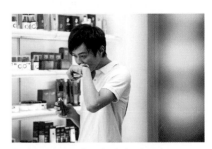

Perfumes are often impulse buys

A large proportion of cosmetic and perfume sales are **impulse buys**. It is no accident that perfumery departments are beside the main entrances to department stores, or right beside access points such as escalators.

Product displays where possible, should be placed in the area where the treatment is delivered. As you use the products, you can discuss and recommend them for the client. If displays are there to see and to take from, the sale can be closed even before the client returns to reception. Although clients can of course change their minds between the treatment area and actually paying, usually once they have the product in their hands they will go on to buy it.

Most small businesses will design and create their own displays using the counter **display packs** provided by the product companies. Some will have a professional **window dresser** to regularly change the window displays for the best effect.

Displays should always be well stocked, with smart undamaged packaging. Eye-level displays are best and ideally should be accessible. Change the display regularly according to the **promotion**, for example UV skin protection skincare products in summer.

Displays must be checked and cleaned regularly – this will usually mean daily. The display from which products are being sold will also need to be regularly dusted, cleaned (testers may drip), and straightened up. Testers need to be checked to make sure they are not sticky and spilt, lids are secure and that no-one has left dirty fingerprints on them.

HEALTH & SAFETY

Testers – maintaining hygiene and preventing cross-infection

Spatulas must be used for reasons of hygiene to avoid clients putting their fingers into pots either when testing or during home use. (You may consider a further retail opportunity of selling spatulas for clients to use at home.)

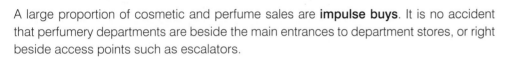

The range of products

It is not enough to stock just a few items and expect clients to fit in with the range you carry: different ranges must be available for each skin type, and a number of specialist products – such as eye gel, skin serums or creams – that will suit all skin types and conditions. You should have a range that meets the needs of the majority of your clients. Make-up and nail polish ranges should be attractive to all ages and diversity of customer. Sales must not be lost because of a lack of product range.

Information provided to the client should be accurate and not false or misleading. Legal action could follow in the case of non-compliance with **consumer protection legislation**.

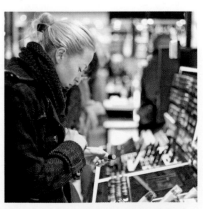

Have a product range to suit each client

REVISION AID

What are the opportunities for a beauty therapist to promote products and treatments?

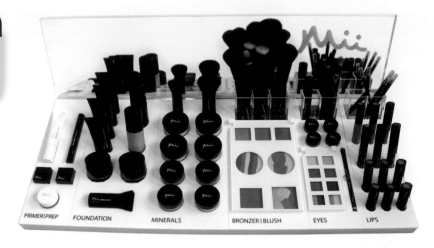

A professional commercial product range

TOP TIP

Kitemark™

The BSI Kitemark™ is a quality mark applied to goods and services that conform to certain standards of quality and safety.

Goods you may see in the workplace with the Kitemark™ logo include financial products, PPE, electrical and IT goods.

Consumer protection legislation

Be familiar with consumer protection legislation relating to the sale of beauty therapy products and services.

Consumer Protection Act (1987) This Act follows European laws to protect the customer from unsafe, defective services and products that do not reach safety standards. It also covers misleading price indications about goods or services available from a business.

It is important, therefore, to only use highly regarded products, purchased from a reliable source and that sufficient information is provided to the client on their correct use. All staff should be trained in using products and maintaining them so they are in consistently good condition. Up-to-date prices for products and services must be available. Local authorities are responsible for protecting consumers. Trading Standards or Consumer Protection Departments check that trading standards and laws are adhered to and investigate any complaint. If proven at fault and an offence has occurred the business may face legal action. For more information about consumer rights, visit www.gov .uk/consumer-protection-rights. Also Citizens Advice at www.citizensadvice.org.uk. This body can refer complaints to local Trading Standards Officers for investigation.

Consumer Safety Act (1978) The Consumer Safety Act (1978) aims to reduce risk to consumers from potentially dangerous products. It outlines the minimum safety standards to be met.

Prices Act (1974) The Prices Act (1974) states that the price of products or services has to be displayed in order to prevent the buyer being misled.

Trade Descriptions Acts (1968 and 1972) The Trade Descriptions Acts (1968 and 1972) prohibit the use of false descriptions of goods and services provided by a business. Products must be clearly labelled. When retailing, the information supplied both in written and verbal form must always be accurate. The supplier must not:

◆ supply misleading information

◆ describe products falsely

◆ make false statements.

ALWAYS REMEMBER

Fake goods

Fake goods are an example of a breach of the Trade Description Act. An offence under consumer protection law.

In addition they must not:

◆ make false comparisons between past and present services

◆ offer products at what is said to be a 'reduced' price, unless they have previously been on sale at the full price quoted for a 28-day minimum

◆ make misleading price comparisons.

The Acts also require accurate information to be included in advertisements.

Resale Prices Acts (1964 and 1976)
Under the provisions of the Resale Prices Acts (1964 and 1976) the manufacturer can supply a recommended retail price (MRRP), but the seller is not obliged to sell at the recommended price.

Supply of Goods and Services Act 1982
This Act provides protection when a contract is agreed for the supply of goods or services. Both may apply in certain circumstances where there is also a service provided in relation to the supply of a product.

Sale and Supply of Goods Act (1994)
This Act amended the previous Sale of Goods Act (1979) but the customers' rights as outlined in 1979 remain unchanged. The Sale and Supply of Goods Act (1994) provides that goods must be as described (as advertised or in a verbal description), of satisfactory quality including fit for their intended purpose, in appearance and finish, free from minor defects and safe and durable. The Act also covers the conditions under which customers can return goods. It is the responsibility of the retailer to correct a problem where the goods are not as described. This may be by refund, credit note, repair or replacement. This Act also applies to online purchases.

Cosmetic Products (Safety) Regulations (2004)
The Cosmetic Products (Safety) Regulations (2004) consolidates earlier regulations and incorporates current EU directives. Part of consumer protection legislation, it requires that cosmetics and toiletries are safe in their formulation and are safe for use for their intended purpose as a cosmetic and comply with labelling requirements.

Data Protection Act (DPA) (1998)
The Data Protection Act (1998) applies to any business that uses computers or paper-based systems to store information about its clients and staff. (See earlier in this Chapter for more information on the DPA.)

Confidential information on staff or clients should only be made available to persons to whom consent has been given.

Clients who have given information need to know how it will be used; otherwise they have a right to withhold it. Information stored must be accurate and up-to-date. It is necessary to register with the Data Protection Registrar who will place the business on a public register of data users. A code of practice is provided which must be complied with. For more information visit http://www.ico.gov.uk.

Consumer Protection (Distance Selling) Regulations (2000)
These regulations, as amended by the Consumer Protection (Distance Selling) (Amendment) Regulations (2005) are derived from a EU directive and cover the supply of goods/services made between suppliers, acting in a commercial capacity, and consumers. They are concerned with purchases made where there is no face-to-face contact, that is, by telephone, fax, Internet, digital television or mail order, including catalogue shopping.

HEALTH & SAFETY

The requirements of the Cosmetic Product Safety Regulations are enforced in the UK by the Cosmetic Products Enforcement Regulations 2013.

Non-compliance can lead to prosecution and imprisonment.

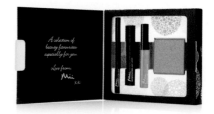

INCLUDES ENCHANT 01

Customers must receive clear information on goods or services, including delivery arrangements and payment, suppliers' details and consumers' cancellation rights, which should be made available in writing. The customer also has a 7 working day cooling-off period where they may cancel their purchase. The point at which the right to cancel services is reached is detailed in the 2005 amendment to the 2000 Regulations.

The Disability Discrimination Act (DDA) (1996) Under the **Disability Discrimination Act (1996)**, as a supplier of goods, facilities and services your workplace has the duty to ensure that clients are not discriminated against on the grounds of disability. It is unlawful to use disability as a reason or justification to:

◆ refuse to provide a service

◆ provide a service to a lesser standard

◆ provide a service on worse terms

◆ fail to make reasonable adjustments to the way services are provided.

From 2004 this includes failure to make reasonable adjustments to the physical features of service premises to overcome physical barriers to access. Service can be denied to a disabled person if justified and if any other client would be treated in the same way. Your employer has a responsibility under the DDA to ensure that you receive adequate training to prevent discrimination in practice, and as such is responsible for your actions. Also they must make reasonable adjustments to the premises to facilitate access for disabled persons.

Insurance

Product and service liability insurance is usually included within public liability insurance, but should be checked with the insurance company. Product liability insurance covers risk, which might occur as a result of the products you are selling.

Informing clients about additional products or treatments

Present information at a pace relevant to the client's knowledge and previous experience. If the information is new this may be slower and more detailed. If the client is receiving a service this information may be provided at the consultation, when discussing the treatment objectives, during service delivery when you have the opportunity to recommend and share advice, or when discussing aftercare. Here you will be able to emphasise the importance of further products and treatments to further improve the service benefits gained. This may be further use of products or services that the client has used before or of those that are new to the client.

TOP TIP

Create your own selling opportunity (often called 'up-selling')

◆ If the client is having a manicure and has weak nails, you could recommend a course of nail treatment services and an appropriate nail strengthener.

◆ If the client is going away on holiday tell them about the special 'holiday package promotion'.

◆ If the client is having an eyelash tint, tell them how quick and simple an eyebrow wax is and the immediate difference it can make to the eye area!

ALWAYS REMEMBER

Avoid offending the client

In the beauty industry you are regularly commenting on an area of the client's skin, hair or nails that requires improvement – which of course you can professionally help with. Initiating a judgement comment should only occur when you have a rapport with the client and you know they will welcome your professional advice.

Choose the most appropriate time to inform the client about any additional products and services.

Communication

Good communication with clients, both verbal and non-verbal, is essential. Communication should be relaxed and informal. Create a rapport, or connection with your client and give your attention fully to the client above any other tasks that may interfere with this. Use your client's name (if known), addressing them by their preferred title: this increases their sense of self-importance and value.

"Remember, it's about the client in front of you – they are paying for your time so become a good listener. You often get to be privy to personal information from your clients but never gossip, with anyone, your client's information is private and should remain as such."

Sam Sweet

◆ At all times remain polite, friendly and respect the client's individual opinions and preference in choice of product. Never be critical as this will break the rapport and also potentially lose the sale!

◆ A client may be already considering purchasing a product or service and the type of questions they ask will signal this. The most common question is 'How much is it?'

◆ Make eye contact, but always consider the diversity of your clients and consider if this is appropriate. To some cultures this body language is deemed intrusive and rude. Observe the client's **body language**: are they interested in what you are telling them? If the client is interested, they will agree with you and their body language will be relaxed yet attentive. There are many customer types: those that are decisive and quick to make a decision, indecisive, chatty, quiet, opinionated, awkward and disbelieving. This should be considered in your approach: it is important that the client gains confidence in you and ultimately your products or service. This will be assisted through your appearance, communication style differentiated for each client and manner.

◆ **Questions** must be specific, requiring detailed responses. You are the expert: show your knowledge. Do not ask the client what sort of skin they have – they are not the expert, and will probably give the wrong answer. Instead, ask detailed questions, such as 'Does your skin feel tight?' (which may indicate dryness), or 'Do you have spots in a particular area?' (which may indicate an oily area). Use open questions. These are questions that may not be answered with yes or no. Open questions usually start with 'why', 'how', 'when', 'what' and 'which'.

TOP TIP

The importance of questioning when selling

Questions may lead to the opportunity to increase the sale of more products or services.

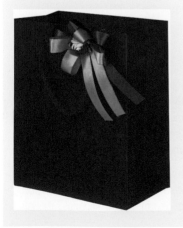
Remember to always make sure the environment is helpful to making the client feel comfortable to ask questions. If necessary take the client to a more private area to discuss their requirements.

◆ **Listen** to your client; this will help you to find out more about them helping you to identify their product or service requirements and personality. Always listen carefully to the answers your client gives: do not talk over their answer when they are speaking or interrupt. Only when they have finished should you give a considered, knowledgeable reply. You may need to ask another question, or you may be able straightaway to direct them to the best product or service for their needs.

◆ Allow time for the client to think about their purchase before a decision is made. Never be pushy or put pressure on the client to purchase.

◆ When a decision is made to purchase, ensure that the client receives sufficient information about the service or products. Explain any specific requirements in their use or application in order that they gain the maximum benefit from them.

◆ In the case of a treatment, make an appointment and provide the client with an appointment card and relevant information to read about the treatment. If the client has made a decision to receive a treatment or purchase a product, sometimes there may be a delay in its availability. Ensure any delay is minimal. Do not be tempted to offer unsuitable alternatives, which are not as suited to the client's needs or service requirements. Inform the client honestly and realistically of their availability. In the case of a product you may be able to give the client a sample to use until the product is available.

◆ If a sale is achieved, be positive – smile, this will help to make the client feel they have made a good decision.

◆ Ask the client if there is anything else they need when closing the sale on the product. Confirm the size of product the client wishes to purchase, explaining any financial benefit of a larger size linked to their selection. This is referred to as up-selling.

◆ Record all sales on the client's record. This is a useful reference point in the future for you and the client to refer back to on products used, samples and treatments received. Follow this up with the client next time you see them to see if they have enjoyed their product or treatment received.

◆ If the client does not wish to proceed with a sale, they will inform you of this but often not the reason why. Acknowledge this and listen to any further conversation to try to find out why.

◆ Learn from this, but it might be that they would like more time to think about it.

◆ Be appreciative, thank the client when they are about to leave even if an enquiry has not resulted in a purchase.

"Be happy, grateful and thankful for your clients. They are your bread and butter and should be treated as such."

Sam Sweet

Promotions

Promotions are another way of informing your clients about products or services that are currently available. They are also a great way of gaining interest in a product or service from a wider or potentially new client group.

ALWAYS REMEMBER

What is the purpose of your promotion?

Sales promotion activities are aimed at promoting products and services.

If it is the intention to promote awareness of the business and what it can offer this is referred to as a **public relation** activity.

Public relation activities are studied at Level 3 when you will be required to co-ordinate such activities. When taking part in any promotional activities when studying at Level 2, consider what went well and identify what could be done better for future activities.

Learn to view things through the client's eyes: this will help you improve the quality and service of everything you do.

TOP TIP

Demonstrations

An effective demonstration will always create sales. Have the product ready to sell, or you could consider giving out vouchers to encourage clients to purchase the product or service later, at a discounted rate.

General benefits of a promotion

◆ Promotional events can create a relaxed, fun social atmosphere where clients can sample different products or services without pressure to purchase. Refreshments may be provided and gift bags of samples to take away. Make sure your engagement with clients ensures they have a great time and the event is a good public relations activity for the business.

◆ A service or product on sales promotion may cost less and therefore be affordable to more clients. Having had the opportunity to use the product or service they may feel it is now a necessity to receive or use.

◆ Clients may take the opportunity of using a product or service because it is on offer at a reduced cost. If they do not like it, it is less of a costly mistake.

◆ Limited editions and sale offers are a way of gaining client interest as the product or service may not be available or on offer at a later date.

◆ The enthusiasm of some clients during a public relation event or sales promotion will motivate others to purchase.

ACTIVITY

Up-selling

When a client purchases skincare products suited to their skin type, what additional products can you recommend, providing an opportunity for up-selling?

Provide further examples of when up-selling opportunities may occur.

TOP TIP

Increasing your clientele

It is important to constantly increase the number of clients visiting the business. A promotional event is an opportunity for existing clients to bring friends with them who you hope will become future clients.

ALWAYS REMEMBER

Promotions

All staff should be aware of any promotions that their business is offering so that they can confidently engage and build on a client's initial interest in a product or service and turn it into a sale.

ACTIVITY

Product and service promotion

Think of different services or products that your workplace offers that are not as popular as they once were. Consider a promotion you could offer to gain client interest. How would this promotion be presented and would any activities be required?

Demonstration

Demonstrating to an audience needs particularly careful planning if the demonstration is to achieve the maximum benefit. Everything required must be available, together with all the relevant literature to be given out to the audience or clients.

TOP TIP

Promotional media

You may wish to have the promotion activity recorded. This may then be used as a video on your website (if available) or shown through a visual display unit in reception to capture a client's interest and generate questions from those who did not attend.

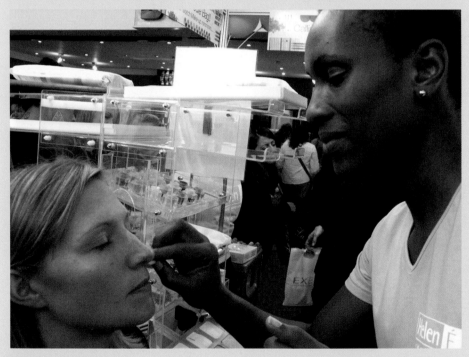

Trade demonstration

Consider all possibilities in your planning. What type of demonstration is required? Will you be working on one client, to demonstrate and sell a product, or demonstrating to a group? Is a range of products or services to be demonstrated, or just one item?

Client suitability

If the client is not interested they will probably not engage with you, and will appear uninterested in what you are saying. If this occurs, go back to the beginning and suggest alternatives to attempt to regain their interest, but avoid pressuring the client. Following discussion about a product or service, you may feel that the client is unsuitable. Tactfully explain to the client why this is. If it is for medical reasons, ask them to seek permission from their GP before the product or service is provided. The expectations of some clients may be unrealistic. If this is the case, patiently and diplomatically explain why and aim to agree to a realistic treatment programme. Remember your legal duty under the **Health and Safety at Work Act (1974)** to take reasonable care to avoid harm to yourself and others.

Single client When demonstrating on a client, have a mirror in front of them so that you can explain as you go along and the client can watch. They can then see the benefit of the product and learn how to use it at the same time. This is a simple but effective way to sell products. Demonstrations may be used to discuss facial skincare or make-up application and removal techniques.

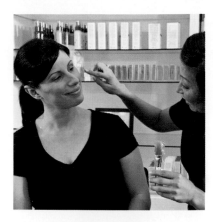

A group The presentation should include an introduction to the demonstrator and the product, the demonstration itself, and a conclusion with thanks to the audience and model. Written **promotional material** can be placed on the seats before the audience arrives, or handed out at an appropriate point during the demonstration; **samples** can be handed around for the audience to try while being discussed.

The demonstration itself must be clear, simple and not too long. The audience *must* be able to see what is being done and hear the commentary. Maximise the impact of the demonstration by giving the audience the opportunity to buy the product immediately.

If this is not possible – because the demonstration is in another room, away from the products or at another venue, not the salon business premises – ensure that members of the audience leave with a **voucher** to exchange for the product. This should offer some incentive, such as a **discount**, to encourage potential buyers to make the effort to come to the salon and buy. Never sell the features and benefits to potential customers, creating the desire for the product, without also giving them the chance to buy it.

Insurance and legal requirements

You must know the health and safety procedures for the venue you are using. This will include:

◆ Fire drill.

◆ Who is responsible for public and staff safety?

◆ Who is responsible for emergencies?

For further information refer to the section entitled *Insurance* earlier in this chapter (within the *Health and Safety in the Workplace* section).

Also, be aware of legislation that applies to you when taking part in a promotional activity.

Marketing to develop the business brand

It is essential that the business develops clear expectations in terms of the supply of its products and services to customers. The aim is to establish a brand image that is instantly synonymous and recognisable for your business. This will influence the choice of products and services offered.

Creating a business brand The business brand says everything about you. It is the impression you make and will encourage clients to choose you for their treatments.

The visual brand is your business name, logo, the font and colours you use for your typeface, advertising, decorating, uniforms, soft furnishings and everything else you can

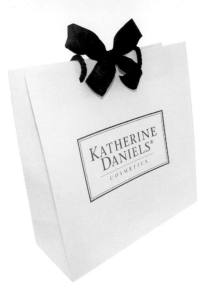

Joyfully wrapped up!

REVISION AID

How can you keep up-to-date with beauty treatments and products that the workplace offers?

TOP TIP

A strong brand will help to attract new clients, build strong relationships with existing clients and keep clients for longer.

see. Where there is a dress code and image associated with personal appearance, it is necessary for this to be consistent at all times.

The brand is also how you sound, what you say in communications such as social media, emails, leaflets and your 'tone of voice'. For example, friendly, warm, competent, happy, etc.

Creating a strong and attractive brand will encourage more clients to choose you.

Create a strong brand image for your business using social media

Social media is free to use, easy to update and reaches a large number of people. Using social media is an effective way to communicate with people for any size of business.

A Facebook page can be the main part of your social media presence. Your other social media presence could include Twitter, Pinterest, Instagram and a range of others. Have a plan and make sure that they work together with the same themes, offers, information and talking points.

Schedule Facebook posts for weekends and evenings. This is a time when most people are looking online.

Have a consistent feed of content, which will keep your clients and followers engaged. Seeing that it is regularly updated makes it more interesting. If they notice that it hasn't been updated for months, they may stop following you.

Photos are the best type of content for social media. Take photos before, during and after treatments to show the results to potential clients. Make sure you have a signed agreement from your clients to use their photos. Ask the client receiving the treatment to share on their own social media page as this will also create greater exposure for your business and the treatments you provide.

Eyelash and brow treatments, lash extensions, nail services, spray tanning and make-up all make good social media content. Bridal and special occasion make-up and nail finishes are especially interesting and make effective before and after photos.

Use hashtags when posting content on Facebook, Twitter and Instagram. Hashtags will allow your content to be seen by other people who may not already follow your page. This could result in new clients. Keep the hashtag words broad in their appeal as this will create greater exposure of your content, for example #Hair #Beauty #Nails. Three to five hashtags work well on images.

Ensure you reply to a client's questions or messages as soon as you can. A quick reply will create a good relationship between you and your followers on social media.

If a complaint is posted, then refer this to the relevant person following your complaints procedure and ask to communicate privately so you can sort it out quickly.

Information systems

Information systems ensure the smooth running of the business and provide data for the manager and external agents as legally required; for example to HMRC (Her Majesty's Revenue and Customs) at the end of the financial year.

Information systems can be manual or computerised. If using a manual system, you will need an index of filing to access information quickly.

There is a wide range of salon software (programmes and electronic information used by a computer) available for all sizes of business. They are valuable business management tools, which work in an integrated way from appointments to stock control and ordering.

Online systems are commonly available to access on most internet enabled devices and are capable of some or all of the following:

◆ point of sale (till) operation

◆ online bookings for clients

◆ stock management: as one item is sold, the remaining stock will be recalculated

◆ scheduling for therapists

◆ business intelligence statistics, e.g. which treatments are most popular, which therapists sell most additional products, which treatments are most profitable

◆ minimum and maximum stock levels calculated

◆ SMS and email lists for marketing and promotions.

Salon software will make administration tasks quicker and more accurate. It can improve customer experience by ensuring treatment bookings are accurate. It will complete time-consuming tasks such as stock taking quickly and accurately. The point of sale (till) provides accurate daily sales and business information.

TOP TIP

Salon software providers

Speak to several salon software providers to see which would best suit different types of business. Research internet forums and advice to support your own judgement.

ALWAYS REMEMBER

Audit stock control

A policy of conducting a stock audit is necessary to ensure the information on your computer system is correct.

Stock control

Stock is the total amount of professional consumables for use on clients during treatments, plus retail products for client purchase, plus other items such as product samples. Information systems should be in place for stock maintenance, which should be accurate, up-to-date and legible. Identified staff should be responsible for:

◆ ordering stock

◆ maintaining stock records and levels

◆ receiving incoming stock and checking deliveries for quality and discrepancy

◆ unpacking stock and locating it in the correct storage/display area.

TOP TIP

Supplier reliability

It is important that your supplier is reliable. An efficient business cannot afford uncertain delivery schedules which, if late, may mean certain stock items will run out, affecting retail and treatment sales and creating client disappointment.

TOP TIP

Reputable and secure websites

◆ Check if the distributor you are purchasing from is listed on a directory of safe suppliers.

◆ A small padlock symbol should be located in the website address bar.

◆ The web address should start with https. The inclusion of the letter 's' after http means secure.

TOP TIP

Stock orders

Some companies require a large minimum set-up order. This means that your money will be tied up in stock. It is important that you are confident that it will sell and will match your client market. Capital should not be tied up unnecessarily and unproductively.

Stock control should link to anticipated needs. Therefore where staff have productivity targets, this should be linked to anticipated stock requirements too.

Where these targets are not met it is necessary to review this to see why. Are more education and training required about the products or services? Does the therapist know how to recommend and promote products and to maximise the opportunities to up-sell? Is the sales expectation understood by all staff?

Salon ordering systems

Stock can be ordered from different places and in different ways. Whatever system is used it should be well managed.

Wholesalers These are cash-and-carry outlets that sell wholesale products to businesses. Most companies offer internet and mail-order purchase facilities.

Representatives from companies Some companies have sales representatives who visit the business and with whom you can place purchase orders. The order is returned to the company to be processed and dispatched. Representatives are useful as they can advise you of new product ranges and promotions that you may wish to take part in, to help increase financial productivity.

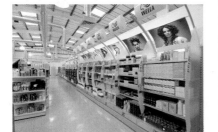

Salon wholesaler's showroom

Online orders Some companies allow orders to be placed online, which can be completed as part of the treatment aftercare advice and recommendation as a point-of-sale transaction. Next day delivery to the client is guaranteed, ensuring service satisfaction and accommodating impulse purchases too.

Ordering stock

When you make an order, the supplier will normally open a credit account for you and provide information on how to order and pay. Cash-and-carry wholesalers do not normally have minimum orders. Mail order and internet companies usually charge postage on small orders. It is important to consider the most cost-effective way to order. When placing an order, ensure sufficient time is allowed to avoid running out of stock.

TOP TIP

Slow stock

Where sales of stock are poor, plan a marketing campaign to encourage its sale.

Principles of stock control Stock levels can only be maintained if accurate records are kept of how much stock the business has. The records will identify retail and professional stock used and what needs to be reordered. Maintaining accurate records means you don't have to count all stock. Importantly, you also avoid running out of stock, especially of popular items, and avoid over-ordering products.

A good **stock-keeping** checklist:

◆ *Anticipate needs.* Stock must be ordered regularly, *before* it runs out. Orders should be placed as stock becomes low so new stock will be arriving as the existing stock is being used or sold. There may be short-term influences on needs, such as seasonal factors. For example, there may be an increased demand for cosmetic UV-screening preparations in summer or following a promotion. Regularly review order levels for stock to anticipate and accommodate demand.

◆ *Check incoming stock.* What has been ordered should be checked against a delivery note when it arrives. The delivery note lists all the items that have been dispatched and any that are to follow, such as items that are out of stock. Never assume that the order received will be correct. Inaccuracies must be reported to the supplier immediately, before countersigning the order and confirming the delivery. Any damaged goods must be dealt with and either returned to the sender or replaced, according to the policy of the supplier. Never return anything without the relevant paperwork or without confirmation from the supplier. Inform your manager of any discrepancies as applicable.

◆ *Rotate the stock.* Stock must be stored and used in rotation, so that new items go to the back of the shelf and older items are used first. This is often referred to as FIFO – 'first in first out'.

◆ *Keep accurate and up-to-date records.* Stock levels may be recorded manually or electronically. Whichever method is used, records must be accurate and updated regularly as per the business policy, usually weekly, but monthly is a necessity. You may identify a training requirement if product use seems high against treatments delivered. If there is stock loss, stock control will be required daily to identify the cause.

ALWAYS REMEMBER

Inadequate 'sloppy' stocktaking procedure

The lack of a robust procedure that results in stock running out can lead to:

◆ loss of sales due to insufficient retail stock or commercial stock to deliver treatments

◆ poor practice, such as borrowing retail stock for commercial use

◆ excessive issue of samples; these should be fairly distributed and relevant to the objective of why they have been provided. For example, to check client skin sensitivity, try a new product the client is unsure of or you are about to receive as a new product line.

TOP TIP

Success of treatments and product ranges

Use data to review the success and popularity of your brands. It may be time to try something new, where sales are low or a marketing campaign is required to refresh interest. Always remember to gain feedback from your clients too.

TOP TIP

Sustainability tip: product use

Use training to ensure staff are not using products excessively during their treatments, with unnecessary wastage.

HEALTH & SAFETY

Duty of care

Employees should be made aware that they can be fined for breaking safety rules.

HEALTH & SAFETY

Damaged stock

Handle broken containers with care as they could cause harm. Before touching them or clearing up, check that the contents are not hazardous, and whether they have spilt. Always dispose of damaged stock safely and quickly.

Manual and computerised stock-control systems
The two main types of stock control systems used to collect and collate stock information are *point-of-sale systems* and *stock-check systems*, which can be manual or computerised.

Point-of-sale systems collect information concerning sales at the time the sale is made. The till will collect the stock information as well as sales information. If it is done manually, the person making the sale has to complete a form, such as a sales bill, which includes stock information.

ISBN 0-333-68902-X

Barcodes

Computers read price tickets coded by means of barcodes printed on the packaging. As the products are sold, the code numbers are read by the computer via a scanning barcode reader, which recognises the product and automatically updates its records. This system is essential for large businesses with a high rate of stock turnover.

BEAUTY WORKS

CASH SALE INVOICE

Date and Tax Point:

Invoice No: 32622

Quantity	Description	Price £	p	
1	Moisturiser (sensitive) – 20 g	12	50	
1	Toner (oily) – 200 ml	9	50	
1	Nail varnish – tropical red	7	50	

The Beauty Garden
Mytown
The Midlands
Tel: 01234 456789

Goods   29.50
VAT   5.90
Invoice Total   £35.40

A typical sales bill

Stock-check systems allow the stock-keeper to refer quickly to the quantity of stock available. If you have a record of how many stock items you started with and what is left, you will know immediately how many you have sold.

With a regular stock check you can set a reorder level. Whenever the quantity of goods falls to a predetermined level, it is time to reorder this product.

A simple stock-check system is the stock record card. Alternatively, stock information is fed into a computer, which analyses the sales details, recalculates stock levels and calculates when to reorder and other details, as required. This provides automated stock-control information and printouts for use when performing manual stock-taking checks.

The stock-taking record needs to show:

◆ a description of the product and its size

◆ how much is in stock

◆ what has been sold and used

◆ what has come in

◆ the minimum and maximum holding levels

◆ the point at which the product is to be reordered.

Precious Skin Care

Ellisons

REP: Susan Green

TEL: 361619

		Min	Max	Mar	Apr	May	Jun
Coral							
Cleanser	500 ml	10	20	5 / 15	10 / 10	12 / 8	9
	200 ml	20	30	22 / 8	20 / 10	19 / 11	20
Toner	500 ml	10	20	10 / 10	11 / 9	9 / 11	10
	200 ml	20	30	20 / 10	20 / 10	21 / 9	19
Moisturiser	250 ml	5	10	5 / 5	6 / 4	5 / 5	4
Cream	50 ml	15	25	12 / 13	16 / 9	15 / 10	11
Night	250 ml	5	10	5 / 5	8 / 2	5 / 5	6
Cream	50 ml	15	25	14 / 11	16 / 9	14 / 11	10

Manual stock-recording system

ALWAYS REMEMBER

Stock records

◆ All stock records can suffer from human error. Make sure that those responsible understand the business system.

◆ Careful records ensure enough stock is held until the next reorder and delivery. Regular supplies of stock keep the stock turning over and reduce the amount of money tied up on the shelf.

Stock rotation

When new stock arrives it must go to the back of the shelf and existing stock should be brought forward: remember the rule of FIFO (first in, first out).

Many products have a shelf life or best before date. This is because they contain the minimum amount of preservatives in their formulation.

Products that have exceeded their shelf life should be disposed of.

If the company updates its packaging, request any stock you hold is replaced to maintain currency of image.

Moving and storing stock

Stock should be taken to the appropriate storage area following checking. This may be into storage, into the retail area or into the treatment area for use within the treatment.

Always take care of yourself when moving goods around the workplace. Do not struggle: get assistance as necessary.

Both employers and employees have a duty to work in as safe and healthy a way as possible. Employees have a responsibility not to endanger their own health and safety, but the employer must ensure that rules are laid down for safe working practices. They must:

◆ train staff in safe working practices

◆ provide safe systems for the handling, transit and storage of all materials.

The legislation to ensure safe working practice when handling resources is the Manual Handling Operations Regulations (1992).

Stock must be easily accessible and products need to be found easily. Place the stock labels towards the front. Remember, the oldest stock should be used first. Therefore, place new stock at the back of the shelves.

REVISION AID

Why is it important to have a stock control system?

HEALTH & SAFETY

Avoid hazards

All packing materials must be tidied away immediately. They are a hazard and might cause accidents.

HEALTH & SAFETY

Stock deterioration

Stock that is deteriorating may change in consistency, look discoloured and the smell may change or become unpleasant. Bacterial or fungal growth may even be seen on the product surface.

Ensure that stock is stored to maintain its quality and shelf life.

Certain substances may require special storage and handling requirements. Legislation relating to the storage and handling of resources is covered by the **Control of Substances Hazardous to Health Regulations (COSHH) (2002)**. All cosmetic products come under the strict legislation of the **Cosmetics Products (Safety) Regulations (2004)**. Written by the Cosmetic, Toiletry and Perfumery Association (CTPA), with the co-operation of the Hairdressing and Beauty Suppliers' Association (HBSA), this piece of legislation consolidates earlier regulations and incorporates European Directives. Part of consumer legislation, it requires that cosmetics and toiletries are safe for use in their intended purpose as a cosmetic and comply with labelling requirements.

Security Security concerns should be taken into consideration to prevent loss of stock through theft. Regular stock checks may identify loss of stock.

◆ The retail area should be designed to be in full view of staff, with a security camera placed where possible for additional security.

◆ Attend to customers looking at and handling retail stock politely and cheerfully, asking them if they require assistance. In most instances the person is genuine, but being attentive and aware at all times can help prevent stock theft and loss.

◆ Retail and product resources should be kept in a secure area, accessed only by those with authority to do so. Some businesses will request stock is signed for.

◆ Open display areas should be stocked with replica 'dummy' products and minimal sample products.

◆ At their induction, all staff should be made aware of the consequence of theft. Theft is often referred to as gross misconduct and may lead to dismissal and prosecution.

Dealing with theft If you suspect a client of stealing and you have reasonable evidence, you have the right to make a citizen's arrest under the Police and Criminal Evidence Act (1984). Theft is a criminal offence. You must know your employer's policy on theft and apprehending a thief.

ASSESSMENT OF KNOWLEDGE AND UNDERSTANDING

Having covered the learning objectives for this chapter test your knowledge and understanding by answering the short questions below.

The information covers:

Workplace procedures and legal requirements

1. What are your main responsibilities under the Health and Safety at Work Act (1974)?

2. Name four different pieces of legislation relating to health and safety in the workplace.

3. What is the purpose of a workplace health and safety policy? What information does it include?

4. Why must regular health and safety checks be carried out in the workplace? Provide five examples of checks you may be required to perform.

5. How would you define an accident? What is the procedure for dealing with an accident in the workplace?

6. Which insurance is the workplace expected to display by law?

7. Treatments should be completed in commercially acceptable time frames. Why is it important to adhere to these?

Workplace skills, values and behaviours

1. What is the importance of professional standards in personal presentation and behaviour? How does this relate to your workplace policy and professional image?

2. Provide five examples of sustainable and environmentally friendly working practices that can be implemented in a beauty salon.

3. How can you keep up to date with beauty products and treatments? Why is this important?

4. Values, skills and behaviours underpin the delivery of all beauty therapy services. Briefly explain the meaning of each term and provide two examples to demonstrate each.

   ◆ Skills
   ◆ Values
   ◆ Behaviours

Health and safety

1. Why is personal conduct important to maintain the health and safety of yourself, colleagues and others? Give three workplace examples of how you comply with this requirement in respect of yourself, colleagues and others.

2. How should you lift a large box from the floor level to place on a work surface? Which legislation applies to safe handling of resources in the workplace?

3. What is a hazard? What hazards may exist in the beauty therapy workplace?

4. What is a risk? What is a risk assessment and why is it carried out?

5. What is a fire drill? What is the emergency fire evacuation procedure in your workplace?

6. What health and safety guidance should be available for reference detailing the correct use, storage and disposal of hazardous substances?

7. The salon policy should include security procedures for staff, clients and visitors. Provide three examples where you apply security procedures in your daily work in the salon.

Hygiene and infection control

1. When carrying out a client consultation, you identify that the treatment cannot be carried out because the client has impetigo, an infectious bacterial skin disorder. What action would you take?

2. Effective sterilisation and disinfection methods prevent cross-infection and secondary infection. What do you understand by the following terms:

   a. sterilisation
   b. disinfection
   c. cross-infection
   d. secondary-infection

3. How should industry codes of practice and ethics be used to implement best practice in health and safety?

4. Why is it important to complete a client record, gain the client's signature and update this at every treatment?

5. What is the purpose of a skin sensitivity patch test, and when should this be completed?

6. Select a treatment of your choice and provide a list of the steps you take from start to finish which demonstrate best health and safety practice and infection control.

Reception duties

1. What are the main duties of the salon receptionist?

2. How should the reception be maintained?

3. What are the important details to record when taking a message?

4. A client complains at reception about a leg wax service they have received. What questions should you ask? What action should you take?

5. What systems may be used in salons to make appointments?

6. Why is it important to inspect the quality and condition of goods before payment is processed?

7. What interpersonal skills are essential in a salon receptionist?

8. A client arrives for a treatment to find there has been a mistake when booking their appointment and it has not been made for them. What action should be taken?

Professional workplace relationships

1. Why are positive relationships with your colleagues important?

2. Why is it important to co-operate with and willingly assist colleagues in the workplace? Provide three examples where you have acted using your initiative to help others to resolve different problems throughout the working day.

3. Sometimes disputes are not immediately resolved leading to poor working relationships which can create a stressful working environment. If you were experiencing relationship difficulties, how would you handle this? When and to whom would you report this?

4. Why are good listening and questioning skills important when you are trying to gain more information to help understand client motivation to have a make-up service, for example?

5. All colleagues should be treated equally. What are the legal requirements that must be applied in the workplace?

6. How can positive relationship be established with clients?

7. How can you identify if a client is dissatisfied with their treatment? How can this be avoided through positive client handling? Answer this question considering the client's treatment journey from their entering the salon to leaving it.

Productivity and development targets

1. Why is it important that you have a good knowledge about the products and treatments available in your workplace?

2. Why is it important to know your strengths and areas for development within your job role?

3. What is the purpose of staff receiving personal productivity and development targets?

4. Why is it important to gain honest feedback about your performance, including positive and negative points, from others?

5. How can continuous training and professional development improve your performance?

6. What sources of information can you access to find out more about the beauty industry and the different career paths?

Selling and promotions

1. Why are retail sales important to the business and its clients?

2. What are the opportunities with your client when you can promote products and treatments?

3. Communication is important when selling. Why is it important to observe the client's body language?

4. As well as directly (face-to-face), what other ways can you make clients aware of the products and treatments available in your workplace?

5. How must retail displays be maintained? Why is this important?

6. State three pieces of legislation that relate to the way products or treatments are delivered to clients that protect their legal rights.

7. How would you define a 'feature' or 'benefit' of a product or treatment?

Marketing to develop the business brand

1. Why must you be aware of current trends in the beauty business?

2. How can you help to promote the business brand on a daily basis?

3. Client feedback is important to ensure you know what your clients thinks about the service and products provided by the business. How is this information gathered and can you think of an example of how feedback has been acted on?

4. How would you know if a product brand is suited to your client?

5. What can you do to raise the profile of a new product range or treatment with your clients?

6. Why is it important to know about the offers and promotions offered by your business?

7. What ways do businesses use to engage with their clients and encourage new clients to visit the business?

Information systems and stock control

1. How does effective and efficient use of resources contribute to the business?

2. Provide examples of where unnecessary wastage of resources within the salon can be avoided?

3. State three key principles of stock control.

4. How can measures be taken to ensure security of stock?

5. Why must accurate stock records be kept?

6. Why must you consider where stock is stored according to the stock item?

7. What information is provided to assist you in the correct storage of stock items?

8. What action should be taken with damaged stock?

2 The Science of Beauty Therapy

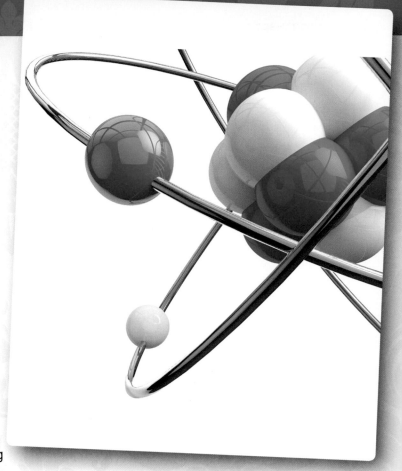

LEARNING OBJECTIVES

This chapter covers the science underpinning the knowledge and understanding for Level 2 treatments. It is divided into three areas for you to learn more about:

◆ Cosmetic science – ingredients and actions of cosmetic products

◆ Anatomy and physiology – the role and organisation of the body

◆ Electrical science – basic knowledge for electrical equipment.

The reason for the study of these areas is to understand how products, electrical equipment and their application affect the skin and underlying structures. Further explanation is provided in each beauty therapy technical chapter.

KEY TERMS

Acid mantle

Adipose tissue

Alternating current (AC)

Anagen

Astringent

Atoms

Blood

Blood vessels

Catagen

Cells

Central nervous system

Circulatory system

Connective tissue sheath

Dermal papilla

Dermis

Direct current (DC)

Elastin

Electric current

Elements

Endocrine system

Erythema

Fibres

Hair

Hair follicle

Hair growth cycle

Hirsutism

Histamine

Homeostasis

Hormones

Hypertrichosis

Inner root sheath

Integumentary system

Insulators

Joint

Keratin

Lanugo hairs

Limbic system

Lipids

Lymph

Lymphatic system

Matter

Melanin

Melanocyte

Motor nerves

Motor point

Muscular system

Nail

Nerve

Neurones

Node (lymphatic)

Oedema

Olfactory system

Outer root sheath

Papillae

Pilosebaceous unit

Repetitive strain injury (RSI)

Sebaceous gland

Sebum

Sensory nerves

Skeletal system

Skin appendages

Superfluous hair

Sweat glands

Telogen

Terminal hairs

Tissues

Vellus hairs

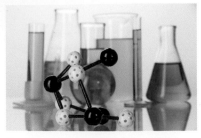

Cosmetic chemistry is the science of selecting ingredients and formulating products for use in beauty treatments.

Cosmetic science

Cosmetic science bases its principles on chemistry, which is the scientific study of *matter* and its chemical changes. Cosmetic chemistry is the science of selecting ingredients and formulating products suitable for use in the beauty industry to achieve a particular objective. As a beauty therapist, it is important to understand the composition and structure of matter, such as the skin and products that are applied to it, and how the skin, **hair** or **nails** change as a result. Also, remember all cosmetic products are made of chemicals.

Matter

Matter is anything that takes up space. It exists in three physical forms: solid, liquid and gas. Matter is made up of chemical **elements**. An element is the basic unit of all matter and is the simplest form of matter that cannot be broken down further.

Atoms are the smallest part of an element that can exist by themselves and possess the element's characteristics. For example, an atom of oxygen has the characteristics of the element oxygen.

ALWAYS REMEMBER

Elements in skin and hair

Carbon (C), oxygen (O), nitrogen (N), sulphur (S) and hydrogen (H) are chemical elements found in the skin and hair.

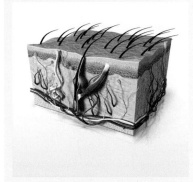

ALWAYS REMEMBER

Periodic table

All known elements are listed in the periodic table with a symbol, usually shorthand letter/s. For example carbon is denoted as C and chlorine is Cl. Elements are divided into gases, liquids and solids. This table arranges the chemical elements in order of their atomic number, usually in rows.

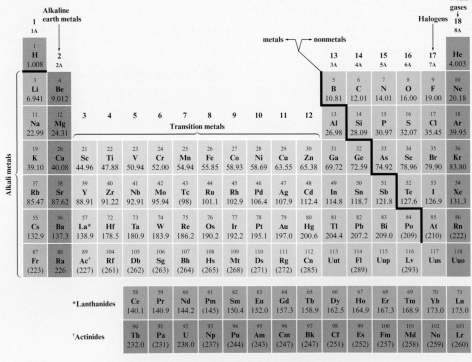

Group numbers 1–18 represent the system recommended by the International Union of Pure and Applied Chemistry.

The entry for hydrogen is shown on the right.

atomic number ——— 1
symbol ——— **H**
atomic mass ——— 1.008

An atom has a nucleus at its centre, which consists of tiny particles called **protons** and **neutrons**. The nucleus is surrounded by other tiny particles called **electrons**. The number and arrangement of these particles may differ.

◆ *Neutrons* have no electrical charge; these are found in the nucleus of the atom.

◆ *Protons* have a small positive electrical charge (+); these are found in the nucleus of the atom.

◆ *Electrons* have a small negative electrical charge (–); these orbit (circle around) the nucleus in energy levels, called electron shells. The electrons are attracted towards the nucleus because it has a positive charge, the opposite to their charge.

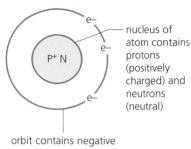
nucleus of atom contains protons (positively charged) and neutrons (neutral)

orbit contains negative electrons constantly moving around the nucleus

Atoms of different elements have different numbers of particles.

The physical state of matter is affected by temperature and pressure. When matter is *solid*, the atoms are tightly packed, and move only slightly. When matter is *liquid*, the atoms have space between them, enabling more movement. When matter is a *gas*, the atoms are widely spaced and can move freely.

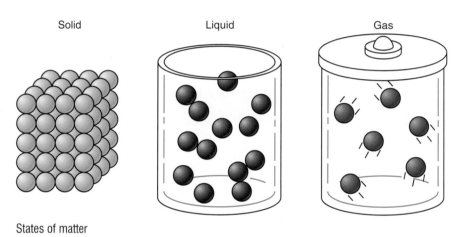

Solid   Liquid   Gas

States of matter

ALWAYS REMEMBER

Solid has a fixed volume and shape, such as a bar of soap.

Liquid has a fixed volume but its shape can change, such as when you dispense a liquid product into a container.

Gas has no fixed volume or shape and takes the shape and volume of its container, such as when using a facial steamer.

ALWAYS REMEMBER

Changing the state of matter

When hot wax (also called hard wax) is heated, its molecules are able to move more freely. The wax becomes fluid as it reaches this stage, called the 'melting point', and the wax can be moulded onto the skin. As it cools, it contracts and returns to a solid state. The excess hairs to be removed become embedded in the wax as it returns to its solid state before removal.

ALWAYS REMEMBER

Stability testing cosmetics product

Cosmetic products are temperature tested to ensure their quality of consistency in different temperature ranges. The cosmetic product is required to meet the intended quality standards and retain its suitability for purpose when stored under appropriate conditions.

When storing cosmetics, always keep them in the environmental conditions recommended by the manufacturer.

When two or more elements combine and react together chemically they form a **compound**. The compound develops its own properties, which are different from the properties of the individual elements. When two elements join to form a compound, the symbols of the elements are combined, such as H_2O, which is the joining of hydrogen and oxygen to form water.

When you join atoms together they form a **molecule**; the smallest particle of an element or compound that retains all the properties of the element or compound.

◆ If the molecule is of an element, the atoms are all the same.

◆ If the molecule is of a compound, the atoms are different, losing their individual identity.

ALWAYS REMEMBER

◆ **Compounds** – formed by a combination of elements; form common chemical substances.

◆ **Organic compounds** – contain the element carbon.

◆ **Inorganic compounds** – do not contain the element carbon.

HEALTH & SAFETY

Volatile liquids

There can be differences in the energy levels of molecules. When they move rapidly at the surface of a liquid they are not attracted by the electrical charge of other molecules and escape, becoming a gas. This is called **evaporation**. Volatile liquids evaporate more easily than others. This is an important part of some treatments where the liquid content of a substance evaporates, creating its therapeutic properties on the skin's surface as it does so. This is an important property of perfume. They are volatile and the perfume molecules reach the nose quickly, where our sense of smell decodes the fragrance.

REVISION AID

What is a compound?

Water is a compound with the formula H_2O. The number 2 means there are two atoms of hydrogen for every one oxygen atom. Together these form a water molecule.

Atoms are held together by a chemical bond. There are three types of bond:

◆ *Covalent bonding*. This type of bond is created when electrons are shared between atoms.

◆ *Hydrogen bonding*. This occurs between a hydrogen atom of one molecule and an other electronegative atom, one that strongly attracts electrons such as nitrogen or oxygen.

◆ *Ionic bonding*. This takes place between atoms of opposite electrical charge.

An atom is charged when it does not have the same number of electrons as protons. The charged atom or molecule is an **ion**.

◆ When an ion has more electrons than protons it is negatively charged and is called an **anion**.

◆ When the ion has more protons than electrons it has a positive charge and is called a **cation**.

Many beauty products are combinations of elements or compounds. These may not combine naturally so are assisted during the chemical formulation of the products.

Cosmetic emulsions

Emulsions are a blend of two liquids that do not normally mix, for example oil and water. This can be oil in water (o/w) or water in oil (w/o). The addition of an emulsifier keeps the emulsion stable. This is called a surfactant. It reduces the surface tension between the two liquids, enabling them to mix. All surfactants have a hydrophilic (water loving) head and a hydrophobic (water hating) tail, which enables the ingredients to mix.

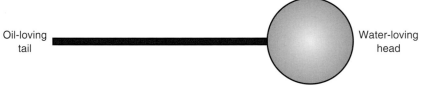

A surfactant molecule

◆ The hydrophilic head binds with the water.

◆ The hydrophobic head binds with the oil.

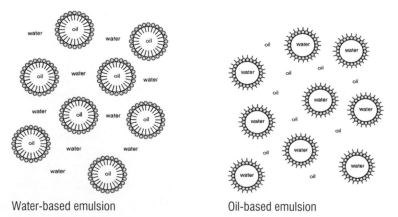

Water-based emulsion   Oil-based emulsion

Oil in water (o/w) emulsions have a greater water content and make the product more lightweight, such as a face lotion or cream. Micro-emulsions are o/w; their formulation of small droplets dispersed evenly through the product and facilitates skin absorption. These are commonly used to deliver essential oils and perfumes into the skin, such as pre-blended body products and moisturisers.

The emulsion's oil content reduces water evaporation from the epidermis, helping to maintain skin hydration. Water in oil emulsions have a greater oil content and are used in cleansing creams and sun creams.

Some finer textured emulsions are termed **multi-phased**. These allow the slow release of a product's active ingredients. Their ingredients successfully combine chemicals that do not readily mix. Their texture provides a smoother application.

Fats and oils used in cleansing agents are known as **lipids**. These need to be dissolved in a solvent or detergent.

Certain ingredients may be used in the formulation of emulsions to assist the transport of other ingredients into the skin. Examples include alpha hydroxy acids (AHA) such as glycolic acid, which alters the skin's oils to assist entry. Liposomes are empty spheres that can be filled with lipid materials, compatible with the lipids of the skin, and are used to transport active ingredients into the skin such as vitamin E. This process is called microencapsulation.

Humectants

Humectants are water-binding agents capable of chemically binding water to themselves and, therefore, retaining water. Natural humectants or lipids are found in the intercellular cement of the epidermis and are known as natural moisturising factors (NMF). They are important in helping the skin retain water to keep it hydrated.

Acids and alkalis

The pH scale   The term 'pH' is an abbreviation for 'potential hydrogen'. It is used to measure the hydrogen-ion concentration of a solution. The pH scale measures whether a substance is acidic, alkaline or neutral. Substances are measured using a scale from 0 to 14.

◆ pH 7 is neutral.

◆ pH 0–6 is acidic.

◆ pH 8–14 is alkaline.

```
     1  2  3  4  5  6  7  8  9  10 11 12 13 14
acidic ◄──────────────── neutral ──────────────► alkaline
```

The skin has a pH of approximately 5.5, which is slightly acidic. Beauty therapy products usually have an acidic pH of around 4 to avoid skin irritation or burns. Neutralisers and buffers are cosmetic chemicals added to alter the pH of chemical ingredients to achieve and maintain the pH required. The alpha hydroxy acid (AHA), glycolic acid, is an example of a chemical buffer.

Treatment of some oily skin conditions may require an acidic pH to support the anti-bacterial properties of the skin. Products that are slightly alkaline may be required when a skin softening effect is necessary to achieve the desired physical result. It is important to use products that have the most suitable pH for the skin type.

Some advanced skincare ingredients may require a neutral pH to keep them stable: examples include peptide proteins. The skin has the ability to return to its natural pH after treatments.

To extend the shelf life of a product it will contain a preservative. This will prevent contamination by the growth of microorganisms, with potential harm to the client. Preservatives are governed by the EU Cosmetics Directive Regulation 1223/2009 and listed accordingly.

Parabens are a type of preservative. They are chemical compounds based on parahydroxybenzoic acid. More than one paraben is often used, working in synergy, to enable smaller quantities to be used overall.

For those clients seeking natural preservatives that are 'paraben-free' there are products increasingly available that contain blends of natural preservatives in their ingredients.

You will see the terms 'organic' and 'natural' used in cosmetic labelling identification.

Organic generally refers to products that have a specific percentage of organic ingredients, which are ethically harvested and not subjected to pesticides, GM, parabens or chemical fertilisers. They are also usually presented in environmentally friendly packaging.

Natural means that it contains ingredients sourced from nature but the production history does not follow the same requirements as that of organic.

HEALTH & SAFETY

Parabens

Medical concerns have been discussed concerning potential side effects of parabens which are popular preservative ingredients used in cosmetics. Alternatives may be required for clients who seek a more natural alternative.

ACTIVITY

Organic and natural products

Select an organic and natural skincare cosmetic. Research how each is able to use the term 'organic' or 'natural' in its production.

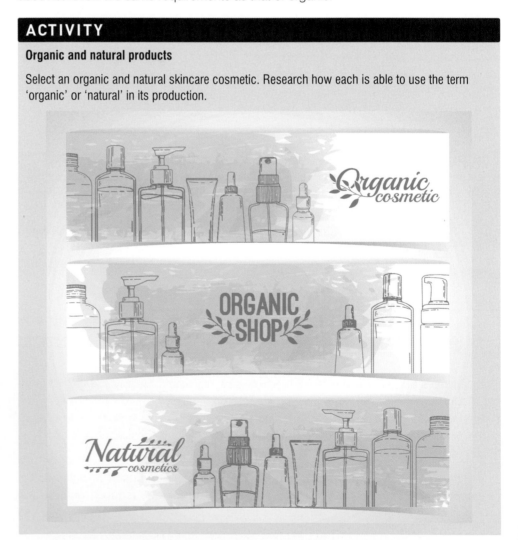

Cosmetic classification

Cosmetics are substances or mixtures. They are classified according to their physical and chemical nature to assist their identification. This includes:

- creams, emulsions, lotions
- gels and oils for the skin
- face masks
- tinted bases (liquids, pastes, powders)
- make-up powders
- perfumes, toilet waters and eau de Cologne
- bath and shower preparations (salts, foams, oils, gels)
- depilatories
- deodorants and antiperspirants

- hair colourants
- make-up and products for removing make-up
- products intended for application to the lips
- products for care of the teeth and the mouth
- products for nail care and make-up
- sunbathing products
- products for tanning without sun
- skin-whitening products
- anti-wrinkle products.

Legislation

The choice of cosmetic products available is vast. In order to safeguard the consumer from potentially harmful ingredients, the packaging should list all the ingredients used in its manufacture. Excessive packaging is increasingly avoided in order to be more environmentally friendly. If this is the case, the container should list this information or it should be provided in an alternative format, for example a label. These ingredients are listed in descending order according to the quantity used, with the highest quantity ingredient listed first. Guidance is provided on presentation from COLIPA (the European cosmetics industry trade association).

A 'best before date' must be provided in any instance where ingredients will deteriorate over time and become a potential safety hazard to the consumer.

Where applicable, storage instructions must be provided so that the product can be kept in optimum conditions for the consumer. Although some products have a long shelf life, they will deteriorate once opened. This information must be shared with the consumer.

HEALTH & SAFETY

Symbols to indicate safety of product use

Once opened, a product will start to perish. In the EU there is a symbol that informs you of the life expectancy for safe use of the product once opened. This is indicated by an open jar with the number of months marked on or under it. It is known as the period after opening or PAO.

All cosmetic products supplied in Europe must comply with the latest EU Regulation 1223/2009 (Cosmetics Regulation) which has been in force since 2013. In the UK, all cosmetic products supplied must comply with the Cosmetics Products (Safety) Regulations of 2008 and the Cosmetic Products Enforcement Regulations 2013.

TOP TIP

Knowledge about your products

It is good practice to be familiar with the ingredients that products contain and their purpose. This knowledge is highly relevant when promoting and answering questions about suitable cosmetic products with your client.

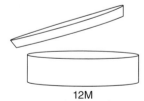

12M

Period after opening (PAO) symbol

ECO TIP

Disposing of cosmetics

If it is necessary to dispose of any products, this should be done responsibly, complying with manufacturer's instructions.

ALWAYS REMEMBER

Cosmetic product definition

In Europe, a cosmetic product is defined in Regulation 1223/2009 as 'any substance or mixture intended to be placed in contact with the external parts of the human body (epidermis, hair system, nails, lips and external genital organs) or with the teeth and the mucous membranes of the oral cavity with a view exclusively or mainly to cleaning them, perfuming them, changing their appearance, protecting them, keeping them in good condition or correcting body odours.' *(EU Regulation 1223/2009, Article 2.1.a)*

Cosmetic safety

HEALTH & SAFETY

Occupational dermatitis

This is classed as an occupational disease and can occur where a person's work involves significant or regular exposure to a known skin sensitiser or irritant.

Safety when handling cosmetics When using certain cosmetic ingredients it is necessary for the beauty therapist to protect their skin. Although the skin has a protective function, contact with some ingredients can lead to skin disorders or occupational diseases.

HEALTH & SAFETY

Care of the skin

Avoid unnecessary prolonged contact with cosmetic ingredients. Always remove a product by washing your hands and drying thoroughly.

When handling certain cosmetics it may be necessary to wear personal protective equipment (PPE).

COSHH guidance on any known irritants should be readily available or obtainable from the supplier on request. Under RIDDOR legislation (regulation 8), employers and the self-employed are required to report cases of diagnosed reportable diseases linked to occupational exposure to specific hazards. This includes occupational dermatitis.

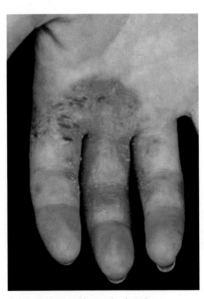

Contact dermatitis on the hands

Suitability for the client It is important to check for allergies when recommending any cosmetic product to your client. Hypo-allergenic products have known allergens excluded from their ingredients, but this is no guarantee that a client will not suffer an allergic reaction. What is important is that you have confirmed suitability prior to application or purchase at consultation. A skin sensitivity patch test is always advisable to check client tolerance to a product and its ingredients in the case of a history of skin sensitivity or known sensitivities. This assessment technique is explained in Chapter 3.

The variety of ingredients used within cosmetics is continuously advancing and it is important to keep up to date with what these are.

Chemical ingredients found in different cosmetic products

Cosmetic ingredient	Effect
acetate	A salt created from acetic acid combined with an alkali.
acids	Substances that have a pH below 7.
alcohol	A common ingredient of cosmetics. For example, alcohol in the form of ethanol is mixed with water for toning lotions. For dry, sensitive skin the alcohol content is reduced or replaced with an alternative such as witch hazel, which is an organic substitute. Alcohol is also used as a preservative.
aldehyde	A compound made of carbon, hydrogen and oxygen, which is used to make other compounds as a solvent.
abrasive	Ingredients that are used to polish a surface and are selected according to the body part to be treated. Those selected for use on skin must be mild to avoid skin irritation, an example being mineral kaolin which is used for its exfoliating action.

(Continued)

Cosmetic ingredient	Effect
alkalis	Substances that have a pH above 7, also referred to as bases; react with acids to form salts.
alpha-hydroxy acids (AHAs)	Naturally occurring mild acids present in fruit and vegetables. They are also chemically manufactured and used in skincare treatments. They can benefit many skin conditions by dissolving the intercellular cement that holds dead epidermal cells together, improving skin appearance and function.
amino	A compound that is present in amino acids; this protein may be derived from plant or animal sources, or synthetically sourced.
antimicrobial	An ingredient used to slow the growth of microorganisms; the type used will depend on whether the product is oil or water based.
antioxidants	Examples include vitamins C and E. These are used to reduce the damage caused by free radicals. Free radicals are unstable atoms that damage healthy cells. They also keep products stable preventing their deterioration.
aqueous	Water-based ingredient.
astringent	An ingredient that cools as it evaporates and tightens the skin. Examples include the alcohol ethanol, and aromatic ingredients such as camphor.
ceramide	A vegetable derived lipid (fat) used for its protective function in anti-ageing products and the treatment of sensitive skin conditions.
chemicals that cause thermal cooling (cryo) reactions	Products that create a constriction effect on the blood vessels of the skin and underlying muscles. These may be mineral based, such as zeolite, with the addition of ingredients that create a thermal cooling effect.
chemicals that cause thermal heating reactions	Products that create a dilative effect on the blood vessels of the skin and underlying muscles.
cocamide MEA	A mild foaming and emulsifying agent, derived and formulated from coconut oil fatty acids.
colourings	Colours added for effect or function. These include dyes, pigments and lakes: ◆ Dyes – soluble in carrier substances, such as water, oil and lipids. They change colour when in contact with the substance they combine with. ◆ Pigments – insoluble powders that provide colour by reflecting some light. ◆ Lakes – inorganic pigments achieved by adding a dye to a salt.
comedogenic	Ingredients such as those from wax and oils can create a build up of dead skin cells causing congestion of hair follicles and leading to the appearance of comedones. Non-comedogenic refers to ingredients that do not cause comedones.
cosmeceutical	Products that are designed to improve skin health and appearance. These are referred to as active ingredients as they chemically cause physiological changes. Alpha Hydroxy Acids are an example.
detergent	An ingredient that emulsifies oil with water and has cleansing properties, such as sodium stearate.
diaphoretics	Substances that create a waterproof action on the skin's surface, which increases the sweating action of the skin as a response. These substances are commonly used in face masks.
dihydroxyacetone	An ingredient found in self-tanning products, which reacts with the amino acids in the skin, creating a tanned appearance.
dimethicone	A silicone oil used as a lubricating and conditioning agent in skin and hair products.
distilled water	A term used when something is heated to remove impurities. Distilled water is water that has been heated, turned to steam and cooled, which separates the impurities from the water.
emollients	Ingredients such as fatty acids and oils that are used to improve skin smoothness and moisture content, preventing water loss, such as jojoba oil.
emulsifying agent	Ingredients that cause oil and water to mix creating an emulsion.
enzyme	Products that activate a process, for example, an enzyme breaks down the protein keratin achieving an exfoliation action.
essential oil	Volatile plant oil, used for its perfume and therapeutic properties.
exfoliators	Ingredients that remove surface dead skin cells, improving the texture and appearance of the skin.
foaming agent	An ingredient that helps create a foam.

(Continued)

Cosmetic ingredient	Effect
glycolic acid	An AHA which helps remove dead skin cells.
humectant	An ingredient that prevents moisture loss from the skin or skincare product by its ability to attract water to itself. This may be a protein compound with the addition of molecules such as glycerine, which is a lipid that can be organically sourced or manufactured.
hyaluronic acid	This occurs naturally in the skin, forming part of the tissue surrounding the collagen and elastin fibres in the dermis. When included in skincare, this ingredient is known as a substantive, which can attach to the surface of the skin to protect and hydrate the surface. As well as assisting skin hydration, it may be injected into the skin as a dermal filler.
hydroquinone	A bleaching ingredient applied at a maximum strength of 2%, used to achieve a skin lightening effect. Activity of melanocytes, the pigment creating cells in the skin, is reduced.
isopropyl alcohol	A highly volatile alcohol.
isopropyl myristate	Oil-like liquid used as a thickening agent and non-greasy emollient in cosmetics.
lanolin	Natural oil derived from sheep's wool and used as an emollient. Its popular use is in hand cream.
magnesium silicate	Chemical compound used as a powder, such as in talcum powder, and as a bulking agent.
mineral oil	Lubricant and emollient derived from petroleum.
minerals	Naturally occurring substances, sourced from the earth, including zinc and titanium oxide, iron oxide and mica. Used in a finely ground form; some pigments are derived from these ingredients: ◆ zinc and titanium – white ◆ iron oxide – brown, green, red and yellow ◆ mica – provides iridescence.
natural oils	Lubricants derived from vegetable plant sources.
nitrocellulose	Derived from plant sources; used in nail polish as a film-forming plastic producing a hard shiny surface.
occlusives	Lipid ingredients that help retain water and protect the skin's surface. Examples include ceramides and linoleic acid.
parabens	Organic acids used as a preservative ingredient.
pearl essence	Used in a variety of cosmetics to achieve a pearlised effect; commonly supplied by the organic compound guanine, derived from fish scales, and bisthmus oxychloride used for its pigment effect, an inorganic compound of bisthmus.
peptides	A protein amino-acid source, derived from plant, animal or synthetic sources. Used in cellular regeneration and anti-ageing products to transfer active ingredients to skin cells.
phthalates	Plasticiser used to prevent brittleness, improving flexibility in products such as nail polishes.
plant extracts	Compounds found in plants; added to cosmetics for their therapeutic benefits.
preservatives	Included to make sure a product remains free from contamination, ensuring their safety and stability. Different preservatives are used according to the product type. A paraben is an example of a preservative.
retinoic acid	An antioxidant and derivative of vitamin A; used in the treatment of acne and to stimulate growth of the epithelial cells and collagen production, reducing the appearance of fine lines. Retinoic acid derivatives are included in skincare in small quantities for hydrating effects.
salycilic acid	Also referred to as beta hydroxy acid, it is a chemical exfoliating product.
silicone	Lubricant oil, chemically combined with silicon and oxygen; used to create a skin-smoothing effect and enhance skin penetration.
sodium chloride	Salt; used as a thickening agent.
sodium lauryl sulphate	Foam and thickness enhancer; used for its cleansing properties.
solvent	A liquid in which a substance dissolves; alcohol is an example of a solvent.
UV screens	Contain organic, carbon-based chemicals, such as 2-ethylhexyl salicylate, which absorbs sunlight and releases the energy as heat, and inorganic chemicals – mineral ingredients such as zinc oxide and titanium dioxide, which create a UV physical block on the skin's surface, reflecting light away from the skin.
vitamins	Commonly vitamins A, C and E are included as antioxidants.

Anatomy and physiology

This section of the science chapter covers the knowledge and understanding of anatomy and physiology requirements for students studying for an accredited foundation course in Beauty Therapy (Level 2). A brief discussion can also be found within each of the chapters where essential anatomy and physiology are identified, using the symbol shown here.

This section explains the basic principles, and structure and function of the following body structural units and systems. You can select the information you need according to the coverage of your course of study.

- the **cells** and **tissues**
- the skin
- subcutaneous layer and **adipose tissue**
- the hair
- the nails
- the eye

- the **skeletal system**
- the nervous system
- the **olfactory system**
- the **endocrine system**
- the **muscular system**
- the heart and **circulatory system**
- the **lymphatic system**.

As a beauty therapist it is important that you have an overview and the necessary understanding of anatomy and physiology for your occupational area, as many of your services aim to affect and improve functioning of different systems of the body. For example, a facial massage will improve blood and lymphatic circulation locally, as you massage the skin's surface. It will also increase cellular renewal by improving nutrition to the living cells and removing dead skin cells. The result is healthier looking skin.

Decisions you make when designing the client's treatment plan will be based on your assessment of the area and recognition of any changes that you feel are not normal and require further exploration as to suitability before treatment delivery.

Anatomy and physiology knowledge and understanding

To help guide you on, the anatomy and physiology, knowledge and understanding requirements for the different technical skills, these are identified in the chart below.

Look for the anatomy and physiology symbol in each technical chapter, which will remind you to check back here for the anatomy and physiology knowledge required.

Anatomy is the structure. Physiology is the function of the body.

Anatomical terminology

Anatomical terminology may be used to describe the location, function and structure of body parts that you will work upon. It is therefore useful to know these terms, as it will assist your understanding of anatomy. You will come across these terms as you read through this and other chapters. The second chart below explains the meaning of each term.

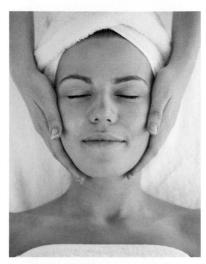

Your treatments affect the physiological functioning of the different body systems in the area being treated

ACTIVITY

Anatomical terminology

Terms used to describe the location, function and structure of body parts that you will work on. Make a sketch of the drawings below and label the following:

- anterior view of the body
- posterior view of the body
- plantar surface of the foot
- dorsal surface of the foot
- muscles which appear superior to the knee
- muscles which appear inferior to the knee.

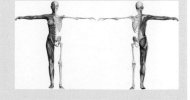

Anatomy and physiology knowledge and understanding requirements for each technical skill.

Topic:	Ear piercing	Self-tanning	Perfumery retail services	Artificial nail enhancements services	Wax depilation	Hand and foot services	Make-up	Eyelash and eyebrow treatments	Facials
Cells and tissues: structure and function	✓	✓	✓	✓	✓	✓	✓	✓	✓
Skin: structure and function	✓	✓	✓	✓	✓	✓	✓	✓	✓
Factors affecting skin condition	✓	✓	✓	✓	✓	✓	✓	✓	✓
Structure and type of hair					✓			✓	
Hair growth and cycle					✓			✓	
Nail structure and function				✓		✓			
Nail growth				✓		✓			
Factors affecting nail health				✓		✓			
Primary muscle groups in parts of the body: types, position, structure and function				✓		✓	✓		✓
Primary bones and joints in parts of the body: types, position, structure and function				✓		✓	✓		✓
Blood circulatory system: structure and function				✓	✓	✓	✓		✓
Lymphatic system: structure and function				✓	✓	✓	✓		✓
Composition and function of blood and lymph				✓	✓	✓	✓		✓
Nervous system: basic principles									✓
Endocrine system: basic principles					✓				✓
Olfactory system and sinuses			✓						✓
External ear	✓								
Basic structure and function of the eye							✓	✓	

Anterior	Front (usually refers to front of the body)	Insertion	Muscle point of attachment (to a bone or body part that moves)
Posterior	Back (usually refers to the back of the body)		
Proximal	Nearest to	Lateral	Side
Medial	Middle	Superficial	Near the surface
Distal	Furthest away	Superior	Above
Origin	Muscle point of attachment (usually part of the muscle that does not move, attached to a bone)	Inferior	Below
		Plantar	Front surface
		Dorsal	Back surface

This chapter discusses the anatomy and physiology of the following:

◆ *Cells*. Microscopic structural units that make-up tissues, organs and the body systems.

◆ *Tissues*. Groups of similar cells that perform a specific function, e.g. a muscle.

◆ *Organs*. A structure made of different tissue types with a specific function, e.g. the skin.

◆ *Systems*. A number of organs and tissues working together to perform a function, e.g. the circulatory system.

Cells

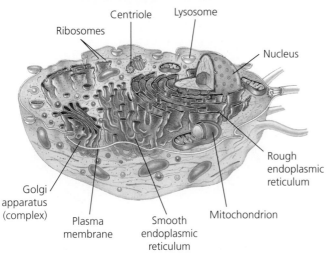

A basic cell

The human body consists of many trillions of microscopic cells. Each cell contains a colourless, clear jelly-like fluid composed of 70% water, called **protoplasm,** which contains various specialised structures, the activities of which are essential to our health. If cells are unable to function properly, a disorder results.

Surrounding the cell is the **cell membrane**, which forms a boundary between the cell contents and their environment. The membrane has a porous surface that allows food to enter and waste materials to leave.

In the centre of the cell is the **nucleus**, which contains thread-like structures called **chromosomes**. These contain the **genes** we have inherited from our parents, making us who we are. The genes are ultimately responsible for cell reproduction and cell functioning.

HEALTH & SAFETY

Cell health

The body's health is subject to the health of its cells; if they are unable to perform their specific functions properly this will result in disease or disorder. You will learn about these later as they will affect if and how you are able to carry out your treatment.

Client health is checked at the initial consultation.

The liquid within the cell membrane and surrounding the nucleus is a gel-like substance called **cytoplasm** containing nutrients necessary for cell growth, reproduction and repair. Scattered throughout this are other small bodies, the **organelles** or 'little organs'; each has a specific function within the cell. Examples of organelles include the following.

◆ Mitochondrion (or mitochondria if plural): the 'power house' of the cell. It produces energy through cellular respiration converting oxygen and glucose to energy, or adenosine triphosphate (ATP) which is the chemical energy needed for cell processes such as muscle contraction.

◆ Ribosomes: produce proteins for growth and repair.

◆ Golgi apparatus: a system of membranes which makes proteins more complex, enclosing them within a capsule that is transported within the cell to be used as energy or removed from the cell.

◆ Lysosomes: secrete enzymes which speed up the rate of a chemical reaction and break down harmful microorganisms (e.g. bacteria) or worn out organelles.

◆ Endoplasmic reticulum: located throughout the cytoplasm, it is a series of canals responsible for the manufacture, storage and transport of substances in the cell. There are two types *rough* and *smooth*, which describe their appearance. Ribosomes are attached to rough endoplasmic reticulum providing its rough appearance.

◆ Centrioles: tiny tubular structures found in pairs which help in the reproduction of new cells.

Chemical reactions take place within the cell. They transform food into energy for cell growth; this is part of what is known as cellular metabolism. Many beauty therapy services aim to stimulate cellular metabolism and cellular regeneration to improve cell function and repair or replace damaged cells.

Cells renew by a process called mitosis, where the cell's nucleus divides, creating two daughter cells, each containing the same genetic information as the parent cell.

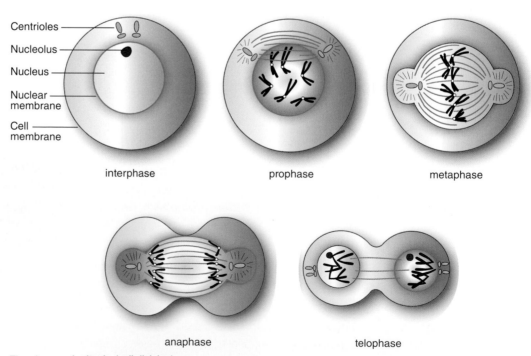

Centrioles
Nucleolus
Nucleus
Nuclear membrane
Cell membrane

interphase   prophase   metaphase

anaphase   telophase

The phases of mitosis (cell division)

Cell division by mitosis is a five phase process: interphase (resting phase), prophase, metaphase, anaphase and telophase.

The chromosomes split into two identical sets within the cell, the cell nucleus also divides. The cytoplasm divides and the cell splits creating two new cells.

Mitosis occurs throughout a person's life. New cells are produced to replace those that have died, with the exception of nerve cells which are not replaced.

Cell division varies dependent upon the cell function. Epithelial cells that form surfaces and linings are renewed and replaced more regularly due to the constant need for repair and physical loss.

REVISION AID

What is a cell?

Tissues

Cells in the body tend to specialise in performing particular functions. Groups of cells that share function, shape, size or structure are called tissues. Tissues, in turn, may be grouped to form the larger functional and structural units we know as organs, such as the heart.

If the tissues are damaged, for example if the skin is accidentally broken, the cells divide to repair the damage – a process called regeneration.

The body is composed of four basic tissue types. These are described in the table.

REVISION AID

How many types of muscle tissue are there?

Types of tissue and general function

Name of tissue	Examples	General functions
Epithelial tissue Epidermis	Epidermis layer of the skin; and mucous membranes.	An uninterrupted layer of cells that forms surfaces and linings of the body's cavities for protection. It can be divided into two types: simple and compound (or stratified) epithelial tissue. Simple is a single layer of cells. Compound or stratified is made of many layers. Epithelial tissues are also classified according to the shape of their cells: squamous (flat), cuboidal (square) and columnar (tall).
Connective tissue cytoplasm collagen fibres nucleus Areolar tissue	**Dermis** layer of skin Areolar tissue-protein fibres, collagen and **elastin**, found in almost every part of the body: Bone Ligaments Cartilage Lymphoid tissue Adipose (fatty) tissue Blood	A structural tissue that supports, separates and connects different parts of the body. The cells forming connective tissue are more widely separated than those forming epithelial tissue and are surrounded by inter-cellular matter which ranges from liquid to solid consistency.

(Continued)

Name of tissue	Examples	General functions
Muscle tissue – There are three different types of muscle tissue: voluntary, involuntary and cardiac (heart). Voluntary also referred to as skeletal is striated or striped in appearance; involuntary also referred to as visceral is smooth and non-striated (striped) in appearance. **Muscle tissue** Skeletal muscle Smooth muscle Cardiac muscle	Voluntary or striated muscle tissue, e.g. skeletal muscles. Involuntary, smooth or non-striated, visceral muscle tissue, e.g. muscles that line blood and lymph vessels, intestinal walls and respiratory walls. Cardiac muscle is found in the heart.	Muscle tissue has the ability to contract and shorten producing movement. Skeletal muscle tissue moves the body and maintains posture. Smooth muscle tissue moves substances through the body in the various vessels or walls in which it is found. Contraction is not under the control of will. Cardiac muscle, although not under the control of will, contains striated muscle tissue.
Nervous tissue	Found in the brain and spinal cord. Neurones (nerve cells) receive and respond to stimuli. Neuroglia, cells that support and protect neurones and are part of nerve impulse transmission.	Nervous tissue carries messages to and from the brain and forms a communication system between different parts of the body, receiving and responding to stimulation, controlling and co-ordinating most body functions and activities.

nerve endings on muscle fibres

direction of nerve impulse in this motor neurone away from CNS to muscle or gland

cell body in CNS

muscle fibre

The skin

As discussed earlier, tissues form larger structural units, referred to as organs. These are made from two or more different types of tissue. Groups of organs that perform common functions are called systems. These are explained later in the chapter. The human skin is an organ – the largest in the body. It is also known as the **integumentary system**, made up of the skin and its accessory parts, the oil and sweat glands, sensory receptor nerves and the hair and nails. The skin provides a tough, flexible covering, providing an effective barrier between the body and the environment. It achieves this through many different important functions:

Functions of the skin

◆ sensation

◆ heat regulation

◆ absorption

◆ protection

◆ excretion

◆ secretion.

In addition, Vitamin D is produced in the skin on exposure to ultra-violet light (UVL) which is required for the body's growth and development.

The pigment melanin is also produced in the skin, providing some protection from UVL.

The skin varies in appearance according to the body area, our ethnicity, gender and age. It also alters from season to season and from year to year, and reflects our general health, lifestyle and diet.

ALWAYS REMEMBER

Did you know?

Although the skin has a waterproof property, it allows approximately 500 ml of water to be lost from the tissues through evaporation every day.

You need to keep your skin hydrated by drinking sufficient water and the application of hydrating skincare serums, lotions, balms and creams. Insufficient hydration and lack of protection can lead to a skin condition called dehydrated skin.

Sensation

The skin is a sensory organ, and the sensations of **touch**, **pressure**, **pain**, **heat** and **cold** are identified by **sensory nerves** called cutaneous receptors in the skin. This information is then sent to the brain for decoding and initiating the appropriate bodily response. It also allows us to recognise objects by their feel and shape and helps prevent injury by alerting us to dangers, including sharp objects and hot surfaces. You should explain the expected sensations at the client consultation, ensuring that they are able to inform you of any unwanted reactions, termed contra-actions. It is important in beauty therapy services that you also check client comfort during treatment to avoid a contra-action.

Heat regulation

Humans have a normal body temperature maintained at 36.8–37°C. Body temperature is controlled in part by heat loss through the skin and by sweating, called thermoregulation. If the temperature of the body is increased by 0.25–0.5°C, the **sweat glands** excrete sweat to the skin's surface. The body is cooled by the loss of heat used to evaporate the sweat from the surface of the skin.

If the body becomes too warm, there is an increase in blood flow into the blood capillaries in the skin. The blood capillaries widen (dilate) and heat is lost through radiation from the skin surface, this is referred to as vasodilation. If the external temperature becomes low and the body needs to conserve heat there is a reduction in blood flow into the blood capillaries in the skin. The blood capillaries become narrower (constrict) so less blood is

ALWAYS REMEMBER

Did you know?

The skin accounts for one-eighth of the body's total weight. It measures approximately 1.5 m² in total, depending on body size. It is thinnest on the eyelids (0.05 mm), and thickest on the soles of the feet (approximately 5 mm).

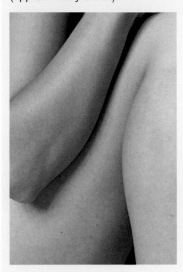

TOP TIP

Functions of the skin

Remembering the word SHAPES will help you remember the functions of the skin:

S   Sensation

H   Heat regulation

A   Absorption

P   Protection

E   Excretion

S   Secretion.

brought to the skin's surface, this is referred to as vasoconstriction. Hair also limits heat loss from the scalp. In addition, when the temperature drops from 36.8°C, the arrector pili muscles in the skin (attached to the hair follicle) contract thereby pulling the skin and create the appearance of 'goose bumps'.

Absorption

Although the skin is structured to protect itself from penetration by harmful substances, absorption may take place through the sweat glands, **hair follicles** and epidermal cells for a beneficial effect. Water and fat-soluble substances such as organic oils are examples of products that can be absorbed by the skin. Certain ingredients are included in the formulation of cosmetics to assist in the transportation of active ingredients into the skin.

Nutrition The skin stores **fat**, which provides an energy reserve.

It is also responsible for producing a significant proportion of our **vitamin D**, which is essential for healthy bones. Vitamin D is created as a positive side-effect of exposure to UV by a chemical reaction when sunlight is in contact with the skin. Although available from exposure to sunlight, most people obtain vitamin D from their diet.

Protection

The skin protects the body from potentially harmful substances and conditions.

- The outer surface is **bactericidal** and **fungicidal**, helping to prevent the growth of harmful microorganisms. This is the combination of dead skin cells, sweat and **sebum** creating an acid surface known as the *acid mantle*. This has a pH of 5.5 to 5.6 dependent upon skin type, condition and body area. It also prevents the absorption of many substances (unless the surface is broken) due to of the structure of the cells on its outer surface, which form a chemical and physical barrier.

- The skin cushions the underlying structures from physical injury. This is assisted by the layer of fat situated below the skin.

- The skin provides a **waterproof coating**. Its natural oil, **sebum**, prevents the skin from losing essential water, and therefore helps to prevent skin dehydration, a condition in which the skin has less moisture in the outer epidermis. This is achieved by the keratinocyte cells which produce keratin, a fibrous protein, to provide protection. They are held together by intercelluar lipids (fats) known as ceramides, which have an important water retention and barrier function.

- The skin contains a pigment called **melanin** produced by melanocyte cells. This absorbs harmful rays of UV light and gives the skin a tanned look.

- The skin uses a warning system to defend against outside invasion. Redness and inflammation of the skin indicate that the skin is intolerant or allergic to something. This may be either an external or internal factor.

Skincare products, including the use of sun protection creams (with a sun protection factor or SPF), are necessary to ensure the skin is adequately protected.

Excretion

Small amounts of certain waste products, such as urea, water and salt, are removed from the body in sweat by a process called excretion. This occurs from sweat glands through pores in the surface of the skin. A client's treatment plan will aim to ensure the skin is kept clean through the appropriate skincare routine. Exfoliation products and face packs are popular specialist treatments applied for their skin cleansing and tightening action.

Secretion

The skin secretes a natural oil called sebum, which is a mixture of fats and waxes. It covers the skin's entire surface except for the palms of the hands and soles of the feet, and helps to protect the skin. As well as its important function in creating the acid mantle, it helps to keep the skin lubricated, supple and intact. Sebum is the skin's natural moisturiser.

The structure of the skin

If we were able to look at a section through the skin using a microscope, we would see two distinct layers: the **epidermis** and the **dermis**. Between these layers is a specialised layer that acts like a 'glue', sticking the two layers together. This is the **basement membrane**. If the epidermis and dermis become separated, body fluids fill the space, creating a **blister**, a small pocket of fluid in the top layer of the skin.

epidermis
basement membrane
dermis
subcutaneous layer

Skin structure

The epidermis

The epidermis is the outer layer of the skin and located directly above the dermis, which is much thicker than the epidermis. It is composed of five layers, with the surface layer forming the outer skin – what we can see and touch. The main function of the epidermis is to protect the deeper living structures from harm from the external environment.

Each layer of the epidermis can be recognised by its shape and by the function of its cells. The main type of cell found in the epidermis is the **keratinocyte**, which produces the protein **keratin**. It is keratin that makes the skin tough, which reduces the passage of substances into or out of the body. It also contains other cells including the melanocytes that produce the skin pigment melanin, and Langerhans cells that assist in the removal of harmful foreign bodies such as bacteria, as part of the immune system, which aims to destroy infection to maintain good health.

The epidermis contains no blood vessels. Nourishment of the epidermis, essential for growth, is received from a liquid called the **interstitial fluid** formed from blood plasma. This acts as a link between the blood and cells.

ALWAYS REMEMBER

Cell renewal: Did you know?

Every five days we shed a complete surface layer of skin. It takes approximately four weeks for the skin to produce a whole new epidermis. About 80 per cent of household dust is composed of dead skin cells. As we age, the cell renewal process slows and many treatment objectives are the stimulation of cell renewal.

Over a period of about four weeks, cells move from the bottom layer of the epidermis to the top layer, the skin's surface, changing in shape and structure as they progress. The process of cellular change takes place in stages:

◆ *The cell is formed at the bottom layer* by division of an earlier cell, a process called **mitosis**.

ALWAYS REMEMBER

Keratin

As well as the skin, hair and nails are also made from keratin.

TOP TIP

Facial schedule and skin cellular renewal

As it takes approximately four weeks for skin cellular renewal and turnover, use this guide to schedule your client's next facial or skin hand or foot treatment. Explain this reason to your client.

REVISION AID

What are cells that are grouped together and perform the same function called?

- ◆ *The cell matures*. It changes structure and moves upwards and outwards, the cell cytoplasm being replaced with keratin, becoming harder and flatter in structure.

- ◆ *The cell dies*. It moves towards the top layer and becomes an empty shell, which is eventually shed from this layer.

ALWAYS REMEMBER

The epidermis

The epidermis is the most significant layer of the skin with regard to the external application of skincare cosmetics and treatments due to their immediate effect on its surface structure and appearance.

REVISION AID

What is mitosis responsible for?

ALWAYS REMEMBER

Psoriasis

Psoriasis is a skin disorder where, cell division occurs much more quickly than normal, termed hyper-keritinisation, resulting in clusters of dead skin cells appearing on the skin's surface.

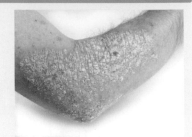

Surface plaques of dead skin, a feature of the skin condition psoriasis.

HEALTH & SAFETY

Allergic reactions

Most people will be unaware that a foreign body has invaded the skin. Sometimes, however, the intolerance of the skin's surface to a substance is apparent. It shows as an allergic reaction, in which the skin becomes red, itchy and swollen. The skin can suddenly develop intolerance to certain substances.

Product ingredients are being sourced all the time that aim to reduce the possibility of skin sensitivity. It is important to keep up to date. However, just because a product is naturally sourced and described as chemical-free, does not mean the client will be tolerant to it.

Skin sensitivity patch testing is essential where recommended by a manufacturer to avoid an allergic reaction and as a legal requirement.

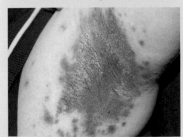

Allergic reaction to antiperspirant

The layers and zones of the epidermis

Five layers or **strata** (the Latin word for layer) make up the epidermis. The thickness of these layers varies over the body's surface.

Each layer is found either in the cell fomation germinative zone or keratinisation zone. before desquamation, where the keratinocyte cells are shed from the skin's surface. This is illustrated and described below.

Desquamation process, shedding of skin cells from the surface

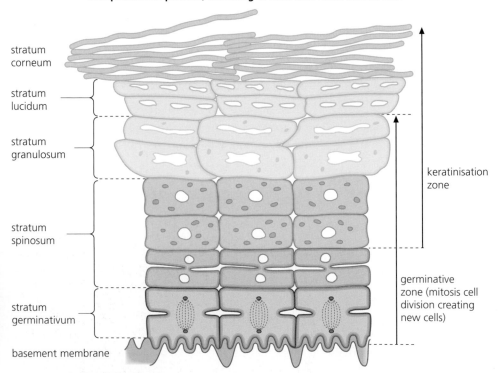

stratum corneum

stratum lucidum

stratum granulosum

stratum spinosum

stratum germinativum

basement membrane

keratinisation zone

germinative zone (mitosis cell division creating new cells)

The layers of the epidermis

The germinative zone
In the layers of the germinative zone the cells are living cells. The germinative zone layers of the epidermis are the **stratum germinativum**, **stratum spinosum** and **stratum granulosum**.

Stratum germinativum The stratum germinativum, or basal layer, is the lowermost layer of the epidermis. It is formed from a single layer of column-shaped cells joined to the basement membrane. These cells divide continuously by mitosis and produce new epidermal cells (keratinocytes).

Stratum spinosum The stratum spinosum, or prickle-cell layer, is formed from two to six rows of elongated cells (they appear long in relation to their width). These have a surface of spiky spines that connect to surrounding cells. Each cell has a large nucleus and is filled with fluid.

Stratum granulosum The stratum granulosum, or granular layer, is composed of one, two or three layers of cells that have become much flatter. The nucleus of the cell has begun to break up, creating what appear to be granules within the cell cytoplasm. These are known as **keratohyaline granules** and later form keratin. At this stage the cells form a new, combined layer.

Two other important cells found in the germinative zone of the epidermis are Langerhans cells and **melanocyte** cells.

◆ *Langerhans cells*. Specialised defence cells found in the epidermis; they absorb and remove foreign bodies that enter the skin and cause an immune response. The cells then move from the epidermis to the dermis below, and finally enter the **lymph** system (the body's waste-transport system) where the foreign bodies are made safe by neutralising them.

◆ *Melanocytes*. Produce the skin pigment melanin, which contributes to our skin colour. About one in every ten germinative cells is a melanocyte. Another pigment, **carotene**, which is yellowish, also occurs in epidermal cells. Its contribution to skin colour lessens in importance as the amount of melanin in the skin increases. There are various forms of the pigment melanin.

Eumelanin is dark brown to black and is found in black and brown skin.

Pheomelanin is red or yellow and is more dominant in lighter skin.

Both types of melanin are often present in the skin. Melanocytes are stimulated to produce melanin by UV rays, and their main function is to protect the other epidermal cells in this way from the harmful effects of UV.

The size and distribution of melanocytes differs according to race. In a white person the melanin tends to be destroyed when it reaches the stratum granulosum layer. With stimulation from artificial or natural UV light, however, melanin will also be present in the upper epidermis.

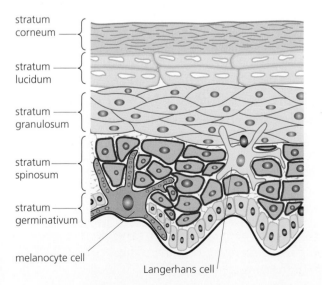

stratum corneum

stratum lucidum

stratum granulosum

stratum spinosum

stratum germinativum

melanocyte cell

Langerhans cell

Location of melanocyte and Langerhans cells

REVISION AID

Which epidermal layer is continuously being shed and replaced?

HEALTH & SAFETY

Sunbathing

If sunbathing, always protect the skin with an appropriate protective sunscreen product according to skin type and natural hair/skin colouring. Ideally refer to the Fitzpatrick classification system discussed in Chapter 3. After UV exposure always use an emollient aftersun preparation to minimise the effects of premature ageing, by rehydrating and soothing the skin.

ALWAYS REMEMBER

Artificial skin tanning

Self-tanning products contain an ingredient called dihydroxyacetone (DHA). This gives the skin an artificial tanned appearance. DHA reacts with the skin's amino acids, chemical protein chains, found in the stratum corneum. The colour is lost gradually through desquamation as the skin's surface cells are shed.

ALWAYS REMEMBER

Desquamation process

When the epidermal cells die they are eventually shed from the skin's surface. This is termed **desquamation** by beauty therapists. Treatments such as exfoliation and the use of alpha hydroxy acids, for example, speed up this process. These treatments can be mechanical, e.g. brush cleansing, or cosmetic, using a humectant containing an abrasive agent, or chemical such as alpha hydroxy acids and retinoids.

HEALTH & SAFETY

Skin cancer

Cancer of a melanocyte is known as melanoma and can spread rapidly to other areas of the body. This is known as metastasis. Careful checks should be made of the skin for signs of change and any unusual looking moles must always be referred for medical attention. See Chapter 3 for more details.

ALWAYS REMEMBER

Cosmetic sunscreens

Many hair, skincare products and cosmetics, including lipsticks and mascaras, now contain sunscreens. This is because research has shown that UV exposure is the principal cause of skin ageing, called photo-ageing, resulting in loose skin and wrinkling. It can also cause the skin and hair to become dry and dehydrated.

Following a service such as exfoliation, the skin's defence mechanisms are reduced. Cosmetic sunscreens should be applied to the area treated before exposure.

In contrast, black skin has larger sized melanocytes throughout **all** the epidermal layers; a level of protection that has evolved to deal with bright ultraviolet UV light. This increased protection allows less UV to penetrate the dermis below, reducing the possibility of premature ageing from exposure to UV light. The more even quality and distribution of melanin also means that people with darker skins are at less risk of developing some types of skin cancers.

Pigmentation can be affected by different factors: medication, genetics and hormonal changes as well as UV exposure. When the skin becomes more pigmented than the surrounding skin, this is termed **hyper-pigmentation**. When the skin becomes lighter than the surrounding types of skin, this is termed **hypo-pigmentation**. When carrying out a make-up application you will identify any areas of uneven pigmentation and select products that will help to provide an even skin tone.

TOP TIP

The Fitzpatrick classification system measures the amount of melanin in the skin. This should equate to the amount of protection required and tolerance it has when exposed to UV light. This assessment should be completed before an artificial UV tanning treatment.

At consultation ask your client a series of questions, allocating a point score. When added up, this provides the Fitzpatrick skin type.

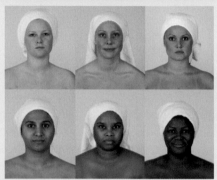

Fitzpatrick skin typing is used to predict the skin's response to UV light and calculates the correct exposure time.

HEALTH & SAFETY

Potential dangers and risks of over-exposure to UV radiation

◆ **Vitiligo:** lack of skin pigment is called vitiligo or leucoderma. It can occur with any skin colour, but is more obvious on a dark skin. Avoid exposing such skin to UV light as it does not have any melanin protection.

◆ **Sunburn:** (termed erythema): if the skin becomes red on exposure to sunlight, this indicates that the skin has been over-exposed to UV. It will often blister and shed itself.

◆ **Keratitis:** inflammation of the cornea (the transparent front of the eye).

◆ **Conjunctivitis:** inflammation of the conjunctiva (the thin skin covering the cornea and eyelids).

◆ **Cataracts:** changes to the lens of the eye, making it opaque.

◆ **Skin cancer:** this is more common in fair-skinned people and those who have suffered episodes of sunburn during childhood. It can take many years to develop.

◆ **Skin ageing:** changes to connective tissues in the dermis make skin less elastic, showing more wrinkles and folds. The epidermis becomes thicker and more leathery. Solar lentigenes occur, also known as liver spots, seen as patches of hyper-pigmentation.

◆ **Allergic reactions:** exposure to sunlight may induce allergic reactions including milaria rubra also known as prickly heat – a prickly, burning sensation accompanied by itchy, red blisters.

ALWAYS REMEMBER

Ultraviolet (UV) rays

UVA are ageing rays penetrating the reticular layer of the dermis.

UVB are burning rays penetrating to the lower layers of the epidermis.

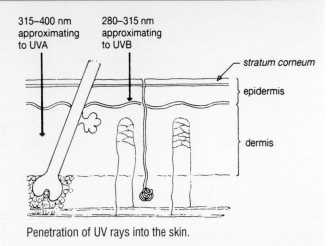

315–400 nm approximating to UVA

280–315 nm approximating to UVB

stratum corneum

epidermis

dermis

Penetration of UV rays into the skin.

TOP TIP

Calluses

Constant friction causes the skin to thicken as a form of protection, developing calluses. You may notice this when performing hand and nail services. A client with a manual occupation may therefore develop hard, rough skin (calluses) on their hands. Calluses are also common on the feet where the skin thickens and becomes dry, such as on the heels.

The skin condition can be treated with an emollient preparation, which will moisturise and soften the dry skin. This may be in the form of a treatment cream or specialised mask.

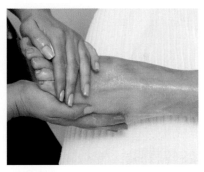

Application of an emollient to the feet

Skin colour also increases when the skin becomes warm. This is because the blood capillaries at the surface dilate, bringing blood nearer to the surface so that heat can be lost. This is called **vasodilation**. If the temperature is cold the blood capillaries become narrower so less blood is brought to the skin's surface to conserve heat, a process called **vasoconstriction**. The skin will then lose colour and appear pale.

The keratinisation zone   The keratinisation zone, or cornified zone, is where the cells begin to die and where finally they will be shed from the skin. The cells at this stage become progressively flatter, and the cell cytoplasm is replaced with the hard protein **keratin**.

Stratum lucidum   The stratum lucidum, clear transparent layer or lucid layer, is only visible in non-hairy areas of the skin such as the palms of the hands and the soles of the feet where the skin is thicker. The cells here lack a nucleus and are filled with a clear substance called **eledin** produced as a further stage of keratinisation.

Stratum corneum   The stratum corneum, cornified or horny layer, is formed from several layers of flattened, scale-like overlapping cells, composed mainly of keratin. The cells combine with fats called lipids, produced by the skin, to create a waterproof barrier.

The cells help to reflect UV light from the skin's surface. Black skin, which evolved to withstand strong UV, has a thicker stratum corneum than white skin.

REVISION AID

How would you describe the difference between the keratinisation zone and the germinative zone of the skin?

The stratum corneum is up to 20 per cent thicker in men than women. Males produce more of the skin's natural oil, sebum, making it appear oilier. They also have less sweat glands.

It takes about three weeks for the epidermal cells to reach the stratum corneum from the stratum germinativum. The cells are then shed by a process called desquamation.

The dermis

The dermis is the inner portion of the skin, situated underneath the epidermis. It is composed of dense connective tissue containing other structures, such as the lymphatic vessels, blood vessels and nerves. It is much thicker than the epidermis (approximately 25 times thicker) and has two distinct layers: the papillary layer and the reticular layer. The dermis cells include fibroblasts, lymphocytes and mast cells.

The dermis is responsible for the elasticity of the skin. It also contains the **skin appendages** – nerves, **blood vessels**, glands and hair follicles and arrector pili muscles.

The papillary layer is nearest to the surface of the dermis and has tiny projections called **papillae**. These contain tactile (touch-sensitive) nerve endings as well as blood and lymph capillaries. The papillae help attach the epidermis to the dermis.

ALWAYS REMEMBER

Papillae ridges

The formation of the papillae ridges in the dermis are unique to each individual, and this provides our fingerprint.

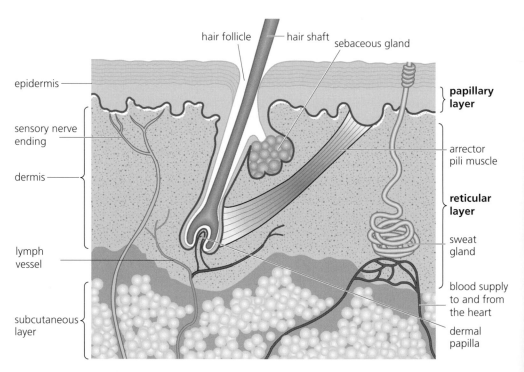

Cross-section of the skin

This part of the dermis also supplies the epidermis above with its nutrition, and removes waste through the associated lymphatic circulation.

The reticular layer Underneath the papillary layer is the reticular layer which contains sweat glands, blood vessels, hair follicles, lymph vessels, the arrector pili muscles and **sebaceous glands**. It also contains a dense network of protein **fibres**. These fibres allow the skin to expand and contract, and to perform intricate, supple movements.

This network is composed of two sorts of protein fibre: yellow **elastin** fibres and white **collagen** fibres. Elastin fibres give the skin its elasticity, and collagen fibres give it strength. The fibres are produced by specialised cells called **fibroblasts**, and are supported and held in a gel called the ground substance. This is a component of connective tissue that has the ability to attract water keeping the fibres hydrated. While this network is strong, the skin appears youthful and firm. As the fibres harden and fragment, however, the network begins to collapse, losing its elasticity. The skin then begins to show signs of ageing.

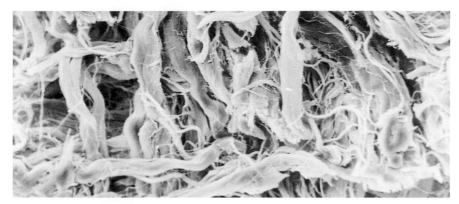

Collagen and elastin fibres in the dermis

Male skin contains more collagen, the skin protein providing strength. Collagen production in females slows at the menopause, which can result in sudden skin ageing. As such, skin ageing appears more rapid in females than males.

A major cause of damage to this network is unprotected exposure of the skin to the environment, especially UV light. Sometimes, too, the skin loses its elasticity because of a sudden increase in body weight, for example at puberty or pregnancy. This results in the appearance of **stretch marks (striations)**, streaks of thin skin that are a different colour from the surrounding skin. On white skin they appear as thin reddish streaks; on black skin they appear slightly lighter than the surrounding skin. The lost elasticity cannot be restored.

Nerve endings The dermis contains different types of sensory **nerve endings**, which register the sensations of touch, pressure, pain and temperature. These send messages to the **central nervous system** and the **brain**, informing us about the outside world and what is happening on the skin's surface. The appearance of each of these nerve endings is quite varied. The sensory nerve endings in the skin cause us to have an involuntary reflex reaction to unpleasant stimuli, thereby protecting the skin from injury.

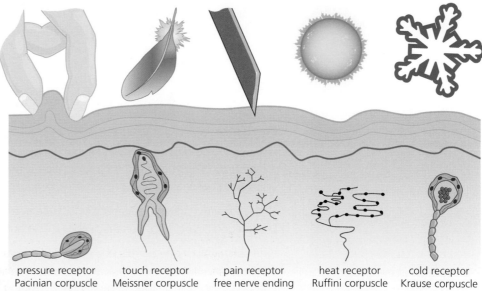

| pressure receptor Pacinian corpuscle | touch receptor Meissner corpuscle | pain receptor free nerve ending | heat receptor Ruffini corpuscle | cold receptor Krause corpuscle |

Sensory nerve endings in the skin

REVISION AID

What are the two main divisions of the dermis?

Growth and repair The body's blood system of arteries and veins brings blood to capillary networks in the skin and takes it away again. The blood carries the nutrients and oxygen essential for the skin's health, maintenance and growth, and takes away waste products.

Repair or healing occurs if the skin becomes damaged. A chemical messenger in the skin, a hormone, called the epidermal growth factor (EGF) initiates this repair. This causes keratinocytes produced in the epidermis to multiply and trigger specific actions of other cells involved. Blood transports repair cells that cover the site of the injury. Behind this, blood cells form a clot, which dries and prevents infection from germs entering the skin. New blood capillaries are formed to support the increased cellular metabolism requirements. Collagen fibres are secreted by fibroblast cells in the dermis. These bind the surface of the wound together. Epithelial cells of the dermis cover the wound underneath the clot. At the same time lymphocytes (a type of white blood cell that plays a key role in the immune system) fight any infection that may be present and indicate to the keratinocyte to slow cell multiplication when the wound is nearly healed. The clot or scab is lost and the cells of the dermis grow upwards until the skin's thickness is restored. When the skin's surface has been broken, a scar may be left at the site of the injury. This initially appears red or purple in colour due to increased blood supply to the area which is initiated during wound healing. When healed the colour fades. If the healing process continues for longer than necessary, excessive scar tissue may be formed.

ALWAYS REMEMBER

Wounds

Wounds are classified according to their depth. The upper papillary layer of the dermis can heal without scarring. If the reticular layer is affected, this may result in raised scarring called hypertrophic scarring; it occurs where there is an increase in collagen production to assist skin healing at the site of the wound. Sometimes you will see pits in the skin, such as in somebody who has suffered from the skin disorder *acne vulgaris,* shown below, where tissue is destroyed during the healing process. This is called an atrophic scar.

It is important that clients are advised not to squeeze or pick blemished areas as this can lead to tissue damage and scarring.

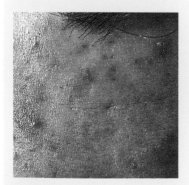

Skin's surface (showing acne vulgaris scarring)

HEALTH & SAFETY

Scars

When the surface has been broken, the skin at the site of the injury is replaced but may leave a scar. This initially appears red, due to the increased blood supply to the area, which is required while the skin heals. When healed, the redness will fade. If the skin's healing process continues for longer than necessary, excess scar tissue will be formed, resulting in a raised scar called a 'keloid scar'. Around 10–15% of all scars may become keloid, but appear more common in people of African and South Indian descent.

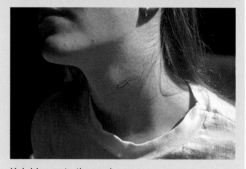

Keloid scar to the neck

Defence As previously discussed the skin's acid mantle is the first defensive action against microorganisms. Within the epidermis and dermis are the structures responsible for protecting the skin from harmful foreign bodies, called pathogens or antigens, and irritants: things that trigger an allergic response.

The epidermis contains Langerhans cells, located amongst the keratinocytes. They collect foreign bodies and transport them to be made non harmful or destroyed by lymphocytes.

One set of cells in the dermis, the **mast cells**, burst when stimulated during inflammation or allergic reactions, and release a chemical substance called **histamine**. This causes the blood vessels nearby to enlarge, thereby bringing more blood to the site of the irritation to limit skin damage and begin repair.

In the blood, and also in the lymph and the connective tissue, is another group of cells: the **macrophages** or 'big eaters'. These play an important role in infection control where they destroy microorganisms and engulf dead cells and other unwanted particles. They play a role in the immune system that protects the body from disease-causing microorganisms.

Collecting waste Lymph vessels are part of the lymphatic system that helps clean the circulatory system. Located in the skin, they carry a fluid called lymph, a straw-coloured fluid similar in composition to blood plasma. Plasma is the liquid part of the blood. It is mainly water, with other dissolved substances and blood cells. It disperses from the blood capillaries into the tissue spaces and helps keep the body stable. Lymph is composed of water, lymphocytes, oxygen, nutrients, **hormones**, salts, urea and waste products such as used blood cells. The waste products are eliminated, and usable protein is recycled for further use by the body. It acts as a link between the blood and the cells.

Improving lymphatic circulation is a popular facial massage technique to assist a sluggish lymphatic circulation, reduce puffiness in the tissues and help in the elimination of waste and toxins.

Control of skin functioning Hormones are chemical messengers transported in the blood. They are secreted from endocrine glands, part of the endocrine system, which is discussed later. They control the activity of many organs in the body, including the cells and glands in the skin. These include **melanosomes**, which produce skin pigment, and the **sweat glands** and **sebaceous glands**.

Hormone imbalance at different times of our life may disturb the normal functioning of these cells and structures, causing various **skin disorders**, for example acne vulgaris during puberty.

Skin appendages Within the dermis are structures called **skin appendages** or skin accessory organs. These include:

◆ sweat glands

◆ sebaceous glands

◆ hair follicles, which produce hair

◆ nails.

Sweat glands **Sweat glands** or **sudoriferous glands,** are composed of **epithelial tissue** – a specialised tissue that lines the gland, extending from the epidermis into the dermis. These glands are found all over the body, but are particularly plentiful on the palms of the hands and the soles of the feet. Their function is to regulate body temperature (thermoregulation) through the evaporation of sweat from the surface of the skin. Fluid loss and control of body temperature are important to prevent the body overheating, especially in hot, humid climates. For this reason, perhaps, sweat glands are larger and more abundant in black skin than white skin as a result of evolution.

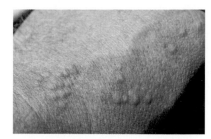

Using something on the skin that the skin is intolerant to can result in an allergic reaction

TOP TIP

Massage benefits

External massage movements and pressure can be applied to the skin to increase the blood supply within the dermis, bringing extra nutrients and oxygen to the skin and to the underlying muscle. At the same time, the lymphatic circulation is increased, improving the removal of waste products that may have accumulated. This is referred to as lymphatic drainage massage.

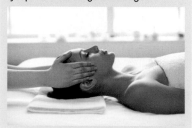

ACTIVITY

The emotions

Emotions, psychological thoughts and feelings, can affect blood supply to the skin: blood vessels in the dermis may enlarge or constrict. Think of different emotions and how these might affect the appearance of the skin.

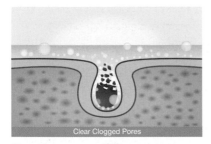

Cleansing action on the pores

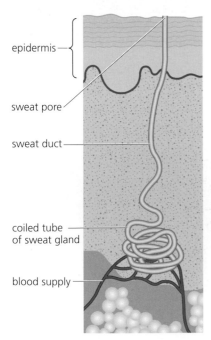

An eccrine sweat gland

(labels: epidermis, sweat pore, sweat duct, coiled tube of sweat gland, blood supply)

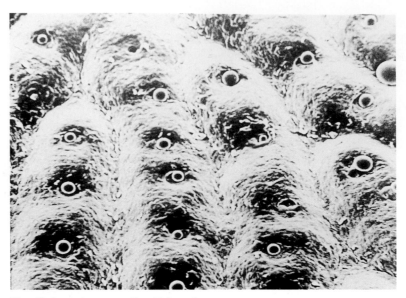

Magnified sweat pores on the skin's surface

There are two types of sweat glands: **eccrine glands** and **apocrine glands**.

Eccrine glands are simple, sweat-producing glands, found over most of the body, appearing as tiny tubes (**ducts**). The eccrine glands are responsive to heat. These are straight in the epidermis and coiled in the dermis. The duct opens directly onto the surface of the skin through an opening called a **pore**.

Eccrine glands continuously secrete small amounts of sweat, even when we appear not to be perspiring. In this way they maintain the body temperature at a constant 36.8°C.

Apocrine glands are found in the armpit, the nipples and the groin area. This kind of gland is larger than the eccrine gland, and is attached to a hair follicle. Apocrine glands are controlled by hormones, becoming active at puberty. They also increase in activity when we are excited, nervous or stressed. The fluid they secrete is thicker than that from the eccrine glands, and may contain urea, fats, sugars and small amounts of protein. Also present are traces of aromatic molecules called **pheromones**, which are thought to cause sexual attraction.

An unpleasant smell – **body odour** – develops when apocrine sweat is broken down by skin bacteria. Good habits of personal hygiene will prevent this.

Cosmetic perspiration control To extend hygiene protection during the day, apply either a deodorant or an antiperspirant. **Antiperspirants** reduce the amount of sweat that reaches the skin's surface: they have an astringent action which closes the pores. **Deodorants** contain an active antiseptic ingredient that reduces the skin's bacterial activity, thereby reducing the risk of odour from stale sweat.

ALWAYS REMEMBER

Skin problems at puberty

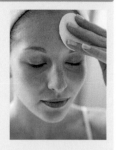

Skin problems are common at puberty when changes in hormone levels cause sebaceous glands to produce excess sebum and the skin's surface becomes oily. Growth of skin bacteria can increase in the sebum, causing inflammation of the surrounding tissues. This can lead to the skin disorder acne vulgaris. The skin should always be kept clean and handled with clean hands.

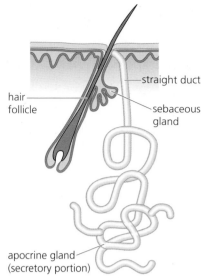

An apocrine gland associated with the hair follicle

Sebaceous glands The sebaceous gland appears as a minute, sac-like organ. Usually it is associated with the hair follicle with which it forms the **pilosebaceous unit**, but the two can appear independently.

Sebaceous glands are found all over the body, except on the palms of the hands and the soles of the feet. They are particularly numerous on the scalp, the forehead, and in the back and chest region. The cells of the glands decompose, producing the skin's natural oil, sebum. This empties directly into the hair follicle. Excess sebum will oxidise, turning black, when in contact with the air. This creates a 'blackhead' appearance, correctly termed comedone. Excess sebum therefore requires removal with an effective cleansing skincare routine.

The activity of the sebaceous gland increases at puberty, when stimulated by the male hormone **androgen**. In adults, activity of the sebaceous gland gradually decreases again. Men secrete slightly more sebum than women; and on black skin the sebaceous glands are larger and more numerous than on white skin.

Sebum is composed of fatty acids and waxes. These have **bactericidal** and **fungicidal** properties, and so discourage the multiplication of microorganisms on the surface of the skin. Sebum also reduces the evaporation of moisture from the skin, and so prevents the skin from drying out.

Acid mantle Sweat and sebum combine on the epidermis, the skin's outer surface, creating an acidic pH film, which is a physical and chemical barrier. This is known as the **acid mantle**, and discourages the growth of bacteria and fungi.

ALWAYS REMEMBER

The lips

Sebaceous glands are not present on the surface of the lips. For this reason the lips should be protected with a lip emollient preparation to prevent them from becoming dry and chapped. To reduce the effect of premature skin ageing it is beneficial for the product to contain UV SPF ingredients.

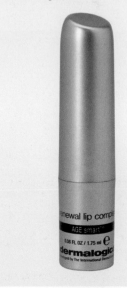

Subcutaneous layer

Situated below the epidermis and dermis is a further layer, the **subcutaneous tissue** hypodermis, subcutis or **fat layer**. It is made up of adipose tissue containing fat cells called adipocytes and areolar tissue (loose connective tissue) containing collagen and elastin fibres. Excess fat that is not used for energy is stored in the adipocyte cells, under the dermis, making the skin appear fuller and thicker. Cellulite is a condition associated with the subcutaneous tissue, which affects the appearance of the skin creating a dimpled surface. It is supplied with a network of capillaries that run parallel to the skin's surface. Also present are nerve fibres,

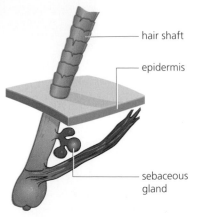

- hair shaft
- epidermis
- sebaceous gland

Sebaceous gland associated with hair follicle, pilosebaceous unit

ALWAYS REMEMBER

Acid mantle care

Avoid chemicals and cosmetic ingredients that can alter the pH of the skin's acid mantle, leading to irritation and reduced barrier protection.

REVISION AID

What is the difference between the sebaceous gland and sudoriferous gland?

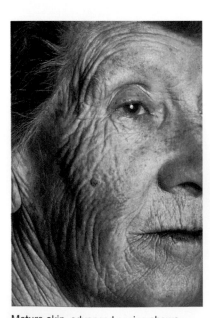

Mature skin, advanced ageing shows wrinkles as a principle skin characteristic

blood and lymph vessels. The thickness of the subcutaneous layer varies according to the body area, and is, for example, very thin around the eyes. This layer is thicker in women than men. The fat layer contributes to the shape of our body.

The subcutaneous layer has a protective function and:

◆ acts as an insulator to conserve body heat

◆ cushions muscles and **bones** below from injury

◆ acts as an energy source, as adipocytes which store fat, are stored in this layer.

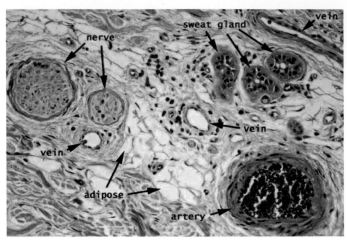

Adipose tissue – the empty-looking structures are adipocytes, or cells storing fat

Skin ageing

The change in appearance of women's skin during ageing is closely related to the altered production of the hormones oestrogen, progesterone and androgen at the menopause.

Mature skin has the following characteristics:

◆ Cellular metabolism slows down the skin's renewal process.

◆ The skin becomes dry, as the sebaceous and sudoriferous glands become less active and reduce in number.

◆ The skin loses its elasticity as the elastin fibres harden, and wrinkles appear due to the cross-linking and hardening of collagen fibres. Females have lower collagen content than males so visible signs tend to be seen faster in women than men. Skin is more easily damaged, with resultant bruising due to less support around its **blood vessels**.

◆ The epidermis grows more slowly and the skin epidermis gets thinner, becoming almost transparent in some areas such as around the eyes, where small veins and capillaries show through the skin. In males this thinning is slower as it is not related to skin changes that occur as a result of the menopause.

◆ Broken capillaries appear, especially on the cheek area and around the nose.

◆ The facial contours become slack as muscle tone is reduced.

◆ The underlying bone structure becomes more obvious, as the fatty layer and the supportive tissue beneath the skin grow thinner. This is obvious around the eye orbits and the chin, cheek and nose areas of the face.

◆ The cartilage tissue reduces noticeably at the end of the nose and support is lost, resulting in a drooping effect.

◆ Blood circulation becomes poor, which interferes with skin nutrition, and the skin may appear sallow.

◆ Due to the decrease in metabolic rate, waste products are not removed so quickly, and this leads to puffiness of the skin.

◆ Patches of irregular pigmentation appear on the surface of the skin, including hyperpigmentation disorders such as lentigines and chloasma, also called melasma.

◆ Reduction in cells including Langerhans cells; the skin can therefore become less sensitive to irritants as we age.

The skin may also exhibit the following skin conditions, although these are not truly **characteristic** of ageing skin:

◆ Dermal naevi may be enlarged.

◆ Seborrhoeic warts may appear on the epidermal layer of the skin.

◆ Verruca filliformis warts may increase in number.

◆ In women, hair growth on the upper lip or chin, or both, may become darker or coarser, due to hormonal imbalance in the body.

◆ Dark circles and puffiness may occur under the eyes.

ALWAYS REMEMBER

Cosmetic moisturisers

Cosmetic moisturisers copy the action of sebum in providing an oily covering for the skin's surface, reducing moisture loss and keeping the skin healthy, soft and supple. Ingredients aim to preserve the hydration and oil content of the skin, absorbed by the surface epidermis, hair follicle, sebaceous gland and sweat glands.

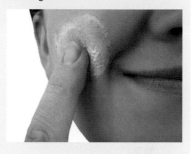

TOP TIP

Alpha hydroxy acids (AHAs)

AHAs are used in many cosmetic products, these can achieve a skin brightening, rejuvenating effect. Mild acids, such as the natural fruit acids are used in face creams that allow the removal of surface dead skin cells by dissolving the intercellular compounds holding them together. A stronger AHA called glycolic acid is used in some anti-ageing preparations to stimulate skin renewal. These are designed to remove the dull outer layer of cells and reveal fresher skin beneath, but continuous use can make the skin sore.

Stronger acids have a shrinking or drying effect on the skin, so care must be taken to apply them in the correct concentrations. Salicylic acid is included in some preparations to remove dead skin cells, such as aftercare products following intimate waxing to exfoliate the skin and reduce the possibility of ingrowing hairs. This is from the group of beta hydroxy acids (BHAs).

AHAs are water soluble while BHAs are lipid soluble and can exfoliate deeper into the skin. They are ideal for the treatment of an acne skin.

YOUNGER SKIN   OLDER SKIN

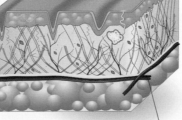

Deep wrinkle

Epidermis

Dermis

Hypodermis subcutaneous layer

Elastin   Collagen

Capillary vessel

Comparison of the structure of younger and older skin

ACTIVITY

The ageing process

Research and find images showing men and women of different ethnicity and at various ages. This can include the hands, which you may treat.

1   Can you identify the visible characteristics of ageing?

2   Does ageing appear to occur at the same rate in men and women and in different ethnicities?

3   Which services could be offered in a treatment plan, the main objectives of which are to treat signs of ageing?

ACTIVITY

Application of hair knowledge

Knowledge of the hair function, structure, type and growth cycle is important to many services offered at Level 2.

Consider why you need this understanding in the following services:

◆ wax depilation

◆ eyebrow shaping

◆ eyelash extensions.

REVISION AID

Where is the subcutaneous layer found? Name two of its functions.

ALWAYS REMEMBER

Did you know?

There are approximately 100 000 hairs on the scalp.

The hair

The structure and function of hair and the surrounding tissues

A hair is a long, slender structure that grows out of, and is part of, the skin. Each hair is made up of dead skin cells, which contain the protein keratin.

Hairs cover the whole body, except for the palms of the hands, the soles of the feet, the lips and parts of the sex organs.

Hair has many functions:

◆ *Scalp hair* insulates the head against cold, protects it from the sun and cushions it against bumps.

◆ *Eyebrows* cushion the brow bone from bumps and prevent sweat from running into the eyes.

◆ *Eyelashes* help to prevent foreign particles entering the eyes.

◆ *Nostril hair* traps dust particles inhaled with the air.

◆ *Ear hair* helps to protect the ear canal. Hair cells in the inner ear send signals to the brain when the head moves; this information is used to help the body maintain balance.

◆ *Body hair* helps to provide an insulating cover (although this function is almost obsolete in humans), has a valuable sensory function and is linked with the secretion of sebum onto the surface of the skin. Terminal hair in the pubic and underarm areas has a purpose to protect the underlying glands and organs.

Hair also plays a role in social communication.

TOP TIP

A strand of hair is stronger than an equivalent strand of nylon or copper. However, repeated chemical treatments weaken the hair. Consider this when booking appointments for services such as lash and brow tinting, chemical eyelash curling and semi-permanent lash extension removal processes. Allow the manufacturer's recommended intervals between each treatment.

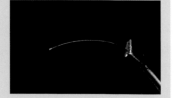

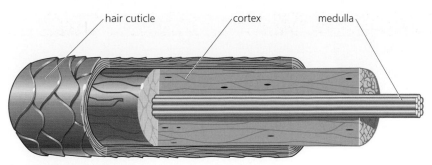

hair cuticle   cortex   medulla

Cross-section of the hair

The structure of hair

Most hairs are made up of three layers of different types of epithelial cells: the **medulla**, the **cortex** and the **cuticle**.

The medulla is the central core of the hair. The cells of the medulla contain soft keratin, and sometimes some pigment granules. Air spaces between the cells allow light to pass through, giving a shiny appearance to the hair. The medulla only exists in medium-to-coarse hair – there is usually no medulla in thinner hair.

The cortex is the thickest layer of the hair, and is made up of several layers of closely packed, elongated cells. These contain pigment granules and hard keratin, giving the hair its strength.

It is the **pigment** in the cortex that gives hair its colour. When this pigment is no longer made, the hair appears white. As the proportion of white hairs rises, the hair seems to go 'grey'. In fact, however, each individual hair is either coloured as before, or white.

The cuticle is the protective outer layer of the hair, and is composed of a layer of thin, unpigmented, flat, scale-like cells. These contain hard keratin, and overlap each other from the base to the tip of the hair.

The parts of the hair and related skin

Each hair is recognised by three parts: the **root**, the **bulb** and the **shaft**:

◆ The root is the part of the hair that is in the follicle.

◆ The bulb is the enlarged base of the hair root.

◆ The shaft is the part of the hair that can be seen above the skin's surface.

Each hair grows out of a tube-like indentation in the epidermis, the **hair follicle**. The walls of the follicle are a continuation of the epidermal layer of the skin.

The **arrector pili muscle** is attached at an angle to the base of the follicle. Cold, aggression or fright stimulates this muscle to contract, pulling the follicle and the hair upright, creating a bumpy appearance on the skin's surface referred to as 'goose bumps'.

The sebaceous gland is attached to the upper part of the follicle. From it, a duct enters directly into the hair follicle. The gland produces sebum, which is secreted into the follicle. Sebum waterproofs, lubricates and softens the hair and the surface of the skin; it also protects the skin against bacterial and fungal infections. The contraction of the arrector pili muscle aids the secretion of sebum.

The **apocrine glands (sweat glands)** are associated with the hairs in the groin area at the top of the thigh and pubic area, and underarm. Their ducts open directly into the hair follicles near to the surface of the skin. These glands, which are under hormonal control, become active at puberty.

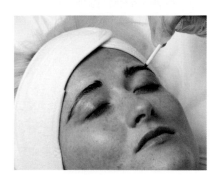

Eyebrow tint

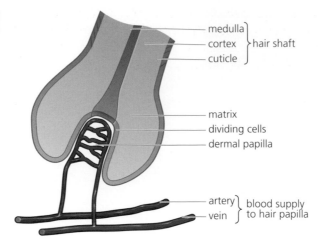

The hair bulb

The **dermal papilla** is connective tissue surrounded by the hair bulb. It provides an excellent blood supply, necessary to provide nutrition and hormones for the growth of the hair. It is not itself part of the follicle, but a separate tiny organ of blood capillaries, which transports blood to the follicle.

The bulb is the enlarged base of the hair root. A gap at the base leads to a cavity inside, which houses the dermal papilla. The bulb contains in its lower part the dividing cells that create the hair. The hair continues to develop as it passes through the regions of the upper bulb and the root.

Cross-section of the skin, hair and hair follicle and its associated structures

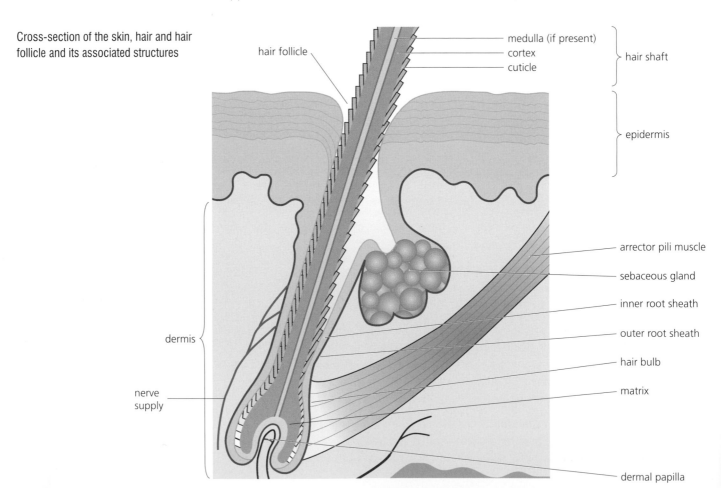

The **matrix** is the name given to the lower part of the bulb, which comprises actively dividing hair germ cells from which the hair is formed. The hair germ cells grow downwards in a column called the **dermal cord**. The dermal cord surrounds the dermal papilla and when this occurs, cellular changes cause a new hair to grow.

The hair follicle
The **hair follicle** extends into the dermis, and is made up of three sheaths: the **inner root sheath**, the **outer root sheath** and the surrounding **connective-tissue sheath**.

The inner epithelial root sheath grows from the bottom of the follicle at the papilla; both the hair and the inner root sheath grow upwards together. The inner root sheath encloses the hair root in three separate layers:

◆ The **cuticle** layer is covered with cuticle cells in the same way as the outer surface of the hair. These cells lock together, anchoring the hair firmly in place.

◆ The **Huxley's** layer is the thickest of the three inner root sheath layers.

◆ The **Henle's** layer is the inner final layer of the inner root sheath composed of a single layer of cells.

The inner root sheath ceases to grow when level with the sebaceous gland.

The outer root sheath forms the follicle wall. This does not grow up with the hair, but is stationary. It is a continuation of the growing layer of the epidermis of the skin.

The **connective-tissue sheath** surrounds both the follicle and the sebaceous gland, providing both a sensory supply and a blood supply. The connective-tissue sheath includes, and is a continuation of, the papilla.

The shape of the hairs is determined by the shape of the hair follicle – an angled or bent follicle will produce an oval or flat hair, whereas a straight follicle will produce a round hair. Flat hairs are curly, oval hairs are wavy and round hairs are straight. As a general rule, curly hairs break off more easily during waxing than straight hairs.

ALWAYS REMEMBER

Broken hairs

When hairs break off due to incorrect waxing technique, they will break at the level at which they are locked into the follicle by the cells of the inner root sheath. This can lead to ingrowing hairs and a poor waxing result.

TOP TIP

The inner root sheath can be seen on hairs removed by both temporary and permanent hair removal techniques by depilation in the anagen stage of hair growth. A white sheath is visible on the part of the hair.

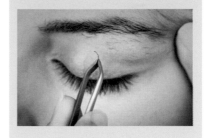

TOP TIP

The type and shape of the hair will influence your choice of waxing product and application technique for waxing. It will also influence your choice of application technique for lash attachment system.

curly	wavy	straight
flat ribbon-like	less oval	round

Hair shapes

REVISION AID

What layer of the hair has a scale-like appearance?

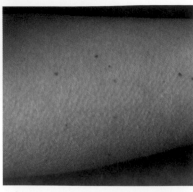

Vellus hair

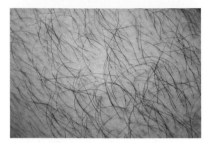

Terminal hair

The nerve supply The number, size and type of nerve endings associated with hair follicles is related to the size and type of follicle. The follicles of **vellus hairs** have the fewest nerve endings; those of **terminal hairs** have the most.

The nerve endings surrounding hair follicles respond mainly to rapid movements when the hair is moved. Nerve endings that respond to touch can also be found around the surface openings of some hair follicles, as well as just below the epidermis.

The three types of hair

There are three main types of hair: **lanugo**, **vellus** and **terminal**.

Lanugo hairs are found on the body prior to birth. They are fine and soft, do not have a medulla, and are often unpigmented. They grow from around the third to the fifth month of pregnancy, and are shed to be replaced by the secondary vellus hairs around the seventh to the eighth month of pregnancy. Lanugo hairs on the scalp, eyebrows and eyelashes are replaced by terminal hairs.

Vellus hairs are fine, downy and soft, and are found on the face and body. They are often unpigmented, rarely longer than 20 mm, and do not have a medulla or a well-formed bulb. The base of these hairs is very close to the skin's surface. If stimulated, the shallow follicle of a vellus hair can grow downwards and become a follicle that produces terminal hairs.

Terminal hairs are longer and coarser than vellus hairs, and most are pigmented. They vary greatly in shape, in diameter and length, and in colour and texture. The follicles from which they grow are set deeply in the dermis and have well-defined bulbs. Terminal hair is the coarse hair of the scalp, eyebrows, eyelashes, pubic and underarm regions. It is also present on the face, chest and sometimes the backs of males.

Hair growth

All hair has a cyclical pattern of growth, which can be divided into three phases: **anagen**, **catagen** and **telogen**.

Anagen is the actively growing stage of the hair – the follicle has reformed, the hair bulb is developing, surrounding the life-giving dermal papilla, and a new hair forms, growing from the matrix in the bulb.

Catagen is the changing stage when the hair separates from the papilla. Over a few days it is carried by the movement of the inner root sheath, up the follicle to the base of the sebaceous gland. Here it stays until it either falls out or is pushed out by a new hair growing up behind it.

This stage can be very rapid, with a new hair growing straight away; or slower, with the papilla and the follicle below the sebaceous gland degenerating and entering a resting stage, telogen.

Telogen is a resting stage. Many hair follicles do not undergo this stage, but start to produce a new hair immediately. During resting phases, hairs may still be loosely held in the shallow follicles.

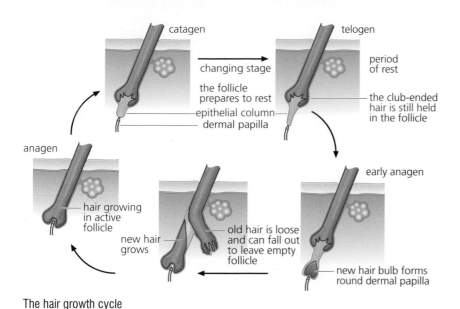

The hair growth cycle

The average time for hair regrowth following temporary methods of hair removal are:

◆ terminal hair – 5–6 weeks

◆ vellus hair – 8–10 weeks.

Speed of growth The anagen, catagen and telogen stages last for different lengths of time in different hair types and in different parts of the body:

◆ *Scalp* hair grows for 2–7 years, and has a resting stage of 3–4 months.

◆ *Eyebrow* hair grows for 1–2 months, and has a resting stage of 3–4 months.

◆ *Eyelashes* grow for 3–6 weeks, and have a resting stage of 3–4 months.

After a waxing service, body hair will take approximately 6–8 weeks to return.

Because **hair growth cycles** are not all in synchronisation, we always have hair present at any given time. On the scalp, at any one time for example, 85 per cent of hairs may be in the anagen phase. This is why hair growth after waxing starts within a few days: what is seen is the appearance of hairs that were already developing in the follicle at the time of waxing.

Types of hair growth **Hirsutism** is a term used to describe a pattern of hair growth that is abnormal for that person's sex, such as when a woman's hair growth follows a man's hair-growth pattern. The hair growth is usually terminal when it should be of a vellus type.

Hypertrichosis is an abnormal growth of excess hair for a person's sex, age and race. It is usually due to abnormal conditions brought about by disease or injury.

Superfluous hair (excess hair) is unwanted hair growth perfectly normal for the age, sex or gender of the person. For example, at certain periods in a woman's life, such as during puberty or pregnancy, terminal hair can form. It usually disappears once the normal hormonal

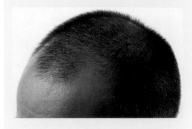
balance has returned. Hair newly formed during the menopause is often permanent unless treated with a permanent method of hair removal, such as electrical epilation or laser service.

Factors affecting the growth rate and quantity of hair

Hair does not always grow uniformly:

- *Time of day.* Hair grows faster at night than during the day.

- *Weather.* Hairs grow faster in warm weather than in cold.

- *Stimulation*. If the area of the skin is stimulated, this can affect skin and hair growth. For example, the wearing of a plaster cast may lead to increased hair growth known as topical hair growth.

- *Hormones*. In women, hairs grow faster between the ages of 16 and 24, and (frequently) during mid-pregnancy and the menopause. Hormone imbalances can lead to excessive hair growth. This is known as **normal systemic** hair growth.

- *Age*. The rate of hair growth slows down with age. In women, however, facial hair growth continues to increase in old age, while trunk and limb hair increases into middle age and then decreases.

- *Gender.* Male pattern baldness affects approximately 50% of all men after 50 years of age.

- *Colour.* Hairs of different colour grow at different speeds. For example, coarse black hair grows more quickly than fine blonde hair.

- *Part of the body*. Hair in different areas of the body grows at different rates, as do different types and thicknesses of hair. The weekly growth rate varies from approximately 1.5 mm (fine hair) to 2.8 mm (coarse hair), when actively growing.

- *Heredity*. Various members of a family may have inherited growth patterns, such as excess hair that starts to grow at puberty and increases until the age of 20–25. This is known as congenital hair growth.

- *Health and diet*. Good health and a varied, balanced diet are crucial factors in the rate of hair growth and appearance. A person suffering from the eating disorder anorexia nervosa will suffer from a fine growth of hair all over the body.

- *Stress*. Emotional stress can cause a temporary hormonal imbalance within the body, which may lead to a temporary growth of excess hair. Trichotillomania is a psychological disorder where the person is unable to stop themselves carrying out a particular action. Commonly this can be to pull out their hair e.g. from their scalp or eyelashes. This condition can become worse in stressful situations.

- *Medical conditions*. A sudden unexplained increase of body hair growth may indicate a more serious medical problem, such as malfunction of the endocrine glands, i.e. ovaries, thyroid gland and adrenal gland; or result from the taking of certain drugs, such as corticosteroids, certain birth control pills and high blood pressure medication. This is known as **abnormal systemic** hair growth.

Alopecia Areata is hair loss from the scalp or on the body in patches. It is commonly related to a disorder of the immune system.

The quantity as well as the type of hair present may vary with race, for example:

- *People of Latin extraction* tend to possess heavier body, facial and scalp hair, which is relatively coarse, dark and straight.

◆ *People of Eastern Asian extraction* tend to possess very little or no body and facial hair growth, and usually their scalp hair growth is relatively coarse, dark and straight. This gives the appearance of greater hair density, but they have a lower hair density than Caucasian, Latin and African–Caribbean people.

◆ *People of Indian and Middle Eastern extraction* tend to have darker, more noticeable hair growth and facial hair growth. The scalp hair is coarse and maybe slightly curled or straight.

◆ *People of Northern European extraction* tend to have light-to-medium body and facial hair growth, with their scalp hair growth being wavy, loosely curled or straight.

◆ *People of African extraction* tend to have little body and facial hair growth, but usually their scalp hair growth is relatively coarse and curled.

Nowadays, people possess mixed characteristics of differing ethnicities affecting hair colour, thickness and shape.

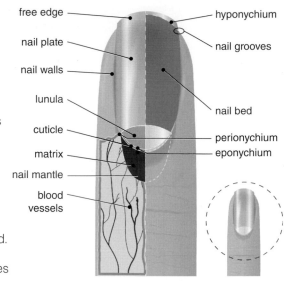

The structure of the nail

The nails

The structure and function of the nail

Nails grow from the ends of the fingers and toes and serve as a form of protection. They also help when picking up small objects. The different parts of the nails and surrounding tissues are discussed below.

As part of your consultation you may look at the appearance of the nail as an indicator of a person's health. You should be able to distinguish between a healthy nail and one suffering from a nail/skin disease or disorder. Certain nail/skin diseases and disorders prevent service. Proceeding would expose you and other clients to cross-infection through contact or it could make the condition worse. Related nail/skin diseases and disorders are discussed in Chapter 3 and Chapter 7.

Nails should be a healthy pink colour, with smooth, supple cuticles. Disease or disorder can show itself in different ways on the nail. If unsure always refer to the client's GP for diagnosis.

ACTIVITY

With a colleague, try to identify the visible structural parts of your nails.

Structure and function of the nail

Nail part	Structure and function
The nail plate nail plate —	Structure: The **nail plate** is composed of compact translucent layers of keratinised epidermal cells called keratinocytes: it is this that makes up the main body of the nail. The layers of cells are packed very closely together with fat but very little moisture. The nail gradually grows forwards over the nail bed, until finally it becomes the free edge. The underside of the nail plate is grooved by longitudinal ridges and furrows, which help to keep it in place. In normal health the plate curves in two directions: ◆ transversely – from side to side across the nail ◆ longitudinally – from the base of the nail to the free edge. There are no blood vessels or nerves in the nail plate: this is why the nails, like hair, can be cut without pain or bleeding. The pink colour of the nail plate derives from the blood vessels that pass beneath it – the nail bed. *Function*: To protect the living nail bed of the fingers and toes.

(*Continued*)

Nail part	Structure and function
The free edge free edge	Structure: The **free edge** is the part of the nail that extends beyond the fingertip; this is the part that is filed. It appears white as there is no nail bed underneath. Function: To protect the tip of the fingers and toes and the hyponychium.
The matrix matrix	*Structure:* The **matrix**, sometimes called the nail root, is the growing area of the nail. It is formed by the division of cells in this area, called mitosis, and is part of the stratum germinativum layer of the epidermis. It lies under the eponychium, at the base of the nail. The process of keratinisation takes place in the epidermal cells of the matrix, forming the hardened tissue of the nail plate. *Function:* To produce new nail cells.
The nail bed nail bed	*Structure:* The **nail bed** is the portion of skin upon which the nail plate rests. It has a pattern of grooves and furrows corresponding to those found on the underside of the nail plate. These interlock, keeping the nail in place, but separate at the end of the nail to form the free edge. The nail bed is liberally supplied with blood vessels, which provide the nourishment necessary for continued growth; and sensory nerves, for protection. *Function:* To supply nourishment and protection.
The nail mantle nail mantle	*Structure:* The **nail mantle** is the layer of epidermis at the base of the nail above the matrix, before the cuticle. It appears as a deep fold of skin. *Function:* To protect the matrix from physical damage.
The lunula lunula	*Structure:* The crescent-shaped **lunula** is located at the base of the nail. These cells gradually harden through keratinisation. It is white, relative to the rest of the nail, and there are two theories to account for this: ◆ Newly formed nail plates may be more opaque (less transparent) than mature nail plates. ◆ The lunula may indicate the extent of the underlying matrix – the matrix is thicker than the epidermis of the nail bed, and the capillaries beneath it would not show through as well. *Function:* None.

(Continued)

Nail part	Structure and function
The hyponychium hyponychium	*Structure*: The **hyponychium** is part of the epidermis under the free edge of the nail. *Function*: To protect the nail bed from infection by preventing dirt and bacteria getting underneath the nail plate by forming a waterproof barrier.
The nail grooves nail groove	*Structure:* The **nail grooves** run alongside the edge of the nail plate. *Function:* To guide the body of the nail plate as it grows forwards over the nail bed.
The perionychium perionychium	*Structure:* The **perionychium** is the collective name given to the nail walls and the cuticle at the sides of the nail. *Function:* To protect the nail bed from infection by preventing dirt and bacteria getting underneath the nail plate by forming a waterproof barrier.
The nail walls nail wall	*Structure:* The **nail walls** are the folds of skin overlapping the sides of the nails. *Function:* To cushion and protect the nail plate and grooves from damage.
The eponychium eponychium	*Structure:* The **eponychium** is the extension of the cuticle at the base of the nail plate, under which the nail plate emerges from the matrix. *Function:* To protect the matrix from infection by preventing dirt and bacteria getting underneath the nail plate by forming a waterproof barrier.

(Continued)

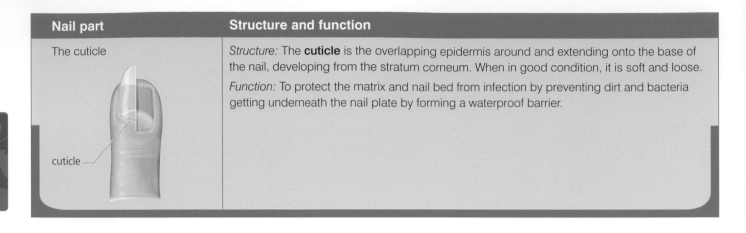

Nail part	Structure and function
The cuticle cuticle	*Structure:* The **cuticle** is the overlapping epidermis around and extending onto the base of the nail, developing from the stratum corneum. When in good condition, it is soft and loose. *Function:* To protect the matrix and nail bed from infection by preventing dirt and bacteria getting underneath the nail plate by forming a waterproof barrier.

ALWAYS REMEMBER

If the nail bed is pink this means the blood circulation to the nail bed is good. Poor health disorders such as respiratory illness and anaemia can affect the appearance of the nail colour, called 'blue nail'.

ALWAYS REMEMBER

Did you know?

Fingernails grow more quickly than toenails. Fingernails grow about 0.1 mm each day or 3 mm to 4 mm per month (4 cm per year); they grow faster in summer than in winter.

REVISION AID

In what ways are nails and hair alike?

Nail growth

Cells divide in the matrix and the nail grows forwards over the nail bed, guided by the nail grooves, until it reaches the end of the finger or toe, where it becomes the free edge. As they first emerge from the matrix the translucent cells are plump and soft, but they get harder and flatter as they move towards the free edge. The top two layers of the epidermis form the nail plate; the remaining three form the nail bed.

The nails' cells die in a process called keratinisation, where the living cells become filled with the protein **keratin** as they mature, losing moisture and becoming hard. No mitotic activity is seen in these cells when this happens.

The nail bed has a pattern of grooves and furrows corresponding to those found on the underside of the nail plate. The two surfaces interlock, holding the nail in place.

Fingernails grow at approximately twice the speed of toenails. It takes about 6 months for a fingernail to grow from cuticle to free edge, but about 12 months for a toenail to do so.

As we age, moisture and fats are lost from the nail and longitudinal ridges can appear on the nail plate.

Nail appearance and growth are affected by internal and external factors and reflect a person's general health. This is discussed in further detail in Chapter 7.

The eye

Basic structure and function of the eye

The eye is positioned in a protective socket formed from the bone of the skull called the orbital cavity. It is cushioned by a layer of fat inside the eye socket and surrounded by a tough outer layer of tissue called the **sclera**, the white part of the eye. The eye is shaped like a ball, and is referred to as the eyeball. It is responsible for providing our vision, collecting light and converting it via nerve impulses, which when received by the brain decode it and inform us what we can see.

The eyeball moves all the time, controlled by six small striated strap-shaped muscles attached to the eyeball and the walls of the orbital cavity. Eye movement is under voluntary control when looking in a particular direction but when looking at differences in distance and in different lighting conditions this is under autonomic control.

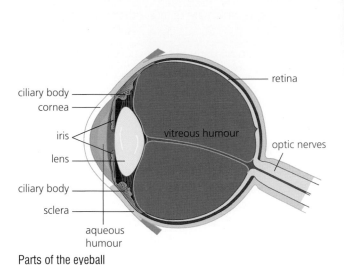

Parts of the eyeball

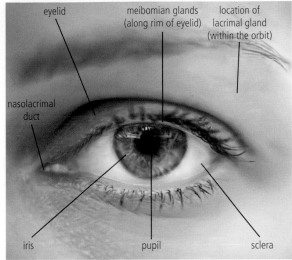

Parts of the eye

The eyeball

The eyeball is made up of a semi-solid clear gel called **vitreous humour,** which gives the eye its shape and keeps structures such as the retina in place. It is made up of two cavities, front and rear, either side of a structure called the lens.

The main structures and their functions are discussed below.

Optic nerves (2nd cranial nerves)   Optic nerves transport the nerve impulses from the eye to the brain.

Retina   The retina is a light sensitive tissue situated in the rear cavity of the eye. It detects light rays and these are transformed into nerve signals that the brain can understand.

Cornea   The cornea is a clear dome-shaped, transparent layer, covering the front part of the eye. It receives light rays and directs them onto the retina.

Lens   The lens is shaped like a disc and is made up of transparent fibres called **crystallins**, which allow light through. The lens focuses the image, enabling us to identify objects at different distances, both near and far.

Iris   The iris is the coloured part of the eye. In the middle of the iris is a hole – the pupil. The iris can adjust the amount of light allowed into the eye by changing the size of the pupil. When the light is bright the pupils contract (go smaller), letting less light into the eye. If the light is dim the pupils dilate (go larger) to allow more light into the eyes.

Pupil   The pupil is a hole that allows light to enter the eye in the middle of the iris.

Aqueous humour   The aqueous humour is a clear, watery fluid found between the cornea and lens. The aqueous humour is found at the front cavity of the eye and helps to give the eye its shape.

Ciliary muscles Ciliary muscles form a ring around the lens and focus light by changing its shape and help in viewing objects which are different distances.

Blood vessels Blood vessels are found in all parts of the eye except the lens and cornea, which are transparent.

Parts of the eye area

The eyelids The eyelids are composed of skin and connective tissue; these movable lids are situated above and below the eye. They protect the eyes from bright light, dust and debris. When we blink, the surface of the eye is cleaned. A membrane lining called the **conjunctiva** lines the eyelids, protecting the cornea and front of the eye. The edges of the eyelids contain numerous sebaceous glands. Some open into the hair follicles of the eyelash hair and some directly onto the edge of the eyelids between the hairs.

Meibomian glands Meibomian glands are modified sebaceous glands, which open directly onto the inside of the edge of the eyelid and secrete an oily substance when blinking that provides a protective film over the conjunctiva. This oily substance also prevents the eyes becoming dry by reducing the evaporation of tears.

The eyelids open and close, either by the voluntary action of opening and closing the eyes or the involuntary action of blinking. The movement is controlled by the contraction of the orbicularis oculi muscle, which closes the eyelid, and the contraction of the levator palpebrae superioris muscle, which opens and lifts the eyelid.

Lacrimal gland The lacrimal gland is situated above the outer corner of each eye in the frontal bone. It secretes tears composed of water, salt and a bactericidal enzyme called lysozyme.

Nasolacrimal duct The nasolacrimal duct drains tears into the nasal cavity.

Eyebrows Eyebrows are short, coarse terminal hairs situated above the bony orbits of the eyes. The eyebrow hair protects the front of the eye from sweat, dust and debris.

Eyelashes Eyelashes are short, coarse terminal hairs situated on the outer portion of the eyelid in rows of three to five. The eyelash hairs protect the eyes from bright light, dust and debris. There are up to 150 lashes on the upper lid and 80 on the lower eyelid. They are between 7 mm and 9 mm in length.

Organ systems

Tissues of the body are grouped to form larger structural units called organs. The human body is made up of organ systems that work together to ensure healthy functioning of the body overall. As well as the skin that we have already discussed, other major organ systems of the body are described on next page.

Organ system	Functions	Diagram
Skeletal	Forms a strong framework, which supports the softer tissues and maintains the shape of the body. Internal organs are suspended from the skeleton, which keeps them anchored in position. Muscles are attached to the bones, which contract and relax allowing movement. Together with the muscles and **joints**, the skeleton allows movement. Many organs are surrounded by a protective cage of bone. Many of the blood cells are made in bone marrow (found inside the bones). The bones of the skeleton that you will need to know are shown. These will be discussed in each technical chapter.	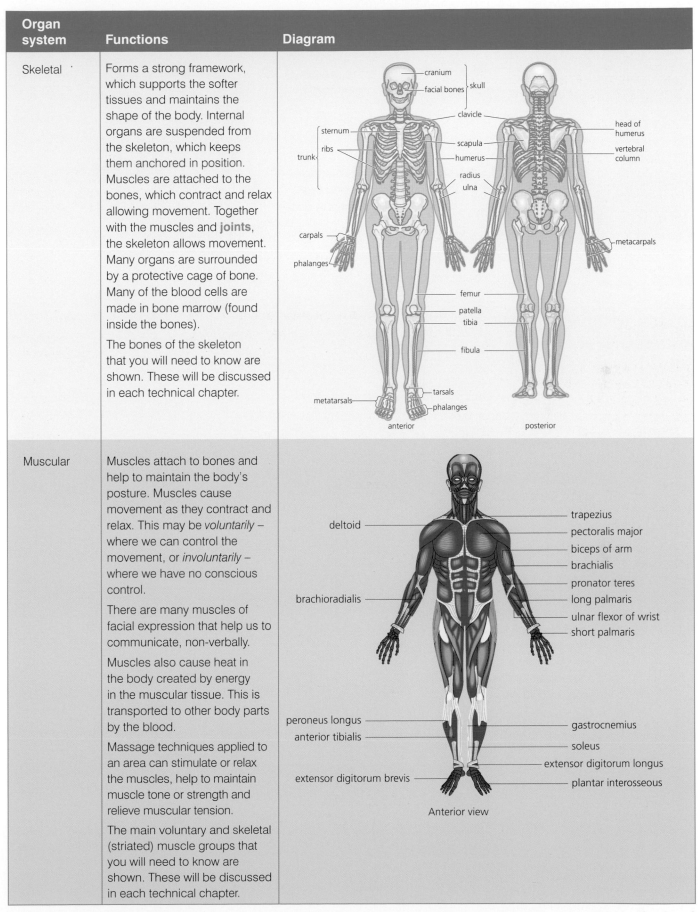
Muscular	Muscles attach to bones and help to maintain the body's posture. Muscles cause movement as they contract and relax. This may be *voluntarily* – where we can control the movement, or *involuntarily* – where we have no conscious control. There are many muscles of facial expression that help us to communicate, non-verbally. Muscles also cause heat in the body created by energy in the muscular tissue. This is transported to other body parts by the blood. Massage techniques applied to an area can stimulate or relax the muscles, help to maintain muscle tone or strength and relieve muscular tension. The main voluntary and skeletal (striated) muscle groups that you will need to know are shown. These will be discussed in each technical chapter.	

(Continued)

Organ system	Functions	Diagram
		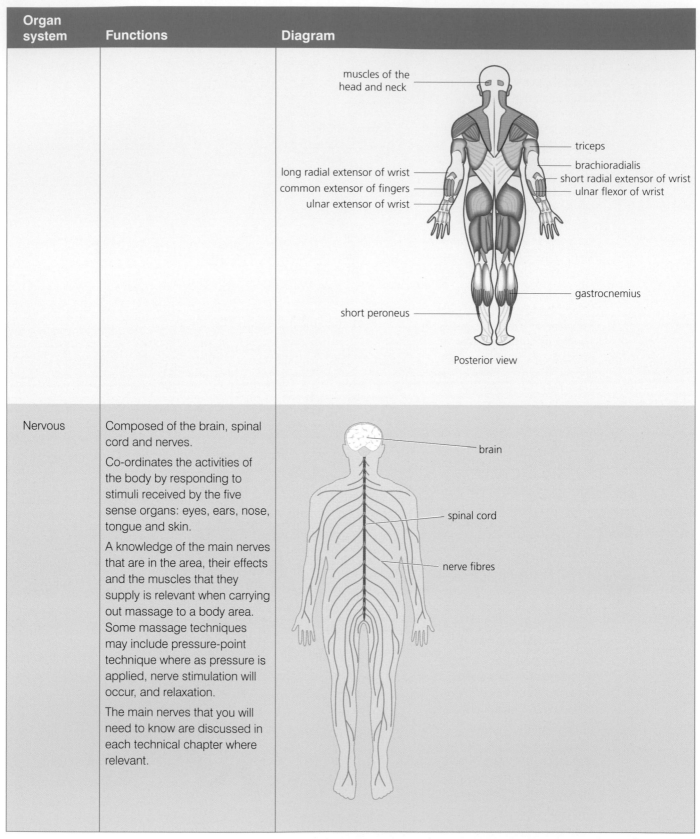 muscles of the head and neck triceps brachioradialis long radial extensor of wrist short radial extensor of wrist common extensor of fingers ulnar flexor of wrist ulnar extensor of wrist gastrocnemius short peroneus Posterior view
Nervous	Composed of the brain, spinal cord and nerves. Co-ordinates the activities of the body by responding to stimuli received by the five sense organs: eyes, ears, nose, tongue and skin. A knowledge of the main nerves that are in the area, their effects and the muscles that they supply is relevant when carrying out massage to a body area. Some massage techniques may include pressure-point technique where as pressure is applied, nerve stimulation will occur, and relaxation. The main nerves that you will need to know are discussed in each technical chapter where relevant.	brain spinal cord nerve fibres

(Continued)

Organ system	Functions	Diagram
Circulatory also known as the cardiovascular system	Transports materials around the body in blood and blood vessels (veins and arteries). The heart (a muscular organ) pumps blood around the body, controlling the transport of materials so that the body can function properly. It supplies oxygen and nutrients, then carries away waste products. Contact with the skin through touch, pressure and heat treatments will stimulate blood circulation in the area. This may cause the skin to become reddened as blood is brought to the area. Hair removal through wax depilation, threading and tweezing causes a protective reaction where blood is brought to the area to repair it and prevent infection. The main arteries and veins that you will need to know are discussed in each technical chapter where relevant.	
Lymphatic system	The lymphatic system is closely connected to the circulatory system. It is made up of lymph **nodes** connected by lymph vessels, carrying lymph fluid. Its primary function is one of protection to remove any harmful bacteria and foreign materials. It also drains excessive fluids which are removed from the body. Massage will improve lymphatic circulation in the area, reducing the appearance of puffiness in the tissues, and removal of waste products and toxins from the muscles. Knowing where lymphatic structures are situated is important to ensure effective massage.	

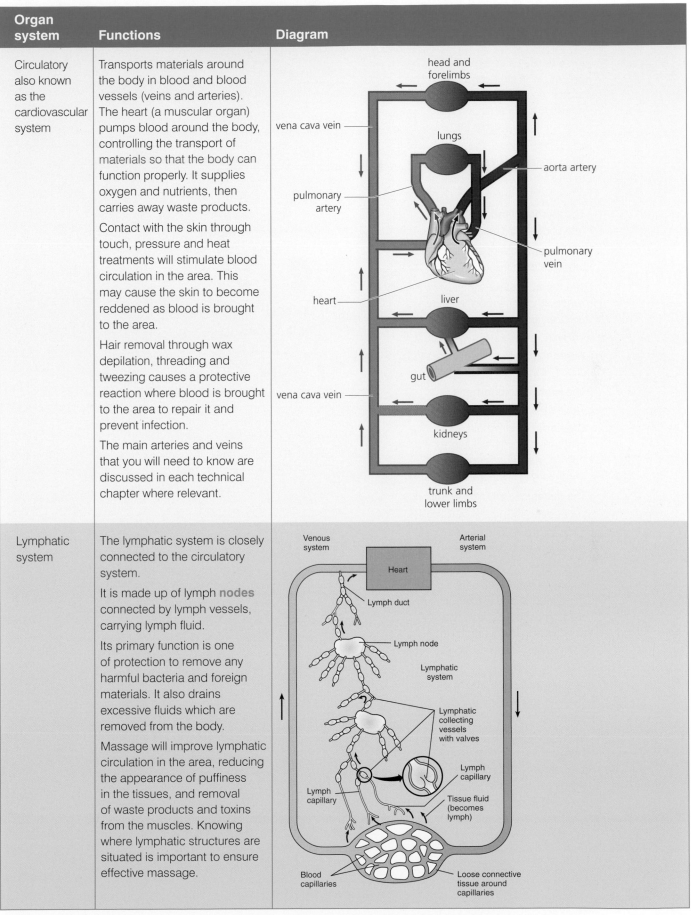

(Continued)

Organ system	Functions	Diagram
Endocrine	Co-ordinates and regulates processes in the body by producing chemicals called hormones, released by endocrine glands into the bloodstream. The **pituitary gland** responds to and controls the activities of other endocrine glands. The **thyroid gland** controls the rate of metabolism. The **parathyroid gland** controls blood calcium levels. The **thymus gland** stimulates lymphoid cells responsible for antibody protection against disease. **Adrenal glands** regulates the stress response. The **islets of Langerhans** control blood sugar levels. **Ovaries** control female productive events including puberty, menstruation, pregnancy and the menopause. The **testes** control male fertility. Hormones control activities such as growth or the development of secondary sexual characteristics. Hormone imbalance affects physical changes in the body, for example the appearance or change in hair type/growth and problematic skin may be hormone related. As a result of hormonal changes in the body the skin ages too. An awareness of the endocrine system and hormones related to health and appearance of the skin is relevant when identifying skin type and condition.	pituitary gland, thyroid gland, parathyroid gland, thymus gland, adrenal glands, islets of Langerhans in pancreas, ovaries (female), testes (male)

The skeletal system

The skeletal system is composed of bones, cartilage, ligaments and tendons. These structures may be felt beneath the skin, where there is less subcutaneous, adipose tissue.

The human skeleton is made up of two parts, the **axial** and **appendicular** skeleton.

The axial skeleton is the central part of the skeleton and is made up of the:

◆ skull – cranium and facial bones

◆ vertebral column or spine – the neck and back

◆ ribs and sternum.

The appendicular skeleton is made up of the bones of the pectoral and pelvic girdles as well as the upper and lower limbs:

◆ shoulder girdle (the clavicle and scapulae bones) and the arms and hands

◆ pelvic girdle and the legs and feet.

Altogether it is made up of 206 individual bones.

Bone structure

When carrying out a massage to the face, head, neck, shoulders, upper chest and back, arms, legs and feet you will feel the underlying bones beneath your hands. Bone is a specialised form of connective tissue, the hardest structural tissue in the body that supports, surrounds and connects different parts of the body.

Bone is a type of connective tissue is made up of water, non-living (inorganic) material including calcium and phosphorus, and living (organic) material such as the cells that form bones, called **osteoblasts**. Bones grow in length by a process called ossification.

There are two main classifications of bone tissue, **compact** and **cancellous** (spongy). Bones are made up of both types of tissue, which varies according to size and function.

Compact bone appears to have no visible spaces and is solid in structure, making it strong and hardwearing. However, under a microscope it can be seen that it is supplied with blood and lymph vessels and nerves, surrounded by concentric circles of bone, where the osteocytes are found.

Cancellous (spongy) bone has many spaces, which contain red and yellow bone marrow. Red bone marrow produces new red blood cells and yellow bone marrow stores fat cells.

Bones are covered with a connective tissue called the **periosteum**, which has an outer layer that provides a protective function and an inner layer that receives a rich blood supply essential for the nutrition of the bone.

Bones can be classified by their shape as: flat; short; irregular; long; and sesamoid.

Flat: strong and light, providing protection and a surface for attachment e.g. scapula, shoulder blade and cranium of the skull.

Short: strong, often as wide as they are long e.g. carpals and tarsals.

Irregular: non-uniform in shape. They provide different functions and their shape relates to their function, e.g. vertebrae, protects spinal cord.

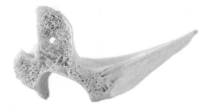

Bone

ALWAYS REMEMBER

Mineral stores

Bone acts as a reservoir for important minerals such as calcium and phosphorus. It also makes new cells for the blood in certain bones, in tissue called bone marrow.

Long: strongest bones of the skeleton, provide movement, form the limbs e.g. humerus bone in the arm femur in the leg, but can also be small such as the phalanges.

Sesamoid: short, irregular bones that develop at a joint in certain tendons e.g. the patella (bone found on the knee) and the pisiform carpal bone.

Examples of these bones are shown here.

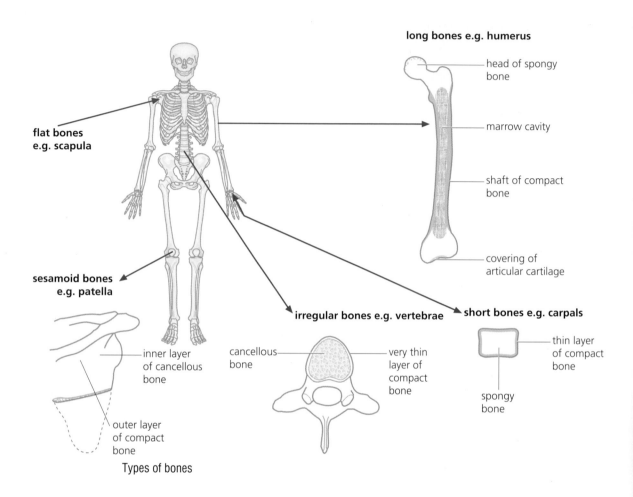

Types of bones

Long bones have a diaphysis or shaft and two extremities called epiphyses. The diaphysis is made of compact bone with a central cavity that contains fatty, yellow bone marrow.

The epiphyses are made of compact bone on the outside and cancellous bone on the inside.

REVISION AID

What is the function of the skeletal system in the body?

Bone movement and joints

The skeleton is made up of many bones to facilitate movement of the body. To enable this each bone is connected to its neighbour by connective tissue. Fibrous connective tissue is used for immovable joints, where the bones fit very tightly together such as those in the cranium of the skull. Fibro-cartilage is used for semi-moveable joints such as those between the bones of the vertebrae. The most common joints are freely moveable. They are called **synovial joints** and are loosely held together by a form of connective tissue called **ligaments**.

Bones get stronger when they are moved regularly by muscles. Load-bearing activity is useful in helping to prevent the bone disease osteoporosis (thinning and weakening of the bone tissue) in older people.

Synovial joints In a typical synovial joint a sleeve-like ligament joins one bone loosely to the next. This forms a fibrous **capsule,** which is flexible enough to allow free movement but strong enough to resist dislocation.

Lining this capsule is the **synovial membrane**, which secretes synovial fluid into the joint. It lubricates the joint, becoming less thick as movement at the joint increases. It also contains phagocytic cells (white blood cells that protect the body by destroying harmful material) to remove debris caused by wear and tear at the joint, and it nourishes the **articular cartilage** that covers the ends of each bone. Articular cartilage provides a smooth coating at the ends of the bones, protecting them from wear by reducing friction.

Extra ligaments may run around the outside of the articular capsule or inside the joint, providing extra strength. Some joints may also contain discs of cartilage to help maintain their stability.

ALWAYS REMEMBER

The body has 206 bones with the important functions of support, protection, movement, blood cell production and mineral storage.

The main support for joints is provided by the muscles that surround them. Very mobile joints such as the shoulder rely heavily on muscles as well as ligaments to hold the joint together. Tendons made of collagen fibres attach muscles to bone. An example is the Achilles tendon, which attaches the calf muscle to the foot at the ankle.

REVISION AID

What is a joint?

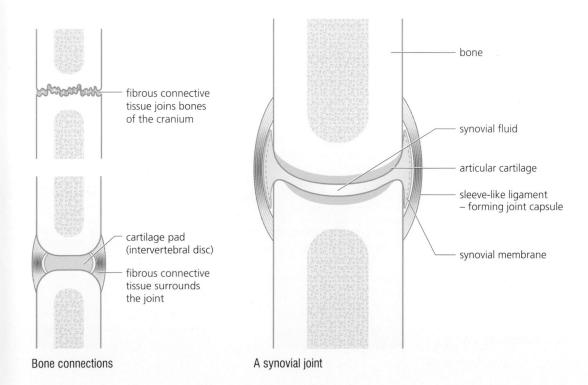

fibrous connective tissue joins bones of the cranium

cartilage pad (intervertebral disc)

fibrous connective tissue surrounds the joint

bone

synovial fluid

articular cartilage

sleeve-like ligament – forming joint capsule

synovial membrane

Bone connections

A synovial joint

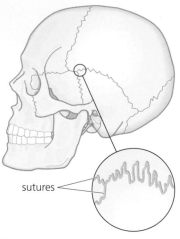

sutures

Sutures

Bones of the head

The bones that form the head are collectively known as the **skull**. The skull can be divided into two parts, the face and the cranium, which together are made up of 22 bones:

◆ The 14 facial bones form the face.

◆ The eight cranial bones form the rest of the skull.

As well as forming our facial features, the facial bones support other structures such as the eyes and the teeth. Some of these bones, such as the nasal bone, are made from **cartilage**, a connective tissue that is softer than bone.

The cranium surrounds and protects the brain. The bones are thin and slightly curved, and are held together by connective tissue. After childhood, the joints become immovable, and are called **sutures**, appearing as wavy lines.

REVISION AID

How many bones form the face?
Name those that form the upper jaw.

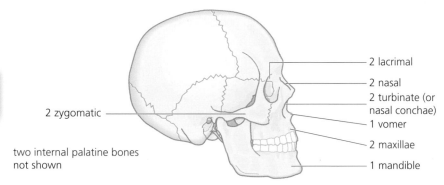

2 zygomatic

two internal palatine bones
not shown

2 lacrimal
2 nasal
2 turbinate (or
nasal conchae)
1 vomer
2 maxillae
1 mandible

Facial bones-lateral view

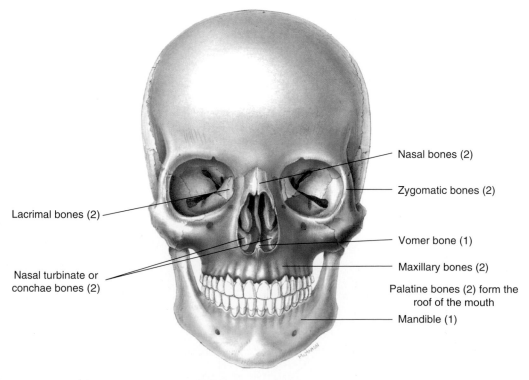

Lacrimal bones (2)

Nasal turbinate or
conchae bones (2)

Nasal bones (2)

Zygomatic bones (2)

Vomer bone (1)

Maxillary bones (2)

Palatine bones (2) form the
roof of the mouth

Mandible (1)

Facial bones-anterior view

Facial bones

Bone	Number	Location	Function
Nasal	2	The nose.	Form the bridge of the nose.
Vomer	1	The nose.	Forms the dividing bony wall of the nose.
Palatine	2	The nose.	Internal bones; form the floor and wall of the nose, the roof of the mouth and bottom of the eye orbits.
Turbinate (Nasal conchae)	2	The nose.	Form the outer walls of the nose.
Lacrimal	2	The eye sockets.	Form the inner walls of the eye sockets; contain a small groove for the tear duct.
Zygomatic (malar)	2	The cheek bones.	Form the cheekbones.
Maxillae	2	The upper jaw.	Fused together to form the upper jaw, which holds the upper teeth.
Mandible	1	The lower jaw.	The largest and strongest of the facial bones; holds the lower teeth and is the only movable bone of the skull.

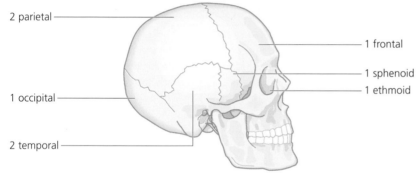

2 parietal

1 frontal

1 sphenoid

1 ethmoid

1 occipital

2 temporal

Bones of the cranium-lateral view

Cranial bones

Bone	Number	Location	Function
Occipital	1	The lower back of the cranium.	Forms the back of the lower skull. Contains a large hole called the **foramen magnum**; through this pass the spinal cord, the nerves and blood vessels.
Parietal	2	The sides of the cranium.	Fused together to form the sides and top of the head (the 'crown').
Frontal	1	The forehead.	Forms the forehead and the upper walls of the eye sockets.
Temporal	2	The sides of the head.	Forms the sides of the head. Provide two muscle attachment points: the mastoid process and the zygomatic process.
Ethmoid	1	Between the eye sockets.	Forms part of the nasal cavities.
Sphenoid	1	The base of the cranium and the back of the eye sockets.	A bat-shaped bone that joins together all the bones of the cranium.

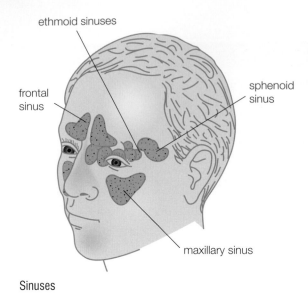

ethmoid sinuses

frontal sinus

sphenoid sinus

maxillary sinus

Sinuses

Sinuses The sinuses are hollow spaces in the facial and cranial bones containing air and lined with a mucous membrane, producing mucus which drains into the nose and keeps the nasal cavities moist and traps bacteria and dirt. The mucous membrane is continuous with the nasal cavities. They can also get blocked by airborne allergens, e.g. pollen, air pollution and chronic drug misuse. They connect with the inside of the nasal cavity through small openings called ostia. The main sinuses are the:

◆ maxillary, in each cheekbone

◆ frontal, either side of the forehead, above the eyes

◆ sphenoid, between the upper part of the nose and between the eyes

◆ ethmoid, behind the bridge of the nose and between the eyes.

The sinuses contain fibres that slow the flow of lymph fluid through them and which enables macrophages to ingest microorganisms that could lead to infection.

Bones of the neck, chest and shoulder

Bone	Number	Location	Function
Cervical vertebrae	7	The neck.	These vertebrae form the top of the spinal column: the **atlas** is the first vertebra, which supports and connects with the skull and allows a nodding movement; the **axis** is the second vertebra, which allows rotation of the head.
Hyoid	1	An irregular U-shaped bone at the front of the neck.	Anchors and supports the tongue.
Thoracic vertebrae	12	Upper and middle back.	The ribcage joins to the thoracic vertebrae and protects the body's vital organs, i.e. heart and lungs.
Clavicle	2	Slender long bones at the base of the neck.	Commonly called the **collar bones**: these form a joint with the sternum and the scapula bones, allowing movement at the shoulder.
Scapula	2	Triangular, flat bones in the upper back.	Commonly called the **shoulder blades**: the scapulae provide attachment for muscles that move the arms. The **shoulder girdle**, which allows movement at the shoulder, is composed of the clavicles and the scapulae.
Humerus	2	The upper long bones of the arms.	Forms a joint with the scapulae: this is called a ball- and-socket joint and allows movement in any direction.
Sternum	1	The breastbone.	Protects the inner organs; provides a surface for muscle attachment and supports muscle movement. The sternum is connected to the ribs by cartilage.
Ribs	12 pairs	Upper body/chest area.	Protects inner organs such as the heart and lungs. The first 7 pairs attach to the sternum. The first 10 pairs attach to the thoracic vertebrae at the back. The 8th–10th pairs fuse with the rib above. The 11th and 12th pairs are called floating ribs as they are unattached at the front.

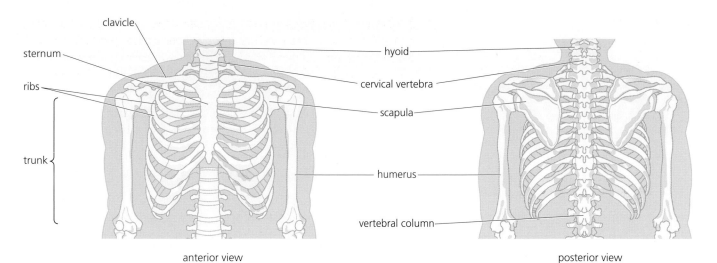

anterior view

posterior view

Bones of the neck, chest and shoulder girdle

Bones of the spine The spine is also referred to as the vertebral column. It is made up of irregular bones that support the skull, protect the spinal cord and give attachment to other bones. It is bound together by powerful ligaments. The curves in each area give the spine an 'S' shape, which helps balance the body's weight. You are required to know the bones of the cervical and thoracic vertebrae.

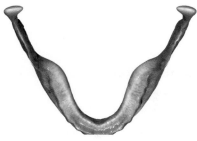

Hyoid bone

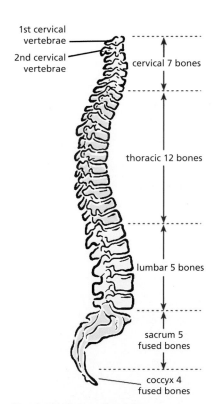

Vertebral column – the spine

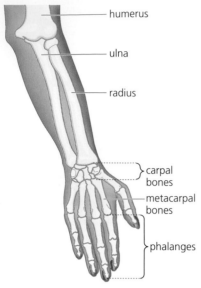

Bones of the hand, wrist and arm

Bones of the hand and arm

The wrist consists of eight small, irregular short **carpal** bones, which glide over one another to allow movement. This is called a **condyloid** or **gliding joint**. There are then five **metacarpal** or metacarpus, long bones that make up the palm of the hand.

The fingers are made up of 14 individual long bones called **phalanges** (the singular of phalanges is **phalanx**) – two in each of the thumbs and three in each of the fingers.

The arm is made up of three long bones: the **humerus** is the bone of the upper arm, from the shoulder to the elbow; the **radius** and **ulna** lie side by side in the lower arm, from the elbow to the wrist.

Having two bones in the lower arm makes it easier for your wrist to rotate. The movement that causes the palm to face downwards is called **pronation**; the movement that causes it to face upwards is called **supination**.

ALWAYS REMEMBER

When carrying out a hand massage and treatments you will move the hand into these positions.

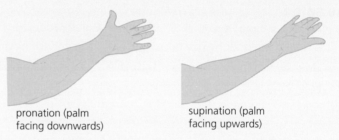

pronation (palm facing downwards)

supination (palm facing upwards)

Hand positions created by wrist rotation pronation and supination of the hand, wrist and lower arm

ALWAYS REMEMBER

Carpal Bones of the wrist

Starting at the thumb side, there are two rows of eight bones:

Upper row

1. Schaphoid   2. Lunate
3. Triquetral   4. Pisiform

Lower row

5. Trapezium   6. Trapezoid
7. Capitate   8. Hamate

ACTIVITY

Identifying bones in the hand

Look very closely at your hand. Can you identify where the bones are? Try feeling the bones with your other hand. How many can you feel?

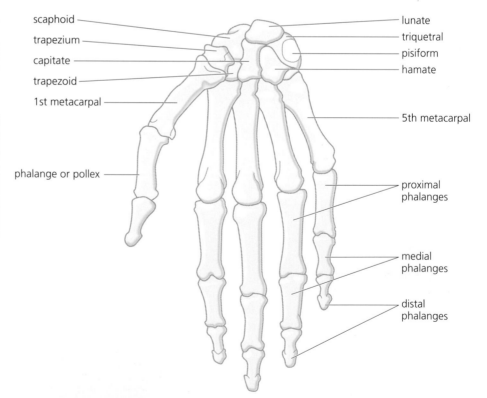

Bones of the hand and wrist

Bones of the foot and lower leg

The foot is made up of seven **tarsal** (ankle) bones, five **metatarsal** (ball of the foot) bones and 14 **phalanges** (toe bones). These bones fit together to form arches, which help to support the foot and to absorb the impact when we walk, run and jump.

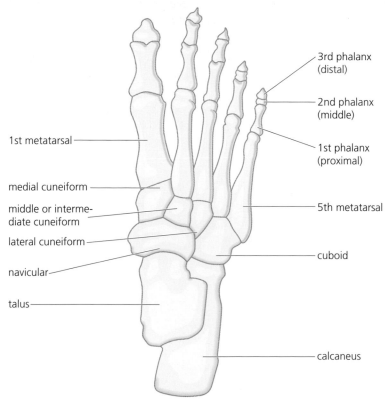

- 1st metatarsal
- medial cuneiform
- middle or interme-diate cuneiform
- lateral cuneiform
- navicular
- talus

- 3rd phalanx (distal)
- 2nd phalanx (middle)
- 1st phalanx (proximal)
- 5th metatarsal
- cuboid
- calcaneus

Bones of the foot

ALWAYS REMEMBER

Bones of the ankle

There are seven bones in the ankle: three cuneiform bones: medial, middle and lateral, navicular, cuboid, talus and calcaneus.

ALWAYS REMEMBER

Anatomical definitions

Medial: towards the midline (middle) of the body.

Lateral: away from the median (middle) line of the body. The outer side of the body.

Remembering this helps you to understand where a bone is by its name.

ALWAYS REMEMBER

Arches

Footprints made by bare feet show that only part of the foot touches the ground. Weight transfers from the heel to the big toe when walking. Feet with reduced arches are referred to as 'flat feet', caused by weak ligaments and tendons.

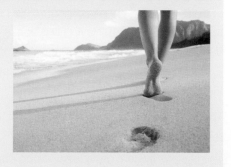

REVISION AID

How many bones form the:

a. wrist

b. hand

c. fingers?

The arches of the foot   The **arches** of the foot are created by the formation of the bones and joints, and supported by ligaments. These arches support the weight of the body and help to preserve balance when we walk on uneven surfaces. Clients with fallen arches may find discomfort when walking, especially longer distances.

The feet are designed to take the body weight. If a client has foot arch problems, they may complain of foot pain. This should be referred to a podiatrist, who will provide professional advice.

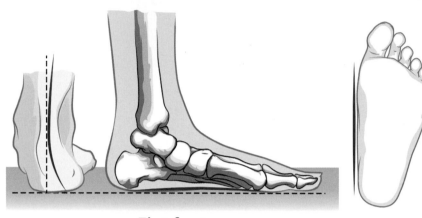

Flat foot

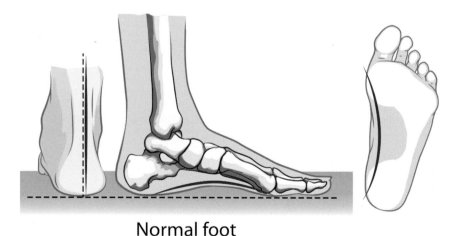

Normal foot

Arches

The bones of the lower leg   The lower leg is made up of two long bones, the **tibia** and the **fibula**. These bones have joints with the upper leg (at the knee) and with the foot (at the ankle). Having two bones in the lower leg – as with the forearm – allows a greater range of movement to be achieved at the ankle.

Above the lower bones of the leg is the thigh bone or femur, which is the longest bone in the body.

The knee bone is known as the patella, a seed-shaped bone classified as a sesamoid bone, which is a small bone located within a tendon.

The skeletal system provides a strong framework upon which muscles contract and relax to create movement.

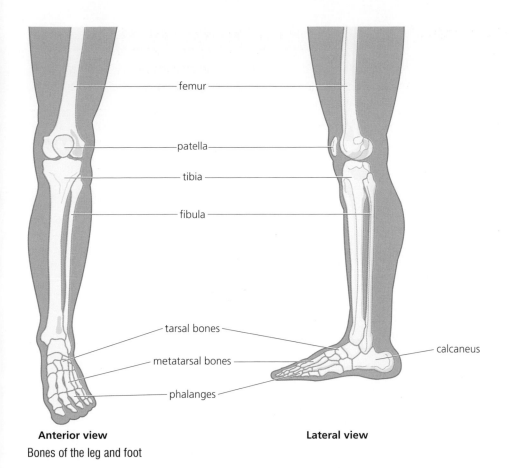

Anterior view   **Lateral view**

Bones of the leg and foot

The muscular system

Muscles are responsible for the movement of body parts. Each muscle is made up of a bundle of elastic fibres bound together in a sheath, the **fascia**. Muscular tissue contracts (shortens) and produces movement. They also enable us to maintain our posture and create heat. When the body temperature falls, an involuntary action of the muscles causes rapid contractions – the shivering action – to make heat.

Muscle tissue has the following properties:

◆ It has the ability to contract or shorten – contractability.

◆ It is extensible (when the extensor muscle in a joint contracts, the corresponding flexor muscle will be stretched or lengthened).

◆ It is elastic – following contraction or extension it returns to its original length.

◆ It is responsive – it contracts in response to nerve stimulation.

Origin and insertion

Skeletal muscle is usually anchored by a strong tendon to one bone. The point of attachment is known as the muscle's **origin**, normally the stationary end of the muscle. The muscle is likewise joined to a second bone: the attachment in this case is called the muscle's **insertion**, the end of the bone that moves. It is this second bone that is moved when the muscle contracts, pulling the two bones towards each other. (A different muscle, on the other side of the bone, has the opposite effect.) Not all muscles attach to bones, however: some insert into an adjacent muscle, or into the skin itself. The muscles with which we are concerned here are those of the face, the neck and shoulders, upper back and chest, arm, hand, lower leg and feet.

ALWAYS REMEMBER

Muscle attachment

Muscles are attached at both ends to ligaments, tendons, bones, skin and even each other. The origin is the part of the muscle that is attached to a stationary bone; the insertion is the other end, which is attached to a moveable part. During muscle contraction this part of the muscle moves.

TOP TIP

Terminology for action

If a muscle has 'flexor' or 'extensor' in front of the muscle name you will know what the action of the muscle is!

Flexor – bends a joint   *Extensor* – straightens a joint

Abduction – 'move away'   *Adduction* – 'move towards'

adduction – muscles pull limb towards body/fingers together to their usual position

abduction – muscles move limb etc. from usual position

extension   flexion

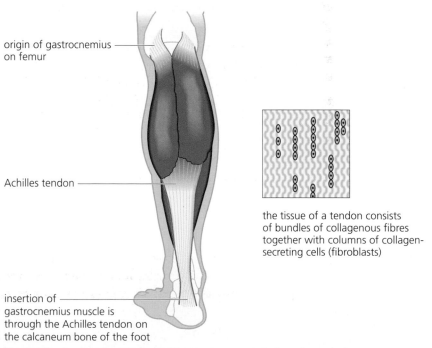

origin of gastrocnemius on femur

Achilles tendon

the tissue of a tendon consists of bundles of collagenous fibres together with columns of collagen-secreting cells (fibroblasts)

insertion of gastrocnemius muscle is through the Achilles tendon on the calcaneum bone of the foot

The Achilles tendon attaches the gastrocnemius muscle to the calcaneum bone

Muscles can also be felt under the skin – those near the surface are called **superficial muscles**. While these are the muscles you can feel when massaging, deeper muscles lying beneath these may be equally important at producing movement. Connective tissue is used to wrap bundles of muscle fibres and to surround the entire muscle. This connective tissue is drawn together at the ends of the muscle to form **tendons**, which attach the muscles to the bones. These are very strong attachments. Tuberosities (thickened and strengthened areas of bone) develop where the muscles are attached.

Muscular activity also increases muscle size – hypertophy – due to an increase in the size of its component fibres. With lack of use, or certain medical conditions, muscles lose their strength and waste away or atrophy.

Muscle tissue

There are different types of muscle that move either involuntarily or voluntarily. Involuntary muscle is made up of smooth or non-striated muscle that we do not control by will (e.g. the part of the eye muscle used when blinking) and striated (having a stripy appearance) or voluntary muscle. These muscles are attached to bones of the skeleton, so are referred to as skeletal muscles and cause movement, which we can control by will.

This type of muscle tissue is made up of many strands of small muscle fibres lying parallel to one another. Each fibre is composed of even smaller strands called myofibrils.

Nerve impulses stimulate muscle tissue to contract. The small fibres pull over each other, shortening the muscle causing it to move at its joint, creating body movement.

How do voluntary muscles contract?
Voluntary muscles contract by a system of sliding filaments. Each myofibril is made up of two types of filament – thin ones composed mainly of a protein called **actin** and thick ones composed mainly of a protein called **myosin**. These filaments partially overlap. When the muscle is stimulated to contract, the filaments pull over each other and overlap more. This shortens the muscle and increases its tension. The more the fibres pull together and overlap (until the actin fibres touch) the more tension is produced. Force increases as the muscle gets shorter and shorter.

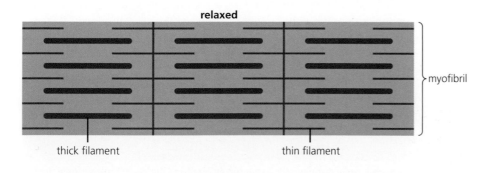

relaxed

thick filament   thin filament

myofibril

contracted

The sliding filament theory of muscle contraction

Voluntary (striated) muscle tissue

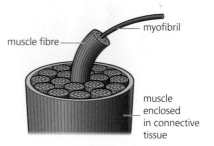

myofibril

muscle fibre

muscle enclosed in connective tissue

Muscle enclosed in connective tissue

Voluntary muscles contract only when stimulated by their nerve supply. Muscle contraction requires energy and this is supplied by tissue respiration taking place inside muscle cells. In this reaction, glucose and oxygen are used to supply the energy, and carbon dioxide and water are released as waste products.

Muscle tone

Muscles never completely relax – there are always a few contracted fibres in every muscle. These make the muscle slightly tense and this partial muscular tension is called **muscle tone**.

Muscle tone helps the body to stand upright and keeps the muscles prepared for immediate action. A slack or flaccid muscle is one with less than normal tone. Sometimes this is due to damage to the nerve supply. A muscle that is not used will become flaccid and then atrophy or waste away. **Flexors** are muscles that bend a limb; **extensors** are muscles that straighten a limb. We can only keep upright if the flexor and extensor muscles of joints are both partially contracted to keep the joints steady.

Disorders of the muscular system

- ◆ *Fatigue.* Lack of response by a muscle to continuous stimulation (i.e. it stops working) due to a lack of oxygen or the build up of lactic acid and carbon dioxide.

- ◆ *Muscle strain.* Injury resulting from over-stretched muscle.

- ◆ *Cramps.* An involuntary complete contraction in a muscle.

- ◆ *Muscular dystrophy.* A disease resulting in progressive degeneration of muscle groups.

- ◆ *Myasthenia gravis.* Chronic muscle fatigue, an autoimmune disorder where the receptors that receive nerve signals in the muscles become unresponsive and weaken.

Facial muscles

Many of the muscles located in the face are very small and are attached into another small muscle or the facial skin. When the muscles contract, they pull the facial skin in a particular way; it is this that creates the facial expression.

With age, the facial expressions that we make every day produce lines on the skin – frown lines. The amount of tension, or **tone**, also decreases with age. When performing facial treatments, the objective will often identify a requirement to maintain or improve the general tone of the facial muscles.

ALWAYS REMEMBER

Look for the term flexor and extensor in the muscle name. This will explain the action it performs.

ACTIVITY

Facial expressions

In front of a mirror, move the muscles of your face to create the expressions that you might form each day.

What expressions can you make? Which parts of your face are moving? Which facial muscles do you think you have contracted to create these expressions?

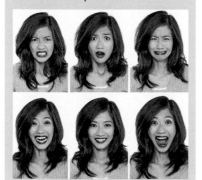

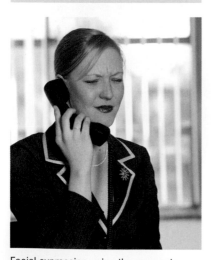

Facial expression using the corrugator muscle, creating a frown expression

TOP TIP

Facial expressions, created through muscles moving the skin around the eyes, cause crows' feet.

To reduce premature formation:

- ◆ Avoid squinting unnecessarily in bright sunlight; wear sunglasses.

- ◆ Have your eyes tested, especially if you feel you are straining your eyes to read.

- ◆ Avoid smoking.

- ◆ If you use a computer screen or other digital device regularly, ensure that you take regular breaks and use features and facilities that reduce glare.

- ◆ Handle the skin around the eye carefully.

- ◆ Use good quality skincare products designed for use around the eye.

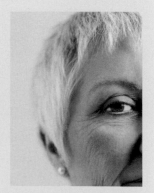

Crows feet

To balance and move the head and facial features, the muscles of the head, face and neck work together.

Muscles of facial expression

Muscle	Expression	Location	Action
Frontalis	Surprise	The forehead.	Raises the eyebrows; causes wrinkling across forehead.
Corrugator	Frown	Between the eyebrows.	Draws the eyebrows down and together.
Orbicularis oculi	Winking	Surrounds the eyes.	Closes the eyelid.
Risorius	Grinning	Extends diagonally, from the masseter muscle to the corners of the mouth.	Draws mouth corners outwards and backwards.
Buccinator	Blowing	Inside the cheeks between the upper and lower jaw.	Compresses the cheeks.
Zygomaticus, major and minor muscles	Smiling, laughing	Extend diagonally from the zygomatic (cheekbone) to the corners of the mouth.	Lifts the corners of the mouth backwards and upwards.

(Continued)

Muscle	Expression	Location	Action
Procerus procerus	Distaste distaste	Covers the bridge of the nose.	Draws down eyebrows and wrinkles the skin over the bridge of the nose.
Nasalis nasalis	Anger anger	Covers the front of the nose and surrounds the nostrils.	Opens and closes the nasal openings.
Levator labii levator labii superioris	Distaste	Surrounds the upper lip.	Raises and draws back the upper lips and nostrils.
Depressor labii depressor labii inferioris	Sulking	Surrounds the lower lip.	Pulls down the lower lip and draws it slightly to one side.
Orbicularis oris orbicularis oris	Pout, kiss, doubt	Surrounds the mouth.	Purses the lip (as in blowing or kissing); closes the mouth.
Triangularis triangularis	Sadness	The corner of the lower lip extends over the chin.	Draws down the mouth's corners.

(Continued)

Muscle	Expression	Location	Action
Mentalis	Doubt	Covers the front of the chin.	Raises the lower lip, causing the chin to wrinkle.
Platysma	Fear, horror	The sides of the neck and chin.	Draws the mouth's corners downwards and backwards.

"Two eyebrows will never be the same and that is because of the muscles below. The side of your face, which is the same as the hand you write with, will be stronger. Ensure the client's facial muscles are relaxed before beginning the treatment as this can alter the shape you are trying to create."

Shavata Singh

ALWAYS REMEMBER

Nerves of the face

Almost all facial muscles are controlled by the 7th cranial or facial nerve, which stimulates their movement.

ACTIVITY

Facial exercises

It is a good idea to provide the client with facial exercises they can practise at home to exercise the muscles! This is relevant when the client's treatment objective is to improve facial skin and muscle tone. For example, tense the muscles of the face, jaw and neck as if trying to push against an object. Repeat 8-10 times, ideally twice per day. Practise these exercises yourself so you will be able to accurately demonstrate them to the client.

REVISION AID

Which muscles compress the cheek, for example when you are blowing?

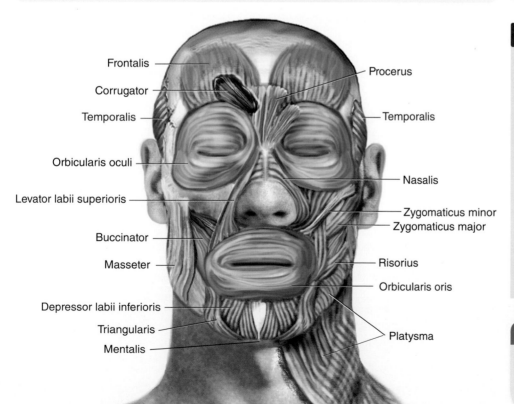

Muscles of the face and neck

"Make sure you know about the facial muscles; they may be small but there are more than 50 of them and keeping them toned helps to maintain a youthful appearance. Facial massage is a useful skill, which will help to maintain the general tone of the facial muscles. You could also encourage your clients to exercise their facial muscles by creating a routine for them."

Charlotte Gabriella Savoury

Muscles of mastication   The muscles responsible for the movement of the lower jawbone (the **mandible**) when chewing are called the muscles of mastication.

Muscles of mastication

Muscle	Location	Action
Masseter	The cheek area: extends from the zygomatic bone to the mandible.	Clenches the teeth; closes and raises the lower jaw.
Temporalis	Extends from the temple region at the side of the head to the mandible.	Raises the jaw and draws it backwards, as in chewing.

Muscles that move the head

Muscle	Location	Action
Sternocleidomastoid	Runs from the sternum to the clavicle bone and the temporal bone; runs down the side of the front of the neck.	Flexes the neck; rotates and lowers the head.
Trapezius	A large triangular muscle, covering the back of the neck and the upper back.	Draws the head backwards and allows movement at the shoulder.
Occipitalis	Covers the back of the base of the skull.	Draws scalp backwards.

Muscles of the upper body

When massaging the shoulder area you will cover the following muscles of the upper body.

Muscle	Location	Action
Pectoralis major	Across the upper chest (underneath the breasts) from the clavicle, sternum and ribs to the top of the humerus, forming the front wall of the axilla.	Used in throwing and climbing to adduct the arm, drawing it forwards and rotating it medially.
Pectoralis minor	Underneath the pectoralis major. Its origin is the third, fourth and fifth ribs and it inserts into the outer corner of the scapula.	Draws the shoulder downwards and forwards.
Deltoid	Over the top of the shoulder from the clavicle and scapula to the upper part of the humerus.	Abducts the arm to a horizontal position; aids in further abduction and in drawing the arm backwards and forwards.

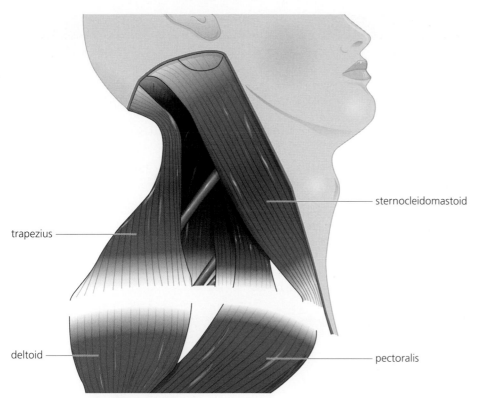

sternocleidomastoid

trapezius

deltoid

pectoralis

Muscles that move the head and upper body

TOP TIP

An adult head weighs about 5 kg; strong muscles of the neck and back are required to allow movement of the head. Remember that these areas will often suffer from tension in the muscles when performing head and neck manual massage.

Adequate support of the head and neck should be provided. Always check client comfort.

ALWAYS REMEMBER

Muscles that move the head assist those of facial expression when communicating, for example nodding the head.

Muscles of the arm and hand

Muscle	Location	Action
Brachioradialis	On the thumb side of the forearm; its origin is at the shaft of the humerus, its insertion is at the end of the radius bone.	Flexes the arm at the elbow.
Flexor carpi radialis	Middle of the forearm.	Flexes and abducts the wrist.
Flexi carpi ulnaris	Front of the forearm.	Flexes and adducts the wrist joint in towards the body.
Extensor carpi radialis	Thumb side of the forearm.	Extends and abducts the hand and wrist.
Extensor carpi ulnaris	Back of the forearm.	Extends and adducts the wrist.
Flexor digitorum tendons	Front of fingers.	Flexes the fingers when contracted.
Extensor digitorum tendons	Back of fingers.	Extends the fingers when contracted.
Flexor pollicis longus	Thumbside of forearm, between the middle of the forearm to the base of the thumb.	Flexion of the thumb and wrist.
Extensor pollicis longus	Thumbside of forearm, from the middle of the forearm to the base of the thumb.	Extension of the wrist and thumb.
Palmaris Longus	Front of forearm.	Flexes wrist.

(Continued)

Muscle	Location	Action
Thenar muscles	In the palm of the hand, below the thumb.	Flexes the thumb and moves it outwards and inwards.
Hypothenar muscles	In the palm of the hand, below the little finger.	Flexes the little finger and moves it outwards and inwards.

REVISION AID

Name three key muscles of the shoulder and lower arm.

ACTIVITY

Observing the tendons

Hold your palm face upwards, with your sleeve pulled back so that you can see your forearm. Move the fingers individually towards the palm. Can you see the tendons moving?

The muscles of the hand and forearm

The hand and fingers are moved primarily by muscles (see table above) and tendons in the forearm. These muscles contract, pulling the tendons, and thereby move the fingers much as a puppet is moved by strings.

The muscles that bend the wrist, drawing it towards the forearm, are **flexors**; other muscles, **extensors**, straighten the wrist and the hand.

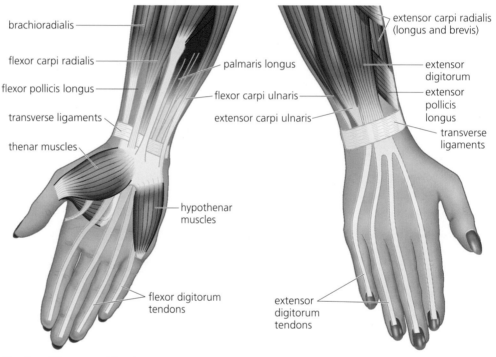

Muscles of the arm and hand

Muscles and tendons of the lower leg and foot

Muscle	Location	Action
Gastrocnemius	Calf of the leg.	Flexes the knee; plantar-flexes the foot.
Soleus	Calf of the leg, below the gastrocnemius (both calf muscles insert through the Achilles tendon into the heel).	Plantar-flexes the foot (flexes and points the toe down) both calf muscles are used to push off, assisting forwards motion when walking and running.
Peroneus longus	Lateral side of the lower leg.	Plantar flexes the foot (flexes and points the toes down). Assists forward motion when walking or running.

(Continued)

Muscle	Location	Action
Tibialis anterior	Front of the lower leg.	Inverts the foot (turns sole inwards); dorsiflexes the foot (flexes and points the toes up); rotates foot outwards; supports the medial longitudinal arch of the foot when walking or running.
Extensor digitorum longus	Lateral side of the front of the lower leg.	Dorsiflexes the foot up at the ankle and extends the toes.
Flexor digitorum longus	Front of lower leg to the toes.	Plantar-flexes foot downwards and inverts the foot; helps the toes to grip; supports the lateral longitudinal arch of the foot.
Extensor hallucis longus	Arises from the middle front surface of the fibula, passing the transverse aspect of the foot and inserting into the big toe.	Extends the big toe.
Flexor hallucis longus	Arises from the back of the lower leg and inserts to the plantar aspect of the foot to the base of the big toe.	Flexes the big toe and pushes the foot off the ground when walking.
Achilles tendon	Attached to the soleus and gastrocnemius down to the heel.	Raises the foot when related muscle contracts.
Extensor digitorum tendons	Tops of toes.	Straightens the toes when related muscle contracts.
Flexor digitorum tendons	Underneath the toes.	Bends the toes when related muscle contracts.

The muscles of the foot and lower leg

The muscles of the foot work together to help move the body when walking and running. In a similar way to the movement of the hand, the foot is moved primarily by muscles in the lower leg; these pull on tendons, which in turn move the feet and toes.

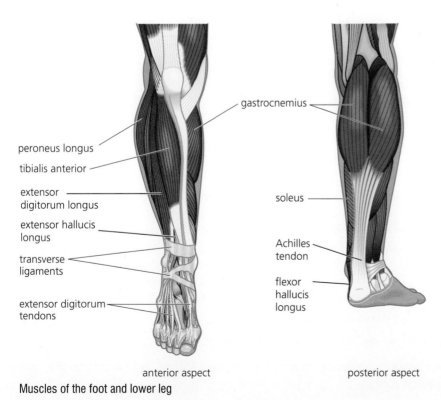

Muscles of the foot and lower leg

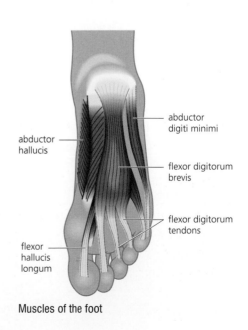

Muscles of the foot

The nervous system

The nervous system informs the body about internal and external conditions affecting it. Information is analysed and signals are sent to cells initiating a response. All systems of the body are controlled and co-ordinated by the nervous system.

Divisions of the nervous system   The nervous system is made up of two main divisions:

◆ Central Nervous System (CNS) – the main control centre of the nervous system.

◆ Peripheral Nervous System (PNS), which is made up of nerves that allow communication from the CNS to the rest of the body.

The autonomic nervous system (ANS), is part of the PNS. It consists of two separate parts: the sympathetic and parasympathetic systems. The sympathetic system increases body activity and processes, whereas the parasympathetic system slows down body activity and processes. In synergy, the ANS aims to ensure equilibrium in the body for healthy, normal functioning.

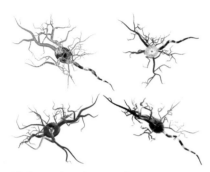

3D illustration of nerve cells

The central nervous system (CNS)

The central nervous system (CNS) consists of:

◆ the brain, protected and surrounded by the skull

◆ the spinal cord, which runs from the brain to the vertebral column and is protected by the vertebral bones.

The CNS co-ordinates the activities of the entire body. Nerves transmit instructions through impulses to all parts of the body in order to stimulate organs to act. It controls voluntary body movement.

The brain is the central communication system, monitoring and controlling the body's activities. It is composed of several parts, each of which performs several functions. Sensations are received, decoded and a response is initiated.

The spinal cord relays nerve impulses to and from the brain and the peripheral nervous system. This helps to maintain the body's internal balance by initiating immediate responses to stimuli.

The peripheral nervous system (PNS)

Cranial nerves   Twelve pairs of cranial nerves emerge from the brain. Some cranial nerves are sensory nerves. The second cranial nerve (the optic nerve) contains only sensory nerve fibres. It supplies the eye and is the nerve of sight. The twelfth cranial nerve is primarily a **motor nerve**. It contains mainly motor fibres and supplies the tongue muscles. (The sensory fibres in this nerve transmit information about the position of the tongue.) Other cranial nerves such as the fifth (trigeminal) nerve are called mixed nerves as they contain both motor fibres (to supply muscles) and sensory fibres (to relay sensations).

Most cranial nerves are named after the body part they control.

The nerves of the peripheral system communicate information to and from the central nervous system (CNS).

Nerves of the face and neck Cranial nerves control muscles in the head and neck region, or carry nerve impulses from the sense organs to the brain. Those of concern to you when performing a facial service are as follows:

◆ The 5th cranial nerve, or **trigeminal**, controls the muscles involved in mastication (chewing) and passes on sensory information from the face, such as the eyes.

◆ The 7th cranial nerve, or **facial**, controls the muscles involved in facial expression.

◆ The 11th cranial nerve, or **accessory**, controls the muscles involved in moving the head, the sterno-cleido-mastoid and trapezius muscle.

5th cranial nerve

This nerve carries messages to the brain from the sensory nerves of the skin, the teeth, the nose and the mouth. It also stimulates the motor nerve to create the chewing action when eating. The 5th cranial nerve has three branches:

◆ The **ophthalmic nerve** serves the tear glands of the eye, the skin of the forehead and the upper cheeks.

◆ The **maxillary nerve** serves the upper jaw and the mouth.

◆ The **mandibular nerve** serves the lower jaw muscle, the teeth and the muscle involved with chewing.

7th cranial nerve

This nerve passes through the temporal bone and behind the ear, and then divides. It serves the ear muscle and the muscles of facial expression, the tongue and the palate. This nerve has five branches:

◆ The **temporal nerve** serves the orbicularis oculi and the frontalis muscles.

◆ The **zygomatic nerve** serves the eye muscles.

◆ The **buccal nerve** serves the upper lip and the sides of the nose.

◆ The **mandibular nerve** serves the lower lip and the mentalis muscle of the chin.

◆ The **cervical nerve** serves the platysma muscle of the neck.

11th cranial nerve

This nerve serves the sternocleidomastoid and trapezius muscles of the neck; its function is to move the head and shoulders.

The nervous system consists of **nerve** cells called **neurones**, with nerve fibres. Neurones are long, narrow and delicate, containing a large central nucleus, and are capable of transmitting messages to other neurones, see images below: 'A sensory neurone receiving information' and 'A motor neurone'.

Nerve fibres are grouped into bundles according to the information they convey. They make contact with the spinal cord through gaps in-between the vertebral bones.

Dendrites are tiny branches of the nerve cell that receive impulses and pass them to the cell body. Axons are long fibres that send impulses away from the cell body.

The PNS consists of nerves that link the various parts of the body with the CNS. When a nerve carries information towards the CNS, it is described as an afferent or sensory nerve. These are found in the dermis of the skin, (responding to touch, pain, pressure and temperature etc.) muscles, tendons and joints, nose, mouth and eye area. They receive information that enables the CNS to make a suitable response.

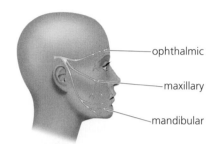

ophthalmic

maxillary

mandibular

5th cranial nerve

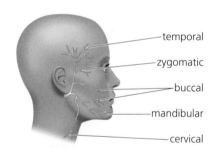

temporal

zygomatic

buccal

mandibular

cervical

7th cranial nerve

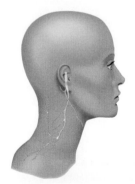

11th cranial nerve

When a nerve carries information away from the CNS, it is described as an efferent nerve or motor nerve. Information is acted on that is sent from the CNS to carry out a particular response, typically muscle movement or the secretion of chemicals from a gland.

Each neurone stimulates up to 2000 muscle fibres depending on the muscle movement to be performed.

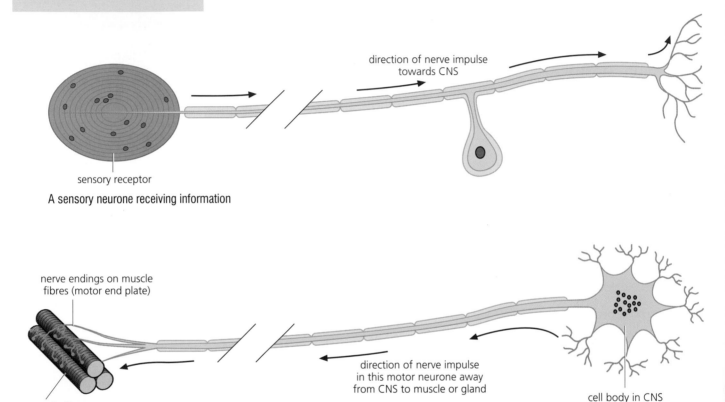

A sensory neurone receiving information

A motor neurone

Passage of impulses from one neurone to another Information passes along neurones to and from the CNS. Inside the CNS, impulses pass from one neurone to another even though individual neurones never touch. When an impulse reaches the end of the nerve fibre a chemical is released. This chemical is called a **neurotransmitter** substance. The chemical passes across a tiny gap and is taken up by an adjacent neurone, generating an electrical impulse in that neurone. The gap between adjacent neurones is called a **synapse**.

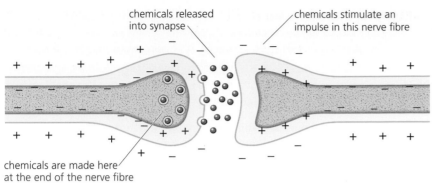

chemicals released into synapse

chemicals stimulate an impulse in this nerve fibre

chemicals are made here at the end of the nerve fibre

Passage of an impulse across a synapse

When neurotransmitters land at their receptor sites they can stimulate or slow down reaction at the receiving cell. Both responses are important to relay the correct message through the nervous system.

Neurones can stimulate muscle fibres to contract. The **motor point** is where a motor nerve enters a muscle. When stimulated by a motor nerve, muscle contraction occurs.

Voluntary and reflex actions

Voluntary actions are always initiated by the brain and we can control these actions. Examples are speaking and walking. A reflex action is a quick, involuntary response to a stimulus. For example, on picking up an unexpectedly hot plate you may automatically drop it. This happens because pain receptors in your hand have been stimulated. Impulses pass via sensory nerve fibres to the spinal cord and are transmitted via relay neurones to motor neurones. Impulses pass to the arm muscles, which are stimulated to contract and the plate is dropped. A reflex involving the spinal cord is called a **spinal reflex**. Impulses will also pass up the spinal cord to the brain so you become aware of what you have done. This may stimulate a secondary response such as yelling 'OW'!

Coughing, sneezing, blinking and swallowing are also reflexes but these are cranial (involving the brain) rather than spinal reflexes.

impulses also pass to brain so you realise what has happened

impulses return via motor neurones to the muscles in the arm causing the hot plate to be dropped

impulses pass to spinal cord via sensory neurones

heat and pain receptors in skin of hand stimulated by hot plate

Diagram of a simple reflex arc

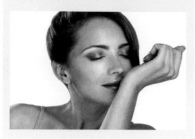

The olfactory system The first cranial nerve is called the olfactory nerve. It is a sensory nerve, giving us our sense of smell. Olfactory receptors are present in the upper nasal passages, which are coated with watery mucus. Some chemicals dissolve in this watery mucus and stimulate the receptors of the sensory cells. Nerve fibres from the receptors join to form the olfactory nerves, which pass through the ethmoid bone into the olfactory bulbs. These lie below the frontal lobes of the cerebrum, the major part of the forebrain.

From the olfactory lobes, nerve fibres run to the olfactory centre of the brain along the olfactory tract. Here, in the olfactory centre, the impulses are interpreted as sensations of smell.

Smells may influence the behaviour of a person. Pheromones are scents given off by animals (including humans) to encourage sexual attention. They may be responsible for male–female attraction and male–male acts of aggression. Food must have a pleasant aroma for us to enjoy it.

The **limbic system** is involved in emotions such as pain, pleasure, anger, fear, sorrow, sexual feelings and affection. It consists of a group of structures that encircle the brain stem. It also plays a part in memory and behaviour. Massage using pre-blended oils takes advantage of this limbic response, using the effects of the aroma of essential oils to produce a range of responses. These may involve feelings of relaxation and wellbeing.

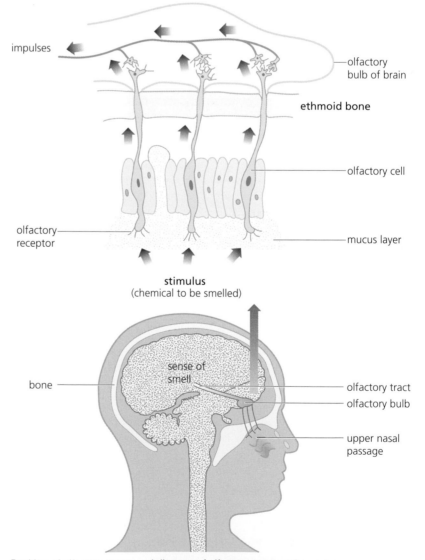

Position of olfactory centre and diagram of olfactory nerve and receptors

The autonomic nervous system

The autonomic nervous system is the division of the peripheral nervous system which controls the involuntary activities of smooth muscle, cardiac muscle and glands. It therefore regulates the size of the pupil, vasodilation and vasoconstriction (see *Flow of blood in arteries* section in this chapter), the heart rate, movements of the gut and the secretion of most glands. There are two divisions, called the **sympathetic** and **parasympathetic**. Many organs receive a supply from each division. **Fibres** from one division stimulate the organ while fibres from the other division inhibit it.

The parasympathetic division is stimulated in times of relaxation. Fibres of this division stimulate digestion and absorption of food.

Although this system is called autonomic, suggesting that we exert no conscious control over its activities, research has shown that transcendental meditation (yoga) seems to inactivate the sympathetic division and has a calming effect on the body.

Disorders of the nervous system

◆ *Multiple sclerosis*. Degeneration of the nervous tissue in the brain and spinal cord causing progressive muscle weakness.

◆ *Neuralgia*. Irritation and inflammation of the nerve, with pain felt along the nerve.

◆ *Stroke*. Interruption of blood supply to the brain, causing loss of function to the body part affected.

◆ *Sciatica*. Inflammation of the sciatic nerve, the longest single nerve in the body. Usually caused by compression of the nerve by a slipped vertebral disc.

◆ *Epilepsy*. Lack of consciousness, which may be accompanied by seizures.

◆ *Bells palsy*. Compression of the facial nerve, causing inflammation and paralysis of one side of the face, which droops.

◆ *Cerebral palsy*. Disorders relating to lack of muscle control, resulting from damage to the developing brain before or during childbirth.

◆ *Migraine*. Severe headache, which may be accompanied by feelings of nausea and vomiting. Flashing lights before the eyes often accompanies the onset of the migraine.

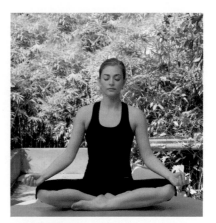

Yoga/meditation

The circulatory system

The circulatory system consists of blood, blood vessels and the heart. It has an essential function to transport nutrients, gases, waste and other materials through every part of the body. Its essential role is to maintain the chemical balance in the body known as **homeostasis**.

The heart

The circulation of blood is under the control of the heart. The heart is a muscular organ the size of a clenched fist that acts as a pump, located behind the sternum in the chest. It keeps the blood circulating through the body's blood vessels.

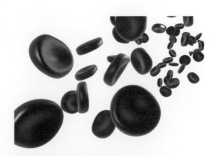

Isolated red blood cells

Blood vessels

There are three main kinds of blood vessel: **arteries**, **veins** and **capillaries**. Arteries are thick, elastic-walled vessels that carry blood away from the heart. Every time the heart contracts to pump blood around the body, the elastic walls become stretched and then recoil. This absorbs and smoothes the surges from the heart and helps to push the blood forwards. This stretching and recoiling is felt as a pulse.

Arteries lead into the main organs where they divide into smaller vessels arterioles, which deliver blood to capillaries. These are the smallest blood vessels. Capillaries are about the diameter of a hair. They are close to all the cells of the body, bringing supplies of oxygen and nutrients and carrying away products from the cells.

The capillary network then reforms into larger vessels called veins to deliver blood back to the heart. The blood flows much more slowly and evenly in veins. They do not pulsate like arteries. The veins often pass through the muscles. Each time muscles contract, veins

Artery and Vein

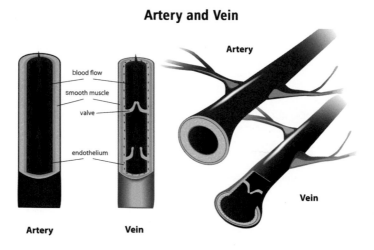

Circulatory system capillary blood flow

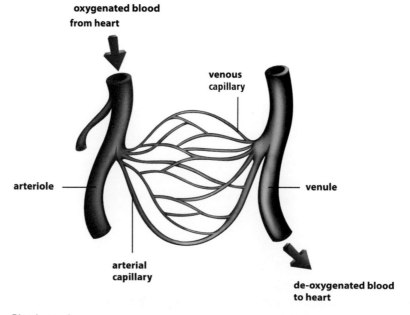

Blood vessels

are squeezed and blood is pushed along. To make sure the blood is squeezed along in the right direction, many veins have valves to stop blood flowing backwards. The veins have much thinner walls than arteries. This means that they are more easily compressed by the muscles they pass through. Veins are divided into smaller vessels called venules and collect blood from capillaries to return to the heart.

Flow of blood in arteries

The flow of blood in the arteries is maintained by blood pressure caused by the forceful contractions of the ventricles of the heart pushing blood into them. Blood pressure is maintained by the elastic walls of the large arteries, which stretch to accept the blood from the ventricles and then recoil to push the blood on its way.

Blood flow through the organs Capillary networks are found through each major organ of the body including the skin.

Blood flow through the skin Normal body temperature is 36.8°C. Blood circulating through the internal organs or through working muscles therefore becomes warm. If the body temperature starts to rise, then allowing blood to pass near the skin surface releases some of this heat to the environment. This will check the rise in temperature. The skin will appear red and may feel warm to the touch.

The blood vessels in the skin are organised so that blood can either flow near the skin surface or can pass through shunt vessels, which lie deeper in the dermis. The skin capillaries are used to help regulate body temperature. If the body temperature begins to drop, then blood flows deeper through the dermis, releasing less heat to the environment. This process of **vasodilation** and **vasoconstriction** is controlled by the autonomic nervous system – nerves control the arterioles that feed the capillary networks through the skin.

Erythema is reddening of the skin caused by dilation of the blood vessels controlling local capillary networks in areas of the skin affected by injury or infection.

blood flow through skin when hot – vasodilation	blood flow through skin when cold – vasoconstriction
blood flows closer to epidermis epidermis	capillaries constricted
shunt vessel constricted	blood flows deep in dermis

Vasodilation and vasoconstriction

Flow of blood in veins

The flow of blood in veins is slower and under less pressure than the flow in arteries. Veins tend to pass through muscles of the body where they can be squeezed so that the blood

REVISION AID
What is the difference between an artery and a vein?

TOP TIP

Blood pressure

Pulse rate relates to the speed of the heartbeat. The strength of the pulse relates to the pressure of blood flow leaving the heart.

Blood pressure increases during activity and decreases during rest.

Relaxing services such as facial massage aim to lower the blood pressure.

TOP TIP

Varicose veins

If your occupation requires you to sit or stand for long periods, you may get swollen feet and ankles or even varicose veins. Keep the blood circulating by exercising those leg muscles.

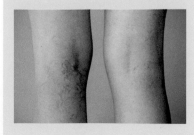

is helped along. This is especially important in the legs, where blood is being returned against gravity.

Varicose veins are a result of incompetent valves that allow blood to flow backwards, stretching and weakening the walls of the vein. The veins on the surface of the leg (and therefore not surrounded by muscle tissue) are the ones most commonly affected as gravity forces the blood back down the leg.

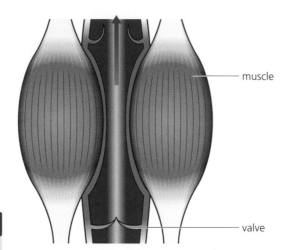

muscle

muscles squeeze the blood in the veins back towards the heart

valve

Control of blood flow by valves

Fluids of the body

All cells need a constant supply of energy and raw materials, and a means of removing waste products.

◆ Epidermal cells need energy to continue dividing, and supplies of raw materials to manufacture new cells.

◆ Muscle cells need energy to contract, and become fatigued if their waste products are not removed efficiently.

◆ Neurones need energy in order to transmit impulses.

The fluids of the body are responsible for delivering whatever the cells require and for removing any waste products. The three principle body fluids are:

◆ blood

◆ tissue fluid

◆ lymph.

Blood

Functions of blood Inside the tissues, some fluid leaks from the capillaries as blood passes through them. When this fluid leaves the capillaries to enter the tissues it becomes tissue fluid.

Blood circulates through the blood vessels (arteries, arterioles, capillaries, venules and veins), collecting oxygen from the lungs and delivering it to the cells of the body.

Blood transports various substances around the body:

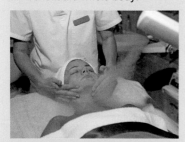

◆ Glucose is carried in the blood to be used by the cells together with the oxygen to supply energy.

◆ Blood supplies other raw materials to build or maintain cells or to manufacture products such as secretions.

◆ Blood carries oxygen from our lungs and nutrients from our digested food to supply energy – these allow the cells to develop and divide, and the muscles to function.

◆ Blood carries waste products such as water, urea and carbon dioxide from the cells and tissues away for removal from the body.

◆ Blood carries white blood cells that produce antibodies that allow the body to prevent or fight disease. It also contains platelets and other substances which help blood to clot and heal injuries.

◆ Blood transports hormones, the body's chemical messengers from endocrine glands, to their target tissue to cause a particular response.

◆ Blood absorbs heat from organs and tissues such as the liver, it helps to maintain the body temperature at 36.8°C: varying blood flow near to the skin surface increases or diminishes heat loss.

The main constituents of blood Blood is an alkaline fluid and consists of the following:

◆ *Plasma.* Constitutes 50 per cent of blood and is a straw-coloured liquid: mainly water with foods and carbon dioxide.

◆ *Red blood cells (erythrocytes).* Constitute 40–50 per cent of blood. These cells appear red because they contain haemoglobin, a protein responsible for their colour, which carries oxygen from the lungs to the body cells.

◆ *White blood cells (leucocytes).* There are several types of white blood cells (lymphocytes, granulocytes and monocytes); their main role is to protect the body by destroying foreign bodies and dead cells, and carry away the debris (a process known as **phagocytosis**).

◆ *Platelets (thrombocytes).* When blood is exposed to air, as happens when the skin is injured, these cells bind together to form a clot. This prevents bacteria entering and reduces blood loss. White blood cells and platelets constitute 1–2 per cent of blood.

◆ *Other chemicals.* Hormones also are transported in the blood – chemical messages to target tissues.

Tissue fluid

This fluid carries essential oxygen and nutrients to the cells. These useful substances are taken up by the cells and exchanged for waste products such as carbon dioxide. Some of the fluid containing waste products will then re-enter the capillaries and be carried by the blood back to the heart.

Lymph

It is not as easy for the fluid to get back into the blood capillaries as it is to leave them, so excess fluid, together with waste products, collects in **lymph capillaries** and is carried

> **REVISION AID**
>
> Which blood vessels are found nearest the skin's surface?

> **ALWAYS REMEMBER**
>
> **Blood transport system**
>
> Blood is made up of a collection of specialised cells suspended in liquid called plasma, supplying the needs of the body's cells and keeping the body healthy. It is transported around the body by a network of vessels (arteries, capillaries and veins) with a length of 90 000 miles.

though lymph vessels. Lymph passes through lymph nodes for processing before it is emptied back into the blood circulation close to the heart.

The diagram illustrates the exchange of blood, tissue fluid and lymph as blood flows through the capillaries.

Exchange of blood, tissue fluid and lymph

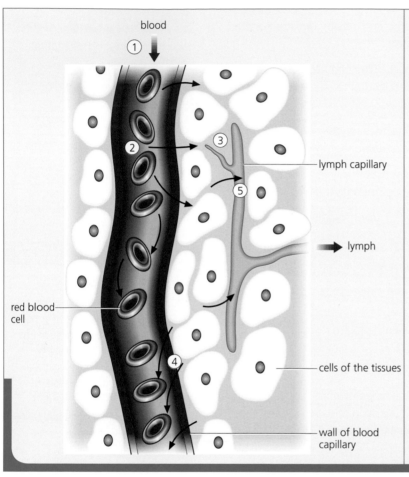

blood

lymph capillary

lymph

red blood cell

cells of the tissues

wall of blood capillary

1. The blood flowing into the capillary network is under high pressure. The liquid part of the blood is forced through the walls of the capillary.

2. Larger proteins and blood cells remain in the capillaries.

3. The fluid has now become tissue fluid. It supplies the cells and removes the waste.

4. Some fluid will be drawn back into the capillaries.

5. Other fluid, together with large molecules like proteins from the cells, is drawn into the very porous lymph capillaries.

Blood supply to and from the head

As previously stated, blood leaving the heart is carried in large, elastic tubes called **arteries**. The blood to the head arrives via the **carotid arteries**, which are connected via other main arteries to the heart. There are two main carotid arteries, one on each side of the neck.

These arteries divide into smaller branches, the *internal carotid* and the **external carotid**. The **internal carotid artery** passes the temporal bone and enters the head, taking blood to the brain. The external carotid artery stays outside the skull and divides into branches:

◆ The **occipital branch** supplies the back of the head and the scalp.

◆ The **temporal branch** supplies the sides of the face, the head, the scalp and the skin.

◆ The **facial branch** supplies the muscles and tissues of the face.

◆ The **posterior auricular** branch supplies the scalp, back and above the ear.

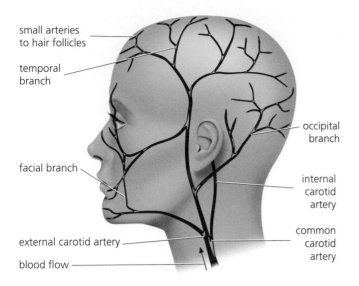

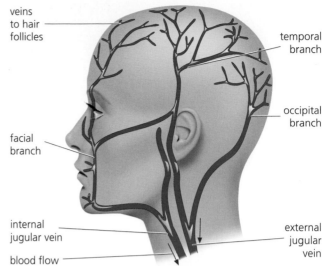

The blood supply to and from the head

These arteries also divide repeatedly; successive vessels becoming smaller and smaller until they form tiny blood **capillaries**. These vessels are just one cell thick, allowing substances carried in the blood to pass through them into the **tissue fluid**, which bathes and nourishes the cells of the various body tissues.

The blood capillaries begin to join up again, forming first small vessels called **venules**, then larger vessels called **veins**. These return the blood to the heart.

Veins are less elastic than arteries and are closer to the skin's surface. Along their course are **valves**, which prevent the backflow of blood.

The main veins are the external and internal jugular veins. The **internal jugular vein** and its main branch, the **facial vein**, carry blood from the face and head. The **external jugular** vein carries blood from the scalp and has two branches: the **occipital branch** and the **temporal branch**. The jugular veins join to enter the **subclavian vein**, which lies above the clavicle.

Blood returns to the heart, which pumps it to the lungs, where the red blood cells take on fresh oxygen and where carbon dioxide is expelled from the blood. The blood returns to the heart and begins its next journey around the body.

Blood supply to and from the arm and hand
The arm and hand are nourished by a system of arteries that carry oxygen-rich blood to the tissues. You can see the colour of the blood from the capillaries beneath the nail: these give the nail bed its pink colour.

The brachial artery supplies blood to the upper arm. This branches into the ulnar and radial arteries, which supply the forearm and fingers. The radial and ulnar arteries are connected across the palm by the superficial and deep palmar arches. These arteries divide to form the metacarpal and digital arteries, which supply the palm and fingers.

Veins of the arms and hands
Veins deliver deoxygenated blood back to the heart. Blood with its oxygen removed appears blue. Veins often pass through muscles. Each time muscles contract, veins are squeezed and the blood is pushed along. Massage is particularly beneficial in this process.

Blood in the digital veins drains blood from the fingers. The palmar venous arches drain blood from the hands. The cephalic and basilic veins drain blood from the forearm.

ALWAYS REMEMBER

Temporal branches

Some of the carotid artery's important temporal branches are:

◆ Frontal: supplies the forehead.
◆ Parietal: supplies the top and sides of the head.
◆ Transverse: supplies the masseter muscle.
◆ Middle temporal: supplies the temples and the eyelids.
◆ Anterior auricular: supplies the front part of the ear.

HEALTH & SAFETY

Capillaries

The strength and elasticity of the capillary walls can be damaged, for example by a blow to the tissues. Broken capillaries are capillaries whose elasticity is damaged and they remain constantly dilated with blood.

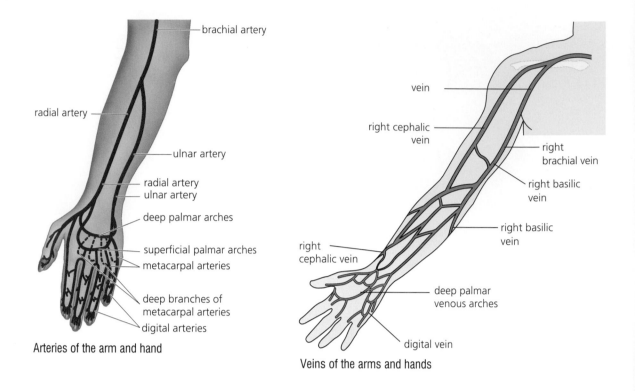

Arteries of the arm and hand

Veins of the arms and hands

Blood supply to and from the foot and lower leg The lower leg and the feet are nourished by a system of arteries that carry oxygen-rich blood to the tissues.

When it is cold, and when the circulation is poor, insufficient blood reaches the hands and feet and they feel cold. Severe circulation problems in the hands and feet may lead to **chilblains**.

The anterior tibial artery supplies blood to the lower leg and foot. The peroneal artery branches off the posterior tibial artery. At the ankle the anterior tibial artery becomes the dorsalis pedis artery. The posterior tibial artery divides at the ankle to form the medial and lateral plantar arteries. The plantar and dorsalis pedis arteries supply the digital arteries of the toes.

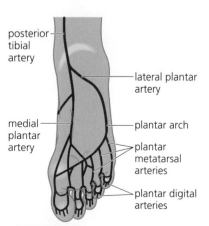

Arteries of the foot

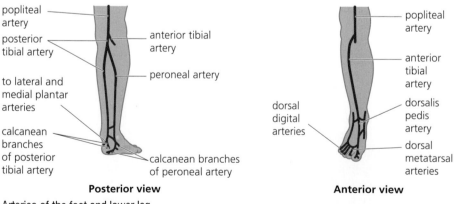

Posterior view

Anterior view

Arteries of the foot and lower leg

The veins of the foot and lower leg The digital veins from the toes drain into the plantar and dorsal venous arch. The dorsalis pedis veins drain to the saphenous vein. The following deep veins drain the lower leg: the posterior tibial vein at the back of the leg; the peroneal vein; and the anterior tibial vein at the front of the leg. The deep tibial veins join to form the popliteal vein.

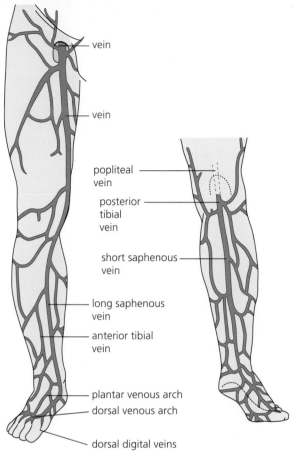

vein

vein

popliteal vein

posterior tibial vein

short saphenous vein

long saphenous vein

anterior tibial vein

plantar venous arch

dorsal venous arch

dorsal digital veins

Anterior view   **Posterior view**

Veins of the foot and lower leg

Disorders of the circulatory system

◆ *High blood pressure (hypertension)*. Blood pressure is higher than normal recommendations. Blood pressure is the force of blood pushing against the walls of blood vessels as the heart forces it around the circulatory system.

◆ *Low blood pressure (hypotension)*. Blood pressure is lower than normal recommendations.

◆ *Thrombosis*. Blood clot in the heart or blood vessels.

◆ *Deep Vein Thrombosis (DVT)*. Blood clot that occurs in the deep veins in the body.

◆ *Phlebitis*. Inflammation of the veins, most commonly the superficial veins.

◆ *Varicose veins*. Caused by an ineffective valve in the vein, which is necessary to prevent blood flowing backwards.

◆ *Haemophilia*. An inability of the blood to clot.

The lymphatic system

The lymphatic system is closely connected to the blood system, and can be considered as supplementing it. Its primary function is defensive: to remove bacteria and foreign materials, thereby preventing infection. It also drains away excess fluids for removal from the body.

The lymphatic system consists of **lymph fluid**, **lymph vessels**, **lymph capillaries** and **lymph nodes** (or glands). You may have experienced swelling of the lymph nodes in the neck when you have been ill.

Unlike the blood circulation, the lymphatic system has no muscular pump equivalent to the heart. Instead, the lymph moves through the vessels and around the body because of movements such as contractions of large muscles. Massage can play an important part in assisting this flow of lymph fluid, thereby encouraging the improved removal of the waste products transported in the lymph.

Massage plays an important role in improving lymphatic circulation

Lymph

Lymph is a straw-coloured fluid, derived from blood plasma, which has filtered through the walls of the capillaries. At this stage it is known as interstitial fluid, becoming lymph when it enters the lymphatic vessels. Contractions of the body muscles push the lymph through a series of one-way valves. The composition of lymph is similar to that of blood plasma, although less oxygen and fewer nutrients are available. In the spaces between the cells where there are no blood capillaries, lymph provides nourishment to the tissue cells and transports away waste products. It also carries **lymphocytes** (a type of white blood cell), which play an important role in the immune system. It can destroy dangerous cells and disease-causing bacteria and viruses directly before it returns to the bloodstream.

Lymph travels only in one direction from body tissues back towards the heart.

Lymph vessels

Lymph capillaries are minute vessels that collect fluid that flows between the cells and tissues – the interstitial fluid – which eventually becomes lymph.

Lymph vessels or lymphatics are similar in structure to veins, having valves at intervals along their length. They collect lymph from the lymph capillaries.

Lymph is squeezed along the vessels by pressure from the muscles they run through. It is important when massaging to make sure movements are compatible with aiding the flow of blood and lymph back towards the heart. **Oedema** is swelling of the tissues, which occurs when fluids accumulate rather than returning to the bloodstream. This can be due to a failure of the circulation or to an imbalance in the composition of the blood. If an operation for breast cancer has included removal of lymph tissue, oedema sometimes affects the arm on that side.

Lymph vessels often run very close to veins, forming an extensive network throughout the body. The lymph moves quite slowly and the valves along the lymph vessels prevent backflow of the lymph.

The lymph vessels join to form larger lymph vessels, which eventually flow into one or other of two large principal lymphatic vessels: the **thoracic duct** (or **left lymphatic duct**) and the **right lymphatic duct.** The thoracic duct receives lymph from the left side of the head, neck, chest, abdomen and lower body; the right lymphatic duct receives lymph

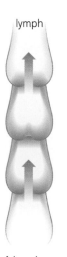

lymph

A lymph vessel

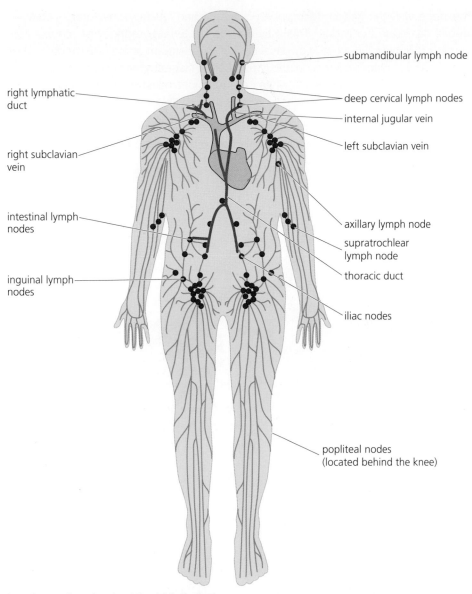

submandibular lymph node

right lymphatic duct

deep cervical lymph nodes

internal jugular vein

left subclavian vein

right subclavian vein

intestinal lymph nodes

axillary lymph node

supratrochlear lymph node

thoracic duct

inguinal lymph nodes

iliac nodes

popliteal nodes (located behind the knee)

Lymph vessels and nodes (glands) in the body

from the right side of the head and upper body. There it connects to one of the subclavian veins at the base of the neck, which in turn empties into the **vena cava**. The lymph is mixed into the venous blood as it is returned to the heart.

Lymph nodes

Lymph vessels take lymph through a series of lymph nodes along their course back to the blood circulation. Lymph nodes are small, oval structures between 1 mm and 25 mm in length.

These are the filtering and storage areas of the lymphatic system. Their purpose is to filter lymph and prevent infection. Surrounded by a capsule, the sinus inside the lymph node contains fibres, which slow the passage of lymph through the node, enabling the detection of foreign particles.

Lymph enters a node through an **afferent** vessel and leaves through an **efferent** vessel.

There are two types of white blood cell present inside the lymph node: **macrophages** line the walls and **lymphocytes** may detach from the lymph nodes and be taken out

REVISION AID

What is lymph?

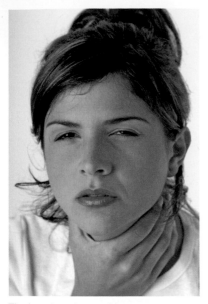

The lymph nodes swell in response to infection. Swollen tonsils will contra-indicate facial treatment.

of the node with the lymph. Macrophages engulf and destroy any foreign particles or debris carried in the lymph. This may include bacteria. Lymphocytes manufacture antibodies to fight pathogens. They pass into the bloodstream along with the circulating lymph. When we suffer an infection, the lymph nodes closest to the site of infection may swell up and become tender as the white cells attempt to destroy the pathogens, such as bacteria or viruses.

Lymph filters through at least one lymph node before returning to the bloodstream. Various groups of lymph nodes drain the different parts of the body.

Lymphoid organs and tissues are part of the system containing large numbers of lymphocytes. Lymphoid tissue includes the tonsils.

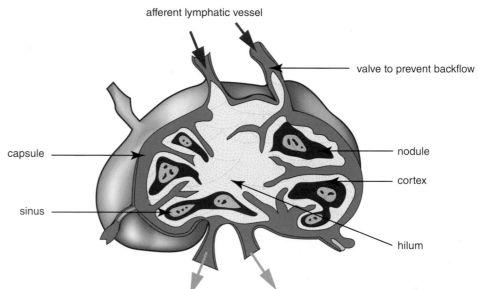

Lymph node structure

TOP TIP

Frontal – Temporal – Parietal Occipital – Mandible (mandibular) – Cervical

Learn and remember these names of the main regions of the head and neck. Not only will this assist you in recalling the names and locations of the bones, it will also help you greatly with the names and locations of muscles, arteries, veins, nerves and lymph nodes.

TOP TIP

When performing massage, the hands should be used to apply pressure to direct the lymph towards the nearest lymph node. This encourages the speedy removal of waste products.

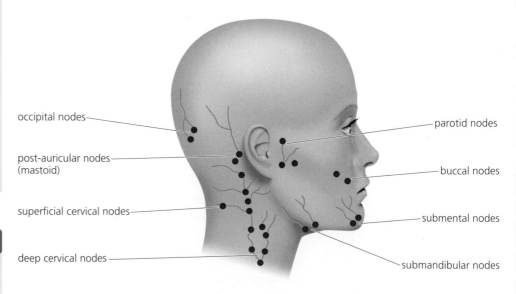

Lymph nodes of the head

◆ The **buccal group** drains the eyelids, the nose and the skin of the face.

◆ The **mandibular group** drains the chin, the lips, the nose and the cheeks.

◆ The **mastoid group** drains the skin of the ear and the temple area.

◆ The **occipital group** drains the back of the scalp and the upper neck.

◆ The **submental group** drains the chin and the lower lip.

◆ The **parotid group** drains the nose, eyelids and ears.

Lymph nodes of the neck

◆ The **superficial cervical group** drains the back of the head and the neck.

◆ The **lower deep cervical group** drains the back area of the scalp and the neck.

Lymph nodes of the chest and arms

◆ The nodes of the armpit area, called axillary nodes, drain various regions of the arms and chest.

Lymph nodes of the legs

◆ The nodes of the legs are situated in the popliteal fossa (the space behind the knee). They are called popliteal nodes. There are also inguinal nodes which are located in the anterior pelvic region.

Disorders of the lymphatic system

◆ *Autoimmune disorders*. Recognised as an inflammatory response created by the lymphatic system. The lymphatic system itself cannot distinguish between foreign bodies (antigens) or its own cells, and attacks them.

◆ *Lymphoedema*. Swelling in the lymphatic tissues from an accumulation of excessive lymph due to poor lymphatic drainage, which can lead to swelling in the limbs.

The endocrine system

While the nervous system uses electrical signals to initiate a response, the endocrine system uses **hormones**. These hormones are essential to the function of different bodily activities.

Endocrine glands secrete chemical messengers called hormones directly into the bloodstream, where they circulate around the body and affect certain organs. The glands are commonly referred to as ductless glands because the hormones are secreted directly into the bloodstream.

The organ affected by a particular hormone is called a **target organ**. The endocrine system works with the nervous system to bring about co-ordination. Hormones tend to be associated with long-term changes, such as growth, rather than the quick response expected from nerve stimulation.

The hypothalamus is the hormone-producing part of the brain and works with the nervous system and endocrine system to regulate the chemical processes in the body to keep them stable. This process is referred to as homeostasis. The hypothalamus links with the pituitary gland, which controls other glands. A low level of hormones detected by the hypothalamus will trigger the pituitary to increase hormone levels released from a 'target' gland.

Many skin and hair disorders are caused by imbalance of hormones within the endocrine system. This is referred to as hypersecretion – too much hormone, or hyposecretion – too little hormone.

REVISION AID

What are hormones?

ALWAYS REMEMBER

Puberty

The skin disorder **acne vulgaris** is caused by inflammation and bacterial infection of the sebaceous glands and hair follicles at puberty, when there is an increased level of male hormones (androgens) in the body. This increases the production of sebum.

Pregnancy

Hyperpigmentation of the skin occurs as a result of hormonal change in the body. Melasma is an example of this, where a hyperpigmented area of skin appears in a mask shape.

Menopause

Oestrogen levels decrease, which slows collagen production, affecting skin strength and elasticity, leading to the formation of wrinkles. Terminal hair growth may also occur in females following the male growth pattern on the upper lip and chin.

Menopausal acne may sometimes be experienced where a reduction in oestrogen causes the androgens to trigger sebum production.

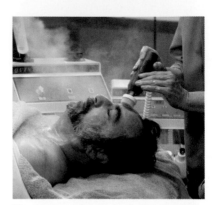

Electrical equipment used within a facial

REVISION AID

Which pieces of equipment do you use that require electricity to power them?

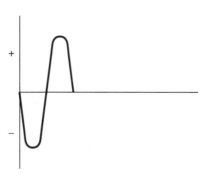

Electric current

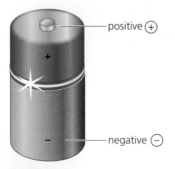

A battery

Electrical science

Electrical treatments produce intensified physiological results in a short period of time compared with those that can be achieved manually.

The aims of electrical treatments used within beauty therapy treatments at level 2 are to:

◆ improve skin condition and function

◆ locally improve blood and lymphatic circulation and drainage.

Different pieces of equipment achieve these aims, which are all powered by an **electric current**. An electric current is created by a flow of electric charge. To understand how an electric charge is created you have to understand the theory of matter, discussed in cosmetic science.

A knowledge of electricity is important so that you always use equipment safely and without harm to yourself or others.

Electric power

Electricity to power beauty therapy treatment using electrical equipment is taken from the 'mains' supply through sockets in the work environment, at 240 volts (an electric measure to register the flow of electric current). Alternatively, a battery might be used to power items of equipment. Certain pieces of larger equipment such as a sauna require a dedicated supply and this must be fitted by a qualified electrician, meeting Government regulations.

Mains electricity is an **alternating current (AC)** moving back and forth. In most countries mains alternates five times each second. This is referred to as a frequency of 50 cycles per second, measured in **hertz** (Hz) (see section on Alternating current later in this chapter).

Batteries

A battery is a device that produces electricity by chemical reactions and delivers a **direct current (DC)**. The stored chemical energy in the battery is converted into electrical energy. The connections of the battery are identified by their polarity – a positive terminal (+) and a negative terminal (−). There is a transfer of electrons between the terminals, which powers the flow of electrons.

positive ⊕

negative ⊖

ALWAYS REMEMBER

Batteries

◆ Dry cell batteries (non-rechargeable) are used for some portable equipment. The cost of running battery-operated equipment is much higher than that of mains operated. Always consider this when purchasing new equipment.

◆ Rechargeable batteries are a preferred option, making a positive environmental choice.

◆ Batteries must be removed once exhausted or they may leak, damaging the equipment.

◆ Always insert the batteries correctly to avoid damage to the equipment.

Electric current

An electric current occurs when there is a flow of charged particles in a **conductor**. A conductor is material that allows the flow of electricity in one or more directions.

The flow of electrons along the wire of an electric circuit between the electrical supply and the appliance is called an electric current. When an electric current flows through a metal wire, a conductor, the electrons pass from atom to atom through the metal. The circuit is the route travelled by an electric current.

Types of electrical current There are different types of currents available and these are used to create different physiological effects in electrical beauty therapy treatments.

You will primarily use an Alternating Current (AC).

Electrical measurement

The pressure creating the flow of electrical current around the circuit is measured in volts (V). Voltage causes the current to flow. The rate of flow of electric current around a circuit when the electrical force or voltage is applied, is measured in amperes or **amps** (A), a measure of electrical strength.

The power or energy used by electrical equipment is measured in **watts** (W) and kilowatts (kW): 1000 watts = 1 kilowatt.

As watts are relatively small units, powerful appliances need several thousands of them. For this reason the larger unit of energy, kilowatt, is used.

In order to transfer the electrical energy, electrical resistance must be reduced and a good conductor of electricity is necessary.

Electrical conductors and insulators

A conductor is a substance that easily transmits an electric current.

Good conductors include metals such as copper, gold and aluminium, and solutions that contain conducting properties such as acids, salts and alkalis, known as **electrolytes** (a compound which in solution conducts an electric current and contains ions).

Good conductors have a nucleus with free electrons that are able to travel. The material has a small resistance, offering little opposition to the moving electrons so that the electric current can pass freely through it. Although electricity passes through a conductor, it has to be forced through it by a battery or the mains supply and as such it offers some resistance.

TOP TIP

Internal batteries

Some items of electrical equipment have specially designed internal batteries. These are charged from the mains supply by a transformer, which reduces the mains voltage, and a rectifier to convert the AC to DC. Such batteries should be fully discharged before they are recharged, otherwise they will fail to operate at their full capacity.

REVISION AID

What do AC and DC stand for?

Poor conductors include rubber, plastic and wood, and are often used to prevent the flow of electrons. They are known as **insulators**. These are materials that have a nucleus with few electrons able to travel so that electricity can only pass through them with difficulty.

Pure water has a high resistance to electricity, but when another compound is dissolved in it, it becomes a good conductor, for example a saline solution, where sodium chloride is dissolved in water.

Fuses
Fuses protect electrical appliances from excess current. Wire in the fuse melts if excessive current occurs. This breaks the electric current. A fuse is fitted in the plug to protect the cable from overheating. It is a cartridge fuse, where the fuse wire is in a glass or porcelain tube.

Some items of electrical equipment also have fuses fitted inside them to give extra protection.

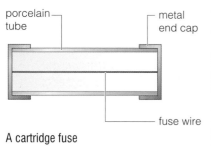

A cartridge fuse

TOP TIP

Typical plug, showing wiring and fuse placement

All plugs must comply with the Plugs and Sockets, etc. (Safety) Regulations 1994. The law regulates safety of electrical plugs, sockets and adaptors for use in the UK.

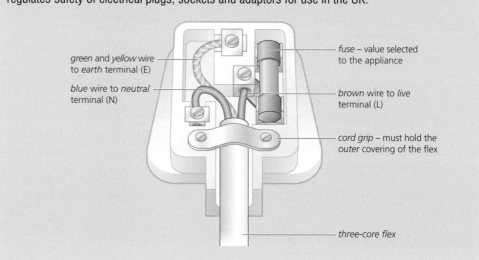

Fuses in plugs are generally 3 amp or 13 amp and have different current ratings:

◆ 3 amp for appliances up to 700 watts

◆ 13 amp for appliances over 700 watts

◆ 5 amp fuses are available for older equipment and are still available to buy.

HEALTH & SAFETY

Moulded plug

All new equipment must be fitted with a 'moulded on' plug on its flex. All plugs must meet British Standard BS 1363 – this will be marked on the back of the plug. This will contain the correct value fuse. Should it blow, it must be replaced with another one of the same value. Should it be necessary to replace the plug, the old one should be cut off, its fuse removed and the plug disposed of.

HEALTH & SAFETY

Fuses and earthing

All electrical appliances must be correctly fused and earthed in accordance with the British Standards Institution (BSI) recommendations. The earth wire in a plug takes away stray electricity should an electrical fault develop in the equipment, reducing the voltage to zero and preventing electric shock as well as protecting the flex and equipment.

Equipment that is not earthed will affect the manufacturer's liability.

REVISION AID

What are the following terms:

a. watts

b. volts?

Electrical equipment in beauty therapy

The following beauty therapy equipment that you will use is powered by electric current. The movement of electrons creates an electrical charge.

◆ **Magnifying lamp** – light is created by passing electricity through a fluorescent glass sealed tube that contains an element and gas that react. The energy created provides ultraviolet light (UV). This light passes through a convex glass lens, one that is fatter in the middle and makes things appear larger.

◆ **UV lamp** – these are used for the application of a gel nail polish finish at the curing stage. The UV lamp design provides UV light at wavelengths between 340–380 nanometres (nm). The UV light reacts with chemicals in the polish called photo-initiators. The wattage of the bulb is limited within a safe range as guided by the manufacturer. This is due to the fact that during polymerisation the chemical reaction that hardens the resin creates heat, which would lead to nail damage if excessive.

LED (Light Emitting Diode/Device) lamp used increasingly for gel polish application is a popular alternative to a UV lamp. The UV reaction occurs in a shorter time, due to the narrower range of UV light used which is at a higher concentration in order for the LED lamp to cure the gel. Traditional UV lamps' rays are in a broader range and are at a lower concentration.

As electricity flows through a conducting metal, energy is created. This energy may be used as follows:

◆ **Facial steamer** – distilled water is heated by conduction from a heating element containing a high-resistance wire, creating steam. This is applied to the face or back, achieving a hydrating and cleansing action as it heats the skin and absorbs surface moisture.

◆ **Paraffin wax** – this is melted and changed to a liquid form by a heating element at a temperature between 45–49 °C. When applied to the skin it solidifies and is used to raise the temperature of the area to which it is applied.

◆ **Wax depilation** – a heating element is used to heat wax to its required temperature.

◆ **Brush cleansing** – an electric motor uses electrical energy to create mechanical movement, which rotates a brush. This is applied to the skin surface for its cleansing action.

◆ **Radiation therapy** using an infrared lamp – a coil of high-resistance wire heats up as electricity is passed though it. A filter applied to the bulb construction allows only infrared and visible red light to pass through it. Gas at low pressure contained

HEALTH & SAFETY

Safety visual checks

Mains-powered equipment should be visually checked regularly. Equipment must not be used if the plug or connector is damaged, the cable has been repaired with tape, is not secure, or internal wires are visible. Discoloured plug casing or cable may indicate overheating. Ensure the equipment is professionally checked by a competent person. Comply with the law Electricity at Work Regulations (1989).

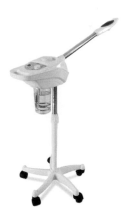

Skin warming equipment

ECO TIP

Consider how you dispose of light bulbs when recycling. Fluorescent lamps are considered hazardous because they contain the element mercury, which is toxic.

within the bulb is used to control light energy. The infrared electromagnetic waves are absorbed by the skin to heat the tissues and prepare them for other treatments such as facial massage.

There are two forms of electricity, **alternating current (AC)** and **direct current (DC)**.

Alternating current

Alternating current (AC) is an interrupted electrical current, which reverses its direction of flow of electrons, flowing first in one direction around the circuit and then the opposite way at a fixed frequency. The **frequency** tells us how many complete cycles occur each second. The unit for frequency is the hertz (Hz). This is used in most equipment used at Level 2.

The width, depth and frequency of electrical impulses can be varied to achieve different effects. This is altered on the machine by selecting the programme or setting. This feature of equipment is used within Level 3 treatments.

Direct current

Direct current (DC) is an electrical current using the effects of polarity. The electrons flow constantly, uninterrupted, in one direction from the positive pole to negative pole. Two electrodes that conduct electricity are necessary: the anode electrode, positive (+ve) – attached to the positive lead, and the cathode electrode, negative (−ve) – attached to the negative lead. Its source is usually a battery.

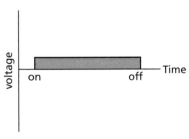

Direct current

Changing the electrical current

The electricity for each electrical treatment can be changed to achieve different effects.

Different components are used in electrical appliances to change the electrical current and the equipment's function:

◆ *Rectifier*. This changes the AC electrical outlet supply to a DC. Electrons are only able to flow in one direction. Batteries produce DC only and AC current is changed to charge batteries of equipment and devices.

Choosing your equipment

Electrical equipment is costly, and careful consideration should be made before purchase. Always:

◆ purchase from a reputable company, whose equipment has proved suitable for its purpose

◆ check that the machine is safe; look for the CE mark, which is awarded only if electrical safety standards have been reached, meeting the provisions of the relevant European Directives and legislation. By affixing the CE mark the manufacturer or supplier who places the product on the market takes on responsibility for the conformity of the product.

The Health and Safety Executive is responsible for enforcing safety standards through the various legislation standards. As well as the Consumer Protection Act (1987). If people are injured by defective equipment they have the right to take legal action.

For further information about your legal responsibilities when using electrical equipment refer to the section entitled 'Health and safety in the workplace' in Chapter 1 The Business of Beauty Therapy.

Also, when choosing your equipment always:

◆ check that it carries a guarantee

◆ ensure you have access to written guidance instructions

◆ consider whether it is financially viable for your business, and the correct size for your work, e.g. if you are freelance, it must be portable

◆ question whether the equipment supplier will support you with marketing and training

◆ ask if a temporary replacement will be provided should the equipment become faulty

◆ ensure you are provided with sufficient accessories. Often accessories may need to be washed or sterilised between clients, therefore have several sets available. This will also reduce wear and tear.

Obviously, care and consideration are necessary when using any piece of equipment to ensure that clients receive safe and effective treatment.

REVISION AID

How do batteries work?

What equipment in the salon uses a battery?

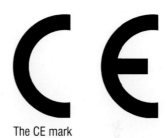

The CE mark

HEALTH & SAFETY

Equipment suppliers should always ensure that instructions are provided with all their equipment. Keep this in a central place for reference. Most are now available electronically.

HEALTH & SAFETY

Refer to the HSE website for guidance on how to comply with legislation to **maintain portable electrical equipment in a low risk environment**. A portable or movable electrical appliance is any item that can be moved.

General electrical safety precautions

The following safety guidelines should always be followed:

◆ Ensure the equipment is at the correct height to use to avoid postural damage or **repetitive strain injury (RSI)**.

◆ Always keep water away from electrical equipment to avoid electrical shock.

◆ Avoid trailing wires, to prevent damage to the machine and personal injury caused by tripping over them.

◆ Check wires are not damaged.

◆ Always check that the intensity controls are at zero before treatment commences, to avoid discomfort.

◆ Check leads are fitted correctly to the equipment before use.

◆ Store and place all equipment on a stable surface.

214 THE FOUNDATIONS OF BEAUTY THERAPY: LEVEL 2

What electrical safety precautions should be taken when carrying out a wax depilation service? Provide at least four examples.

◆ Always perform a skin sensitivity test to ensure the client can indicate their physiological tolerance to the treatment, for example waxing treatment will require a thermal skin sensitivity test.

◆ Position equipment so that the dials are clearly visible.

◆ Check the performance of the equipment on yourself where appropriate before use on a client, to make sure it is in good working order. This is reassuring for the client too.

◆ Sufficient plug sockets should be provided to avoid overloading and possible fire.

◆ Wires should not become twisted or this can lead to poor electric circuitry and breakage of the wires. Consider storage to keep all accessories in optimum condition.

◆ Clean the equipment with products suitable to the finish of the product or damage could occur to the finish, e.g. visibility to read gauges and settings features.

TOP TIP

Sustainability tip

Unplug equipment when not in use. This not only saves energy but also avoids a trip hazard in the workplace.

TOP TIP

Exhibitions

Trade exhibitions are ideal places to view equipment, talk directly to the suppliers and compare benefits and costs with other suppliers in order to make the best choice to meet your needs and budget.

HEALTH & SAFETY

Electrical fires

A fire extinguisher must be available to deal with electrical fires. This will usually be CO_2 colour-coded black or a dry powder type, colour-coded blue.

HEALTH & SAFETY

Put safety first at all times

Do not:

◆ use equipment from a socket where the mains lead is likely to be overstretched

◆ use a twisted, torn flex or cable

◆ handle plugs or sockets with wet hands; remember water is a good conductor of electricity and may result in electric shock

◆ overload a socket.

HEALTH & SAFETY

Equipment testing intervals

◆ A maintenance plan must be in place for all portable electrical equipment.

◆ Training and information should be provided to all employees in order to carry out regular visual safety checks.

◆ The person assigned to carry out inspection and test for equipment that is considered broken, has been repaired or requires a routine safety check, should be identified. This must be a competent person, which means having suitable training, skill and knowledge for the task to prevent injury to themselves or others.

Legal requirements

The **Electricity at Work Regulations (1989)** imposes duties on employers and self-employed persons to comply with specific health and safety regulations within their control and responsibility. Electrical equipment must be safe; equipment must therefore be regularly inspected by a qualified electrician. Accurate records listing the date of inspection, the test results and next test date must be available for inspection by the Environmental Health Officer (EHO).

The **Health and Safety at Work Act (1974)** sets out minimum safety standards and states that:

◆ all equipment should meet safety standards, be regularly checked and be in good working order. Keep an equipment maintenance log for this purpose.

◆ consideration of handling and application of equipment is the responsibility of the employer to avoid possible employee injury, and adequate training should be given.

◆ trailing leads should not pose a threat to the welfare of employees or clients.

Disposal of equipment

If you have to dispose of a piece of electrical equipment this should be done safely. This may be at your local waste recycling department or alternatively, if purchasing a new piece of equipment, the supplier may take your old equipment for recycling. If the equipment contains a battery, this is termed hazardous waste and should be disposed of appropriately in compliance with the **Hazardous Waste Regulations**. Disposal of electrical equipment is governed by **The Waste Electric and Electronic Equipment (WEEE) Regulations 2013**. Further information is available at www.hse.gov.uk.

ASSESSMENT OF KNOWLEDGE AND UNDERSTANDING

Having covered the learning objectives for this chapter test your knowledge and understanding by answering the short questions below.

The information covers:

◆ Cosmetic science

◆ Anatomy and physiology

◆ Electrical science

Cosmetic science

1. a. What is pH?
    b. What is its relevance to the beauty therapist?

2. a. What is matter?
    b. Describe two different states of matter you may work with when using cosmetic cleansing products. Provide examples.

3. How should cosmetics be stored?

4. a. What is a volatile liquid?
    b. Provide an example that you may work with.

5. What is an emulsion?

6. What ingredients may be beneficial when treating an ageing skin?

7. What is the difference between organic and natural ingredients?

Anatomy and physiology

1. The skin has three main layers what are they called?

2. Name the layers of the epidermis shown in the image below numbered 1-5. Which layer is continuously being shed and what is this process called?

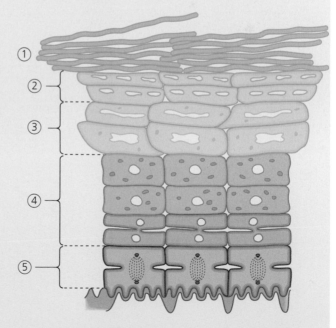

3. List six main functions of the skin. Explain for one how this function is achieved.

4. How would you recognise a combination skin? Explain which gland is responsible for creating the difference in appearance in each facial area for this skin type.

5. What is the skin pigment called that is responsible for creating the tanned appearance of the skin on exposure to UVL?

6. Describe the structure of the dermis and label the features and structures located in the dermis shown below.

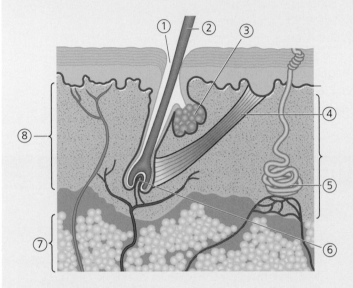

7. What is thermo-regulation and how is this regulated by the body?

8. Name two protein fibres found in the reticular layer of the skin, and describe their appearance and function.

9. How do lifestyle factors affect the skin's appearance and condition? Discuss two examples.

Hair structure, type and growth

1. Referring to the cross section of the hair follicle in the skin below, briefly describe the name and function of each numbered area.

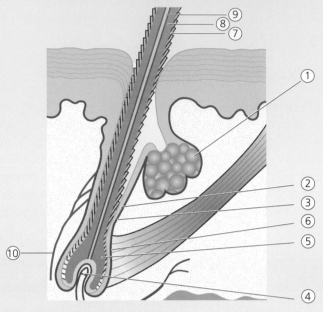

2. What is the function of hair?

3. What is the soft downy hair on the face called?

4. What is the protein found in hair that is also found in skin?

5. What is the function of the dermal papilla in relation to the hair?

6. What are the names of the different stages of the hair growth cycle?

7. What happens to the hair at each stage of the hair growth cycle?

8. What relevance has a knowledge of the hair growth cycle for a wax depilation service?

9. What is the difference in time between the hair growth cycle anagen to telogen for scalp hair and eyebrow hair?

Nail structure, function and growth

1. Referring to the cross-section of the nail structure below, briefly describe the name and function of each of the numbered areas.

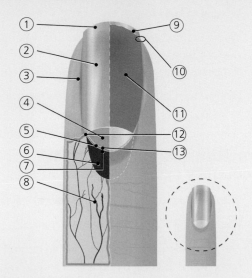

2. What is the function of the nail plate? How is this function achieved?

3. In which part of the nail structure do the cells divide to form the nail plate?

4. As the nail cells grow forward they harden; what is this process called?

5. How long does it take for the fingernail to grow from cuticle to free edge?

Structure and function of the skeletal system

1. What are the main functions of the skeleton?

2. What is the function of bone?

3. What attaches bones to different parts of the body?

4. On the diagram of the cranium name the bones numbered 1–8.

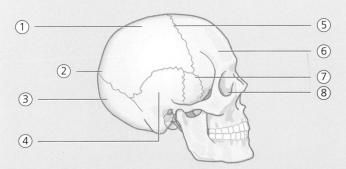

5. Name three facial bones to which you may apply contouring products during make-up.

6. Name the facial bone or bones that form the

   ◆ forehead

   ◆ nose

   ◆ cheekbones

   ◆ jawbone.

7. On the diagram of the bones of the neck, chest and shoulder name the bones and their functions (items 1–7).

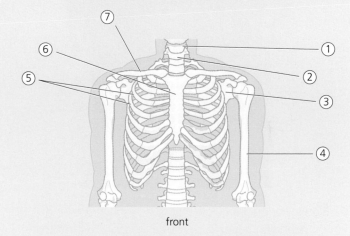

front

8. The wrist is made up of eight small carpal bones which glide over one another to allow movement. Name them.

9. Name the bones that form the lower leg, and what type of bones they are.

Structure and function of the muscular system

1. What are the main functions of skeletal muscle tissue?

2. What happens when muscles contract?

3. What structure attaches a muscle to a bone?

4. On the diagram of the muscles of the face, name muscles 1–6. What are the actions of these muscles?

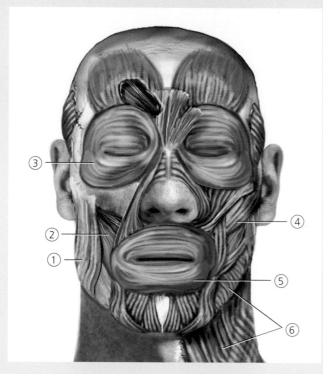

5. On the diagram below of muscles that move the head and upper body, name muscles 1–4. What are the actions of these muscles?

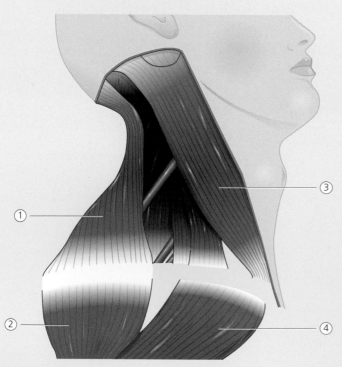

6. What is the collective name for the group of muscles that bend the wrist, drawing it towards the forearm?

7. What is the collective name for the group of muscles that straighten the wrist and the hand?

8. What is muscle tone?

9. With age, the facial expressions that we make every day produce lines on the skin - frown lines. What happens to the tone of the muscles with age?

10. What effect does massage have on the tone of muscles?

Structure and function of the circulatory system

1. What are the functions of the circulatory system?

2. What are the main constituents of blood?

3. The circulation of blood is under the control of the heart, which pumps blood around the body. On the illustrations below label the arteries that transport blood to the head, and veins that return blood from the head.

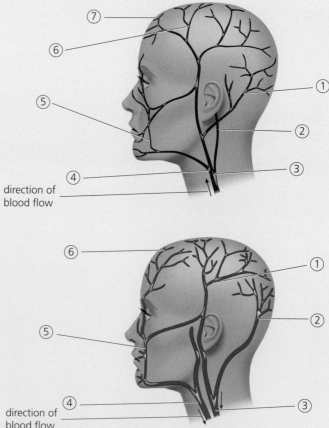

4. Name three different types of blood vessels in the circulatory system and explain their appearance and function.

Structure and function of lymphatic system

1. What is the main functions of the lymphatic system?

2. What are the main constituents of lymph?

3. What is the function of lymph nodes or glands?

4. On the diagram of the head, name the lymph nodes numbered 1–5.

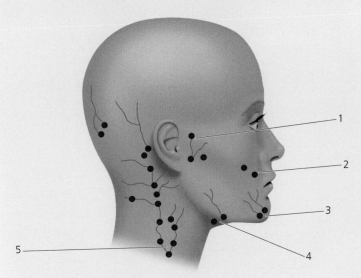

5. How does massage affect the circulation and exchange of blood and lymph? How does this benefit the skin and underlying structures?

Structure and function of the nervous system

1. The nervous system transmits messages between the brain the other parts of the body. There are two main divisions. What are they called?

2. What is the central nervous system composed of?

3. What is the difference between sensory nerves and motor nerves?

4. To what are the main sensory nerve endings in the skin receptive?

5. How many pairs of cranial nerves emerge from the brain?

6. Those of concern to the beauty therapist when performing facial massage are the 5th, 7th and 11th cranial nerves. What is the function of the:

   ◆ 5th, known as trigeminal nerve?
   ◆ 7th, known as the facial nerve?
   ◆ 11th, known as the accessory nerve?

7. Name the main branches of the 7th cranial facial nerve, numbered 1–5 in the diagram.

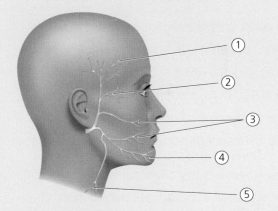

Electrical science

1. What is electricity?

2. What is the difference between a conductor of electricity and an insulator?

3. What is the difference between AC and DC?

4. What does a rectifier do?

5. What is your responsibility under the Electricity at Work Regulations Act?

6. Provide five examples of best health and safety practice when working with electrical equipment.

3 Consultation Practice and Techniques

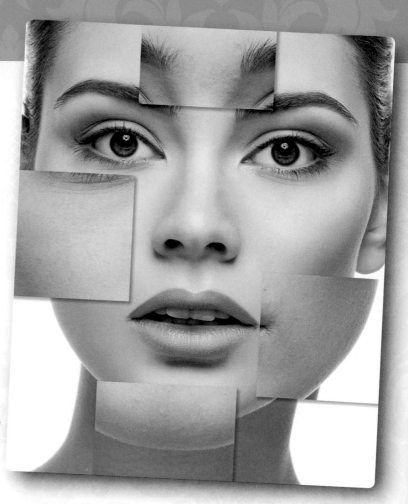

LEARNING OBJECTIVES

This chapter covers the consultation process to be carried out before every treatment. It covers diseases and disorders of the skin, eyes, hair and nails that you may encounter. These will influence whether it is professionally appropriate to proceed with the treatment or not. You will learn more about:

◆ How to assess the client for make-up, facial, hair removal, eye and nail treatments.

◆ The range of assessment techniques to be used.

◆ How to use the consultation process to identify, advise and agree the most appropriate treatment or product to meet the needs of your client.

◆ How to prepare and monitor treatment plans based upon consultation information.

◆ The factors you need to consider with your client before treatment and product selection, such as skin type/condition, lifestyle, health, cost and time commitment.

◆ Performing pre-treatment tests.

◆ Diseases and disorders including bacterial, parasitic, viral and fungal that may prevent or restrict treatment.

KEY TERMS

Allergen

Bacteria

Client record

Consultation

Contra-action

Contra-indication

Data Protection Act

Diagnostic assessment

Fluid retention

Fungal infection

Fitzpatrick scale

Medical history

Hair analysis

Hyper-pigmentation

Hypo-pigmentation

Muscle tone

Nail analysis

Non-pathogenic

Open questions

Parasite

Patch test

Pathogenic

Posture

Pigmentation

Skin allergy

Skin analysis

Skin conditions
(sensitive,
dehydrated, mature,
congested)

Skin disease

Skin disorder

Skin sensitivity test

Skin tone

Skin types (normal, dry,
oily, combination)

Treatment plan

Virus

WHEN PROVIDING CLIENT CONSULTATIONS YOU WILL BE REQUIRED TO

◆ Follow relevant legislation, workplace requirements and manufacturer's instructions for consultation and record keeping.

◆ Gather personal information from your client to assist identifying the treatment objectives.

◆ Use excellent verbal and non-verbal communication skills through the consultation to engage effectively with the client and ensure understanding and satisfaction.

◆ Use different consultation and assessment techniques to correctly identify your client's treatment requirements.

◆ Use products, tools and equipment that will assist you.

◆ Take the necessary actions, and record this on the treatment record where a contra-action, contra-indication or treatment modification is required.

◆ Provide relevant advice and recommendations to support your client's service requirements.

◆ Ensure your client agrees to and understands the objectives of their treatment plan.

◆ Carry out this service at every client visit and for every treatment to inform, gather further information and update the treatment plan.

INTRODUCTION

Consultation is referred to in each technical chapter and is required to be provided before any treatment delivery and retail product selection. An effective consultation is an essential component affecting the success and client satisfaction of every treatment.

Professional image, outstanding customer care and excellent communication skills are required to ensure you develop a positive relationship with your client and fully understand their requirements and any constraints before any treatment is delivered or retail product is sold.

Once you understand the client's requirements, consider any associated contra-indications, you can agree the treatment plan with the client and ensure it matches their needs.

When the client becomes established, you can then use the consultation to inform them about further products and treatments using more technical language to develop their understanding.

The consultation follows a structured format to ensure that all information required is obtained, it meets legal requirements and will assist in gaining client confidence and satisfaction.

Assessing the client's needs and preparing treatment plans

Consultation and plan for treatments

Through the **consultation** process, you assess and agree the needs of the client and identify the most suitable treatment to create their **treatment plan**. As a beauty therapist, you will be performing many different treatments and advising on the use of professional retail products for the face and body. The objectives of these treatments will include the following aims:

◆ to improve facial skin type and condition, function and appearance through facial and make-up services

◆ to improve facial muscular condition and tension or tone

◆ to improve the condition of the nails and skin through hand, foot and nail services

◆ to enhance the appearance of the eyes through the application of make-up techniques and eye services

◆ to enhance facial and body appearance through temporary hair removal

◆ to improve blood and lymphatic circulation in the treatment area

◆ to aid relaxation, reduce symptoms of stress, and improve feelings of wellbeing.

The client should always receive a thorough consultation before treatment. This will confirm the treatment requirements, and enable you to decide on their suitability and whether the treatment needs to be modified in any way. Some clients may have **contra-indications**, problematic symptoms that prevent or restrict treatment. In some instances medical referral to the client's GP is required, or consent to treat received (i.e. there is no objection to the client having treatment) before the treatment may proceed. Personal information is collected from the client using verbal and written questioning techniques. When suitability is confirmed, you will then carry out further manual and visual assessment techniques, which will inform how you should apply or modify your treatment application. At this stage you may require the client to remove specific clothing to assess the area to be treated. The client should be informed of the reason for this and their privacy and modesty considered at all times.

The consultation service can be offered independently so that the client can find out more about a treatment before they commit to booking it. This is also the case when giving advice on treatment products. This is also necessary if any skin sensitivity, thermal and tactile **patch tests** are recommended and the results of these are required before treatment proceeds. The consultation should be carried out as part of every client treatment.

"Have a tester unit available for clients to try and feel the product for themselves."

Daniella Norman

Your conduct should be appropriate to the situation and professional at all times. Professional boundaries for conduct should be known and understood. Your client will usually adapt their behaviour in accordance with yours. This is important. Never place yourself in a situation where your behaviour could be considered unprofessional or inappropriate. Follow your workplace procedure for safeguarding staff if ever you are made to feel uncomfortable when interacting with a client.

Consultation assessment techniques

Often there may be an underlying cause for the main treatment requirement that is not immediately obvious and will only become apparent through:

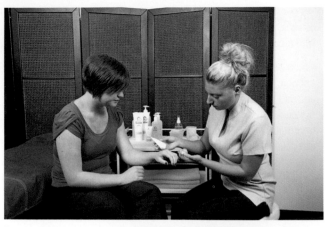

◆ questioning techniques using verbal and written communication

◆ observation and **diagnostic assessment**

◆ **skin analysis** to learn more about the skin type, condition and cause

◆ **nail analysis** to learn more about appearance, condition and cause

Demonstrating recommended treatment products to the client

◆ **hair analysis** to learn more about appearance, hair type, growth and cause.

Questioning techniques It is necessary to gain information from your client by asking a series of questions before the treatment plan can be finalised. Ideally, this must be carried out in a private area and not the open salon space to maintain client confidentiality. All resources you may require should be available in this area. You should ensure that the client is comfortable before you proceed. The consultation notes should be recorded on paper or electronically on a computerised record. This record when signed by yourself and the client confirms client understanding, agreement and consent for the proposed treatment. Always follow your workplace requirements, and ensure the accuracy of the information recorded and compliance with record keeping. Any ill effect from the treatment could be deemed negligent on your part, resulting in legal proceedings and a requirement for compensation. The consultation notes and treatment plan record provides a historical reference and should always be completed in full.

For the treatment of minors, that is anyone under the age of 16 years, the responsible parent/guardian must be present throughout the treatment. Written or signed consent is also required before the treatment stating that they are happy for the treatment to go ahead, a record of which must be available. Each salon will have their own policy and procedures for treating minors.

All information gained from the client is confidential: the client must be made aware of how the information is to be used and it should be stored in a secure area following their treatment. Information must be up to date. This requirement is enforced through the **Data Protection Act** (1998) – legislation designed to protect the client's privacy and confidentiality. Non-compliance may result in legal action by the client.

> ## TOP TIP
>
> **Treatment of minors**
>
> A parent or guardian present at all times during treatment ensures that they witness all interaction with the minor. Inform a colleague if treating a minor as you may need them to be in close proximity.
>
> For any treatment delivered to a minor, you must consider if it is in their wellbeing to receive the treatment. You may limit treatment of minors to those such as facials and hand treatments.
>
> Always comply with government legislation related to the welfare and safety of children.

ALWAYS REMEMBER

Data Protection Act (1998)

The Data Protection Act requires anyone who processes personal data to inform the Information Commissioner's Office (ICO) of how you will use this information. For advice, contact the Information Commissioners' Office at www.ico.org.uk. It also provides specialist advice on data sharing.

When completing your client consultation you may seek their permission and consent to use their personal data for the purpose of their treatment and any future treatment.

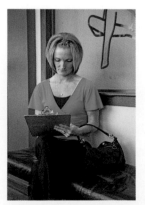

Client answering personal questions relating to their health and current skin care programme

The client should understand the reason behind all questions asked and feel comfortable when answering them. As such, they should be asked in a sensitive and supportive manner. At all times avoid unnecessary technical terms, choosing commonly understood words to ensure the client understands. Using 'open' questions will encourage the client to give more than a one-word response of 'yes' or 'no'.

Always listen attentively to your client as well as demonstrating that you are interested. Ensure you do not miss anything that may affect your treatment or product choice. Good face to face and eye contact will help ensure you understand the client's body language. Remember that a person's body language can be saying something quite different from their spoken words!

Consider the diversity of your client's needs Book sufficient time to carry out the consultation. Depending upon the assessment techniques to be used this may take up to to 15 minutes. The consultation should always be completed within a commercially specified time. The benefit of this time is that it allows you to get to know your client and for them to get to know you too. This will enable you to build a professional rapport with them and gain essential information to inform the treatment plan. As a result of this process, the client should gain confidence in you and, at the same time, understand their part in any procedures they must follow in relation to the treatment including after-care advice and recommendations.

Health It is a requirement to question the client about their health and any medication being received. Where a health contra-indication is identified, a suitable alternative treatment should always be considered. Specific contra-indications to each treatment are identified in the relevant chapter.

Consider any disability, which includes sight, hearing, mobility, mental health and learning disabilities. This can be confirmed tactfully when making a telephone appointment. Ask if they need any particular assistance in respect of their treatment. Examples are discussed below.

Sight impairment Always check first if help is required. Introduce yourself by name, before starting any communication. Remember how, on occasions, peoples' voices can sound similar. Escort the client to the consultation area. Explain this and lightly touch the person on their arm or shoulder, and allow the person to take your arm as you guide them to the area, providing verbal instructions about the environment. It may be necessary to complete the records for them on their behalf, but always ask what assistance is required. Body language remains important as it affects the tone of words, which assists communication.

Hearing impairment Position yourself, facing the client, in an area of adequate light to assist lip/speech reading. Remove any unnecessary background noise, such as music. Speak clearly, using short words and sentences. Use facial expressions and body language to assist communication, but without exaggeration, to avoid visible alteration to your lips and speech.

Make good use of any visual aids. Do not speak when referring to any written information.

Check the client's understanding regularly. Only obtain the client's signature when the client confirms understanding.

Physical disability Ensure that the area where the consultation is to be completed is accessible, considering wheelchair access and mobility issues. During the consultation, position yourself at the client's level so you are able to communicate face to face. Ensure a stable surface is provided when written information is required. By law, all reasonable adjustments should be made to provide a service in the least restrictive way.

Always question your client as you would any other client, to ensure that their treatment meets their expectations, and consider any suggestions for future improvement.

Mental health The category of mental health is broad including depression, anxiety, forgetfulness and eating disorders. Ensure descriptions and instructions are straightforward. Access to written information, such as aftercare instructions, may be useful depending on the context. Many of the treatments will be of benefit if ethically appropriate. For example, many provide beneficial side-effects of relaxation and wellbeing plus social interaction.

Certain medications may result in a skin side-effect such as dryness, photo sensitivity or pruritus and may require GP consent before treatment.

Learning disability Depending on the learning disability keep language simple avoiding technical words that can be confusing. The communication method of consultation is an ideal way to reassure and engage with the client as it is delivered in a one to one, face to face setting without distractions. Allow time for the other person to respond to questions. Do not assist or interrupt their response.

In written communication, it may be more suitable to use a larger font size. Visual aids may be used to enhance understanding.

In some instances it may be necessary to ask a parent or guardian for their advice so that the way you proceed with the consultation and following treatment ensures the client gains maximum benefit from the treatment. The parent or carer may also need to sign on behalf of the client to confirm agreement to the treatment.

User friendly information
When designing or discussing information, keep things clear and concise. Avoid technical jargon. Clients with dyslexia, for example, have difficulties with words and may misunderstand unfamiliar words. They may find text difficult to read such as black on white. Provide lots of opportunities to discuss the content of your consultation. Avoid small print. Use colour to break up information and present text using bullet points, avoiding long, descriptive sentences.

Cultural diversity
We have discussed the important adaptation of verbal and non-verbal communication to assist in your consultation, but always consider cultural diversity. Whilst Western cultures use eye contact as an important way of demonstrating engagement with the other person and confidence, this interpretation differs for other cultures. Middle Eastern countries use static, prolonged eye contact to communicate sincerity. Females avoid eye contact with non-family males as it could communicate romantic interest.

Asian cultures avoid eye contact to communicate respect to figures of authority. An example would be to look downwards whilst the other person is speaking. Static, prolonged eye contact is avoided.

African and Latin American cultures may view static, prolonged eye contact as confrontational and disrespectful.

Consider your communication style at all times. Position yourself also so that you respect other people's personal space. Different cultures will have varying preferences on what is deemed appropriate for proximity to another person.

Unnecessary contact with the client should also be avoided. However, as part of the consultation, assessment techniques will require tactile and visual assessment. You should explain this.

When English is not your client's first language, speak normally and avoid exaggerating words but avoid technical terms too. Keep your language simple, use short sentences and commonly understood words that will be familiar. Images, demonstrations of equipment on yourself and visual aids will be useful to assist understanding. Allow sufficient time to complete the documentation required to inform the treatment plan. Your consultation may take longer to ensure that the client is confident with the content.

TOP TIP

Body language

Observe your client during the consultation, their facial expression often will indicate how they are feeling.

TOP TIP

Informing others of customer care requirements

Make a note on your client's record of the best way to communicate or carry out their treatment to meet the workplace service standards. This will assist other colleagues in the workplace when dealing with this client.

REVISION AID

What is the purpose of the consultation?

ALWAYS REMEMBER

Affordability

Never make assumptions about what the client can afford. Usually the client will indicate to you what they are prepared to spend.

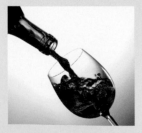

Suitability for treatment

Suitability for treatment If, after the consultation, you are unsure of the client's suitability for treatment, tactfully explain to the client why this is and, if medically related, ask them to seek permission from their GP before the treatment is given. Some clients' expectations may be unrealistic. If this is the case, tactfully explain why and aim to agree to a more realistic treatment programme.

Finally, you must tactfully confirm with the client that they can commit to the time required to receive the treatments and if the total cost is manageable.

ALWAYS REMEMBER

Consultation and Treatment planning

Designing an effective consultation and treatment plan includes:

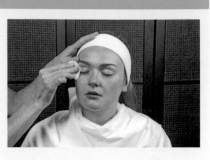

◆ collecting and recording personal information about the client

◆ checking client suitability for treatment

◆ asking questions to identify the specific treatment objectives

◆ listening and responding appropriately to client responses

◆ providing opportunity throughout for the client to ask questions

◆ identifying any treatment modification

◆ carrying out consultation assessment techniques

◆ advising the client of a suitable, realistic, treatment plan to meet their treatment objectives

◆ ensuring the client can commit to the time and financial requirements.

Client wellbeing The wellbeing of clients should always be at the forefront of any decision to proceed with treatment following consultation. On occasions during the consultation assessment you are the person who may notice any unusual **pigmentation**, lump, bump or swelling. Always refer any client to their GP when you notice anything unusual, without causing alarm.

This recommendation is supported by the British Association of Dermatologists, who have produced a mole and skin check guide. The recommendation is to keep an eye on any changes to moles on the skin.

During the consultation, question the client to gain both general and specific personal information related to the treatment.

Lifestyle factors After questioning, consider whether the client's current lifestyle habits have contributed to the condition:

◆ *Alcohol.* Alcohol is a toxin (poison) and deprives the body of its vitamin reserves, especially vitamins B and C, which are necessary for a healthy skin, resulting in premature ageing. Alcohol also dilates the blood vessels, specifically arterial capillaries. This can lead to facial flushing. It also causes skin dehydration as it has a diuretic action stimulating the production of urine. The toxic effects of certain chemicals in alcohol damage the liver in different ways and can lead to **skin conditions** such as jaundice, yellowing of the skin caused by a build-up of a pigment called bilirubin in the blood and tissues. An excess of toxins in the body can result in poor elimination of waste products, which means they remain in the tissues and along with fluid retention, result in puffiness and a sluggish circulation. In addition, alcohol is high in calories and it has no essential nutritional value. Excess calories are stored as fat in the adipose layer of the skin and around body organs.

◆ *Smoking*. Smoking interferes with cell respiration and slows down the circulation. This makes it more difficult for nutrients to reach the skin cells and for waste products to be eliminated. As such, the skin looks dull with a tendency towards open pores. The skin is also slower to heal. Cigarette smoking also releases a chemical that destroys vitamin C. This interferes with the production of collagen and elastin and contributes to premature ageing of the skin. Nicotine is also a toxic substance. This can cause contraction and weakening of the blood vessels in the skin leading to the appearance of broken capillaries (telangiectasia).

When providing nail services, you may notice the skin of the hands and feet feel dry and cold, and the skin of the hands can sometimes be stained as a result of contact with the cigarette ingredient nicotine.

◆ *Recreational drugs*. Drugs are chemical substances that affect homeostasis – the regulation and maintenance of balance of the internal systems of the body. Drugs enter the blood and are transported to the cells, affecting the body in different ways. This can lead to **skin disorders** caused by side-effects of the drugs such as dry skin, premature ageing, skin rashes and infections from scratching the skin.

◆ *Stress*. Stress can occur any time a person becomes pressurised. The symptoms of stress are seen in many different forms, including insomnia, poor digestion, headaches, muscular tension, and skin disorders such as psoriasis and eczema. Nervous habits such as nail biting may become worse, leading to the nail disorder onychopagy. The skin can appear dull, tension in muscles can restrict blood flow leading to poor nutrition in the area, resulting in skin congestion and facial tension lines. If someone is suffering from stress, they may drink more alcohol and smoke more cigarettes, causing further stress to the skin and body systems. Women under considerable stress may have excessive hair growth due to high levels of the hormone adrenaline, which also stimulates androgen production or hair loss due to poor circulation. Also, there is an increase in the release of the hormone cortisol, which can lead to blemishes including the skin disorder acne vulgaris. At the consultation stage, try to determine if the client is suffering from symptoms of stress. Very often the client will offer this information and the treatment objective will be to induce relaxation through its therapeutic effect.

◆ *Diet*. A nutritionally balanced diet is vital to the health of the body and the appearance of the skin. Nutrition, good or bad has a significant impact on the appearance of the skin. A healthy diet contains all the nutrients we need for energy, health and growth. Calories are the measure of energy derived from food and drink. The amount of calories required varies according to body height and physical activity undertaken. Excess energy is stored and can lead to weight gain. Poor quality nutrition can lead to feeling lethargic, and skin allergies and disorders are, in part, the result of a poorly balanced diet. Nutritional content of the diet can lead to creation of free radicals.

Free radicals are created from weak molecules that have split and are unstable. To correct this they attempt to gain an electron from a stable atom, which then becomes unstable and this process can continue creating further free radicals. The effect can lead to tissue damage and increase the effects and signs of ageing including wrinkling and slackness of the skin.

Diet can affect hair growth. People suffering from the eating disorder anorexia nervosa become very thin and undernourished. It is quite common to see excessive hair growth all over the face and body. This is a result of a shutdown in the ovaries, reducing the oestrogen levels and stimulating the circulating androgens.

TOP TIP

Food and exercise diary

Encourage the client to keep a food diary if they need to consider the quality of their nutrition. Good and poor patterns can become evident. However, you should take care not to give out advice but refer your client to a qualified nutritionist.

ALWAYS REMEMBER

Vitamins

Foods high in vitamins C, E and beta-carotene act as excellent anti-oxidants which neutralise free radicals. Vitamins can be sourced in the diet. For example:

◆ **Vitamin C** is found in a wide variety of fruit and vegetables, such as peppers, broccoli, sweet potatoes, oranges and kiwi fruit.

◆ **Vitamin E** is found in nuts, seeds, spinach, vegetables, sardines and egg yolks.

◆ **Beta-carotene** is turned into **Vitamin A** and is sourced from yellow and green vegetables and yellow fruit, e.g. mango and carrot.

You will notice the use of antioxidants in beauty products such as:

◆ **Vitamin A:** retinoic acid, Retin-A used to assist cellular regeneration and stimulate collagen.

◆ **Vitamin C:** ascorbic acid for cellular regeneration and skin brightening.

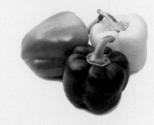

REVISION AID

Why must you communicate with a client in a professional manner?

The nails may show characteristics of the nail plate that indicate nutritional deficiencies. For example, white nails and koilonychia (spoon shaped nails) are an indicator of iron deficiency.

Lack of water can lead to skin dehydration. Drinks such as alcohol and those containing caffeine such as tea, coffee and energy drinks can make this worse.

ALWAYS REMEMBER

A healthy diet

Your body works hard to keep you healthy, diet is important.

The NHS Eatwell guide provides useful tips and recommendations that your client could refer to. www.nhs.uk/Livewell/Goodfood/Pages/the-eatwell-guide.aspx

Example Advice for a client – eight guidelines for a healthy diet:

1 Enjoy your food.
2 Eat a variety of different foods.
3 Eat the right amount to maintain a healthy weight.
4 Eat plenty of starchy and high-fibre foods.
5 Avoid eating too much saturated fat.
6 Avoid eating too much sugary food.
7 Ensure you get sufficient vitamins and minerals in your food.
8 If you drink alcohol, keep consumption within recommended unit limits.

ALWAYS REMEMBER

Ageing skin treatment considerations

As the skin ages it will be necessary to advise the client that the results achieved will be limited; it will take longer to achieve the optimum effect.

ALWAYS REMEMBER

Ageing

Intrinsic ageing is the natural, inevitable changes that take place in the skin due to deterioration of the physiological functioning of the skin.

Extrinsic ageing is how the skin ages in response to exposure to external factors such as UV light, resulting in photo-ageing.

◆ *Health*. The diagnosis of the client's health is important before considering any treatment plan. Medication and ill health can contra-indicate certain treatments or be a contributory cause of the problem. Certain prescribed drugs, such as anabolic steroids, can also cause superfluous hair. The nails can sometimes indicate illness or side-effects of medication being taken through visible physical characteristics. Always confirm the client's general health while completing the consultation.

◆ *Ageing*. This occurs as an result of our genes, our health and other contributory lifestyle factors such as exposure to environmental conditions, quality of diet, smoking etc. At the consultation you may discuss such negative factors on the ageing process with the client. With ageing, there is a decrease in bone density (osteoporosis) so that bones become brittle and are easily fractured. Exercise and a diet containing plenty of calcium-rich foods can guard against this. The change in appearance of women's skin during ageing is closely related to the altered production of the hormones oestrogen, progesterone and androgen during the menopause. The skin loses its elasticity, becomes drier, appears thinner, expression lines deepen and the facial contours become slack. Male skin will exhibit these signs of ageing but thinning of the skin is gradual and the skin is already 25% thicker in males than females. Ageing is closely related to collagen content which decreases with age. Male skin has a higher collagen content which affects skin thickness. Oestrogen deficiency in menopausal female skin affects fibroblast production of collagen in the dermis, and will result in thinning of skin. Treatments that accelerate the skin's natural functioning by nourishing and firming are recommended.

The nails become ridged vertically and may suddenly split at the free edge, usually centrally. This is a sign of age similar to a wrinkle on the face. Due to less natural fats and moisture the nail may become brittle and growth slows whilst thickening of the toenail nail plate occurs.

◆ *Exposure*. Unprotected exposure to the environment allows evaporation from the epidermis, which results in a dry, dehydrated skin condition. UV exposure causes premature ageing of the skin as the UVA rays penetrate the dermis. Free radicals – are also formed that can cause skin cells to degenerate. These molecules disrupt the production of the collagen and elastin that give skin its strength and elasticity. Environmental pollutants such as lead, mercury and aluminium can accumulate in the body, where they attack protein in the cells. The skin should always be protected. Advise the client on suitable skincare and cosmetics that offer maximum protection. Antioxidant nutrients in the form of vitamins C, E and beta-carotene are beneficial in that they reinforce the effects of the skincare routine and treatment plan.

Central heating creates an environment with low humidity and this causes moisture loss from the skin leading to a dry, dehydrated skin condition. Air conditioning creates water loss from the skin and dries the mucous membranes leading to dry, irritated eyes which can be a problem for contact lens wearers. The effect on skin cells is that the skin too can become dry, reddened and irritated. Conditions such as eczema and psoriasis can become worse.

◆ *Pregnancy*. Clients may feel they need pampering during pregnancy. It is a time when the body undergoes significant bodily changes, which can cause sensitive and pigmented skin, stretch marks, **fluid retention**, insomnia, nausea, constipation and backache. Caution is needed in the choice of treatments, but there are many treatments available that may be of significant help to the client. Pigmented skin on the face is termed 'melasma' or a 'pregnancy mask' as it appears centrally on the face. Pigmentation disorders can be reduced with the use of sun block. Superficial effleurage massage technique can assist with reducing non-medical oedema by increasing lymphatic drainage.

TOP TIP

UV exposure

UV exposure is a primary cause of skin ageing referred to as photo-ageing. Noticeably the skin will be affected by reduced elasticity, dryness or UV-related pigmentation disorders such as solar lentigo. Recommend the client wears suitable UV protection at all times. You may apply a suitable product with an SPF for the client to experience at the end of a facial or hand treatment.

ALWAYS REMEMBER

Collagen, elastin and hyaluronic acid

Collagen fibres provide skin with strength and elastin fibres provide elasticity.

Collagen accounts for up to 75 per cent of the weight of the dermis; elastin accounts for 5 per cent.

Collagen helps provide a plump, youthful appearance to the skin. Gaining in popularity as a cosmetic product ingredient is hyaluronic acid (HA), a clear, sugary substance naturally made in the body, which helps maintain moisture levels. The molecules, once too big to penetrate the skin, have been now manufactured by the cosmetic industry to enable this, by changing their molecular structure. HA can attract water and has the capacity to retain it too, making the skin appear fuller and plumper.

HEALTH & SAFETY

Pregnancy care

Miscarriage is most likely during the first 3 months of pregnancy. Regular monitoring of the client's health is important before every treatment, as medical conditions may occur, such as changes in blood pressure and diabetes.

Modification of the treatment may be required. Explain the reason for this, e.g positioning of the client during wax depilation treatment. Recommend the client contacts their midwife to ensure they are happy for treatments to proceed. Also, only perform treatments that the client feels comfortable with.

ALWAYS REMEMBER

Client advice

If the client's expectations from the treatment are unrealistic, tactfully advise them why. An example may be lash extension application technique if it is unsuitable for the client's natural lashes.

Remember, always consider alternative treatments that can be offered, which will support the client in achieving their treatment goal.

If a client is unhappy with your decision, involve other relevant staff as necessary.

Always aim to swiftly resolve any issue to a satisfactory conclusion.

Suitable questions for consultation and assessment

Sample questions	Relevance of information to you
What is your treatment need? (e.g. hair removal, improved facial **skin tone**, improved nail condition)	This helps you to understand the client's treatment goal. Is this realistic for this client? The beauty therapist can consider appropriate treatments and products to use.
Which area requires treatment?	Never presume the area to be treated! The treatment area may require an intensive approach through selection of different products and treatments in order to achieve maximum results. The duration of treatment and cost may be increased, requiring discussion and agreement, e.g. a course of treatment to encourage improvement in nail condition and nail growth.
What treatments have you received previously? Were you satisfied with the treatment results? If not, why? (A client may be nervous of wax depilation treatments because of a previous bad experience.)	Discuss the benefits of the treatment choice you are able to offer to meet their needs. When necessary, reassure the client and regain their confidence in the treatment demonstrated through your knowledge and professionalism.
Are you undergoing any current treatment to the area? (e.g. temporary methods of hair removal, restylane injections, current skincare routine.)	You may find that the area of treatment has become worse through neglect or inappropriate application methods or techniques. You may not be able to treat the area because of conflict with other services received. Advise the client accordingly. You will be able to assess how knowledgeable and confident the client is in the use and types of treatments and products.
Related lifestyle factors (these are discussed in more detail below).	These factors will directly affect the client's health, general appearance and wellbeing.
What is your occupation/domestic situation?	The client's occupation or domestic situation may be stressful or contribute to the condition. Discuss relevant advice and recommendations as appropriate.
Are there any external factors that may limit your commitment to the treatment programme or use of additional products?	The client's domestic situation or employment hours may present restrictions to the programme required.
Describe your diet (this is highly relevant to the nail and skin condition).	Is the client's diet healthy and balanced? If not, discuss a healthy alternative relevant to their needs. Food should be eaten from a wide variety of food groups as recommended by the Food Standards Agency in their Eat Well guide. More information at www.food.gov.uk/. Take into consideration any special dietary requirements.
Do you take part in any leisure activities?	Are these offering an effective means of relaxation? Offer suggestions where relevant, such as relaxation techniques within the limit of your qualification.
Do you smoke?	Smoking has a detrimental effect on health and can lead to premature ageing and wrinkling of the skin. The colour of the skin often looks dull. Tactfully discuss those issues relevant to the characteristics observed.
Check the client's suitability for treatment – the client may have known contra-indications or previous related **contra-actions**.	The client's health may contra-indicate treatment, e.g. **medical history**, current medication, recent operations, allergies to products or positive reaction to a **skin sensitivity patch test**, etc. Explain the reason and offer alternatives.
Inspect the treatment area and question the client if there are any evident conditions that cause concern.	There may be visible contra-indications to treatment application. The treatment may require modification to accommodate contra-indications which restrict treatment, e.g. varicose veins in the area when performing wax depilation.
Suggest a realistic treatment plan and discuss attendance, period of time and cost.	You need to know if the client can commit themself to the plan, in terms of time and cost.
Question the client to ensure they understand all aspects of the treatment plan, e.g. objectives.	This should provide an opportunity to answer relevant questions and will ensure client satisfaction.

Diagnostic assessment

Specific diagnostic assessment procedures will enable you to identify any underlying condition or cause, which may be creating or contributing to the condition identified. These are discussed in relation to the face, hair and nails.

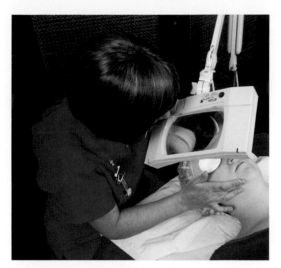

Skin being viewed to determine skin type and condition using a magnifying lamp whilst manually assessing skin texture and tone

Facial skin analysis

Following facial cleansing and toning to remove excess sebum, make-up and dead skin cells, inspect the skin's surface using a magnifying lamp looking at the face, neck and upper chest area. Protect the client's eyes from the light and use visual and touch diagnostic techniques to analyse skin type and condition.

The magnifying lamp is a safe and practical way to superficially inspect the skin's surface before treatments such as facial and eyebrow shaping treatments. In addition, the Wood's lamp may be used, which is a UVA lamp with an optical filter that blocks out visible light. It is able to identify skin type, sun damage and photo-ageing in the deeper layers of the skin. The colour it produces indicates the various skin conditions present.

Assessing skin type The skin's basic structure does not vary from person to person in health, but the physiological functioning of its different features does and this gives us different **skin types**.

The skin types are categorised according to sebaceous gland activity:

◆ **Normal** – usually observed on young skin, it has an even balance of oil and water secretions. Skin texture is soft and supple, with little imperfection. Pores are small with even colour.

◆ **Oily** – due to over activity of sebum production, this type is prone to open pores, comedones, pustules and papules. The surface of the skin appears shiny and texture is often thick and coarse. This skin type is more prevalent in teenagers as a response to hormonal changes taking place in the body.

◆ **Dry** – due to under-activity of sebum production and often lacking in moisture too, resulting in visible flaky areas on the skin's surface. Skin appearance is dull with an even texture but will often feel tight, especially following contact with water. The skin is prone to the formation of broken capillaries and sensitivity.

◆ **Combination** – this is the most common skin type which has the characteristics of an oily skin in the T-Zone (forehead, nose and chin) and normal/dry in the cheek area. However, it can be a combination of any skin type and condition.

In addition the skin is affected by environmental influences externally, and health and lifestyle internally, these affect the **skin condition**. Examples include sensitive, mature, congested and dehydrated.

◆ **Sensitive**-recognised by its high colouring, which flushes easily and feels warm to the touch. Often dilated capillaries will be present. Care must be taken handling this skin type as it may also have a tendency to become sensitive to products being used.

◆ **Mature**-as part of the ageing process, physiological activity slows resulting in a reduction in sebum production, the skin becomes less hydrated, drier and more lined. Contours are visibly slacker and the skin texture takes on a crepe-like appearance.

◆ **Congested**-skin texture and appearance is uneven with excess surface dead skin cells, raised lumps and the presence of comedones, pustules and papules.

◆ **Dehydrated** skin's tissues are lacking in water moisture. This results in a dull appearance, where fine lines are visible. The skin will often feel tight, is easily irritated, making it feel itchy.

Skin also reflects general health and responds quickly to any changes. This must be taken into consideration. For example, hormonal changes at puberty or in pregnancy may cause the sebaceous glands to become more active, resulting in oilier skin. During this time, the treatment routine must, therefore, be altered to suit the skin's needs. However, when the hormonal balance is settled, the skin type may change completely.

Assessing skin tone   A healthy young skin will probably have good **skin tone** and will be supple and elastic. This is because the collagen and elastin fibres in the skin are strong. The skin loses its strength with age as collagen production slows and elasticity is reduced. Poor skin tone is recognised by the appearance of facial lines and wrinkles. To test skin tone, gently lift the skin at the cheeks between two fingers, gently pinch and then let go. If the skin tone is good, the skin will spring back to its original shape. The longer it takes to return to its original position the poorer the skin tone. This manual test can also be used to test for tissue hydration. If the skin is dehydrated, when squeezed the skin will have a crepe-like appearance.

Pigmentation   As well as using the magnifying lamp, pigmentation can be viewed with a Wood's lamp (black light). This assesses damage at deeper levels in the skin.

Colours reflected by the Wood's lamp	Skin condition
Yellow	Oily
Blue-white	Normal
Brown	Pigmentation and sun damage
Pink-orange	Oil
Red	Inflamed or sluggish skin
Violet	Dehydration

REVISION AID

How would you describe skin type?

TOP TIP

Assessing skin hydration levels using equipment

Equipment is available that can assess the hydration level of the skin by analysing how effectively current is passed through the tissues, providing a value for hydration. This enables the correct diagnosis of the skin's needs and choice of therapeutic ingredients.

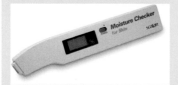

Moisture checker machine

REVISION AID

What is the relevant legislation that covers the protection of client data?

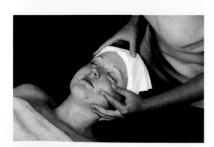

Testing skin tone

Touching the skin to assess skin texture and temperature Stroking the skin will help to inform your assessment of skin type/condition. Identify how the skin feels: oily, rough, smooth or dry. Areas of congestion may feel lumpy indicating papules, pustules or milia. Some types of skin will become warm and reddened when handled and are termed touch sensitive. This will influence how the skin is to be handled, products to be selected and how the skin may react to treatment. This can be explained to the client.

Assessing circulation Apply pressure to the area and wait for the colour to return. If this occurs immediately, circulation is healthy. The longer it takes indicates that circulation is sluggish and there may be capillary damage in the area.

Assessing muscle tone Observe the facial contours when the client is semi-reclined on the treatment couch. Poor **muscle tone** will be recognised by slack facial contours. The treatment aim will be to improve local circulation, metabolism and strengthen the muscles by shortening them, which will tighten and firm the muscles and contours. Facial exercises that the client can perform at home can be recommended.

A healthy diet, applications of appropriate facial skincare products and an effective skincare routine, and delivery of a supportive professional treatment plan all help to maintain the health of the skin, its underlying structure and delay the effects of ageing. Findings from the questioning techniques, analysis and diagnostic procedures should be recorded on the **client record**. Techniques used at consultation should be reviewed regularly, sometimes at each stage of the treatment plan according to the objectives to be achieved to confirm positive progress has been made and the client is satisfied. Sample treatment plans are shown later in this chapter for facial treatment, nail services and wax depilation.

Body fat The amount of body fat stored underneath the skin in the subcutaneous layer will depend upon the weight of the client. This will make a difference to the body and facial contours.

Advise the client on the modifications of any treatment applications and of any retail products recommended. Often the cost of the treatment will include the supporting home skin care preparations. It is important to demonstrate how these should be used.

Stretch marks (striations) Stretch marks appear on the skin as long, faint scars. They occur as a result of the skin tearing beneath the surface, in the dermal layer. Stretch marks are permanent and are caused by fluctuations in body weight as the skin stretches with weight gain, for example, during pregnancy. They are commonly seen on the breasts, abdomen, inner upper arm and inner thigh. This should be considered when performing treatments such as massage and wax depilation over these areas because the skin has less elasticity and is more fragile.

TOP TIP

Stretch marks

If a client has stretch marks, treatments that stretch the skin further will be contra-indicated, for example skin-stretching massage manipulations. A healthy, balanced diet is important – low levels of zinc, vitamins B6 and C are thought to contribute to the formation of stretch marks. The application of skin toning products can also be suggested.

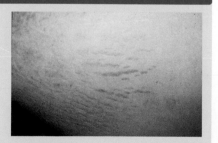
Stretch marks

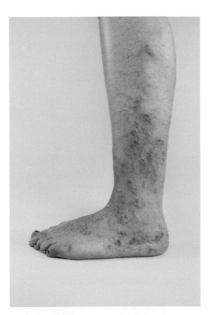

Varicose veins

Fluid retention Tissue fluid can accumulate, causing swelling (oedema). You must ascertain if this has a medical or non-medical cause. This will be determined at the consultation stage.

Normal swelling can occur around the ankles if a person stands for long periods, and is common during pregnancy. It is common before menstruation, affecting the abdomen and breasts. Fluid retention can also be caused by allergies and a diet with excessive processed foods, high salt intake and insufficient water. To test for fluid retention, press the client's skin. If it remains indented and does not immediately spring back, this is a sign of fluid retention.

Fluid retention in the face is often caused by poor hydration, leading to dehydration. It can also be caused by poor lymphatic circulation where excess fluid appears in the spaces between the adipose tissue.

Varicose veins Veins have valves to prevent backflow as they carry blood under low pressure back towards the heart. An occupation requiring you to sit or stand for long periods may lead to varicose veins, a condition where the veins' valves have become weak and have lost their elasticity. The area appears knotted, swollen and bluish/purple in colour. Where varicose veins are present, treatments that put further pressure on the weakened vein will be unsuitable. Pressure should be reduced when performing a lower leg massage as a part of a pedicure service and the area should be avoided when carrying out a wax depilation treatment.

Pre-treatments tests In line with the manufacturer's recommendations and legal requirements, certain treatments require a pre-treatment test to be applied to the skin before treatment is given. In some instances this occurs before each treatment. Re-test if there is a change in the medical health of the client, or an interval between treatments.

Test patch thermal This is used before a service where heat is applied to the skin to assess tolerance to temperature. Examples include depilation waxing and paraffin waxing which is used in hand and nail treatments.

Skin sensitivity patch test This is used to assess skin tolerance to potential allergens. It includes artificial eyelash extension adhesives and permanent tint. Where a client has known allergies or a history of allergies, a **skin sensitivity test** may be required in advance to assess suitability of products used within the treatment or service. Manufacturers will often state if a skin sensitivity test is required when using their products and how and when this is to be carried out.

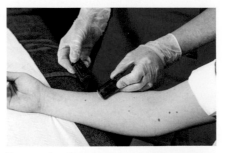

Test patch – thermal, to assess skin nerve stimuli response to heat

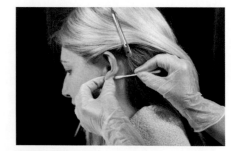

Skin sensitivity test – test to assess skin tolerance to potential allergens

A sample client treatment plan record: FACIAL

Date		Beauty therapist	
Title	First name	Surname	Date of birth (D.O.B.) Female Male
			(client age group) This will allow you to classify the client and health of the skin for this age. It also provides a reference for when clients share the same name, and whether permission is required e.g. treatment of minors.
Address Contact details are important for marketing purposes and, when necessary, to change appointment bookings. The client will often have a preference for which is the most suitable method of contact; make a record of this.		Postcode	

Email address	Landline	Mobile phone number

IDENTIFY YOUR STATUS, ARE YOU:

☐ A member ☐ A guest ☐ A client ☐ None of these

If your business is set in a leisure/spa club you may wish to find out the following information which may influence your treatment plan choices.

Name of doctor	Doctor's address and phone number

HEALTH AND WELLBEING

Related medical history (check for any conditions that may restrict or prevent treatment application)

If the client has any known medical condition which is not listed below, they must inform you of this as it may prevent or restrict treatment application.

Are you taking any medication? (This may affect the appearance of the skin, or treatment area, skin sensitivity or reaction to the treatment.)

CONTRA-INDICATIONS WHICH PREVENT TREATMENT OR REQUIRE MEDICAL REFERRAL

☐ bacterial infection (e.g. impetigo)
☐ viral infection (e.g. herpes simplex)
☐ fungal infection (e.g. tinea corporis)
☐ parasitic infection (e.g. pediculosis and scabies)
☐ eye infections (e.g. conjunctivitis)
☐ watery eyes
☐ systemic medical condition e.g. blood pressure
☐ severe skin condition (e.g. psoriasis if skin is broken and inflamed)
☐ ongoing chemotherapy or radiotherapy treatment
☐ undiagnosed lumps, bumps or swellings
☐ certain types of cancer e.g. skin cancer in area

CONTRA-INDICATIONS WHICH RESTRICT TREATMENT OR REQUIRE TREATMENT ADAPTION
(Service may require adaptation)

☐ cuts and abrasions   ☐ bruising and swelling
☐ recent scar tissue   ☐ eczema
☐ skin allergies   ☐ diabetes
☐ styes   ☐ hyperkeratosis

SKIN TYPE

☐ oily   ☐ normal
☐ combination   ☐ dry

SKIN CONDITION

☐ sensitive   ☐ dehydrated
☐ mature   ☐ congested
☐ young

SKIN CONDITION CHARACTERISTICS

☐ milia   ☐ comedones
☐ broken capillaries   ☐ ingrowing hairs
☐ pustules   ☐ papules
☐ open pores   ☐ hyper-pigmentation
☐ hypo-pigmentation   ☐ dermatitis papulosa nigra
☐ keloids   ☐ hyperkeratosis
☐ pseudo folliculitis

A sample client treatment plan record: FACIAL (continued)

FACIAL PRODUCTS

- ☐ eye make-up remover
- ☐ cleanser
- ☐ toner
- ☐ eye make-up remover
- ☐ exfoliator

- ☐ masks (setting and non-setting)
- ☐ massage medium
- ☐ moisturiser
- ☐ specialist skin products (e.g. eye cream/gel)

Following skin analysis record on the illustration below skin condition characteristics found and in which numbered areas they appear.

1 _____
2 _____
3 _____
4 _____
5 _____
6 _____
7 _____

EQUIPMENT

- ☐ magnifying light
- ☐ skin warming device

MASSAGE TECHNIQUES

- ☐ effleurage
- ☐ petrissage
- ☐ tapotement
- ☐ frictions
- ☐ vibrations

ASSESSMENT TECHNIQUES VISUAL CHECK

- ☐ skin type
- ☐ skin condition
- ☐ skin elasticity and muscle tone
- ☐ sun damage
- ☐ skin reaction and sensitivity
- ☐ evidence of cosmetic surgery
- ☐ aesthetic non-medical procedures e.g. botox

MANUAL CHECK

- ☐ skin temperature
- ☐ pinch test (to assess elasticity and hydration)

Beauty therapist signature (for reference)

Client signature (confirmation of details and consent for treatment)

TREATMENT ADVICE

Consultation – provided at the first treatment or as an independent service – this service will take 15 minutes.

Full facial treatment – this service will take 60 minutes (1 hour).

TREATMENT PLAN CONTENT

What are the client's main concerns and treatment results required?

What is the client's current skincare programme?

Find out:

- ◆ what products the client is currently using to cleanse and care for the skin of the face and neck
- ◆ how the products are applied and removed
- ◆ regularity of use
- ◆ client satisfaction with their skincare routine and products used.

A sample client treatment plan record: FACIAL (continued)

Explain:

◆ how the products used should be correctly applied and removed

◆ if the products are not suitable, explain why

◆ if the regularity of application is sufficient/appropriate.

◆ how to recognise a contra-action to the treatment or products used.

Confirm the most appropriate treatment for your client, what is involved and products to be used. Record these as treatment notes. Treatment notes for your client should be updated at each visit and for every treatment. This will include a check on the medical health and related updates.

Ensure the client's records are up-to-date, accurate, signed by the client and beauty therapist and fully completed following the treatment. Non-compliance may invalidate insurance.

Note: any contra-action (adverse/unwanted) skin reaction; if any occur what action has been taken?

AFTER

Record:

◆ specific facial areas and conditions treated

◆ any modification to treatment application that has occurred, e.g. less pressure applied over the cheek area when working on a sensitive skin with broken capillaries

◆ any contra-actions and actions taken

◆ what products have been used in the facial treatment

◆ the effectiveness of treatment; did you achieve what you planned for and agreed at the consultation?

◆ any product samples provided (review client satisfaction with their use at the next appointment).

Advise on:

◆ product application and removal in order to gain maximum benefit from product use

◆ use of make-up and other services such as UV exposure, self tanning treatment following facial treatment

◆ recommended time intervals between each treatment

◆ the importance of regular or a course of facials to maintain and improve skin condition and appearance.

RETAIL AND FURTHER TREATMENT OPPORTUNITIES

Advise on:

◆ promotional treatment offers

◆ future progression of the facial treatment plan

◆ skincare products that would be suitable for the client to use at home and which support achievement of the treatment plan objectives

◆ up-selling – further suitable products or treatments that you have recommended that the client may or may not have received before.

Note: any purchases made by the client and any samples provided – follow their effectiveness and the client's satisfaction with their use up at the next appointment.

EVALUATION

Record:

◆ comments on the client's satisfaction with the treatment

◆ how the treatment can be progressed to maintain and advance the treatment results in the future.

HEALTH AND SAFETY

Advise on:

◆ avoidance of activities, other treatments or products that may cause a contra-action

◆ action to be taken if an unwanted skin reaction occurs (contra-action).

Record relevant details of the consultation and advice and recommendations for future reference.

A sample NAIL SERVICES client treatment plan record

Date	Beauty therapist name

Client name	Date of birth (identifying client age group)
Home address	Postcode

Email address	Landline phone number	Mobile phone number

Name of doctor	Doctor's address and phone number

Related medical history (conditions that may restrict or prohibit treatment application)

Are you taking any medication? (this may affect the sensitivity of the skin to the treatment)

CONTRA-INDICATIONS REQUIRING MEDICAL REFERRAL

(preventing nail services)

☐ bacterial infections (e.g. paronychia)

☐ viral infections (e.g. warts)

☐ fungal infections (e.g. tinea unguium, tinea pedis)

☐ parasitic infections, (e.g. scabies)

☐ severe nail separation

☐ severe eczema and psoriasis

☐ severe bruising

☐ severe skin conditions

☐ diabetes

☐ severe skin disorders (e.g. eczema) or conditions (e.g. psoriasis)

CONTRA-INDICATIONS WHICH RESTRICT TREATMENT

(treatment may require adaptation)

☐ minor nail separation   ☐ undiagnosed lumps or

☐ product allergies   swellings

☐ recent scar tissue   ☐ minor eczema and psoriasis

☐ severely damaged nails ☐ severely bitten nails

☐ broken bones   ☐ minor bruising or swelling

☐ recent fractures   ☐ minor cuts or abrasions
   and sprains

☐ broken capillaries or varicose veins

☐ moles

☐ circulatory conditions (e.g. phlebitis)

PRODUCTS, TOOLS AND EQUIPMENT

☐ nail and skin treatment tools

☐ abrasives (e.g. buffing cream)

☐ cuticle softeners

☐ nail and skin products

☐ nail conditioners (e.g. cuticle cream/oils)

☐ skin conditioners (e.g. hand or foot cream)

☐ nail, skin and cuticle corrective treatments (e.g. paraffin wax)

☐ consumables

HAND AND NAIL TREATMENTS

☐ warm oil hand mask   ☐ thermal mitts

☐ paraffin wax   ☐ exfoliators

FOOT TREATMENTS

☐ paraffin wax   ☐ thermal booties

☐ foot masks   ☐ exfoliators

NAIL FINISH

☐ light colour   ☐ French manicure

☐ dark colour   ☐ buffing

COURSE OF TREATMENT

	Date	Date	Date
☐ improvement of skin	_____	_____	_____
☐ condition products	_____	_____	_____
☐ improvement of nail condition products	_____	_____	_____

NAIL, CUTICLE AND SKIN CONDITION

Nails

☐ healthy   ☐ brittle   ☐ split

☐ dry   ☐ weak   ☐ bitten (onychophagy)

☐ ridged (horizontal or longitudinal)

Nail shape

☐ oval   ☐ claw

☐ tapered   ☐ fan

☐ square   ☐ pointed

☐ squoval

Cuticle

☐ healthy   ☐ split   ☐ overgrown

☐ dry   ☐ hangnails   (pterygium)

Skin

☐ healthy   ☐ dry   ☐ hard

MASSAGE MEDIUMS

☐ creams   ☐ oils   ☐ lotions

Beauty therapist signature (for reference)

Client signature (confirmation of details)

A sample NAIL SERVICES client treatment plan record (continued)

TREATMENT ADVICE

Consultation – provided at the first treatment or as an independent service – *allow up to 15 minutes.*

Preliminary sections of the treatment plan have not been included; client details, history, contra-indications, products and services etc.

Manicure – *allow 45 minutes.*

Pedicure – *allow 45 minutes.*

Specialised skin/nail conditioning treatment – *allow up to 60 minutes.*

TREATMENT PLAN

Record relevant details of your service, advice and recommendations provided for future reference.

Include:

- details that may influence the client's nail condition, such as their occupation, footwear, hobbies, e.g. running, which may damage the toe nails
- the products the client is currently using to care for the skin of the hands, feet and nails, and the regularity of their use
- the client's satisfaction with these products.

Confirm the most appropriate treatment for your client, what is involved and products to be used. Record these as treatment notes for your client. These should be updated at each visit and for every treatment. This will include a check on their medical health and related updates.

Ensure the client's records are up-to-date, accurate, signed by the client and beauty therapist and fully completed following treatment. Non-compliance may invalidate insurance.

DURING

Discuss:

- relevant nail and skin treatment procedures (e.g. how to file the nails correctly).

Guidance on how to care for the nails and skin including lifestyle factors and time management tips to ensure a routine can be established.

Note:

- any contra-action (adverse, unwanted) reaction, if any occur during or after the nail service.

If this is a follow-up appointment discuss the progress and success of the suggested advice and recommendations.

AFTER

Record:

- results of service
- any modification to service application that has occurred
- what products have been used in the service
- what skin and nail treatments have been used
- the effectiveness of treatment; did you achieve what you agreed at the consultation?
- any product samples provided (review their success at the next appointment).

Advise on:

- product application in order to gain maximum benefit from product use
- specialised products following the service for home use
- general skin/nail care and maintenance
- care of the foot structure, e.g. bones, arches and joints of the foot within your responsibility
- the recommended time intervals between each nail service
- the importance of a course of treatment to improve nail/skin conditions.

A sample NAIL SERVICES client treatment plan record (continued)

RETAIL AND FURTHER TREATMENT OPPORTUNITIES

Advise on:

- special treatment/product offers
- progression of the treatment plan for future appointments
- products that would be suitable for the client to use at home to care for the skin and nails and which support achievement of the treatment plan objectives
- recommendations for further services and treatments
- up-selling further products or treatments that the client may or may not have received before.

Note:

- any purchase made by the client.

Remember to follow up their effectiveness at the next appointment.

EVALUATION

Record:

- comments on the client's satisfaction with the service
- if unsatisfactory results are achieved, the reasons why
- how you may alter the treatment plan to achieve the required results if applicable.

HEALTH AND SAFETY

Advise on:

- appropriate necessary action to be taken in the event of an unwanted skin or nail reaction occurs (contra-action)
- recommendations for correct product use
- the importance of compliance with recommendations, e.g. professional removal of gel polish finish.

Sample WAX DEPILATION client treatment plan record

Date	Beauty therapist name		
Client name		Date of birth Male Female	
		(identifying client age group) Relates to health of the skin for this age and cause of hair growth. It also provides a reference when clients share the same name, and whether permission is required, e.g. treatment of minors.	
Home address		Postcode	
Email address	Landline phone number		Mobile phone number
Name of doctor	Doctor's address and phone number		
Related medical history (Conditions that may cause hair growth, restrict or prohibit treatment application)			
Are you taking any medication? (This may affect the hair growth, sensitivity and skin reaction following treatment.)			

CONTRA-INDICATIONS WHICH PREVENT SERVICE OR REQUIRE MEDICAL REFERRAL	*CONTRA-INDICATIONS WHICH RESTRICT SERVICE OR REQUIRE SERVICE ADAPTATION*
☐ bacterial infection (e.g. impetigo, conjunctivitis)	(Treatment may require adaptation.)
☐ viral infection (e.g. herpes simplex/warts)	☐ cuts and abrasions ☐ mild eczema/psoriasis
☐ fungal infection (e.g. tinea corporis)	☐ bruising and swelling ☐ broken bones

Sample WAX DEPILATION client treatment plan record (continued)

☐ severe skin conditions

☐ infectious skin conditions

☐ diabetes

☐ severe varicose veins

☐ phlebitis

☐ deep vein thrombosis

☐ client is undergoing chemotherapy or radiotherapy treatment

☐ thin and fragile skin

☐ known allergies to products and ingredients, e.g. rosin found in adhesive plasters and wax

TEST CONDUCTED

☐ thermal patch test, self   ☐ thermal patch test, client

☐ client skin sensitivity test patch

WAX PRODUCTS

☐ hot wax

☐ warm wax

PREVIOUS METHODS OF HAIR REMOVAL

☐ tweezing   ☐ shaving

☐ depilatory creams   ☐ electrical depilatory

☐ abrasive mitt   ☐ light-based hair reduction

☐ threading   ☐ electrical epilation

☐ self tan   ☐ recent fractures

☐ skin disorders   ☐ recent scar tissue

☐ heat rash   ☐ hyperkeratosis

☐ sunburn   ☐ skin and product allergies

☐ hairy moles   ☐ circulatory conditions

☐ skin tags   ☐ infected ingrowing hairs

                        ☐ medication affecting the skin, blood or immune system

AREAS TREATED FOR HAIR REMOVAL

(Treatment may require adaptation.)

☐ eyebrows   ☐ chin

☐ upper lip/face   ☐ full leg

☐ half leg   ☐ underarm

☐ bikini line

HAIR TYPE

☐ Vellus   ☐ Terminal

SKIN TYPE

☐ normal   ☐ oily

☐ dry   ☐ combination

SKIN CONDITION

☐ sensitive   ☐ mature   ☐ dehydrated

Beauty therapist signature (for reference)

Client signature (confirmation of details)

TREATMENT ADVICE

*SERVICE TIMINGS**

Half leg wax – *allow 30 minutes*   Eyebrow wax – *allow 15 minutes*

Full leg wax – *allow 50 minutes*   Facial wax   top lip or chin – *allow 10 minutes*

Bikini wax – *allow 15 minutes*   top lip and chin – *allow 15 minutes*

Underarm wax – *allow 15 minutes*

*Waxing timings may differ according to the wax depilation system used. Always allow slightly longer when using hot wax.

Discuss what methods of hair removal the client has been using, for how long and their success.

TREATMENT PLAN

Consultation – provided at the first treatment or as an independent service – allow up to 15 minutes.

Record relevant details of your service and advice and recommendations for future reference.

Ensure the client's records are up-to-date, accurate, signed by the client and beauty therapist and fully completed following service treatment. Non-compliance may invalidate insurance.

Sample WAX DEPILATION client treatment plan record (continued)

DURING

Monitor:

♦ client's reaction to treatment to confirm suitability.

Note:

♦ work techniques including direction and angle of hair removal, wax temperature checks

♦ skin reaction to treatment

♦ success of hair removal

♦ necessity to change wax or working technique

♦ any contra-action (adverse/unwanted) reaction, if any occur and what action has been taken.

AFTER

Record:

♦ results of treatment, e.g. success of hair removal and skin reaction

♦ any modification to treatment application that has occurred

♦ what products have been used in the wax removal treatment

♦ the effectiveness of treatment

♦ any samples provided (review their success at the next appointment).

Advise on:

♦ use of aftercare products following wax removal treatment

♦ maintenance procedures

♦ the recommended time intervals between treatments.

RETAIL AND FURTHER TREATMENT OPPORTUNITIES

Advise on:

♦ promotional treatment and retail product offers

♦ products that would be suitable for the client to use at home to care for and maintain the treatment area (these include body exfoliation and moisturising skincare products, and hair retardants that slow hair regrowth)

♦ recommendations for further treatments

♦ up-selling further products or treatments that the client may or may not have received before.

Note:

♦ any purchase made by the client – follow up their effectiveness at the next appointment.

EVALUATION

Record:

♦ comments on the client's satisfaction with the service

♦ if poor results are achieved, note the reasons why

♦ how you may alter the service plan to achieve the required treatment results in the future, if applicable. This may include change to waxing technique/wax depilation product or other hair removal system.

HEALTH AND SAFETY

Advise on:

♦ how to care for the area following service to avoid an unwanted reaction

♦ avoidance of any activities, other treatments or product application that may cause a contra-action

♦ appropriate **necessary action** to be taken in the event of an unwanted reaction (contra-action).

Skin diseases and disorders

Like any organ of the body, the skin is at risk of developing diseases or disorders. As a beauty therapist you must be able to distinguish a healthy skin from one suffering from any disease or disorder. Certain skin disorders and diseases prevent or contra-indicate a beauty treatment. Moreover, treatment would expose the beauty therapist, colleagues and clients to the risk of cross-infection or could make the condition worse. It is therefore essential that you are familiar with skin, hair and nail diseases and disorders including infections with which you may come into contact at work. You need to know which diseases and disorders are a risk to yourself and which are not, as well as the correct action to take.

Although you may be able to recognise the symptoms of these conditions by their appearance, remember you are not qualified to diagnose. In the instance of an undiagnosed condition, this should always be referred to the client's GP without causing alarm. Also, remember that you cannot always see the symptoms of a disease or disorder. There are sensations that are *felt*, such as itching, heat and pain.

Many disorders though, are not harmful and a beauty treatment can have both psychological and/or physiological benefit for the client.

Your knowledge of skin structure and function will enable you to provide the most appropriate advice, recommendations, treatments and products for each client. These are discussed below with relevant diseases, disorders and parasitic conditions. Further information can also be found in each treatment chapter.

Many disorders and diseases will share characteristics in terms of their texture, colour, size and shape. We are able to classify these as lesions.

There are primary and secondary lesions.

Primary lesions have the following characteristics:

◆ They are a different colour from the surrounding skin.

◆ They appear raised in relation to the surrounding skin.

Secondary lesions follow the primary lesion, they:

◆ exhibit changes to the skin as a result of the process of skin repair.

ALWAYS REMEMBER

Skin lesions

A visible change to the skin's appearance in texture, colour and shape is referred to as a lesion. It is important to recognise the different types of skin lesions. A harmless lesion is a bruise; a harmful lesion would be a malignant melanoma or skin cancer. Lesions can indicate disorder or disease.

Primary lesions, are those that are a different colour than the surrounding skin, or are raised. Primary lesions include papules, pustules, vesicles and macules.

A secondary lesion, occurs generally as a result of the primary lesion, examples include scale, scab and scar.

REVISION AID

Why are skin sensitivity tests carried out?

Primary skin lesions

Figure	Name of Lesion	Description	Typical size	Examples	Can you proceed?
	Vesicle	An area of skin that is a different colour containing clear fluid. It is located within or slightly below the epidermis and is commonly referred to as a *blister*.	Less than 0.5 cm	Herpes simplex, herpes zoster	No
	Bulla	Similar to the vesicle but larger.	Greater than 0.5 cm	Contact dermatitis, large second-degree burns, bulbous impetigo, blister	No
	Papule	Small, solid skin elevation; doesn't contain fluid but may develop pus, a sign of infection.	Less than 0.5 cm in diameter	Warts, acne vulgaris	Yes, depending on the, type, number of lesions and the severity
	Tubercle	Abnormal, rounded, solid lump larger than a papule, located above, within or under the skin. Whilst solid and elevated, however, it also extends deeper than papules into the dermis or subcutaneous tissues.	0.5 to 2 cm	Cyst	
	Pustule	Elevated lesion that becomes filled with pus and cellular debris. Raised, inflamed, papule with white or yellow centre containing pus in the top of the lesion.	Usually less than 0.5cm in diameter	Acne vulgaris, impetigo, furuncles, carbuncles, folliculitis, boil	No
	Tumour	External swelling varying in size, shape and colour.	Greater than 2 cm	Carcinoma (such as advanced breast carcinoma); not basal cell or squamous cell of the skin	No
	Macule	A flat skin lesion where the skin is a different colour to the surrounding skin. This may be an area of redness (erythematous), no pigmentation (hypo-pigmentation) or darker pigmentation (hyper-pigmentation).	Less than 1 cm	Freckle (ephelide), or an area where a pustule/papule has healed	Yes
	Wheal	Itchy, swollen lesion that usually has irregular borders. It is usually only temporary and on the skin for a few hours.		Insect bite or a hive, urticaria, contact with product allergens	No

Secondary skin lesions

Figure	Name of Lesion	Description	Examples	Can you proceed?
	Scar	Lighter or darker coloured, slightly raised mark on the skin following an injury or healed lesion.	Mark left following skin healing with the production of new connective tissue in the dermis	Yes (if the scar has healed and, as a guideline, is older than six months)
	Crust	An accumulation of dead skin cells, blood, pus, and epidermal debris. Crusting is usually yellow or brown in colour and moist in texture.	Scab	No
	Ulcer	Open lesion on the skin affecting the epidermis as well as part, or all, of the dermis; accompanied by loss of skin depth and possibly weeping of tissue fluids or pus.	Open wound	No
	Scale	Visibly thickened stratum corneum layer of the epidermis, without substantial depth, where dry, white scales appear on the skin's surface.	Dermatitis, psoriasis	Yes (as long as the skin is not broken)
	Fissure	A split in the skin's epidermal surface that may go into the dermis.	Cracked lips or skin on the hands or feet	Yes (but avoid area as it may be sensitive)
	Excoriation	Lesion resulting from scratching or scraping.	Mark left after a superficial skin injury	No (or avoid as long as skin is not broken)

Microorganisms leading to disease and disorder are discussed below.

Bacterial infections

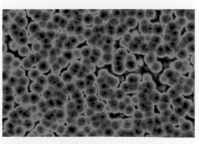

Microscopic bacteria

Bacteria are minute single-celled organisms of varied shapes. Large numbers of bacteria inhabit the surface of the skin and are harmless **(non-pathogenic)**, with some playing an important positive role in the health of the skin. Others, however, are harmful **(pathogenic)** and can cause disease.

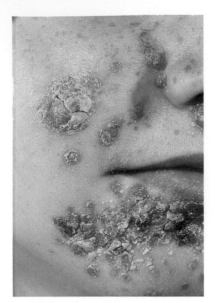

Impetigo

Impetigo An inflammatory disease of the surface of the skin, usually appearing on exposed areas.

Infectious? Yes.

Appearance: Initially the skin appears red and feels itchy. Small, thin-walled blisters appear, which burst and form honey-coloured crusts. Untreated, small pus-filled ulcers can occur with a dark thick crust that can lead to scarring.

Site: The commonly affected areas are the nose, the mouth and the ears, but impetigo can occur on the scalp and limbs.

Treatment: Medical – usually an antibiotic or an antibacterial ointment is prescribed containing corticosteroids such as hydrocortisone as the infection can spread quickly.

Conjunctivitis or pink eye Inflammation of the conjunctiva, the mucous membrane that covers the eye and lines the eyelids. The cause can also be viral.

Infectious? Yes.

Appearance: The skin of the inner conjunctiva of the eye becomes inflamed and the eye becomes very red and feels sore, with the sensation of itchiness and feels as if grit is in the eye. Water and pus may exude from the area, leaving a sticky coating on the lashes.

Site: The eyes, either one or both, may be infected.

Treatment: Medical – usually an antibiotic lotion is prescribed. However, in some cases medical treatment will not be necessary and the infection will heal independently.

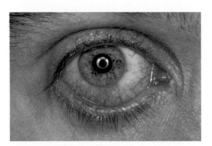

Conjunctivitis or pink eye

Hordeolum or styes

Infection of the sebaceous glands of eyelash hair follicles. It can be an effect of blepharitis (inflammation of the eyelids).

Infectious? Yes, if the bacteria comes into contact with someone else's eye, this might lead to cross-infection.

Appearance: Small red, inflamed lumps containing pus, a sign of infection.

Site: The inner rim of the eyelid.

Treatment: Medical – usually an antibiotic is prescribed.

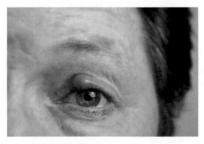

Hordeolum or styes

Furuncles or boils Infection affecting the hair follicle.

Infectious? Yes.

Appearance: A localised red lump appears around the hair follicle; this then develops a core of pus, yellowish-white fluid formed in infected tissue. Scarring of the skin often remains after the boil has healed.

Site: The back of the neck, the armpits and the buttocks and thighs are common areas, but furuncles can occur anywhere.

Treatment: Medical – antibiotics may be prescribed to help control infection.

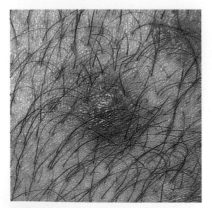

Boil (localised red lump surrounding a hair follicle indicating infection)

Carbuncles Infection of several hair follicles.

Infectious? Yes.

Appearance: A hard, round abscess, larger than a boil, which oozes pus from several points upon its surface. Scarring often occurs after the carbuncle has healed.

Site: In particular where there is friction, such as the back of the neck or on the thighs. However, they can occur anywhere.

Treatment: Medical – usually involving incision of the skin, drainage of the pus, and a course of antibiotics.

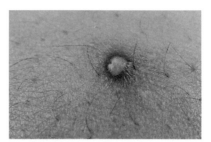
Carbuncle

Paronychia Infection of the skin tissue surrounding the nail (the nail fold). If left untreated the nail bed may also become infected.

Infectious? Yes.

Appearance: Swelling, redness and pus appears in the nail fold and in the area of the nail wall.

Site: The skin surrounding the nail plate.

Treatment: Medical – usually a course of antibiotics. Incision and drainage of pus is necessary if it collects in the skin next to the nail plate.

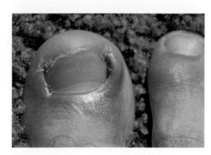
Paronychia

Viral infections

Viruses are minute bodies, too small to see even under an ordinary microscope. Viruses invade healthy body cells and multiply within the cell: in due course the cell walls break down, releasing new viral particles to attack further cells, spreading the infection.

Herpes simplex This is commonly referred to as a cold sore and is a recurring skin condition, appearing at times when the skin's resistance is lowered through ill health or stress. It may also be caused by exposure of the skin to extremes of temperature or to UV light.

Infectious? Yes.

Appearance: Inflammation of the skin occurs in localised areas. As well as being red, the skin becomes itchy and small vesicles appear. These are followed by a crust, which may crack and weep tissue fluid.

Site: The mucous membranes of the nose or lips; herpes simplex can also occur anywhere on the skin generally.

Treatment: There is no specific treatment and they usually clear in 7–10 days. A proprietary brand of anti-inflammatory antiseptic drying cream is usually prescribed. This must be applied in the early stages of the condition when a tingling, itching sensation is experienced.

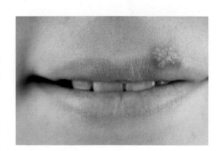
Herpes simplex

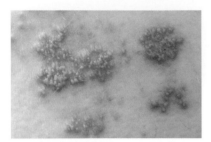

Herpes zoster or shingles

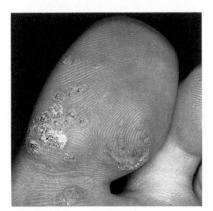

Verrucas

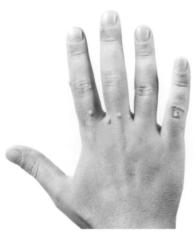

Warts on the hand

Herpes zoster or shingles Herpes zoster or shingles is caused by the same virus that is responsible for chickenpox. In this painful disease, the virus attacks the sensory nerve endings and is thought to lie dormant in the body and be triggered when the body's defences are lowered.

Infectious? Yes.

Appearance: Redness of the skin occurs along the line of the affected nerves. Blisters develop and form crusts, leaving purplish-pink pigmentation.

Site: Commonly the chest and the abdomen.

Treatment: Medical – usually including anti-viral medicines. Calamine lotion can soothe the irritation. If there are complications with bacterial infection, antibiotics will be prescribed.

Verrucas or warts Small epidermal skin growths. Warts can be raised or flat, depending upon their position. There are several types of wart: plane, common and plantar.

Infectious? Yes.

Appearance: Warts vary in size, shape, texture and colour. Usually they have a rough surface and are raised. If the wart occurs on the sole of the foot it grows inwards, due to the pressure of body weight.

Site:

◆ plane wart (flat wart): the fingers, either surface of the hand, face or legs

◆ common wart (verruca vulgaris): the face, hands, elbows and knees

◆ plantar wart (verruca): the sole of the foot and toes.

Treatment: Sometimes verrucas and warts can clear on their own. Medical – using acids, e.g. salicylic acid, solid carbon dioxide, cryotherapy or electrocautery.

Infestations

An infestation is where animal **parasites** invade and live off the host's tissue to gain all their nutrients.

Scabies or itch mites (Sarcoptes scabiei) A condition in which an infestation of tiny parasitic mites burrow beneath the skin and invade the hair follicles. The mites feed on tissue and fluid as they burrow into the skin.

Infectious? Yes.

Appearance: Initially, minute papules and wavy greyish lines appear, where dirt has entered the burrows. Secondary bacterial infection may occur as a result of scratching the skin.

Site: Usually seen in warm areas of loose skin, such as the webs of the fingers, under the fingernails and the creases of the elbows.

Treatment: Medical – an anti-scabetic lotion containing an insecticide.

Pediculosis capitis or head lice
A condition in which small lice infest scalp hair.

Infectious? Yes.

Appearance: The lice cling to the hair of the scalp. Eggs are laid, attached to the hair close to the skin. The lice bite the skin to draw nourishment from the blood; this creates irritation and itching of the skin, which may lead to secondary bacterial infection.

Site: The hair of the scalp.

Treatment: Medical – an appropriate medicated insecticidal lotion or rinse.

Pediculosis pubis or pubic lice
A condition in which small lice parasites infest body hair.

Infectious? Yes.

Appearance: The lice cling to the hair of the body. Eggs are laid, attached to the hair close to the skin. The lice bite the skin to draw nourishment from the blood; this creates irritation and itching of the skin, which may lead to secondary bacterial infection.

Site: Pubic hair.

Treatment: Medical – an appropriate insecticidal lotion.

Pediculosis corporis
A condition in which small parasites live and feed on body skin.

Infectious? Yes.

Appearance: The lice cling to the hair of the body. Eggs are laid, attached to the hair close to the skin. The lice bite the skin to draw nourishment from the blood; this creates irritation and itching of the skin, which may lead to secondary bacterial infection. Where body lice bite the skin, small red marks can be seen.

Site: Body hair.

Treatment: Medical – an appropriate insecticidal lotion.

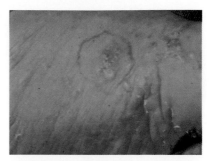
A scabies burrow ringed

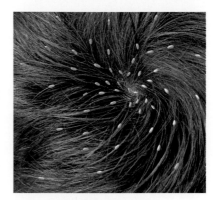
Pediculosis capitis or head lice

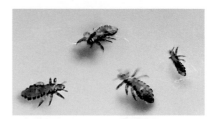
Head lice

ACTIVITY

Infection prevention and control

Risks from infection need to be controlled, just like any other health and safety concern.

◆ Identify the hazard.
◆ Assess the risks.
◆ Control the risks.

1   Identify different ways in which infection may be transferred in the workplace.

2   Provide examples of how can you control and prevent the risk of cross-infection in the workplace.

Fungal diseases

Fungi are parasitic plants which may be microscopic in size. They are dependent upon a host for their existence. Fungal diseases of the skin feed off the waste products of the skin. Some fungi are found on the skin's surface; others attack the deeper tissues. Reproduction of fungi is by means of simple cell division or by the production of spores.

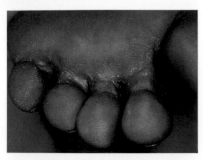

Tinea pedis or athlete's foot

Tinea pedis or athlete's foot   A common fungal foot infection.

Infectious? Yes.

Appearance: The skin can appear white and spongy-looking. Small blisters form, which later burst. The skin in the area can then become dry, crack and peel, giving a scaly appearance.

Site: Commonly affects the webs of skin between the toes.

Treatment: Thorough cleansing of the area. Medical application of fungicides. Untreated, infections such as bacterial infections may occur. It can also lead to infection of the toe and fingernails.

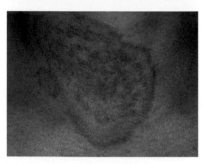

Tinea corporis or body ringworm

Tinea corporis or body ringworm   A **fungal infection** of the skin.

Infectious? Yes.

Appearance: Small scaly red patches, which spread outwards and then heal from the centre, leaving a ring.

Site: The trunk of the body, the limbs and the face.

Treatment: Medical – using a fungicidal cream. Oral anti-fungal medication is necessary if there are several infection sites.

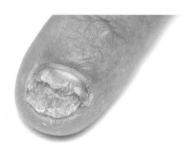

Tinea unguium or ringworm of the nail plate

Tinea unguium or onychomycosis   Fungal infection of the fingernails.

Infectious? Yes.

Appearance: The nail plate is white and opaque. Eventually the nail plate becomes brittle, can crumble and separates from the nail bed.

Site: The nail plate.

Treatment: Medical application of fungicides.

Pityriasis versicolour or tinea versicolour (sun fungus)   A fungal infection which interferes with the ability of melanocytes to produce melanin.

Infectious: No.

Appearance: Small patches of skin, either lighter or darker than the surrounding skin.

Site: Commonly affects the trunk, neck, upper arms and back.

Treatment: Medical application of fungicides.

Sweat (sudoriferous) gland disorders

Prickly heat or milaria rubra   Acute inflammatory disorder of the sweat glands caused when the skin sweats more than normal and the sweat glands become blocked. The trapped sweat then causes skin irritation.

HEALTH & SAFETY

Nail enhancements and nail fungus

Nail enhancements can increase the risk of developing a fungal infection. This is due to the natural nail plate being roughened. If not maintained correctly, moisture can collect between the artificial nail and the natural nail plate, which provides ideal growth conditions for fungi.

It is essential that the client understands the importance of complying with the aftercare advice and recommendations provided.

Infectious: No.

Appearance: A rash of small red, raised spots accompanied by a prickling and itching sensation.

Site: Usually worse in areas covered by clothing as this can cause further skin irritation.

Treatment: Skin cooling agent such as calamine lotion and antihistamine tablets may be prescribed to reduce skin irritation.

Anhidrosis An inability to sweat normally. As sweating is a cooling mechanism, this creates a danger because the body is incapable of naturally cooling itself.

Infectious: No.

Appearance: Absence of sweat on the skin's surface.

Site: Affects different areas of skin on the body, or all of the skin.

Treatment: Medical referral to establish underlying cause.

Hyperhidrosis Excessive perspiration which can cause distress to the client and interfere with everyday activities. There is no identifiable cause. It can affect one in every 100 people.

Infectious: No.

Appearance: Excessive sweat on skin's surface.

Site: Affects skin surface of whole body or specific parts.

Treatment: Medical referral to establish underlying cause. This condition may be treated with botulinium injections.

Sebaceous gland disorders

The sebaceous glands produce sebum, the skin's natural oil, which has bactericidal and anti-fungal properties. This helps to keep the skin healthy and also to prevent the skin from drying out. The following are sebaceous gland disorders.

Milia Keratinisation of the skin over the hair follicle occurs, causing sebum to accumulate in the hair follicle. This condition usually accompanies dry skin.

Infectious? No.

Appearance: Small, hard, pearly-white cysts.

Site: The upper face or close to the eyes.

Treatment: The milium may be removed by the beauty therapist (if qualified to do so) or by a GP, depending on the location. A sterile microlance is used to pierce the skin of the overlying skin epidermis and thereby release the milium.

Advanced beauty facial treatment Microdermabrasion may be used to avoid their development. Also, retinoid creams may be applied, which remove the outer epidermal layers.

Comedones or blackheads Excess sebum and keratinised cells can block the opening of the hair follicle.

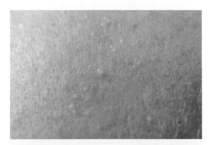

Milia

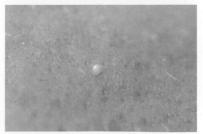

Extracted milia

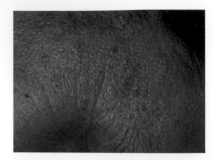

Comedones or blackheads

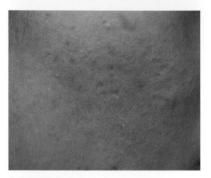

Seborrhoeic skin

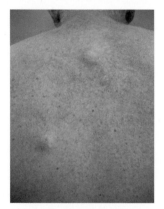

Sebaceous cyst

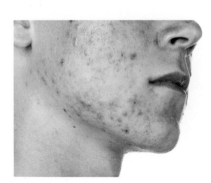

Acne vulgaris

Infectious? No.

Site: The skin on the face (the chin, nose and forehead), the upper back and chest.

Treatment: The area should be cleansed, and a pre-heating treatment such as an electrical steam treatment should be given to relax the opening of the hair follicle; a sterile comedone extractor should then be used to remove the blockage. Recommend a regular cleansing treatment and use of appropriate skincare products such as exfoliating treatments and facial masks to control the production of further comedones.

Seborrhoea

Excessive secretion of sebum from the sebaceous gland, resulting in excessively oily skin. This skin disorder usually occurs during puberty, as a result of hormonal changes occurring in the body.

Infectious? No.

Appearance: The follicle openings enlarge and excessive sebum is secreted. The skin appears coarse and oily; comedones, pustules and papules are present.

Site: The face and scalp. Seborrhoea may also affect the back and the chest.

Treatment: The area should be cleansed to remove the excess sebum. Deep-cleansing treatments that help the skin to heal, such as exfoliation, steaming and setting masks which cleanse the skin may be suggested. Medical treatment may be required. This would use locally applied steroid creams.

Steatomas, sebaceous cysts or wens

Localised pockets or sacs of sebum, which form in hair follicles or the sebaceous glands in the skin. The skin opening becomes blocked and the sebaceous gland becomes enlarged, appearing as a lump on the skin.

Infectious? No.

Appearance: Semi-globular in shape and ranging in size, the tissue in the area may feel hard or soft. The cysts are the same colour as the skin, or red if secondary bacterial infection occurs. A comedone can often be seen at the original opening of the hair follicle.

Site: If the cyst appears on the upper eyelid, it is known as a **chalazion** or **meibomian cyst**. If it appears on the scalp it is known as a **pilar cyst**.

Treatment: Medical – often a GP will remove the cyst under local anaesthetic. Small inflamed cysts can be medically treated with steroid medications or antibiotics.

Acne vulgaris

Hormone imbalance in the body at puberty influences the activity of the sebaceous gland, causing an increased production of sebum. The sebum may be retained within the sebaceous ducts, causing congestion and possibly leading to bacterial infection of the surrounding tissues.

Infectious? No.

Appearance: Inflammation of the skin, accompanied by comedones, pustules, papules and possibly cysts. Scarring of the skin can be associated with this skin disorder following skin healing after bacterial infection.

Site: Facial acne vulgaris commonly affects the skin on the face, nose, chin and forehead. Acne vulgaris may also occur on the chest and back.

Treatment: Medical – oral antibiotics may be prescribed, as well as antibiotic skin preparations. Other preparations that may be prescribed aim to unblock the skin and destroy bacteria. With medical approval, regular salon treatments may be given to cleanse the skin deeply, and also to stimulate the blood circulation to promote healing of the skin.

Pigmentation disorders

Pigmentation of the skin varies according to the person's genetic characteristics. In general the darker the skin, the more pigment (melanin) is present, but some abnormal changes in skin pigmentation can occur.

◆ **Hyper-pigmentation** is caused by increased pigment production, seen as darker areas or patches of skin.

◆ **Hypo-pigmentation** is caused by loss of pigmentation in the skin, seen as lighter areas of the skin or white patches.

The following disorders relate to changes in pigmentation in the skin.

Ephelides or freckles
Multiple, small hyper-pigmented areas of the skin. Exposure to UV light (as in sunlight) stimulates the production of melanin, intensifying their appearance.

Infectious? No.

Appearance: Small, flat, pigmented areas, darker than the surrounding skin.

Site: Commonly the nose and cheeks. Freckles may also occur on the shoulders, arms, hands and back.

Treatment: Freckles may be concealed with cosmetics. A sun block or high sun protection factor (SPF) sunscreen should be recommended, to prevent them intensifying in colour.

Lentigo (plural: lentigines)
Hyper-pigmented areas of skin, slightly larger than freckles. Lentigo simplex occur in childhood. Actinic (solar) lentigines occur in middle age as a result of sun exposure.

Infectious? No.

Appearance: Brown, slightly raised, pigmented patches of skin, of variable size.

Site: The face, hands and shoulders.

Treatment: Application of skin lightening and cosmetic concealing products.

Chloasma or liver spots
Concentrated melanin, hyper-pigmentation almost completely caused by long term UV skin exposure.

Infectious? No.

Appearance: Flat, smooth, irregularly shaped and sized pigmented areas of skin, varying in colour from light tan to dark brown. Chloasma are larger than ephelides and can appear suddenly. They are more apparent in clients over 40 years of age.

Site: The back of the hands, forearms, upper chest, temples and forehead.

Treatment: A barrier cream or a total sun block will reduce the risk of the chloasma increasing in size or number.

Dermatosis papulosa nigra
Often called flesh moles, characterised by multiple benign, small brown to black hyper-pigmented papules, common among black-skinned people.

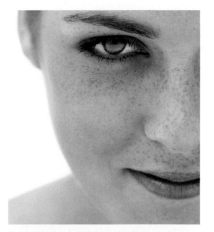
Ephelides or Freckles

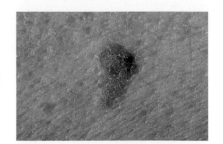
Lentigo

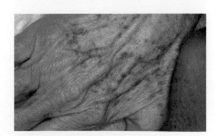
Chloasma or liver spots

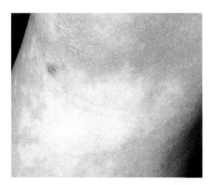

Vitiligo or leucoderma

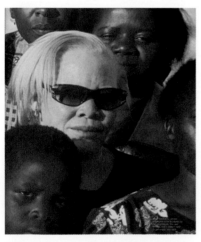

Albinism in someone of African race

Infectious? No.

Appearance: Raised pigmented markings resembling moles.

Site: Usually seen on the cheeks and forehead, although they may appear on the neck, upper chest and back.

Treatment: Medical – medication or surgery. Cosmetic concealment.

Vitiligo or leucoderma Patches of completely white skin that have lost their pigment or which were never pigmented.

Infectious? No.

Appearance: Well-defined patches of white skin, lacking pigment.

Site: The face, the neck, the hands, the lower abdomen and the thighs. If vitiligo occurs over the eyebrows, the hairs in the area will also lose their pigment.

Treatment: Camouflage cosmetic concealer can be applied to give even skin colour, or skin staining preparations can be used on the de-pigmented areas. Care must be taken when the skin is exposed to UV light, as the skin will not have the same protection in the areas lacking pigment and a total sunblock is required.

Albinism The skin is unable to produce the normal melanin pigment, and commonly the skin, hair and eyes are all affected.

Infectious? No.

Appearance: The skin is usually very pale and the hair is often white, but this will depend upon the amount of pigment in the area. The eyes may also be very pale blue or pink dependent upon the pigment present, and are extremely sensitive to light.

Site: The entire skin.

Treatment: There is no effective treatment. Maximum skin protection is necessary with an SPF of 30 or above when the client is exposed to UV light, and sunglasses should be worn to protect the eyes.

Vascular disorders

Erythema An area of skin where there is an increase in blood to the area causing the blood capillaries to dilate. The cause can be due either to injury or inflammation as the body's immune system responds to infection or irritation.

Infectious? No.

Appearance: The skin appears red.

Site: Erythema may affect one area (locally) or all of the skin (generally).

Treatment: The cause of inflammation should be identified. In the case of a **skin allergy**, the client must not be brought into contact with the irritant again. If unknown, refer the client to their GP.

Rosacea Excessive sebum secretion combined with a chronic inflammatory condition, caused by dilation of the superficial blood capillaries. Their appearance is referred to as telangiectasis.

Infectious? No. The cause is unknown.

Appearance: The skin becomes coarse, the pores enlarge and the cheek and nose area becomes inflamed, sometimes swelling and producing a butterfly pattern. Blood circulation slows in the dilated capillaries, creating a purplish appearance. Pustules and papules may also be present in severe cases.

Treatment: Medical – usually including antibiotics.

The condition is aggravated by stress and some foods that create a vasodilative effect, such as alcohol and spicy food.

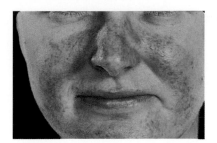
Rosacea

TOP TIP

Vascular circulatory skin disorder

If there is a vascular skin disorder, avoid overstimulating the skin or the problem will become more noticeable and the treatment may cause further damage. Carry out a patch test to check skin tolerance and reaction to treatment.

Dilated capillaries or telangiectasis Blood capillaries near the surface of the skin that are permanently dilated.

Infectious? No.

Appearance: Small red visible blood capillaries.

Site: Areas where the skin is neglected, dry or fine, such as the cheek area.

Treatment: Dilated capillaries can be disguised using a cosmetic concealer, which will contain pigments to counteract the redness dependent upon skin colour. They can also be permanently removed using advanced electrical epilation techniques with diathermy or lasers.

Naevi There are two types of naevus of concern to beauty therapists: vascular and cellular.

◆ Vascular naevi are skin conditions in which small or large areas of skin pigmentation are caused by the permanent dilation of blood capillaries. Examples include spider naevi, naevi vasculosis and capillary naevi.

◆ Cellular naevi or moles are skin conditions in which changes in the cells of the skin result in skin malformations. Examples include malignant melanomas, junction naevi, dermal naevi and hairy naevi.

Spider naevi or stellate haemangiomas Dilated blood vessels, with smaller dilated capillaries radiating from them.

Infectious? No.

Appearance: Small red capillaries, radiating like a spider's legs from a central point.

Site: Commonly the cheek area, but may occur on the upper body, the arms and the neck. Spider naevi are usually caused by an injury to the skin.

Treatment: Spider naevi can be concealed using a camouflage cosmetic, or treated by a qualified beauty therapist using advanced electrologist techniques with diathermy or lasers.

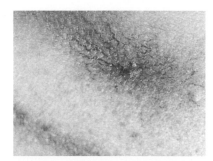
Spider naevi or stellate haemangiomas

Naevi vasculosis or strawberry marks Red or purplish raised marks, which appear on the skin at birth.

Infectious? No.

Appearance: Red or purplish lobed mark, of any size.

Site: Any area of the skin.

Treatment: About 60 per cent disappear by the age of six years. Treatment is not usually necessary; concealing camouflage cosmetics can be applied if desired. A sunblock is also recommended.

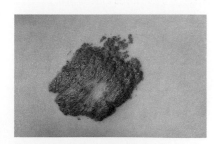
Naevi vasculosis or strawberry marks

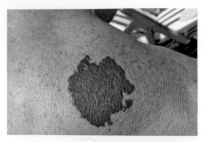
Capillary naevi or port-wine stains

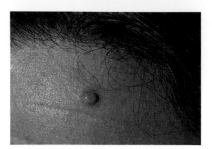
Benign naevi

Capillary naevi or port-wine stains Large areas of dilated capillaries, which contrast noticeably with the surrounding areas.

Infectious? No.

Appearance: The naevus has a smooth, flat surface.

Site: Some 75 per cent occur on the head; they are probably formed at the foetal stage. Naevi may also be found on the neck and face.

Treatment: Camouflage cosmetic products can be applied to disguise the area.

Evolution involves comparing a mole to those that are considered normal on the individual (the appearance of our moles is unique to each of us).

Always remember that this is only a guide. A dermatologist will be able to make a qualified judgment.

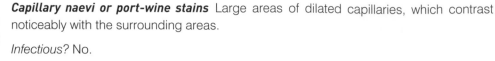

TOP TIP

Naevi numbers and skin colour

A white skin normally has up to four times as many naevi as black skin.

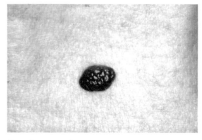
Junction naevi

Junction naevi
Localised collections of naevoid cells that arise from the mass production locally of pigment-forming cells (melanocytes).

Infectious? No.

Appearance: In childhood, junction naevi appear as smooth or slightly raised pigmented marks. They vary in colour from brown to black.

Site: Any area.

Treatment: Camouflage cosmetics can be used to conceal the area and the application of sunblock can prevent further pigmentation or skin darkening.

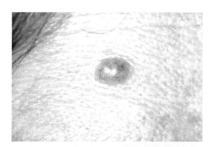
Dermal naevi

Dermal naevi
Localised collections of naevoid cells.

Infectious? No.

Appearance: About 1 cm wide, dermal naevi appear smooth and dome-shaped. Their colour ranges from skin tone to dark brown. Frequently, one or more hairs may grow from the naevus.

Site: Usually the face.

Treatment: None.

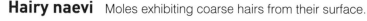

Hairy naevi
Moles exhibiting coarse hairs from their surface.

Infectious? No.

Appearance: Slightly raised moles, varying in size from 3 cm to much larger areas. Colour ranges from light to dark brown.

Site: Anywhere on the skin.

Treatment: Hairy naevi may be surgically removed where possible, and this is often done for cosmetic reasons. Hair growing from a mole should be cut, not plucked: if plucked, the hairs will become coarser and the growth of further hairs may be stimulated.

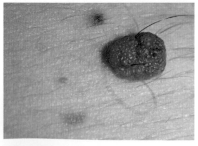
Hairy naevi

Skin disorders involving abnormal growth

Here we will look at skin disorders where cellular reproduction is abnormally increased, referred to as hypertrophy.

Psoriasis Patches of itchy, red, flaky skin, the cause of which is unknown. Psoriasis is often hereditary.

Infectious? No. Secondary infection with bacteria can occur if the skin becomes broken and dirt enters the skin. This may occur due to scratching.

Appearance: Red patches of skin appear, covered in waxy, silvery scales. Bleeding will occur if the area is scratched and scales are removed.

Site: Common areas are the elbows, knees, lower back and the scalp, but it can occur anywhere.

Treatment: There is no known treatment. Some relief can be found from hydrating oils and coal tar based preparations. Medication including steroid creams can bring relief to the symptoms. Medically administered UV treatment is also found to be beneficial.

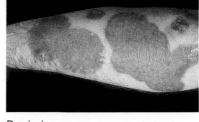
Psoriasis

Seborrhoeic or senile warts Raised, pigmented, benign tumours occurring in middle age.

Infectious? No.

Appearance: Slightly raised, brown or black, rough patches of skin. Such warts can be confused with pigmented moles.

Site: The trunk, the scalp and the temples.

Treatment: The warts can be cauterised where the tissue is destroyed by a GP using heat or cold, or an electrologist using advanced techniques.

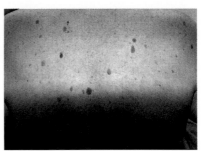
Seborrhoeic or senile warts

Verrucae filliformis or skin tags Skin tags appear as threads projecting from the surface of the skin.

Infectious? No.

Appearance: Skin-coloured threads of skin 3–6 mm long.

Site: Mainly seen on the neck and the eyelids, but may occur in other areas such as under the arms and groin.

Treatment: Medical – removal using cauterisation where the tissue is destroyed using heat or cold, diathermy, either by a GP or an electrologist using advanced techniques.

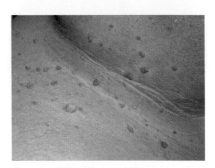
Verrucae filliformis or skin tags

HEALTH & SAFETY

Skin tags

Skin tags often occur under the arms and in the groin area. If present, take care when carrying out a wax depilation treatment in this area: do not apply wax over skin tags. If the hair is long, trim the hair instead of waxing over skin tags.

Xanthomas Small yellow growths appearing on the surface of the skin, made up of lipid deposits.

Infectious? No.

Appearance: A yellow, flat or raised area of skin.

Site: Commonly the eyelids, but can occur anywhere on the body.

Treatment: Medical – the growth is thought to be connected with certain medical diseases, such as diabetes or high or low blood pressure; sometimes a low-fat diet can correct the condition.

Keloids Keloids occur following skin injury and are overgrown abnormal scar tissue that spreads, characterised by excess deposits of the protein **collagen**. To avoid skin discoloration the keloid must be protected from UV exposure.

Infectious? No.

Appearance: The skin tends to be red or purple, raised, shiny and ridged. The area will fade over time.

Site: Located over the site of a wound or other lesion. Common sites include ear lobes, sternum area and upper shoulders.

Treatment: Medical – by drug therapy, such as cortisone injections, or surgery.

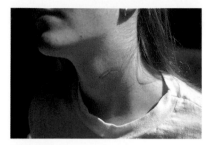

Keloid scar

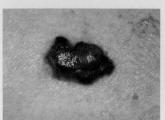
Skin cancers

Excessive skin exposure to UV light is the main cause of skin cancer.

Malignant melanomas or malignant moles Rapidly growing skin cancers, usually occurring in adults, the least common form of skin cancer.

Infectious? No.

Appearance: Each melanoma commences as a bluish-black mole, which enlarges rapidly, darkening in colour and developing a halo of pigmentation around it. It later becomes raised, bleeds and ulcerates. Secondary growths will develop in internal organs if the melanoma is not treated.

Site: Usually the lower abdomen, legs or feet.

Treatment: Medical – always recommend that a client has any mole checked if it is changing in size, structure or colour, or if it becomes itchy or bleeds.

Melanoma detection You should always be vigilant in checking a client's moles in the treatment area to note any change. The 'Guidance images for moles' table following shows healthy normal moles and melanomas.

Check the characteristic of the mole using the A, B, C, D and E mole check. The difference between a normal mole and melanoma are identified through the characteristic as follows:

A—asymmetry   D—diameter

B—border   E—evolution (changing in appearance)

C—colour

Guidance images for moles

Normal mole	Melanoma	Sign	Characteristic
		Asymmetry	When half of the mole does not match the other half, not symmetrical.
		Border	When the border (edges) of the mole are ragged or irregular.
		Colour	When the colour of the mole varies throughout.
		Diameter	If the mole's diameter (breadth) is larger than a pencil's eraser.

Squamous cell carcinomas or prickle-cell cancers Malignant growths originating in the epidermis.

Infectious: No.

Appearance: When fully formed, the carcinoma appears as a raised area of skin.

Site: Anywhere on the skin.

Treatment: Includes surgical removal, also radiotherapy (treatment with X-ray) or treatment with drugs as necessary.

Basal cell carcinomas or rodent ulcers Slow-growing malignant tumours, occurring in middle age, the most common form of skin cancer.

Infectious? No.

Appearance: A small, shiny, waxy nodule with a depressed centre. The disease extends, with more nodules appearing on the border of the original ulcer.

Site: Usually the face.

Treatment: Includes surgical removal, also radiotherapy (treatment with X-ray) or treatment with drugs as necessary.

Skin allergies

The skin can protect itself to some degree from damage or invasion. Mast cells detect damage to the skin; if damage occurs, the mast cells burst, releasing the chemical histamine

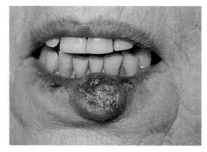

Squamous cell carcinomas

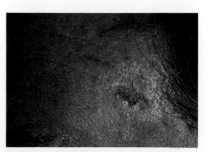

Basal cell carcinomas

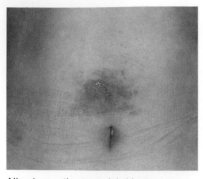

Allergic reaction to a nickel button

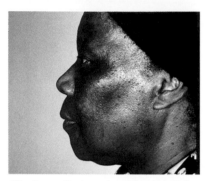

Allergic reaction to an ingredient in hair dye

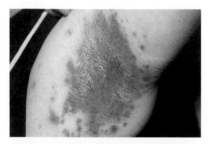

Allergic reaction to an antiperspirant

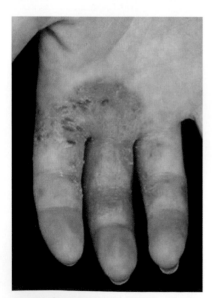

Contact dermatitis on the hands

into the tissues. Histamine causes the blood capillaries to enlarge, giving the reddening we call 'erythema'. The increased blood flow carries materials in the blood that tend to limit the damage and begin cellular repair.

If the skin is sensitive to and becomes inflamed on contact with a particular substance, this substance is called an **allergen**. Allergens may be animal, chemical or vegetable substances, and they may be inhaled, eaten or absorbed following contact with the skin. An allergic skin reaction appears as irritation, itching and discomfort, with reddening and swelling (as with nettle rash). If the allergen is removed, the allergic reaction subsides.

Each individual has different tolerances to the various substances we encounter in daily life. What causes an allergic reaction in one individual may be perfectly harmless to another.

Here are just a few examples of allergens known to cause allergic skin reactions in some people:

◆ metal objects containing nickel

◆ sticking plaster

◆ rubber

◆ lipstick containing eosin dye

◆ nail polish containing formaldehyde resin

◆ scalp hair and lash and brow tints

◆ lanolin, the skin moisturising agent

◆ detergents that dry the skin

◆ foods – well-known examples are peanuts, cow's milk, lobster, shellfish and strawberries

◆ plants such as tulips and chrysanthemums.

HEALTH & SAFETY

Allergies

You may suddenly become allergic to a substance that has previously been perfectly harmless. Equally, you may over time cease to be allergic to something.

Infection following allergy

Following an allergic skin reaction in which the skin's surface has become itchy and broken, scratching may cause the skin to become infected with bacteria.

Dermatitis An inflammatory skin disorder in which the skin becomes red, itchy and swollen. There are two types of dermatitis. In *primary dermatitis* the skin is irritated by the action of a substance on the skin, and this leads to skin inflammation. In *allergic contact dermatitis* the problem is caused by intolerance of the skin to a particular substance or group of substances. On exposure to the substance the skin quickly becomes irritated and an allergic reaction occurs.

Infectious? No.

Appearance: Reddening and swelling of the skin, with the possible appearance of vesicles.

Site: If the skin reacts to a skin irritant outside the body, the reaction is localised. Repeated contact with the allergen will lead to a general hypersensitivity. If the irritant gains entry to the body, it will be transported in the bloodstream and may cause a general allergic skin reaction.

Treatment: Moisturising cream can be used to help prevent drying of the skin. Personal protective equipment (PPE) should be worn in the case of an occupational hazard. For example, single use disposable non-latex (synthetic) powder-free gloves should be worn to avoid developing contact dermatitis due to the hazards in the nature of the work, such as contact cleaning chemicals. When an allergic dermatitis reaction occurs, the only 'cure' is the absolute avoidance of the substance. Steroid creams such as hydrocortisone are usually prescribed, to soothe the damaged skin and reduce the irritation.

HEALTH & SAFETY

Occupational disease

Occupational **skin diseases** can occur because of the type of work you undertake on a daily basis. Dermatitis is a skin condition caused by contact with an irritant or if you develop an allergy to a substance. Never ignore guidance that shows the skin may be sensitised or irritated by contact. Always care for the skin and wear the relevant PPE as instructed.

HEALTH & SAFETY

Recognising symptoms of skin, hair and nail diseases and disorders

If you are uncertain whether or not you should treat the client, don't! Tactfully refer them to their GP before going ahead with the planned treatment. Remember, you are not qualified to diagnose medical conditions.

Eczema Inflammation of the skin, the cause of which is unknown, but is often hereditary and can be related to contact with an irritant.

Infectious? No.

Appearance: Red, dry and cracked. The skin will often feel itchy. The area affected may appear darker after the skin improves. This is especially noticeable in darker skin.

Site: Commonly the face, the neck and at the inner creases of the elbows and behind the knees, but can occur anywhere.

Treatment: Refer the client to their GP. Eczema may disappear if the source of irritation is identified and removed. Steroid cream may be prescribed by the GP to reduce swelling and irritation and special diets to avoid food triggers may help. If the area is small and the skin unbroken, the treatment may go ahead; just avoid contact with the area.

HEALTH & SAFETY

Record any known allergies

When completing the consultation, always ask whether your client has any known allergies. Be aware that product formulations change, therefore check the suitability of ingredients. Record any allergies on the client's personal details.

Urticaria (nettle rash) or hives A minor skin disorder caused by contact with an allergen, either internally (food or drugs) or externally (for example, insect bites).

Infectious? No.

Appearance: Erythema with raised, round whitish skin wheals (red, swollen markings). In some cases the affected area can be accompanied by an intense burning or itching

HEALTH & SAFETY

Broken skin

If the skin is broken with any skin disorder that is not infectious e.g. eczema, treatment is contra-indicated as the skin may become infected; referred to as secondary infection.

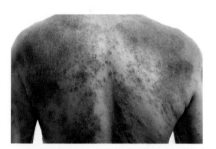
Eczema on the back

HEALTH & SAFETY

Hypoallergenic products

The use of hypoallergenic products reduces the risk of skin contact with likely irritants. Select these products for clients with skin allergies and hypersensitive skin.

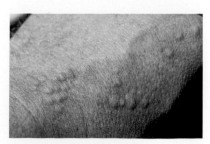
Urticaria (nettle rash) or hives

REVISION AID

Why must you gain signed consent from your client before you carry out a treatment?

sensation, a condition known as **pruritis**. Pruritis is a *symptom* of a disease (such as diabetes), not a disease itself.

Site: At the point of contact.

Treatment: Antihistamines may be prescribed to reduce the itching. The visible skin reaction usually disappears quickly, leaving no trace. Complete avoidance of the allergen 'cures' the problem.

ASSESSMENT OF KNOWLEDGE AND UNDERSTANDING

Having covered the learning objectives for this chapter, test what you need to know and understand by answering the following short questions below.

1. What is the reason for carrying out a consultation before starting every beauty therapy treatment?

2. a. What does the facial skin analysis confirm to the beauty therapist?
   b. Why does it follow the consultation?

3. What questions and diagnostic procedures may you include when assessing your client's needs for:
   a. facial treatments?
   b. nail services?

4. What equipment may assist you when carrying out a skin analysis?

5. Why should lifestyle factors be discussed with the client at the consultation?

6. At consultation, what contra-indications mean that a beauty therapy treatment may not proceed and that treatment may be restricted? Provide **five** examples for each.

7. How should all records be stored following consultation in order to comply with the Data Protection Act (1998)?

8. What sort of information would be included when preparing a client treatment plan?

9. In what ways might you be required to adapt your consultation to meet the diverse needs of clients that you could be treating? Provide **three** examples.

10. Describe the different communication techniques that you would need to use when performing a client consultation.

11. Why is a client's current home care beauty routine an important part of discussions that take place at consultation?

12. Why is it necessary to discuss post treatment advice and further treatment recommendations at the consultation stage?

NOTES

4 Facials

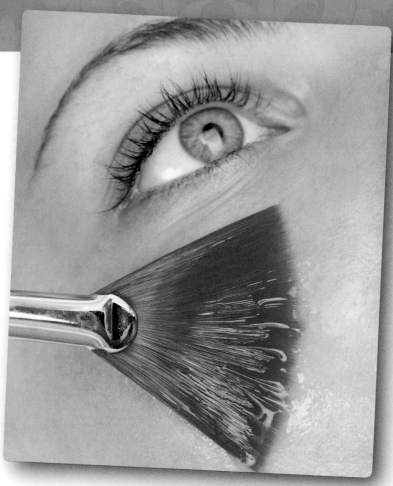

LEARNING OBJECTIVES

This chapter covers how to provide facial treatments. Different techniques and products are applied to improve or maintain the health of the skin and its underlying structures. You will learn more about:

◆ Facial treatment: purpose and effects.

◆ The key elements of facial treatments, including cleansing, toning, exfoliating, skin warming, extractions, massaging, masks, specialised skin products and moisturising.

◆ The sequence and techniques of facial application.

◆ Maintaining safe, effective methods when working.

◆ The information that must be obtained at the consultation including outcomes of the skin analysis and any skin sensitivity patch tests to ensure the client's suitability for treatment and their welfare.

◆ The different tools, products and equipment that may be applied during a facial to meet the required treatment objectives.

◆ How to select the most appropriate products and equipment, and modify your treatment application to achieve the treatment objectives.

◆ How to provide advice and recommendations to your client including further services and additional products, to further improve and maintain a healthy skin condition.

KEY TERMS

acid mantle
advice and
  recommendations
antioxidant
cleanser
comedone removal
consultation
contra-action
contra-indication
dermis
effleurage

epidermis
equipment
exfoliation
extraction
express facial
eye make-up remover
facial products
facial treatment
frictions
lifestyle factors
magnifying light

masks
massage
massage medium
moisturiser
muscle tone
nutrition
petrissage
skin analysis
skin colour
skin conditions
skin sensitivity patch test

skin tone
skin type
skin warming device
specialised skin products
steam treatment
subcutaneous layer
tapotement
toning lotion
towel steaming
treatment plan
vibrations

WHEN PROVIDING FACIAL TREATMENTS YOU WILL BE REQUIRED TO

◆ apply environmental and sustainable working practices

◆ follow relevant laws and manufacturers' instructions

◆ use different consultation and assessment techniques to correctly identify your client's needs

◆ use products and equipment that will enhance the required results

◆ adapt the treatment to meet your client's physiological and psychological* requirements (where needed)

◆ take the necessary actions where a contra-action, contra-indication or treatment modification is required

◆ provide relevant advice and recommendations to support your client's treatment objectives

◆ identify opportunities to promote further products and services that will be of benefit to your client.

INTRODUCTION

A facial treatment personalises the application of different techniques using the hands, tools and equipment, and scientifically formulated products with key ingredients to maintain and improve the health and appearance of the skin.

Facials are commonly provided in businesses which offer make-up, beauty therapy and spa services. The objectives, however, will slightly differ. A facial offered before make-up will aim to ensure the skin is in optimum condition to show the make-up at its best effect, with products serving to enhance the appearance of the client's skin, e.g. providing luminosity and minimising imperfections such as skin pigmentation. A beauty therapy business may offer a range of different facials to meet the time demands of the client's lifestyle, skin conditions and possible skin disorders associated with:

◆ each skin type

◆ the care the skin has previously received

◆ individual characteristics

◆ ethnicity, gender and age-related requirements.

Dealing with people in a polite, efficient manner and using good communication and questioning skills to find out exactly what they require from the facial, forms an important part of this technical treatment.

*If your client is tense your reassurance, choice of mask, massage techniques and speed of application, for example, can be modified to induce relaxation.

Caring for the skin

 The necessary anatomy and physiology knowledge for this subject is listed in the checklist in Chapter 2.

At the consultation, lifestyle, health and wellbeing are reviewed to see if there are improvements that can be made or considered by the client. Premature ageing is accelerated by poor nutrition and other factors related to lifestyle. If the skin is to function efficiently it must be cared for both internally and externally.

Internally, a nutritionally balanced diet is vital to the health and appearance of the skin. Nutrition is the study of the chemical substances the body obtains from food needed for health and growth. The digestive system is responsible for breaking down our food into nutrients that the cells can use. A healthy diet contains all the essential nutrients. These are carried to the skin in the blood, where they nourish the cells in the processes of growth and repair.

A number of skin allergies and disorders are in part the result of poor **nutrition**, caused by a poorly balanced diet, including highly processed food, caffeine, alcohol and a lack of essential nutrients.

A balanced diet prevents malnutrition (undernourishment) and vitamin/mineral deficiencies. The following food triangle diagram illustrates the different food groups.

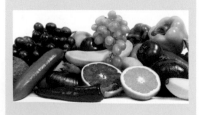
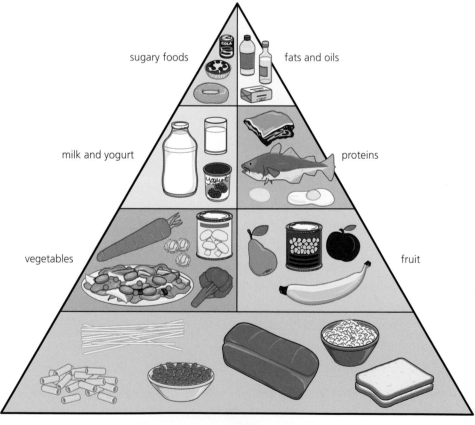

Healthy living food pyramid – basic guide to food quantities that make up a balanced healthy diet

The daily recommended amounts to be consumed are:

Fats/oils	1 serving*
Fruit	2–4 servings
Milk and yoghurt	2–3 servings
Proteins	2–3 servings
Starch	6–11 servings
Sugar	1 serving*
Vegetables	3–5 servings
*use scarcely	

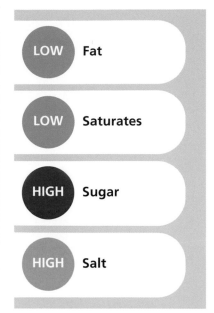

A traffic light system of food package labelling shows information on the nutritional content of foods to inform healthy food choices. There are six principal groups of nutrients:

Carbohydrates Carbohydrates provide energy quickly. They are either simple sugars or starches that the body can turn into simple sugars.

Food sources: Carbohydrates are found in fruit, vegetables, milk, grains and honey.

Fats Fats provide a concentrated source of energy, and are also used in carrying certain vitamins around the body. Fat is stored in the body around organs and muscles and under the skin. However, if too much fat is deposited under the skin, the elastic fibres may be damaged by the expansion of the adipose tissue. Fat is also used in the formation of sebum, the skin's natural lubricant.

Food sources: Although this is not always evident, fats are present in almost all foods, from plants and from animals.

HEALTH & SAFETY

Vegan diets

Proteins are composed of many smaller units called *amino acids*. Animal protein sources contain all the amino acids essential to health. A *vegetarian* consuming dairy food will likewise obtain all the essential amino acids. A *vegan*, however, must be careful to eat an adequate quantity and variety of vegetables and other foods, in order to be sure that they receive all the amino acids they need.

Vegans must take vitamin B_{12} as a vitamin supplement or eat foods fortified with B_{12}, such as some cereals, as this vitamin only occurs naturally in animal-derived foods.

Proteins Proteins provide material for the growth and repair of body tissue, and are also a source of energy. Severe protein deficiency in children gives the skin a yellowish appearance, known as **jaundice.**

Food sources: Proteins are found in meat, fish, eggs, dairy products, grains and nuts.

Minerals Minerals provide materials for growth and repair and for regulation of the body processes. The major minerals are calcium, iron, phosphorus, sulphur, sodium, potassium, chlorine and magnesium. Of these, the most important to the skin is iron. A pale, dry skin may indicate **anaemia**, caused by a shortage of iron.

Food sources: Fruit and vegetables; iron is found in liver, egg yolks and green vegetables.

HEALTH & SAFETY

Quick weight loss diets and the effect on skin

Inform your clients about the danger of very low-fat, low-carbohydrate or low-protein diets: these can deprive the body of the nutrients it needs for growth, repair and energy. A nutritionally balanced diet is always best.

TOP TIP

Antioxidant foods

As we know, antioxidants are essential to maintain the health of the skin, fighting the damaging effects of free radicals in your body. Vitamins A, C and E and the mineral selenium all have good antioxidant properties. These can be found in significant amounts in the following foods: blueberries, kale, strawberries, spinach, avocado and broccoli.

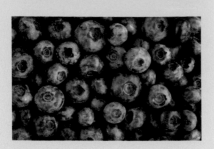

ACTIVITY

Vitamins

How do each of the following vitamins benefit the skin's appearance and its function: A, B, C and E?

HEALTH & SAFETY

Weight loss

If you lose weight too quickly, your skin may sag and wrinkle. A healthy, steady weight loss plan should be followed, drinking the recommended amount of water to ensure the skin remains hydrated.

Vitamins Vitamins regulate the body's processes and contribute to its resistance to disease. Vitamins are divided into two groups, according to whether they are soluble in water or in fat:

◆ the fat-soluble vitamins are A, D, E and K

◆ the water-soluble vitamins are B and C.

The vitamins most important to the condition of the skin are vitamins A, B_2, B_3, C and E.

Vitamin A Essential for the growth and renewal of skin cells. Insufficient vitamin A in the diet leads to **hyperkeratinisation** (production of too much keratin). This causes blockages in the skin tissue. The skin becomes rough and dry, and eye disorders such as styes may occur.

Food sources: Vitamin A is found in red, yellow and green vegetables, and in egg yolk, butter and cheese.

Vitamin B_2 Vitamin B_2 (also called **riboflavin**) helps to break down other foodstuffs, releasing energy needed by cells to desquamate and function efficiently. A deficiency of vitamin B_2 causes the skin at the corners of the mouth to crack.

Food sources: Vitamin B_2 is found in brewer's yeast, milk products, leafy vegetables, liver and whole grains.

Vitamin B_3 Vitamin B_3 (also called **niacin**) has the same function as vitamin B_2, but is also vital in the maintenance of the tissues of the skin.

Food sources: Vitamin B_3 is found in meat, brewer's yeast, nuts and seeds.

Vitamin C Vitamin C (also called **ascorbic acid**) maintains healthy skin and is important for the production of collagen, providing tone and elasticity. A lack of vitamin C causes the capillaries to become fragile, and haemorrhages of the skin, such as bruising, may occur. Severe deficiency results in **scurvy**.

Food sources: Vitamin C is found in fruit and vegetables.

Vitamin E Vitamin E is found in most foods. It is an antioxidant and helps prevent premature skin ageing. It helps to rehydrate the skin, calms inflammation, helps healing and maintains healthy skin.

Food sources: Vitamin E is found in most foods. The richest sources are vegetable oils, cereal products, eggs and meat.

HEALTH & SAFETY

Effects of dehydration

Sufficient water consumption means that we avoid being dehydrated, which can lead to symptoms such as headaches, tiredness and loss of concentration.

In hot weather or following active physical exercise more water must be consumed.

Dehydration is recognised on the skin surface when the skin is lightly pinched as crepey, fine lines.

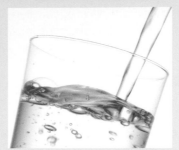

At the end of a facial treatment offer the client water, reminding them that this is to help toxin removal and for hydration.

TOP TIP

Detoxification for the skin

Detoxification aims to cleanse the body and remove toxins. The body is equipped to cleanse itself through its organs – the kidneys, liver and colon. Drinking more water, eating a nutritionally balanced diet high in fibre will support the body to achieve this.

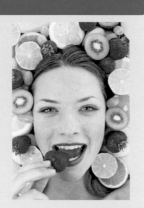

When requiring a detox as a result of the negative internal and external factors discussed, the skin may feel itchy and appear dry, dull, ashy grey in colour and with signs of congestion such as blemishes.

Many skincare products, often containing antioxidants, will have *detox* in the name of the product.

Water Water forms about two-thirds of the body's weight, and is an important component both inside and outside the body cells. Water is essential for the body's growth and maintenance. It helps remove waste from the body through urine and sweat and regulates temperature. Water must be regularly replaced through the diet. At least one and a half litres of water should be drunk every day, to avoid dehydration of the body and the skin. Aim to drink 6–8 medium glasses daily.

Food sources: Water is also a constituent of many foods, including fruit and vegetables.

Fibre Fibre is a type of carbohydrate, however it is not broken down into nutrients, but it is very important for effective digestion.

Food sources: Fibre is found in fruit, vegetables and cereals.

Threats to the skin

Internal

Alcohol Following alcohol consumption the heart rate increases. This causes the blood vessels to expand, called vasodilation. Alcohol deprives the body of its vitamin reserves, especially vitamins B and C, which are necessary for a healthy skin. Alcohol

HEALTH & SAFETY

Alcohol Related Liver Disease (ARLD)

Excessive alcohol consumption can lead to ARLD. The liver is the organ responsible for removing alcohol from the body. This may lead to liver damage, seen as:

- yellow skin, called jaundice; this is harder to observe on a darker skin colour but the eyes become yellow also
- itchy skin
- skin swelling, called oedema
- skin bruising, which will occur more easily.

TOP TIP

Increase hydration when consuming alcohol

A glass of water should ideally be drunk between each alcoholic beverage, the purpose being to increase hydration. However, avoid exceeding the recommended units per day to avoid accelerating the ageing process.

Tactfully discussing alcohol consumption at consultation will inform you if any visible facial characteristics may be attributed to this.

TOP TIP

Caffeine

Advise your clients to replace tea with herbal infusions and to drink decaffeinated coffee (in moderation) rather than regular coffee. Caffeine is a diuretic, causing increased urination and loss of water leading to dehydration.

HEALTH & SAFETY

Illegal drug classification

Illegal drugs are categorised as class A, B or C. Class A drugs are the most harmful. Common signs of recreational drug misuse include skin blemishes, bruising, dull skin, self-inflicted wounds caused by scratching and needle marks.

HEALTH & SAFETY

Smoking

Smoking depletes the body of vital nutrients, preventing their absorption. If you are a smoker, it is essential that you have a diet high in vitamin C.

ACTIVITY

Causes of stress

1 Can you think of everyday situations that can trigger stress?

2 How do you react physically when put in a stressful situation?

3 How can you create a relaxing environment for your client?

also tends to dehydrate the body as it attempts to remove alcohol in urine, including the skin, the body's largest organ. Skin conditions such as acne rosacea, eczema and psoriasis are often aggravated by the consumption of alcohol. Over time the results of excessive alcohol consumption lead to premature ageing, seen as visible redness caused by vasodilation, thread veins and dark skin under the eyes.

Caffeine
Coffee, tea, cocoa and soft, fizzy, high-energy drinks contain a mild stimulant drug called **caffeine**. This is mildly addictive. In moderate doses, such as two or three cups of coffee per day, caffeine is safe. If you drink too much, however, caffeine can cause nervousness, interfere with digestion, block the absorption of vitamins and essential minerals, such as calcium and iron, dehydrate and spoil the appearance of the skin, stimulating skin ageing.

Drugs
Drugs are chemical substances that affect the way our body performs. When they enter the body they are transported throughout the body in the blood. Recreational drugs are taken because they cause a particular effect or sensation, which may feel good initially. Long term, they are harmful and addictive. Most affect the blood pressure and heart rate, causing facial flushing. Stimulants, for example, can cause sweating, shaking and headaches. Heroin, in the class of drug called *narcotics*, ravages the skin, causing chronic dryness and premature ageing.

Smoking
The skin of a smoker will appear dry, dehydrated and often thickened. Vertical lines will often be seen around the lips, caused by contraction of the skin and underlying muscles beneath it. Smoking interferes with cell respiration and slows down the circulation. This makes it harder for nutrients and oxygen to reach the skin cells and for waste products to be eliminated. Skin conditions such as acne and eczema are often aggravated and become worse. Cigarette smoking also releases a chemical that destroys vitamin C. This interferes with the production of collagen, and thereby contributes to premature wrinkling. Nicotine is a **toxic** substance – a poison!

Medication
Certain medicines taken by mouth can cause skin dehydration, oedema – swelling of the tissues – (this may for example be caused by steroids) or irregular skin pigmentation (sometimes caused by the contraceptive pill). During the initial **consultation** with the client, find out whether they are taking any medication – and take this into account in your diagnosis and **treatment plan**. However, you should check any changes to the client's medical history or medication being taken each time you carry out a treatment.

Stress
The skin responds to stress by releasing hormones, which cause vasodilation and increase perspiration from the sudoriferous glands. Mast cells release histamine. Stress is also shown in the face as tension lines where the facial muscles are tight. This impedes blood and lymph circulation, causing a sluggish skin condition and poor facial nutrition. Sensitivity and irritation are signs of stress, and can lead to redness, itchiness and dry patches or blemishes.

A person suffering from stress usually experiences disturbed sleep or sleeplessness (**insomnia**). Sleep is an important time, when the cells of the body repair and regenerate. Discuss sleep patterns with your client. Ideally a person should have between 6 and 9 hours sleep every night. Lack of sleep causes the skin to become dull and puffy, especially the tissue beneath the eyes, where dark circles also appear. Too *much* sleep can also cause the facial tissue to become puffy – because the circulation is less active, body fluids collect in the tissues.

Often when suffering from stress, a person may make unhealthy life choices, e.g. increasing smoking and alcohol consumption. This leads to the production of free radicals, which damage healthy skin cells, leading to skin ageing.

Stress and anxiety are often the underlying cause of certain skin disorders. Some skin conditions, such as boils and styes, appear at times of stress; others, such as psoriasis, eczema and dermatitis may become much worse. At the consultation, try to determine whether the client is suffering from stress: if they are, make sure that the salon treatments have the additional benefit of promoting relaxation.

External

As well as looking after the skin from the *inside*, by diet, it needs care from the *outside* – it must be kept clean, and it must be nourished.

With normal physiological functioning, the skin becomes oily and sweat is deposited on its surface. The skin's natural oil (**sebum**) can easily build up and block the natural openings, the hair **follicles** and **pores**: this may lead to congestion, blockages and infection. Facial cosmetics can also affect the health of the skin; if not correctly removed as recommended, they may cause cosmetic congestion. This is often as a result of the ingredients they contain such as waxes and oils which have comedogenic properties, causing comedone formation. Skincare treatments help to maintain and improve the functioning of the skin.

How the skin responds and ages in relation to exposure to external factors is called *extrinsic ageing*.

Ultraviolet light Although ultraviolet (UV) has been identified as a hazard to skin, it also has some *positive* effects. One of these is its ability to stimulate the production of **vitamin D**, which is absorbed into the bloodstream and nourishes and helps to maintain bone tissue. UV light also activates the **pigment melanin** in the skin, and thereby creates a **tan**. Many people feel better when they have a tan, as it gives a healthy appearance.

UV light is divided into different bands. The most important to skin tanning are UVA and UVB. **UVA** stimulates the melanin in the skin to produce a rapid tan, which does not last very long. UVA penetrates deep into the **dermis** where it can cause premature ageing of the skin. **Free radicals** – highly reactive molecules that cause skin cells to degenerate – are also formed. These molecules disrupt production of collagen and elastin, the fibres that give skin its strength and elasticity. Reduced elasticity leads to wrinkling.

HEALTH & SAFETY

Sun tanning

Never wear perfume, cosmetic products or deodorants either in natural sunlight or in artificially produced UV. The chemicals in these products can sensitise the skin, causing an allergic skin reaction and skin pigmentation.

UV can penetrate water to a depth of 1 metre, so even when swimming you need to wear a sunscreen.

HEALTH & SAFETY

UV exposure

UV is most intense between 11 am and 3 pm, when the sun is at its highest. Recommend clients are safety aware if exposing the skin to sunlight between these times. A high SPF or sun block should be worn to minimise skin damage.

UVB stimulates the production of vitamin D. Melanin activation by UVB produces a longer-lasting tan than that produced by UVA. UVB is partially absorbed by the atmosphere – it has a shorter wavelength than UVA – and only 10 per cent reaches the dermis. UVB causes thickening of the stratum corneum, which reflects UV away from the skin's surface. UVB causes **sunburn**: the skin becomes red as the cells are damaged, and the skin may blister. UVB is also implicated in skin cancers, especially malignant melanoma.

The relaxing, warming effect of the sun is caused by the **infrared (IR)** light which achieves a sedative relaxing effect on the nerve endings.

Although black skin has a high melanin content, which absorbs more UV and allows less to reach the dermis, it is not fully protected against the UV and still requires additional protection.

Chemical skin protection, or sunscreens, are designed to absorb UV light (UVA and UVB), reducing the rate of skin ageing in all skin types. Various sunscreens are available, classified by number according to their sun protection factor (SPF). This is the amount of protection that the sunscreen gives you from the sun. An SPF of at least 15 is recommended in winter and 30 in summer. The application of the sunscreen extends your natural skin protection, allowing you to stay in the sun for longer without burning. For example, if normally you can be in the sun for 10 minutes before your skin begins to go red, a sunscreen with an SPF of 10 will allow you 10 × 10 minutes (i.e. 100 minutes) of safe exposure in the sun. Always check the expiry date of sunscreens, they only have a shelf life of 2–3 years.

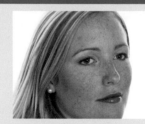
Artificial UV light produced by sunbeds, used for cosmetic skin tanning, also causes premature ageing. Most sunbeds use concentrated UVA, which causes dermal tissue damage resulting in lines and wrinkles.

It may take years to see the effects of the dermal damage caused by unprotected UV exposure, but once they have occurred the effects are irreversible. UVA rays are present all year round. UV rays can pass through glass so, on a daily basis, a person may be exposed to more UV than they think. To prevent premature ageing and skin disease, cosmetic preparations containing sunscreens should be worn at all times.

Climate Sebum, the skin's natural grease, provides an oily protective film over the surface of the skin that reduces evaporation. Despite this, unprotected exposure of the skin to the environment allows evaporation from the **epidermis**, which results in a dry, dehydrated skin condition.

The climate has several effects on the skin:

◆ *Sebum production* When the skin is exposed to the cold, less sebum is produced. The skin has reduced protection, allowing moisture to evaporate.

◆ *Perspiration* In very hot weather more moisture is lost as **perspiration**: perspiration increases to cool the skin and regulate the body's temperature.

◆ *Humidity* Moisture loss from the skin is also affected by the humidity (water content) of the surrounding air. In hot, dry weather humidity will be low, so water loss will be high. In temperate, damp conditions humidity will be high, so water loss will be low.

ALWAYS REMEMBER

Occupation and lifestyle factors

At the consultation, find out what the client's occupation or hobbies are; this will guide you further as to their likely skincare requirement. A client who spends a lot of time outside, for example, will have different treatment needs from the one who spends a lot of time inside in terms of skin protection requirements and ways of achieving this.

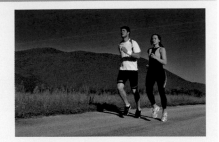

◆ *Extremes of temperature* Alternating heat and cold often leads to the formation of **broken capillaries**. These appear as fine red lines on white skin, and as discoloration on black skin.

◆ *Stratum corneum* The cells of the stratum corneum multiply with repeated unprotected exposure to the climate, as the body's natural defence.

The damaging effects caused by the climate can be reduced by using protective skincare preparations such as moisturisers. These spread a layer of oil over the skin's surface, reducing evaporation.

Environmental stress and pollution
Further causes of moisture loss include harsh alkaline chemicals such as detergents and soaps – which remove sebum from the skin's surface – and air conditioning and central heating.

Environmental **pollutants** such as lead, mercury, cadmium and aluminium can accumulate in the body. One result is the formation of dangerous chemicals that attack proteins in the cells. Such pollutants find their way into food through polluted waters, rain and dust. To protect the body, always wash vegetables thoroughly, and eat a diet rich in vitamins C and E.

Air pollution, involving carbon from smoke, chemical discharges from factories, and fumes from car exhausts, should be removed from the skin by effective cleansing. Absorption of these pollutants is reduced by the application of a **moisturiser**: this forms a barrier over the skin's surface.

HEALTH & SAFETY

Protecting the skin from pollution

There are many components to air pollution. Car exhaust fumes, for example, release nitrogen oxide and volatile organic compounds. These react with sunlight to form ozone, a highly reactive form of oxygen. This can penetrate deep inside the skin and damage the cells' DNA (their main component), which can lead to skin cancer. Also, accelerated skin ageing is the result of free radical damage caused by unstable molecules, which affect the skin's elasticity. Moisturisers may contain antioxidants and can be promoted with the benefit of neutralising free radicals or helping them to be removed from the skin before skin damage is caused.

ECO TIP

Environment and humidity

Central heating creates an environment with humidity similar to that of the desert. Unless you use an emollient, the loss of moisture from the skin will cause it to develop the characteristics of a dry, dehydrated skin condition.

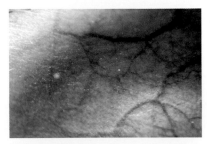

Broken capilliaries seen on a white skin

TOP TIP

Ashiness

A black skin can sometimes appear ashen, with patches of skin becoming grey and flaky. This is caused by sudden changes in temperature combined with low humidity, which can cause the skin to lose moisture. The use of an exfoliant and skin moisturiser will help in alleviating this problem.

ACTIVITY

Geographical variations

Consider the effects of climate on the skin. Name four different geographical locations, research and state the humidity level and climate you would expect at each location.

Think of the probable effects on the skin. What treatments by a beauty therapist might be needed in each country?

Skincare treatments

As a beauty therapist you have the professional knowledge and expertise to help each client improve the appearance, function and condition of their skin by the application of appropriate skincare treatments and products. The facial skin treatments you can provide include:

- consultation and skin analysis
- eye and skin cleansing
- exfoliation
- application of **skin-warming devices**
- **extraction** of comedones, commonly known as 'blackheads'
- manual **massage** techniques applied to the face, neck, chest and shoulders
- the application of face **masks**
- the application of **specialised skin products** e.g. eye creams, eye gels, neck creams, serums, acne products and lip balms
- moisturiser.

You cannot change the underlying skin type, which is genetically determined, but you can keep the physiological characteristics of each skin type in check.

Skin types

The basic structure of the skin does not vary from person to person, but the physiological functioning of its different features does; it is this that gives us **skin types**, recognised by specific visible characteristics.

The first and most important part of a **facial** treatment is the correct diagnosis of the skin type. This is carried out at the beginning of each facial service. You must choose the correct skincare products and facial services for the client's skin type. This assessment is called a **skin analysis**.

Basic types

There are four main skin types:

- normal
- dry
- oily
- combination.

Normal skin Normal skin is often referred to as **balanced**: the water and oil content is constant, it is neither too oily nor too dry. When young, this skin type seldom has any problems, such as blemishes, therefore, it is often neglected. Neglect causes the skin to become dry, especially around the eyes, cheeks and neck, where the skin is thinner.

A normal skin type in adults is rare. It has these characteristics:

◆ The pore size is small or medium.

◆ The moisture content is good.

◆ The skin texture is smooth and even, neither too thick nor too thin.

◆ The colour is healthy (because of good blood circulation).

◆ The skin elasticity is good, when young.

◆ The skin feels firm to the touch.

◆ The skin pigmentation is even with melanin evenly distributed.

◆ The skin is usually free from blemishes.

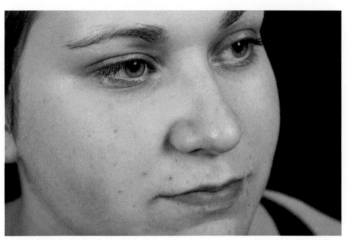

Normal skin

Dry skin Dry skin is lacking in either sebum or moisture, or both. Because sebum limits moisture loss by evaporation from the skin, skin with insufficient sebum rapidly loses moisture. The resulting accompanying skin condition is described as **dehydrated**. This is discussed later and can accompany any skin type but is commonly related to a dry skin.

Dry skin has these characteristics:

◆ The pores are small and tight.

◆ The moisture content is poor.

◆ The skin texture is coarse and thin, with patches of visibly flaking skin.

◆ There is a tendency towards sensitivity (broken capillaries often accompany this skin type).

◆ Premature ageing is common, resulting in the appearance of fine lines leading to deeper wrinkles, seen especially around the eyes, mouth and neck.

◆ Skin pigmentation may be uneven.

◆ Milia, commonly referred to as whiteheads, are often found on this skin type around the cheek and eye area.

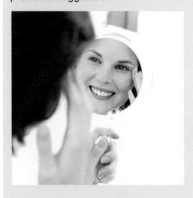

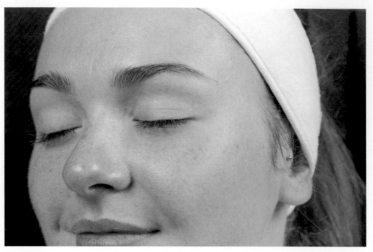

Dry skin

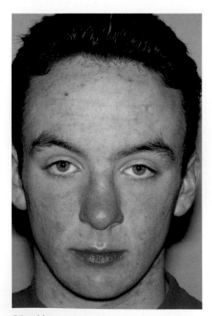

Oily skin

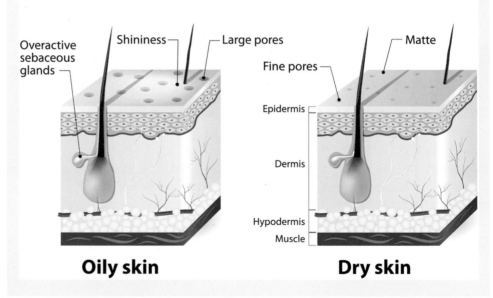

Oily skin   **Dry skin**

Oily skin In oily skin the sebaceous glands become very active at puberty, when stimulated by the male hormone **androgen**. An increase in sebum production often causes the appearance of skin blemishes. Sebaceous gland activity begins to decrease when the client is in their twenties.

Oily skin has these characteristics:

◆ The pores are enlarged.

◆ The moisture content is high.

- The skin is coarse and thick.

- The skin is sallow in colour, as a result of the excess sebum production; dead skin cells become embedded in the sebum, and the skin has sluggish blood and lymph circulation.

- The **skin tone** is good, due to the protective effect of the sebum.

- The skin is prone to shininess, due to excess sebum production.

- There may be uneven pigmentation.

- Certain skin disorders may be apparent – comedones, pustules, papules, milia or sebaceous cysts.

Acne vulgaris and **seborrhoea** are skin disorders that occur when the skin becomes excessively oily due to the influence of hormones. Treatment of these skin disorders should be carried out to control and reduce sebum flow.

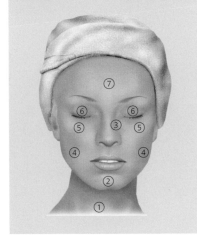
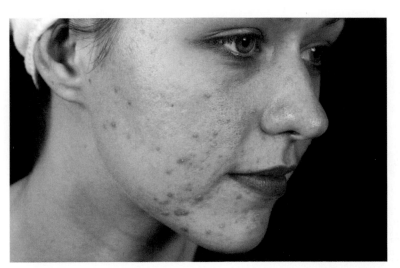

Acne vulgaris

Combination skin Combination skin is partly oily and partly dry. The oily parts are generally the chin, nose and forehead, known as the **T-zone**. The upper cheeks may show signs of oiliness, but the rest of the face and neck area is usually dry.

Combination skin is the most common skin type. It has these characteristics:

- The pores in the T-zone are enlarged, while in the cheek area they are small to medium.

- The moisture content is high in the oily areas, but poor in the dry areas.

- The skin is coarse and thick in the oily areas, but thin in the dry areas.

- The skin is sallow in the oily areas, but can show sensitivity and high colour in the dry areas and in the oily areas if harsher treatment products are used.

- The skin tone is good in the oily areas, but poor in the dry areas.

- There may be blemishes such as pustules and comedones on the oily skin at the T-zone but remember the combination can occur anywhere.

- Milia and broken capillaries may appear in the dry areas, commonly on the cheeks and near the eyes.

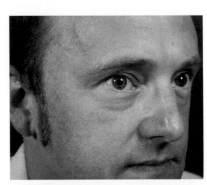

Combination skin

Additional skin conditions

While looking closely at the skin, further **skin characteristics** may become obvious. The skin may be:

- ◆ sensitive
- ◆ dehydrated
- ◆ young
- ◆ mature.

Sensitive skin Sensitive skin usually accompanies a dry skin type, but not always. The characteristics of sensitive skin are these:

- ◆ The skin may show high colouring as it is easily irritated.
- ◆ There are usually broken capillaries in the cheek area.
- ◆ The skin feels warm to the touch.
- ◆ There is superficial flaking of the skin.
- ◆ The skin may show high colouring and tightness after skin cleansing, if it is sensitive to pressure.

In black skin, instead of the redness shown by white skin, irritation shows up as a darker patch.

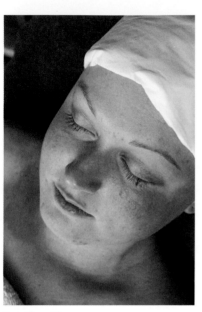

Sensitive skin

TOP TIP

Associated considerations when treating sensitive skin types

Use hypoallergenic products – these do not contain any of the known common skin sensitisers such as perfume that can cause skin irritation.

Skin that is sensitive may also be allergic to certain substances such as adhesives that may be used in artificial eyelash application.

Recommend avoiding lifestyle factors that can make sensitive skin worse. These include alcohol, smoking, poor diet and stress.

Allergic skin Allergic skin is irritated by external **allergens**, including chemicals in some cosmetics. The allergens inflame the skin and may damage its protective function. At the consultation, always try to discover whether the client has any allergies, and if so, to what.

The allergies of most concern to you as a beauty therapist are those caused by substances applied to the skin. You must be aware of such substances and avoid their use. Contact with an allergen, especially if repeated, may cause skin disorders such as eczema or dermatitis (see Chapter 3, where skin diseases and disorders are dealt with in more detail).

Dehydrated skin Dehydrated skin is skin that has lost water from the skin tissues. The condition can affect any skin type, but most commonly accompanies dry or combination skin types. The problem may be related to the client's general health. If they have recently been ill with a fever, for example, the skin will have lost fluid through sweating. If they are taking medication, this too may cause dehydration, as may drastic dieting. In many cases the dehydration is caused by working in an environment with a low humidity, or in one that is air-conditioned. You must try to discover the cause, and provide both corrective treatment and advice.

HEALTH & SAFETY

Sensitive skin

When treating a sensitive allergenic skin, choose a skincare product that does not contain common allergens such as mineral oil, alcohol or lanolin. Such screened products are usually referred to as *hypoallergenic* or *dermatologically* tested.

The characteristics of dehydrated skin are as follows:

◆ The skin has a fine paper-like, orange-peel effect caused by its lack of moisture.

◆ There may be superficial flaking.

◆ Fine, superficial lines are evident on the skin.

◆ Broken capillaries are common.

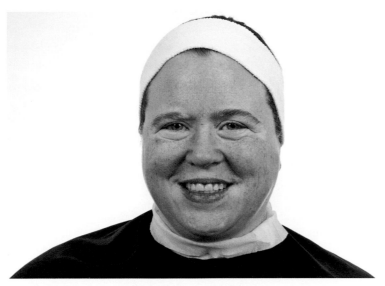

Dehydrated skin

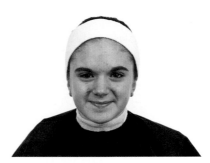

Young skin

The age of the skin

Having identified the skin type, you must classify the age of the skin. This can vary between people of different race because of evolution, which may delay the visible signs of ageing due to differences in sebaceous gland and melanin activity in skin.

Often the age of a client will relate to skin problems that are evident. A young client, for example, may have skin blemishes such as comedones, pustules and papules. These disorders are caused by over-activity of the sebaceous gland at puberty, when the body is developing its secondary sexual characteristics and is responsive to hormonal changes. It is at this time that the skin disorder acne vulgaris is most likely to occur, due to the hormonal imbalance. The skin of clients aged over 25 years, however, is generally termed **mature skin**.

You should also consider the client's skin appearance, texture, skin tone and **muscle tone** in relation to their age. A young skin will probably have good skin tone, and the skin will be supple and elastic. This is because the collagen and elastin fibres in the skin are strong. Poor skin tone, on the other hand, is recognised by the appearance of facial lines and wrinkles.

A healthy young skin will also have good muscle tone, and the facial contours will appear firm. With poor muscle tone, the muscles becomes slack and loose.

The change in appearance of women's skin during ageing is closely related to the altered production of the hormones oestrogen, progesterone and androgen and the effects of change and imbalance. In addition, the effects of **lifestyle factors** such as health, environmental and hereditary factors may be in evidence. Significant changes occur as a person enters their forties to fifties, which can be observed as the following characteristics.

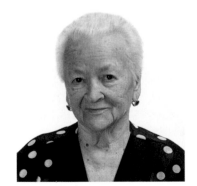

Mature skin

- The skin becomes dry, as the sebaceous and sudoriferous glands become less active.

- The skin loses its elasticity as the elastin fibres harden, and wrinkles appear due to the cross-linking and hardening of collagen fibres.

- The epidermis grows more slowly, as mitosis slows, and the skin appears thinner, becoming almost transparent in some areas such as around the eyes, where small veins and capillaries show through the skin.

- Broken capillaries appear, especially on the cheek area and around the nose as vascular walls weaken.

- The facial contours become slack as muscle tone is reduced.

- The underlying bone structure becomes more obvious, as the fatty layer and the supportive tissue beneath the skin grow thinner.

- Blood circulation becomes poor, which interferes with skin nutrition, and the skin may appear sallow.

- Due to the decrease in metabolic rate, waste products are not removed so quickly, and this leads to puffiness of the skin.

- Patches of irregular pigmentation appear on the surface of the skin, such as lentigines and chloasmata.

The skin may also exhibit the following skin conditions, although these are not truly *characteristic* of an ageing skin:

- Dermal naevi may be enlarged.

- Sebhorrheic warts may appear on the outer epidermal layer of the skin.

◆ Verrucal filliformis warts (skin tags) may increase in number.

◆ Hair growth on the upper lip or chin, or both, may become darker or coarser, due to hormonal imbalance in the body.

◆ Dark circles and puffiness may occur under the eyes.

In addition the following skin conditions may be present:

Moist skin Moist skin appears moist and feels damp: this is due to the over-secretion of sweat. You cannot correct this skin condition, which is often caused by some internal physiological disturbance such as a hormonal or metabolic imbalance.

Advise the client to use lightweight cleansing preparations. The client should avoid skin-toning preparations with a high alcohol content; these would stimulate the skin, causing yet further perspiration and skin sensitivity. They should avoid highly spiced food, and be aware that alcoholic or hot drinks will cause dilation of the skin blood capillaries, thereby increasing the skin's temperature.

Puffy skin Sometimes referred to as oedematous skin is, and appears, swollen and puffy: this is because the tissues are retaining excess water. The condition may be caused by a medical disorder, or may be a side-effect of medication. Hot weather can cause temporary swelling of the tissues, as can local injury to the tissues. Poor blood circulation and lymphatic flow may cause puffy skin, too; this is often seen around the eyes. In this case the condition may benefit from gentle massage around the eye area. Tissue fluid retention in the facial skin may be caused by inactivity, an incorrect diet, such as one that includes too much salt or the drinking of too much alcohol, tea or coffee and insufficient water.

Unless you are quite sure about the cause of the oedema, always seek permission from your client's general practitioner (GP) before treating the skin.

The sex of the client

Men have a more acidic skin surface than females and the stratum corneum is thicker on males than females. However, males have coarse facial hair, termed terminal hair and shaving daily removes cells of the stratum corneum before they are ready to desquamate naturally. This can sensitise and dry the skin, especially if aftershave lotions with a high alcohol content are directly applied. Cleansers are available which help shaving. A moisturiser should always be applied to protect the skin, ideally containing a sun protection factor (SPF). These may be formulated to treat the skin following shaving.

The collagen content of the skin is different in men and women. Collagen and sebum production falls in menopausal women, related to hormonal changes and causing skin ageing. Skin does not appear to age as quickly in males as females because collagen, elastin and sebum production are not subjected to the same hormonal changes as women, remaining constant. The skin of males typically feels firmer.

Often the main reason males choose to have a facial is for relaxation and wellbeing, to improve the appearance of the skin, and increasingly for the anti-ageing benefits. Typically, the skin will require cleansing to remove dead skin cells and congestion, exfoliation and hydration. Related products to achieve these effects may be priorities when discussing home skincare. Specialised skin treatment products such as eye care are popular.

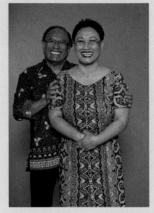
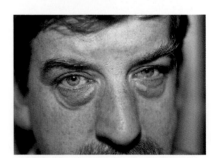

Puffy skin

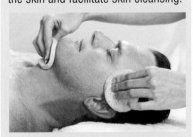

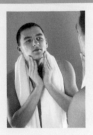

Differences in skin

Although there is no difference between skin functions such as sweat and sebaceous gland activity in white and black skin, the amount of pigment, called *melanin*, varies, resulting in different skin and hair colour.

There are two forms of the melanin pigment: *eumelanin*, produced in black and brown **skin colours**, and *pheomelanin*, found in lighter skins. Both forms of pigment can be present together but the amount of each can vary.

People who originate from hot countries and are nearer the equator have the same number of melanocytes as those from cooler countries, but they are larger and transfer more melanin to the keratinocytes and have a darker skin pigment. This is because the UV is very intense and the skin requires more protection. Those who originate from cooler countries have smaller melanocytes and a lighter skin pigment. The pigmentation of the skin is the result of millions of years of evolution. Also, the skin of people of mixed ethnicity will display a combination of those characteristics related to their origin.

Black skin   The skin colour is dark brown and ranges in tone to almost black. As black skin is exposed to UV light it becomes darker.

Care must be taken when dealing with blemishes on darker skins as scars may occur as the skin heals. The scars may become keloids, scarring that becomes enlarged and projects above the skin's surface. Even minor scratches may result in keloid formation.

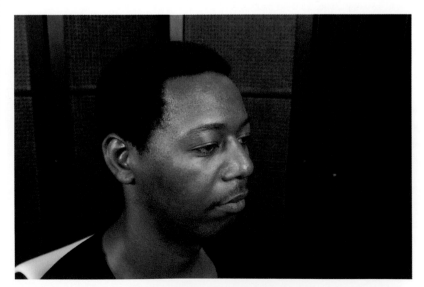

Hyperpigmentation (uneven patches of skin tone that are darker than the surrounding skin) may also occur with exposure to UV light. It is more common in darker skinned people due to increased melanin. Hyperpigmentation most commonly occurs following skin inflammation, such as acne vulgaris. Keloids may become hyperpigmented if exposed to the sun in the early stages of their formation.

Vitiligo (a type of hypopigmentation or loss of skin pigment) is a considerable problem when it occurs in dark skin, as it is very obvious. Cosmetics may be applied as a corrective technique.

Hair colour is usually dark brown to black. Male clients may have a tendency towards *pseudo folliculitis*, an inflammatory skin disorder. This occurs as the hair is coarse and curly and has a tendency as it grows out of the skin to curl back and re-enter it, becoming ingrown. This foreign object in the skin becomes irritated and inflamed. Hyperpigmentation may also accompany this condition.

Dermatosis papulosis nigra, also called flesh moles, can occur. These are brown or black hyperpigmented markings, resembling moles, usually seen on the cheeks. Their cause is unknown but they are sometimes found to be hereditary. They also occur more frequently in women than men.

ALWAYS REMEMBER

Skin pigmentation

Hyperpigmentation and **hypopigmentation** can affect the skin of any race.

Chloasma or 'liver spots' are an example of hyperpigmentation and are commonly seen as dark brown marks on the backs of the hands. These occur as a result of skin damage caused by sun damage, skin trauma or hormonal imbalance.

Freckles or ephelides are another example of hyperpigmentation. These become darker when the skin is exposed to the sun.

Prescription creams containing hydroquinone bleach and laser treatment may be used to lighten the skin by reducing the amount or production of melanin in the skin. Care must be taken using hydroquinone bleach on black and Asian skin as hypopigmentation and skin allergy can occur and can only be medically prescribed.

Increasing in popularity are botanical brighteners, derived from plants, such as liquorice root, to remove the pigmented surface cells and serum. Also, exfoliants including alpha hydroxy acids and beta hydroxy acids which lighten areas of pigmentation.

ALWAYS REMEMBER

Skin and UV defence

Very dark skin offers up to 30 times more protection against the sun than lighter skin. However, UV protection is still required.

Asian The skin colour has a light to dark tone due to increased melanin, with yellow undertones. There is a tendency towards uneven pigmentation with hyperpigmentation appearing as dark patches of skin, and scarring can appear following skin inflammation. Dermatosis papulosis nigra can occur. In women there is a normal tendency towards superfluous facial hair.

Hair colour is dark brown to black.

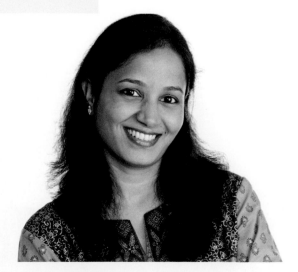

White The skin colour appears white to pink. This skin has fewer melanin granules and so less defence in the presence of UV light; sun damage results in skin burning and premature ageing. White skin has a tendency to show freckles (ephelides), as a result of uneven melanin distribution in the skin. Vascular disorders such as broken capillaries are also more obvious on a white skin. Scarring following blemishes will be observed as pink marks on the skin.

Hair colour is usually fair, red or brown.

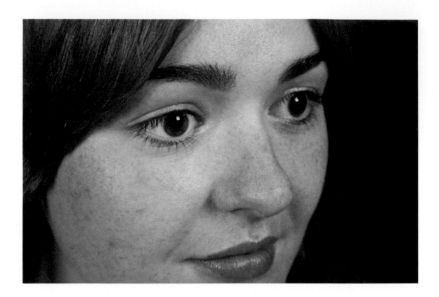

Oriental The skin colour has more melanin present and has a yellowish tone. Oriental skin is usually oily and prone to hyperpigmentation. Blemishes should be treated with caution as hyperpigmentation and scarring could result due to increased levels of melanin. Female skin generally appears smooth and has little facial hair.

Hair colour is usually mid-brown to black.

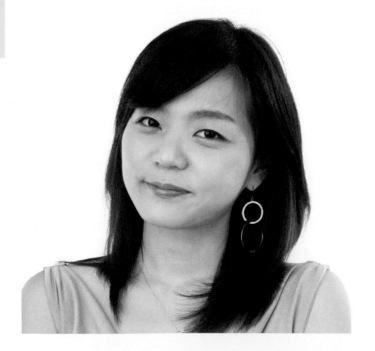

INDUSTRY ROLE MODEL

DANIELLA NORMAN Education Operations Manager and Acting Education Department Manager, Dermalogica UK and Ireland

What makes a good beauty therapist? Our hands! In a touch-starved society, a professional skin therapist's ability to offer 'safe touch' is one of the things that makes our industry unique. It's vital we are connected to the treatment process through our hands for a truly outstanding client experience.

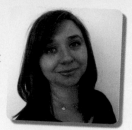

Preparation for facial treatment

Beauty workplaces differ in floor space available and how much of that is allocated to each beauty treatment. There may be one or several facial treatment work areas. If only one room is available, it is important that the range of **facial treatments** offered can be performed safely and hygienically, in a clean, efficient and relaxing environment.

Remember to always:

◆ consider and conform with all related health and safety legislation throughout the treatment

◆ implement all hygiene, health and safety requirements as identified in the National Occupational Standards (NOS)

◆ refer to the Health and Safety Executive (HSE), manufacturers' guidelines and Habia website to keep up-to-date with current health and safety practice

◆ follow industry hygiene, health and safety workplace practices throughout the treatment from preparation to completion.

For more information on general legal hygiene and safety practice that you are legally obliged to implement refer to Chapter 1 Business of Beauty.

The following equipment guidelines describe the basic preparation of the work environment for facial treatment.

Products, tools and equipment

Each facial work area should have the following basic **equipment** below. Further products, tools and equipment relevant to other stages of the facial are also discussed within the chapter.

Basic equipment:

◆ **Couch or beauty chair** with an adjustable **back rest**, for the comfort of both the client and the beauty therapist. If possible, purchase a couch that also has an adjustable **leg rest**, as this enables you to be flexible with service delivery providing other treatments such as pedicure. The couch should be wide enough and sufficiently sturdy to accommodate people of different heights and weights. It should be made of flame-retardant upholstery and of a medical grade non-permeable material covering to provide durability and allow for hygienic cleaning. Hydraulic couches are useful as they can be adjusted in height to enable the client to position themselves on the couch with ease; ideal for clients with limited mobility access. This is also an important consideration for you too, to ensure comfort and avoidance of unnecessary strain whilst working. If you are a

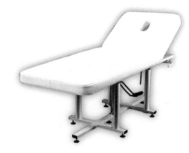

Hydraulic treatment couch

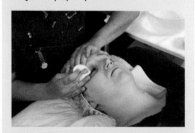

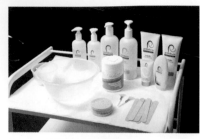

A prepared and organised trolley, ready for a facial treatment

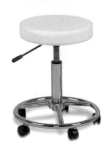

Beauty stool

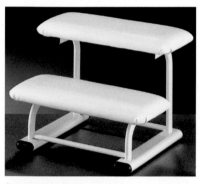

Step-up stool

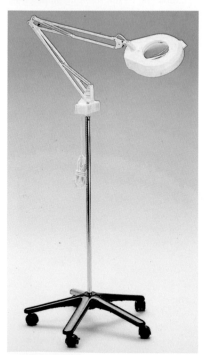

Floor-standing magnifying lamp

freelance beauty therapist you will require a lightweight, portable and durable beauty couch. These couches are also useful to have when carrying out demonstrations at a different location. Remember it must be upholstered to meet health and safety requirements and have an adjustable back rest feature.

TOP TIP

Equipment trolleys

Equipment trolleys come in many different designs. Select one with enough storage for everything you need; drawers are particularly useful. Some models have restraining bars to prevent objects sliding off the trolley. The trolley should have securely fixed easy-glide castors, which can ideally be locked into a fixed position.

◆ **Equipment trolley** To store and display all the necessary equipment and products. This must be easy to clean.

◆ **Beauty stool** The stool should be covered in a fabric similar to that covering the couch. It may or may not have a back rest; in some designs the back rest is removable. For the comfort of the therapist, it should be adjustable in height; to allow mobility, it should be mounted on castors, which may be locked as a safety feature.

◆ **Step-up stool** To assist clients as necessary to position themselves on the couch.

◆ **Magnifying lamp** The magnifying lamp is available in three models: floor-standing, wall-mounted and trolley-mounted.

◆ **Skin warming device** such as a facial steamer and warm towel heater. A **facial steamer** is a piece of electrical equipment that heats water to boiling point. The steam created is safely directed at the skin to warm the skin for its cleansing and physiologically stimulating effect.

◆ **Warm towel heaters** are used to prepare hot steam towels. These are used to soften and warm the skin and remove excess facial skincare products from the skin's surface.

Towel heater

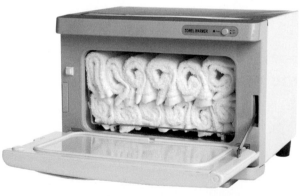

◆ **Covered waste bin** A covered waste bin should be placed unobtrusively within easy reach. It should be ideally foot operated, to minimise contamination, and lined with a heavy duty disposable bin liner.

◆ **Headband** A clean headband should be provided for each client. Use either a material headband/hair net that can be washed or disposable. Male clients with very short hair may prefer not to wear a headband.

HEALTH & SAFETY

Containers

Bottles and other containers should be clean, in good repair and clearly labelled. This is important for reasons of hygiene and professional appearance.

Bottles should not be refilled unless this is permissible and hygiene requirements are met to prevent contamination. Suppliers may offer discount for a refill service. This should be considered when selecting your supplier.

Remember, select recyclable packaging that is less harmful to the environment in its production. Recycling packaging codes will inform you of this.

◆ **Skincare products** The trolley should carry a display of facial care products to suit all skin types and conditions.

◆ **Disinfecting fluid** in which to place small sterilised equipment such as eyebrow tweezers and facial extraction tools.

◆ **Spatulas** Several clean spatulas should be provided for each client. One should be used in tucking any stray hair beneath the headband, if used. Others will be used in removing products from their containers and for applying products to the skin. These may be wooden, sourced from well-managed forest sources, or biodegradable plastic.

◆ **Cotton wool** There should be a plentiful supply of both damp and dry cotton wool, sufficient for the treatment to be carried out. Dry cotton wool should be stored in a covered container; damp cotton wool is usually placed in a clean bowl prepared for each client.

◆ **Cotton buds** These are ideal for removing make-up from the contour of the eye.

ECO TIP

Cotton wool

It is bad practice to leave the client in order to fetch more cotton wool, the client is paying for your time! It is also bad practice to prepare too much and be wasteful – resources cost money!

Pre-shaped cotton wool discs are ideal for facial services. Alternatively, cut high-quality cotton wool into squares (6 cm × 6 cm).

High-quality cotton wool has anti-fleecing properties, so the fibres do not roll and shed on to the skin. Select organic, fairtrade cotton wool made from 100% cotton as an ethical choice. These may be Soil Association approved, meaning artificial pesticides are not used in production, resulting in a less harmful effect on the environment.

◆ **Disposable paper tissue roll** To hygienically protect work surfaces.

◆ **Tissues** Facial tissues should be large and of a high quality. They should be stored in a covered container.

◆ **Towel drapes** A large towel may be used to cover the client's body, and a small hand towel draped across the client's chest and shoulders. Dependent upon the temperature of the work environment, a cotton sheet or lightweight quilt/blanket may be appropriate for the client's comfort – confirm requirements with each client.

◆ **Towel** A clean towel should be available for you to wipe your hands on as necessary.

◆ **Bowls** To store dry and damp cotton wool.

TOP TIP

Towel storage

Wall-mounted towel racks save storage space. Some couches also offer storage space, which serve to heat towels when required for your client's treatment to enhance their comfort.

ECO TIP

Sustainable towels

Towels can be made from renewable sources such as wood fibre. These towels are disposable and easily decompose. This saves energy and time as there is no need to launder.

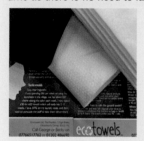

ECO TIP

Facial tissues

Paper manufacturing is harmful to the environment as timber from trees and a significant amount of energy is used to produce it. Recycled paper should be considered for your facial tissues, but these will need to be tested to ensure they will be comfortable for the client.

◆ **Gown, robe or wrap** A clean gown should be provided for each client as necessary.

◆ **Facial sponges, facial mitts or towels** These are used to remove facial products from the skin during service. They are particularly useful when working on a male client where cotton wool would collect on coarse facial hair.

◆ **Mirror** A clean hand mirror should be available for use in consulting with the client before, during and after their service.

◆ **Container for jewellery** A container may be provided in which the client can place their jewellery if they need to remove it prior to treatment. Follow your salon workplace policy in respect of removal and security of client possessions. Some salons state that clients keep their possessions with them when removed and are, therefore, responsible for them.

Environmental and sustainable working practices

When carrying out facial treatments consider the following points.

◆ Ensure equipment purchased is reliable as this will avoid early replacement.

◆ Locally sourced, manufactured products should be used wherever possible.

◆ Recycle as much as you can and wherever possible.

◆ Consider using packaging that can be recycled and refilled.

◆ Be efficient when working with your resources in order to minimise waste. For example, dispense only the amount of product required and inform the client of this when retailing a product.

◆ Reduce energy usage wherever possible by switching off equipment at the mains when not in use and turning off lights when safe to do so (such as during facial massage).

◆ Candles may be used as an alternative, but once again consider ethically, organically sourced products.

◆ Turn off water immediately when the necessary amount has been provided; never leave taps running unnecessarily.

◆ Use 'eco-disposables' which include towels, couch covers, sheets and gowns which are biodegradable and recyclable. This avoids the use of energy during laundry. If not available use economy wash cycles and natural, environmentally-friendly detergents.

◆ Choose products that do not include recognised harmful ingredients such as microbeads which are in exfoliants.

The work area should always be prepared and maintained throughout the day, ready for further treatments.

Client care, consultation and communication

Treatment information to provide to client at initial point of interest

The following points are important for the receptionist to consider when booking a client for a facial treatment.

◆ When a new client makes an appointment for a treatment, always allocate extra time for the consultation beforehand.

◆ **Treatment timing** Explain to the client how long they should allow for the appointment. For example, if a client is seeking an **express facial** treatment including a basic skin cleansing and mask treatment, allow 30 minutes; if they are a new client allow 60 minutes so that there is time for the consultation and completing the treatment plan. If it is necessary to complete facial extractions and to carry out other specialised treatments, allow 45 minutes to 1 hour. For a full facial treatment without consultation, allow 1 hour.

◆ Depending on the facial treatment to be carried out, the client may need to remove some clothing; inform them of this. A **gown**, wrap or robe is usually provided for the client to wear for modesty, especially in a spa or hotel environment where they may need to move through different areas from a changing room. Always consider client modesty and privacy, which must be maintained at all times.

◆ If the client is new to the treatment, it is important to discuss briefly what will be involved so that they will know what to expect. A business website can also be used to provide such information.

◆ If the client informs you of poor health, or is taking medication that may affect their skin condition, it may not be possible to treat them until the medical condition has been treated by their GP, or they have no objection to treatment proceeding. Tactfully check client suitability for facial treatment; this may involve seeking guidance from others.

◆ If there is a history of skin sensitivity and allergies to treatment products, it may be necessary for the client to receive a **skin sensitivity patch test**. This should be carried out 24–48 hours before treatment is received.

Client arrival

Clients should never be kept waiting on arrival for their appointment, unless there is an unavoidable reason.

On arrival the client treatment plan **record** may start to be completed; this may be completed by the salon receptionist. Record the client's personal details, such as their name, date of birth and address and if qualified to, check that there are no contra-indications to the facial treatment.

The beauty therapist will add further information to the record at the consultation and during treatment in relation to information provided by the client, any modifications required and in relation to the results obtained.

If a client is a **minor**, under the age of 16 years of age, it is necessary to obtain signed written consent before teatment is carried out. It is also necessary that the parent or guardian is present when the treatment is given.

Before carrying out *any* facial treatments, you must consult with the client to determine their treatment needs and to discuss the services that are available – referred to as the consultation.

Consultation is a service that should also be offered separately: there should be no pressure on the client to receive or book a treatment following the consultation. Excellent communication skills should be used at consultation to ensure your judgements on the needs of the client are correct.

TOP TIP

Identifying a contra-indication requiring referral

Follow a sequence when performing the consultation. Inform the client of the purpose of information required and assessment techniques used.

At the stage when you confirm client suitability, after questions about medical health and assessment of the skin/skin analysis, this then allows you to discuss your findings.

You can proceed or if unsure there are two options:

1 Seek guidance from a senior staff member by discussing your findings. It may be possible that you can proceed.

2 Explain to your client that you want them to get the best from their treatment and experience appropriate client care. As you are unsure as to their suitability in the particular area, it is a requirement to ensure their suitability and that there is no medical objection to treatment.

By doing this, you are keeping to policy procedure, being professional and tactful, without diagnosing or causing alarm.

ALWAYS REMEMBER

Compliance with the Data Protection Act (1998)

Ensure all client records are stored securely, with only those staff who have the client's permission able to access them.

ALWAYS REMEMBER

You should never simply pass a form to a client and ask them to fill it out. This information is important so you can ensure it is safe to proceed with the treatment, identify if any modifications are required and obtain all the information you need to provide the most relevant treatment plan.

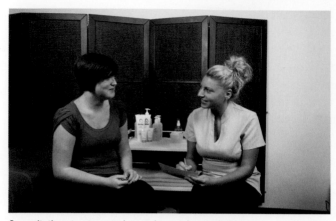

Consultation, treatment plan and record completion

Consultation

Carry out the consultation in a private area. This should take place when the client first meets you. Findings should be reviewed at every follow-up treatment to identify any changes that require consideration, and again whenever a new treatment is to be carried out.

The consultation is the time when you can assess whether the client is actually suited to the treatment. You must check for contra-indications, and must not carry on if there are any – this is to safeguard yourself, the client and, in the case of a client with a contagious skin disorder, other clients and colleagues who would be at risk of cross-infection. Remember, you are not qualified to diagnose a contra-indication. Always refer the client to their GP without causing unnecessary cause for concern.

Question the client about what their skin needs are, their present skincare routine, preferences in product formulation, allergies, their general lifestyle and health. Listen carefully to their responses to guide you in your assessment of what would be most suitable.

Your knowledge of facial treatments and advice on skincare products will build rapport with a new client and gain client confidence. Explain what is involved with each part of the facial treatment, its purpose and effects, and in the case of a nervous client, sensations to be experienced. Inform the client how long it takes and give further advice and recommendations, including additional products and services and how these will benefit the client.

The client is likely to ask which is the most suitable treatment or product for them, and you must advise them as to which would best meet their needs.

Make the client aware of the cost of the individual treatment – or treatment programme – so that they can decide whether or not to undertake the financial commitment and if they have time to commit to what is involved. Recommended time intervals between treatments should also be discussed.

> "A thorough consultation will ensure you target your client's skin priorities, giving them the results they want and allowing you to identify any lifestyle triggers contributing to their skin condition."
>
> *Daniella Norman*

ALWAYS REMEMBER

Affordability

Never make assumptions about what the client can afford. Usually the client will indicate to you what they are prepared to spend.

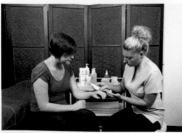

Discussing and demonstrating skincare product usage

> "Customers can be more motivated by how you communicate, not necessarily by what you are saying. Speak with passion and authenticity. Know your product and have a thorough understanding of how the skin works. Only then can you be credible and give prescriptive treatments and home care that deliver results."
>
> *Daniella Norman*

The diversity of your clients should be considered and this is discussed in Chapter 3 Consultation practice and techniques.

Visual aids may be used to explain aspects of the treatment. You could demonstrate some of the products, i.e. exfoliation product, directly on your own skin or theirs, usually the back of the hand. Marketing literature may also be available to refer to.

Invite the client to ask questions during the consultation. By the end, they should understand fully what the proposed treatment involves.

The client may receive the treatment immediately if suitable following the consultation, or go away to consider the suggestions.

During the consultation, details are recorded on the client's treatment plan record. You can fill this in as you speak to them, without diverting your attention away from them. A sample treatment plan record is located in Chapter 3 Consultation and assessment techniques.

REVISION AID

Why is it important to keep a record of a client's treatments?

ALWAYS REMEMBER

Treatment modification

Always adapt or modify your facial treatment to accommodate your client's needs and the objectives required. Examples of facial treatment modification include:

◆ enabling access for a client with a physical disability

◆ how the consultation and communication would accommodate the requirements of a client with a hearing impairment

◆ altering the pressure or choice of facial massage techniques to suit the client's skin type, condition and muscle tone

◆ altering the distance and application of steam heat to take into account skin sensitivity and skin type

◆ providing an express facial, targeting specific areas for maintenance or improvement.

HEALTH & SAFETY

Previous facial treatment history

Check if a client has received any advanced specialist facials such as micro-dermabrasion or chemical peels. These treatments involve removing the surface epidermal cells from the skin, which may cause it to be sensitive. Ensure that you check at consultation if the client has been receiving any injectable treatments such as botox, and if so what and when. Seek guidance as necessary from a senior colleague to confirm client suitability.

ACTIVITY

Recognising contra-indications that prevent or restrict treatment

List **six skin disorders** and **six skin diseases** in a chart.

Briefly describe how you would recognise the features of each.

Which would it be inappropriate to treat and **prevent** treatment?

Which would **restrict** treatment and require treatment modification?

For further information on contra-indications refer to Chapter 3, Consultation practice and techniques.

Contra-indications

The consultation and then skin analysis will draw your attention to any contra-indications or conditions that require special consideration, care and attention. A note is usually provided on the client treatment record for recording any contra-indications.

Remember that not all contra-indications are visible.

The following contra-indications are relevant to *all* facial treatments and prevent the treatment from being carried out:

◆ systemic medical conditions

◆ **severe skin condition**, such as active acne vulgaris

◆ **skin disease**, requiring medical referral, such as impetigo

◆ **severe bruising** in the area

◆ **cuts and abrasions**, if open – wait until the condition has healed

◆ **bone fracture**, if recent – wait for 6 months

◆ **bacterial infection,** e.g. furuncle (boil)

◆ **fungal infection**, such as tinea corporis (body ringworm)

◆ **viral infections**, such as herpes simplex (cold sore) and warts

◆ **parasitic conditions**, such as scabies

◆ **inflammation or swelling** of the skin

◆ **scar tissue in area of treatment**, if recent, avoid – wait for 6 months before treatment proceeds in area

◆ **eye infection**, such as conjunctivitis.

Diseases and disorders are illustrated and discussed in Chapter 3.

Further contra-indications are listed elsewhere in this chapter that are specific to additional aspects (e.g. steaming) of facial treatment.

Following the consultation, the client's answers will indicate to you what is required, and what is achievable, from the facial treatment.

When finalising the most suitable treatment plan:

◆ explain what is involved in each stage of the treatment, how long it takes, and what aftercare advice and home care recommendations are required (if relevant)

◆ explain the benefits of the products to be used and how these will benefit the client's treatment requirements. You can present these key products to the client.

◆ if the client has a budget, design a treatment programme within the client's budget, which will meet their needs

◆ discuss any activities, services or products that should be avoided following treatment application

◆ explain any contra-actions that may occur and action to be taken in the event of an unwanted reaction to treatment.

This allows the client to:

◆ discover what you can offer to meet their needs

◆ ask questions, and receive honest professional advice concerning the most appropriate choice of skincare treatment/product

◆ decide how much they are willing to spend

◆ decide if they wish to proceed with the treatment plan or amend it in any way.

You should ensure that the client fully understands and is realistic about what the proposed treatment involves and what can be achieved.

Preparing the client

When the service plan has been agreed, prepare and position the client for treatment. The client should remove outer clothing and be provided with a modesty robe.

1 Wash your hands before preparing the client for treatment.

2 Explain how the client should position themselves. Assist and position the client on the treatment couch. Ensure the client is comfortable and relaxed. Cover the client with a clean, large bath towel or alternative suitable covering. If necessary, drape a small hand towel across their shoulders. Ensure the client is warm and relaxed throughout the treatment.

3 If a facial, neck and shoulder massage is to be given, ask the client politely to remove her arms from her bra straps in preparation: explain that this avoids unnecessary disturbance later.

4 Fasten a clean hairnet or headband around the client's hairline. Some male clients with short hair may prefer not to wear a headband. Position the headband so that it does not cover the skin of the face. If using a facial steamer, you may protect the hair with a small towel to stop it getting damp.

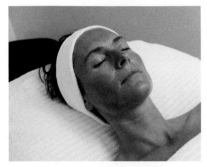

Client prepared for a facial treatment

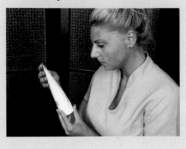
5 After preparing the client, wash your hands: this demonstrates to the client your concern to work hygienically.

The skin should than be cleansed prior to completing a more detailed skin analysis where you can correctly assess and diagnose the skin type and associated conditions.

Choice of products selected will be decided upon from the information you have gained so far.

All **facial products** and equipment should be used with due regard to health and safety following manufacturer's instructions.

Cleansing

Skin cleansing is essential in promoting and maintaining a healthy skin. There are various cleansing preparations to choose from; basically their action is the same in each case:

◆ to gently exfoliate dead skin cells from the stratum corneum, exposing younger fresher cells and improving the skin's appearance

◆ to remove make-up if worn, dirt and pollutants from the skin's epidermal surface, reducing the possibility of skin blemishes and irritation

◆ to remove excess sweat and sebum from the skin's surface, reducing congestion of the skin and the subsequent formation of comedones, milia, pustules and papules

◆ to prepare the skin for further treatments.

Cleansing products

A **cleanser** is required that will remove both oil-soluble and water-soluble substances without drying the skin. Oil is capable of dissolving grease; water will dissolve other substances. Usually, therefore, a cleanser is a combination of both oil and water.

Oil and water do not combine: if you simply mix the two together they separate again, with the oil floating on the top of the water. If the two substances are shaken together vigorously, however, one substance will break up and become suspended in the other. The result is known as an **emulsion**. The addition of a surfactant increases the solubility of both oil in water and water in oil. Detergent is an example of a surfactant. A surfactant has a **hydrophilic head** and a **hydrophobic tail**.

The hydrophilic head binds with the water in the emulsion and the hydrophobic tail will bind with the oil. Surfactants cleanse the skin by clinging to the skin's oils and debris, which can then be washed away.

Emulsions are used in many cosmetic preparations. They are either:

◆ **oil-in-water** (O/W) – minute droplets of oil, surrounded by water

◆ **water-in-oil** (W/O) – minute droplets of water, surrounded by oil.

To give the emulsion stability, and to stop it separating out again, an **emulsifier** is added.

Various cleansing preparations are available to the beauty therapist, with formulations designed to suit the different skin types. They include:

- cleansing milks
- cleansing creams
- cleansing balms
- cleansing lotions
- facial gel or foaming cleansers
- eye make-up removers.

Whichever cleanser is chosen, it should have the following qualities:

- it should be formulated and contain ingredients to treat the skin type and condition it has been designed for
- it should cleanse the skin effectively, without causing irritation
- it should remove all traces of make-up, skin debris, bacteria, oil and pollutants
- it should feel pleasant to use
- it should be easy to remove from the skin
- ideally, it should be pH-balanced.

The skin is naturally slightly acidic: it has an **acid mantle**. Alkalis strip the skin of its protective film of sebum, making it feel dry and taut. To avoid skin irritation it is preferable to use a product that matches the acid mantle, a product with a pH of 5.5–5.6.

Cleansing milks

Cleansing milks are usually oil-in-water emulsions, with a relatively high proportion of water to oil, making the milk quite fluid and light in its consistency. Water may not be required to be used in conjunction with them because the oil acts as the solvent, rather than the surfactant detergent.

Cleansing milks have these specific treatment uses:

- treating normal to dry skin that is prone to sensitivity
- treating sensitive skin.

Cleansing creams

Cleansing creams have a relatively high proportion of oil to water, making the emulsion thicker and richer in its consistency than cleansing milks. The high oil content allows the product to be massaged over the skin surface without dragging the skin's tissues. The cream is also more effective in removing grease and oil-based make-up from the skin.

Cleansing creams have these specific treatment uses:

- removing facial cosmetics
- can be used to provide a deep cleansing massage
- treating normal to very dry skin.

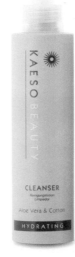

Skin cleanser

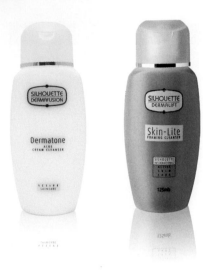

Cleansing lotion and foaming cleanser

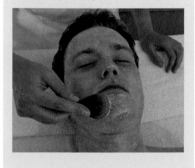

Cleansing balms   Cleansing **balms** are usually lightweight cleansers rich in organic oils that quickly transform from a solid balm to a fluid. They moisturise and improve the texture of the skin while cleansing.

Cleansing balms have these specific treatment uses:

◆ moisturising, non-drying effect

◆ improvement of skin texture

◆ suitable for all skin types except oily.

Cleansing lotions Cleansing **lotions** are solutions of detergents in water. They do not usually contain oil, and are therefore unsuitable for the removal of facial cosmetics.

Cleansing lotions have these specific service uses:

◆ cleansing a normal to combination skin type

◆ treating oily skin (where a high oil content could aggravate the skin, causing yet further sebum production).

Medicated ingredients may be included in a cleansing formulation: these are only suitable for oily, congested, pustular skin types.

If the client has a mature, normal or combination skin, a cleansing lotion may not be effective because of the reduced oil content. A mature skin benefits from oil content to compensate for reduced sebum production.

Facial gel or foaming cleansers Facial **gel** or **foaming cleansers** usually contain a mild detergent that foams when mixed with water. Additional ingredients are selected for the treatment of different skin types. These cleansers are quick to use and afford a suitable alternative for the client who likes to cleanse their face with soap and water. If the client wears an oil-based make-up, advise them to use a cleansing cream first to remove make-up thoroughly before using this cleanser.

Facial foaming cleansers have a general application:

◆ treating most skin types except very dry or sensitive skin

◆ particularly suitable for oily and combination skin due to their formulation, which effectively removes sebum without drying the skin.

Cleansing bars   Although it is efficient as a cleanser, **soap** is usually considered unsuitable for use on the skin. It has an alkaline pH, which disturbs the skin's natural acidic pH balance. Soap strips the skin of its protective acid mantle, leaving insoluble salts on the skin's surface. The skin may be left feeling itchy, taut and sensitive.

Cleansing bars are a milder alternative to soap, and are specially formulated to match the skin's acidic pH of 5.5–5.6. They are less likely to dry out the skin. These are available for retail use, and would not be used for professional use.

Cleansing bars have this specific application:

◆ treating oily to normal skin that is not sensitive.

TOP TIP

Eye make-up remover as an eye treatment

Many eye make-up removers are also eye treatments. If your workplace uses a commercial product in this way apply it to the dampened eye pads used during **mask treatment** and explain the benefits to the client. This may also assist your retail sales, as the client may wish to purchase some for home use.

TOP TIP

Maintenance of artificial lashes

For clients who enjoy wearing semi-permanent lashes, recommend a suitable non-oily make-up remover that will maintain the longevity of the artificial lashes.

Eye make-up remover   Eye tissue is a lot thinner than the skin on the rest of the face. It readily puffs up if aggravated by oil-based cleansing preparations, and becomes very dry if harsh cleansing preparations are used.

To remove make-up from this area, use an **eye make-up remover**. This product cleanses the eyelid and lashes, gently emulsifying the make-up. It also conditions the delicate skin. Formulated as a lotion or a gel, it is designed to remove either water-based or oil-based products (or both) from the eye area. As semi-permanent lashes have increased in popularity it is important to have an eye make-up remover that is suitable to apply in this area.

Oily eye make-up removers have these specific treatment uses:

◆   treating clients who wear waterproof mascara

◆   removing wax or oil-based eyeshadow.

Non-oily eye make-up removers have these applications:

◆   treating clients with sensitive skin around the eyes

◆   treating clients who wear contact lenses

◆   treating clients who wear semi-permanent artificial eyelashes.

HEALTH & SAFETY

Hygiene when cleansing the eye area

Never use the reverse side of the cotton wool pad – this is unhygienic.

Never use the same piece of cotton wool to cleanse both eyes, use a separate piece for each eye to avoid cross-infection.

Cleansing treatment

There are usually two manual processes involved in the cleansing routine: *the superficial cleanse* and the *deep cleanse*.

The superficial cleanse uses lightweight cleansing preparations to emulsify surface make-up, skin debris, dirt and grease. This is followed by the more thorough deep cleanse, in which a suitable product, e.g. a heavier cleansing cream, may be applied to the face. The high percentage of oil contained in the cream formulation allows the cream to be massaged over the skin's surface without evaporation of the product. However, the product formulation should suit the skin type and condition so a cleansing balm may be preferable.

"Our body and our hands are vital to how we make a living, so take care of them! Ensure you pay special attention to your posture during treatments and commit to doing daily hand exercises and stretches to avoid injuries and strains."

Daniella Norman

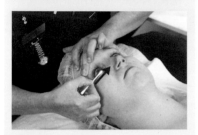
STEP-BY-STEP: SUPERFICIAL CLEANSING

Each part of the face requires a special technique in the application and removal of the cleansing product, considering the area, skin thickness and condition, and the structures below: A suggested cleansing routine follows:

- the eye tissue and lashes
- the lips
- the neck, chin, cheeks and forehead.

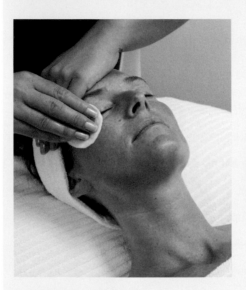

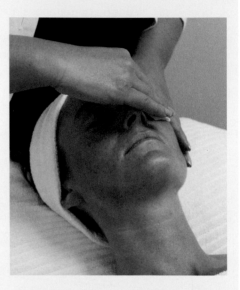

1 Wash your hands.
Ensure that the client's contact lenses are removed if worn.
Gloves may be worn if the client has coarse facial hair which may cause skin irritation to the hands.

Cleanse the eye area, using a suitable eye make-up remover. If the client is not wearing make-up this product can still be used as they are formulated for cleansing the delicate eye area. Each eye is cleansed separately. Your non-working hand lifts and supports the eye tissue and muscle while the working hand applies the eye make-up remover.

Eye make-up remover is applied directly to a clean, damp piece of cotton wool. Stroke down the length of the upper eyelashes, from base to points.

2 Next, cleanse the eye tissue in a sweeping circle, outwards across the upper eyelid, circling beneath the lower lashes towards the nose. This follows the direction of the muscle fibres of the orbicularis oculi eye muscle. Explain the importance of support and direction of application of the cleansing product to the client.

Repeat, replacing the cotton wool until the eye area and the cotton wool show clean.

Sometimes a cleansing milk is used to remove eye make-up. In this case, apply a little of the product to the back of one hand. The ring finger is then used to apply the cleansing lotion to the lashes.

Use damp cotton wool to remove the emulsified product.
Repeat the cleansing process until the eye area is clean.
A cotton bud may be used under the lower lashes to ensure last traces of make-up are removed.

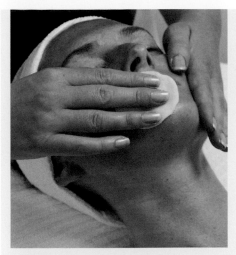
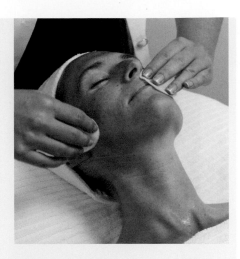

3 Cleanse the lips, preferably with a cleansing lotion, as this readily emulsifies the oils or waxes contained in lipstick if worn.

Support the left side of the client's mouth. With the working hand, apply product directly to damp cotton wool and sweep across the upper lip, from left to right; and then across the lower lip, from right to left.

Remove excess cleanser from the lips. Support the corner of the mouth; using a clean damp piece of cotton wool wipe across the lips.

Repeat the cleansing process as necessary, until the lips and the cotton wool show clean.

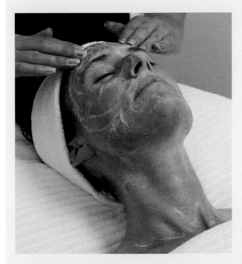

4 Select a cleansing product to suit your client's skin type.

Place the product into one hand – sufficient to cover the face and neck, and to massage gently over the surface of the skin.

Clasp the fingers together at the base of the neck, and unlink them as you move up the neck.

Clasp the fingers together again at the chin, drawing the fingers outwards to the angle of the jawbone.

Stroke up the face, towards the forehead, with your fingertips pointing downwards and your palms in contact with the skin.

Using a series of light circular movements with your fingertips, gently massage the product into the skin, beginning at the base of the neck and finishing at the forehead. This massage technique is known as petrissage.

If the client is wearing facial make-up, it is usual to perform the superficial cleanse twice to ensure all cosmetics are effectively removed.

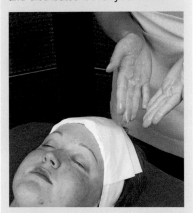

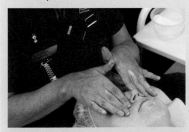

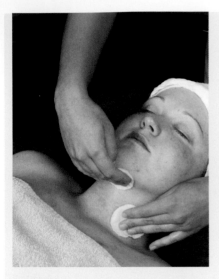
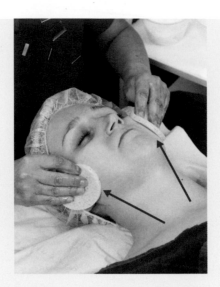
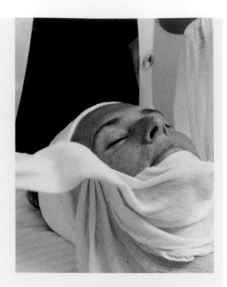

5 Remove the cleanser thoroughly with clean damp cotton wool, facial sponges, facial mitts or hot towels, simultaneously stroking over the skin surface, upwards and outwards from the neck, over the face towards the hairline.

Repeat this process as necessary, using clean cotton wool, if used, each time. Facial sponges and mitts will require regular rinsing with clean, warm water. The facial towel is unwrapped and its surface stroked over the skin to remove all trace of facial cleanser.

TOP TIP

Sponges are ideal when working on males with coarse terminal facial hair type skin. Coarse, terminal hairs will cause the cotton fibres in cotton wool to drag.

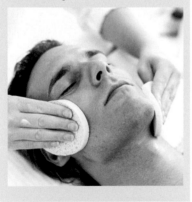

HEALTH & SAFETY

Pressure application

Reduce pressure when working over areas where the skin tissue is thinner, this includes the *hyoid bone* at the throat and bony prominences such as the *zygomatic bone* (the cheekbone) and the *frontal bone* (the forehead).

Pressure must always be *upwards* and *outwards*, to avoid dragging the facial skin and underlying muscles.

ALWAYS REMEMBER

Facial muscles

Unlike the muscles of the body, which attach to bones, most of the facial muscles are attached to the facial skin itself. You should therefore avoid stretching the skin unnecessarily – if you do, you may also stretch the facial muscles and contribute to premature ageing.

REVISION AID

What is the correct way to use an eye make-up remover?

ALWAYS REMEMBER

Thorough cleanser removal

Check that the eyebrow hair and the skin, underneath the nose and beneath the chin are free of product; it is easy to overlook some cleansing product in these areas.

STEP-BY-STEP: DEEP CLEANSING

The deep cleanse follows and involves a series of **massage techniques,** which reinforce the cleansing effect achieved with the cleansing product. Blood circulation is increased to the area; this has a warming effect on the skin, which relaxes the skin's natural openings, the hair follicles and pores. This aids the absorption of cleanser into the hair follicles and pores, where it can dissolve make-up if worn, sebum, sweat and skin debris.

There are various deep-cleansing sequences; all are acceptable if carried out in a safe, hygienic manner, and achieve the desired outcomes – a fresh, clean skin surface. Here is one sequence for deep cleansing.

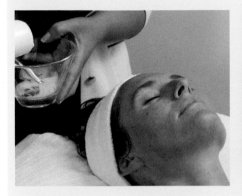

1 Select a cleansing medium to suit your client's skin type. The procedure for application is the same as that for the superficial cleanse.

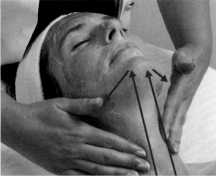

2 Stroke up either side of the neck, using your fingertips. At the chin, draw the fingers outwards to the angle of the jaw, and lightly stroke back down the neck to the starting position.

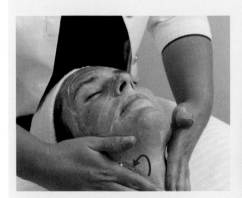

3 Apply small circular petrissage manipulations over the skin of the neck.

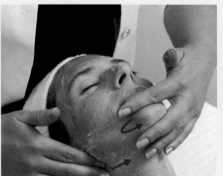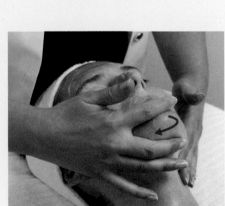

4 Draw the fingertips outwards to the angle of the jaw. Rest each index finger against the jawbone (you will be able to feel the lower teeth in the jaw). Place the middle finger beneath the jawbone. Move the right hand towards the chin where the index finger glides over the chin; return the fingers beneath the jawbone, to the starting position. Repeat with the left hand.

Repeat step 4 a further five times.

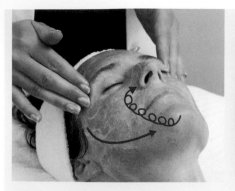

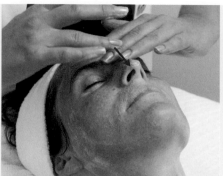

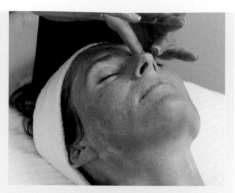

5 Apply small circular manipulations, commencing at the chin, working up towards the nose and finishing at the temples. Slide the fingers from the temples back to the chin.

Repeat step 5 a further five times.

6 Position the ring finger of the right hand at the bridge of the nose. Perform a running movement, sliding the ring, middle and index fingers off the end of the nose. Repeat immediately with the left hand.

Repeat step 6 a further five times with each hand.

7 With the pads of the ring fingers, trace a circle around the eye orbits. Begin at the inner corner of the upper brow bone, slide along to the outer corners of the brow bone and continue the circle around and under the eyes, returning to the starting position.

Repeat step 7 a further five times.

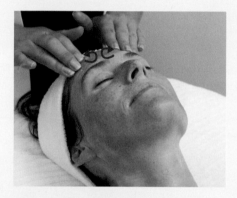

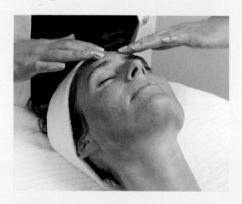

8 Using both hands, apply small circular petrissage manipulations across the forehead.

Repeat step 8 a further five times.

9 Open the index and middle fingers of each hand and perform a criss-cross friction manipulation movement over the forehead.

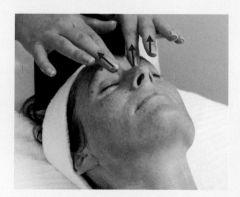

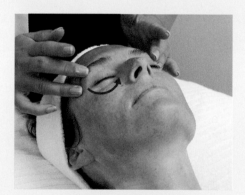

10 Slide the index finger upwards slightly, lifting the inner eyebrow. Lift the centre of the eyebrow with the middle finger. Finally, lift the outer corner of the eyebrow with the ring finger. Slide the ring fingers around the outer corner and beneath the eye orbit.

Repeat step 10 a further five times.

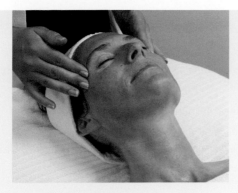

11 With the finger pads of each hand, apply slight pressure at the temples. This indicates to the client that the cleansing sequence is complete.

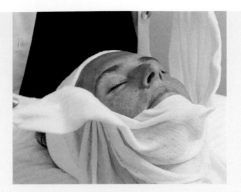

12 Remove the cleansing cream from the skin, using damp cotton wool, facial sponges, facial mitts or towels.

Toning

After the skin has been thoroughly cleansed it is then toned with an appropriate toning lotion.

Toning products

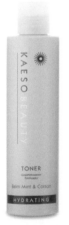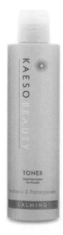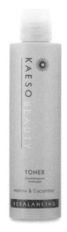

Toning lotions remove from the skin all traces of cleanser, skin debris, oil and skincare products. The toning lotion's main action is as follows:

◆ It produces a cooling effect on the skin when the water or alcohol in the toner evaporates from the skin's surface. (When a liquid evaporates it changes to a gas, which takes energy. In the case of toner, the energy is taken from the skin, which therefore feels cooler.)

◆ It creates a tightening effect on the skin, because of a chemical within the toner called an astringent. This causes the pores to close, thereby reducing the flow of sebum and sweat onto the skin's surface.

◆ It helps to restore the acidic pH balance of the skin. Milder skin toners have a pH 4.5–4.6; stronger astringents disturb the pH more severely, and may cause skin irritation and sensitivity.

ECO TIP

Water usage

Avoid leaving taps running unnecessarily. For example, when rinsing facial sponges, fill a bowl with water and immerse to dampen.

Think of other initiatives on how to achieve economical water usage in the workplace.

If your workplace has a water meter you can see how much is being used and what savings a change of practice can make.

World Water Day is an initiative from the United Nations, which takes place on 22 March each year.

REVISION AID

What is the name of the muscle used to open and close the eyes?

TOP TIP

Toning lotions

All toning lotions have some astringent effect on the skin, but those that contain relatively high alcohol content are actually marketed as astringents.

Do not use toning lotions that contain more than 20 per cent alcohol on dry skin – they may cause skin irritation.

Avoid the excessive use of astringent on oily skin – the astringent will dehydrate the skin, and it will then produce more sebum.

There are three main types of toning lotions, the main difference being the amounts of alcohol they contain. They include:

◆ bracers and fresheners

◆ tonics

◆ astringents.

Specialised ingredients are added to the toners, which add moisture, control oil and have anti-inflammatory properties.

Skin bracers and fresheners Skin **bracers** and **skin fresheners** are the mildest toning lotions: they contain little (10 per cent) or no alcohol. They consist mainly of purified water, with floral extracts such as **rose water**, for a mild toning effect. They may contain a humectant, such as glycerine to prevent moisture loss from the skin.

Skin bracers and fresheners are recommended for:

◆ dry, delicate skin

◆ sensitive skin

◆ mature skin.

"Know your product! Attend product training and try the products yourself. Personal experience will highlight your credibility when discussing home care recommendations, such as how the product feels and its specific skin benefits to improve the client's skin."

Daniella Norman

Skin tonics Skin **tonics** are slightly stronger toning lotions containing up to 20 per cent alcohol. Many contain a little of some astringent agent such as orange flower water.

Skin tonics are recommended for:

◆ normal skin.

Astringents **Astringents** are the strongest toning lotions; they have a high proportion of alcohol, 30–60 per cent, which can be very drying. They may contain antiseptic ingredients such as witch hazel or tea tree oil; these are for use on blemished skin, to reduce the growth of bacteria and promote skin healing. Strong astringents can cause the skin to become dry and irritated if there is any skin sensitivity, so care must be taken.

Astringents are recommended for:

◆ oily skin with no skin sensitivity

◆ problematic, mild acne vulgaris in young skin.

Toning lotions that are suitable for oily skin are becoming increasingly available and rely upon their botanical formulations to control sebum flow and promote skin healing.

ECO TIP

Botanical organic formulations

Botanical (derived from plants) organic beauty products are increasing in popularity, as the number of clients who are concerned about health and wellbeing and the environment increases.

The Soil Association developed the Cosmetics Organic Standard (COSMOS) in 2010 in order to authenticate products in the organic beauty market.

To comply, a product must have:

◆ no animal testing

◆ no genetically modified (GM) products

◆ no synthetic colours or fragrances

◆ no silicone oils or derivatives

◆ less waste and pollution.

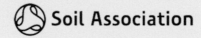

TOP TIP

Home application of toner

For home use, advise the client to apply toning lotion using dampened cotton wool; this is more economical. This tip may be more problematic for male clients due to their short coarse hair, where a spray toner may be suitable or a '2 in 1' facial cleanser and toner preparation.

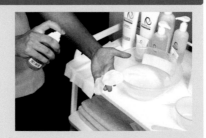

STEP-BY-STEP: APPLICATION

Toning lotion may be applied in several ways. Whichever method you choose, it should leave the skin thoroughly clean and free of grease. Remember to always follow the manufacturer's instructions.

The most popular method of application is to apply the toner directly to two pieces of clean damp cotton wool, which are wiped gently upwards and outwards over the neck and face, avoiding the delicate eye tissue.

Alternatively, the toner may be applied under pressure atomised as a fine spray. This produces a fine mist of the toning lotion over the skin. If using this method, always protect the eye tissue with cotton wool pads and hold the spray about 30 cm from the skin, directing the spray across the skin in a sweeping movement. This is preferable when treating a male client, where the cotton wool application technique would be unsuitable as the cotton wool would collect on facial hair.

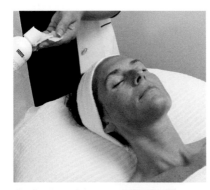

Application of toner to damp cotton wool

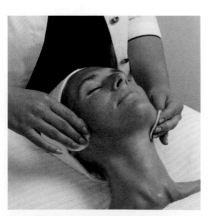

Application of toner to the skin using damp cotton wool

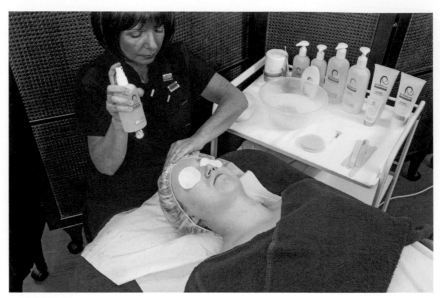

Application of toner to the skin using a spray atomiser

To produce a stimulating effect, the toning lotion can be applied to dampened cotton wool in each hand: hold these firmly at one corner, and gently tap the cotton wool over the skin surface.

Blotting the skin

After applying toning lotion, immediately blot the skin dry with a soft facial tissue to prevent the toner evaporating from the skin's surface (which would stimulate the skin). Alternatively you can make a small tear in the centre of a large facial tissue for the client's nose. Place the tissue over their face and neck, and mould it into position to absorb excess moisture.

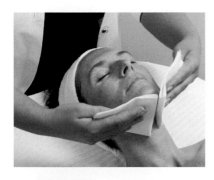

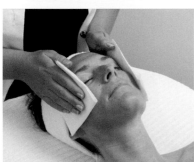

Blotting the skin with large facial tissues

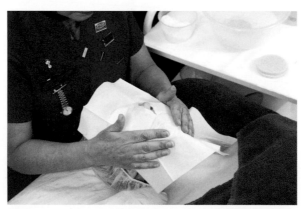

Tearing a nose hole for client comfort, when facial blotting

Alternatively, blot over the face with large facial tissues as shown.

When skin is thoroughly cleansed and toned a thorough skin analysis can occur inspecting all areas of the face and neck using a magnifying lamp. The lamp provides a bright fluorescent light, so if the room is dimly lit, there is no need to switch on the room light. A Wood's, lamp may be useful for inspecting the deeper skin layers. Protect the client's eyes with damp cotton wool pads. For more detail, refer to Chapter 3 Consultation Practice and Techniques.

Performing skin analysis

Now the skin is clean, check for evidence of:

◆ skin type

◆ characteristics of skin condition

◆ evenness of skin colour and uneven pigmentation

◆ signs of premature ageing against chronological age; this may require further investigation to establish factors affecting the skin

◆ skin sensitivity, which may be related to product or touch sensitivity following contact with the skin during cleansing.

Perform a manual test for skin tone, dehydration and circulation.

Ask further open questions as required and update your findings on the treatment record.

Based upon your observations – you may now need to modify products or treatments that you previously selected in your treatment plan.

The skin's surface will be magnified, enabling you to comment further and note any characteristics of skin type and skin conditions requiring attention. Record these on their treatment record.

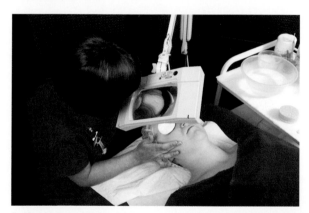

Performing a skin analysis using a magnifying lamp, manually touching the skin's surface to assess for hydration and texture

Moisturising

Although discussed here as the final stage of the facial treatment, when carried out at home as part of the client's skincare routine it follows cleansing and toning.

The skin depends on water to keep it soft, supple and resilient. Two-thirds of our body is composed of water and the skin is an important reservoir, containing about 20 per cent of the body's total water content. Most of the fluid is in the lower layers of the dermis, but it circulates to the top layer of the epidermis, where it evaporates.

The skin protects its water content in these ways:

◆ Sebum keeps the skin lubricated, and reduces water loss from skin.

◆ The skin cells have **natural moisturising factors**, a complex mix of substances that are able to fix moisture inside the cells.

◆ A cement of fats (lipids) between the skin cells forms a watertight barrier.

The natural moisture level is constantly being disturbed. The application of a cosmetic **moisturiser** helps to maintain the natural oil and moisture balance by locking moisture into the tissues, offering protection and hydration.

The basic formulation of a moisturiser is oil and water to make an oil-in-water emulsion. The water content helps to return lost moisture to the surface layers and reduces the oiliness of the product. The oil content may be obtained from many sources but its aim is to moisturise the skin and prevents moisture loss from the surface of the skin. Examples of oils include ceramides, stearic acid and linoleic acid. Often a **humectant**, such as **glycerine** or **sorbitol**, is included: this attracts moisture to the skin from the surrounding air and stops the moisturiser from drying out. Hyaluronic acid is increasingly popular as a humectant which attaches to the surface of the skin as its molecular size is too large to enter the skin. If a humectant is included, less oil is used in the formulation: this results in a lighter cream. Occlusive agents may be included to prevent water loss but may lead to cosmetic congestion, examples include silicone and stearic acid.

Moisturiser also has the following benefits:

◆ It protects the skin from external damage caused by the environment.

◆ It softens the skin and relieves skin tautness and sensitivity.

◆ It plumps the skin tissue with moisture, which minimises the appearance of fine lines.

◆ It provides a barrier between the skin and make-up cosmetics.

◆ It may contain additional ingredients that improve the condition of the skin such as vitamin E and jojoba, which are effective antioxidants, collagen to provide strength, and anti-inflammatories such as aloe vera or lavender to reduce redness and calm the skin.

◆ It may contain SPF UV filters, which protect the skin against age-accelerating sunlight.

Moisturisers are available for wear during the day or the night. These are available in different formulations, to treat all skin types and conditions.

The finish they leave on the skin will indicate their suitability to skin type, so a moisturiser for a dry skin will leave a moist, hydrated finish, whilst a moisturiser for an oily skin will often leave a matt finish.

Moisturisers are applied at the final stage of the facial when the skin is clean and toned, providing a protective barrier.

Moisturisers for daytime use

Moisturising lotions Moisturising lotions contain up to 85–90 per cent water and 10–15 per cent oil. They have a light, liquid formulation, and are ideal for use under make-up.

Moisturising lotions have these specific applications:

◆ oily skin

◆ young combination skin

◆ dehydrated skin

◆ normal skin.

Moisturising creams **Moisturising creams** contain up to 70–85 per cent water and 15–30 per cent oil. They have a thicker consistency, and cannot be poured.

Moisturising creams have these specific applications:

◆ mature skin

◆ dry skin.

STEP-BY-STEP: APPLYING MOISTURISER

Moisturiser is applied after the final application of toning lotion. If the moisturiser is being applied before make-up, use a light formulation or skin primer alternative so that it does not interfere with the adherence of the foundation.

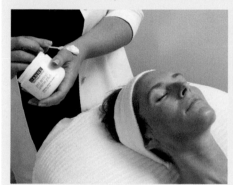 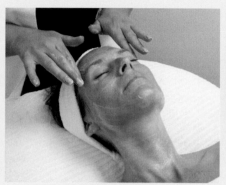 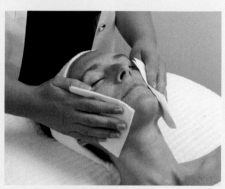

1 Remove some moisturiser from the container, using a disposable spatula or disinfected plastic spatula if required. Place the product on the back of the non-working hand and then take it on the fingertips of your working hand.

2 Apply the moisturiser in small dots to the neck, chin, cheeks, nose and forehead. Quickly and evenly spread it in a fine film over the neck and face, using light upward and outward stroking movements.

3 Blot excess moisturiser from the skin using a facial tissue.

ACTIVITY

Moisturiser content

Collect information on different moisturisers from various skincare suppliers. List the key ingredients and their effects plus the features and benefits of the different products. How do costs vary and why? You could visit local beauty salons, retail stores or beauty wholesale suppliers, or research professional skincare companies online.

Clients will often request detailed information about products and their ingredients. If you are knowledgeable, this will gain client confidence and trust.

HEALTH & SAFETY

Fluid moisturisers

If the moisturiser is very fluid, apply it directly to the fingertips of the non-working hand – it would run if applied to the back of the hand.

ALWAYS REMEMBER

Animal testing

Some clients will question if a product is tested on animals as they may have an ethical objection to this practice. Companies can inform you if they do or do not test their products on animals and often companies who do not test their products on animals will display this information on the packaging. The Leaping Bunny is the only internationally-recognised certification for cosmetics, personal care and household product brands which are not tested on animals. The entire supply-chain monitoring system is audited by Cruelty Free International to check that companies meet their strict criteria.

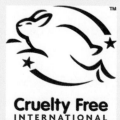

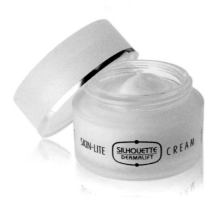

Skin lightening cream to lighten uneven skin tones

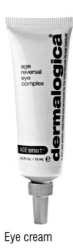

Eye cream

Moisturisers for night-time use

Moisturisers are applied to the skin in the evening, after the skin has been cleansed, toned and blotted dry.

An emulsion **night cream** with a higher proportion of oil is the most effective for application in the evening: by this time the surrounding air is dry and warm, which encourages water loss from the skin; the oil seals the surface of the skin, preventing this water loss.

A small amount of **wax** (such as beeswax) may be included in the formulation: this improves the *slip* of the product, making it easier to apply and helping its skin-conditioning effect.

Specialist skin treatment products

In addition to basic skincare products, **specialist skincare treatment products** are available to target improvement for specific facial areas.

Neck creams The neck can become dry as it is exposed to the weather, often without the protection of a moisturiser. As a client ages, the collagen molecules in the dermis become increasingly cross-linked; they are then unable to retain the same volume of water, and the skin loses its plump appearance.

The formulation for a **neck cream** is similar to that for a night cream; it also contains various skin conditioning supplements, such as collagen or vitamin E, which help maintain moisture in the stratum corneum.

Encourage your client to include the neck in their cleansing routine, applying facial moisturiser to the neck during the day and either a night cream or specially formulated neck cream in the evening. Recommend that they always apply the neck cream gently in an upward and outward direction, using their fingertips.

To improve the appearance of the neck, good posture is important. If the client is round-shouldered the head often drops forwards, putting strain on the muscles of the neck. This causes tension in the muscles, which become tight and painful. Correct the client's posture, and advise them to lightly massage the neck when applying the throat cream to relieve tension and improve circulation to the area.

Eye creams The eye tissue is very thin and readily becomes very dry, emphasising fine lines and wrinkles (**crow's feet**). Special care must be taken when applying products near this area: it contains a large number of **mast cells**, the cells that respond to contact with an irritant by causing an allergic reaction.

Eye cream is a fine cream formulated specifically for application to the eye area. A small quantity of the product is applied to the eye tissue using the ring finger of one hand, gently stroking around the eye, inwards and towards the nose. Support the eye tissue with the other hand. Do not apply the product too near to the inner eyelid or you will cause irritation to the eye. It is important to demonstrate correct quantity and application with your client.

Eye gel Eye gel is usually applied in the morning: it has a cooling, soothing, slightly astringent effect. (This is caused partly by the evaporation of the water in the gel, and partly by the inclusion of plant extracts such as **cornflower** or **camomile**.) As an eye gel serum formulation this can be applied at night and also used as a treatment mask if recommended by the manufacturer.

Eye gel is recommended for all clients, but especially for those suffering with slightly puffy eye tissue. It may also be applied following a facial service, to normalise the pH of the skin.

Eye gel may be applied with a light tapping motion, using the pads of the fingers. This will mildly stimulate the lymphatic circulation in the area and help to reduce any slight swelling.

Serums Serums are chemicals used to revitalise the skin. They are supplied in **ampoules**, sealed glass or plastic phials that prevent the content from evaporating and losing their effectiveness. Serums may be specifically formulated to be used as an alternative to a moisturiser or added to enhance the effects of it. They can be specific to the requirements of your skin and skin type. For example, following ill health, a serum may be applied to revitalise the skin including anti-oxidants and essential oil active ingredients. Serums are usually applied for 7–28 days as a skin tonic course for the treatment of different skin types and conditions.

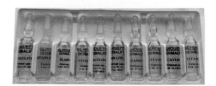

Serums supplied in ampoules

Lip products Products designed to reduce dryness and firm the skin around the lips, reducing the appearance of visible lines. The result aims to smooth, firm and even plump the lip line, reducing the appearance of visible lines caused by lifestyle factors such as smoking and stress. It is advisable to apply the product to the lips in a stimulating, patting motion with the ring finger.

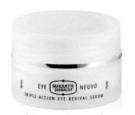

Lip product

Blemished skincare preparations Professional products are available for the client to apply specifically to blemishes such as pustules and papules. Benzoyl peroxide is an example of a product ingredient that dries and promotes healing of skin blemishes. The skincare aims to purify the skin while keeping it hydrated.

After cleansing, the skin may be exfoliated.

Exfoliation The natural physical process of losing dead skin cells from the stratum corneum of the epidermis is called **desquamation**. **Exfoliation** is a salon technique used to accelerate this process, which the client may use at home too. It is normally carried out after the skin has been cleansed and toned, and before further facial treatments. Facial steaming usually follows facial exfoliation.

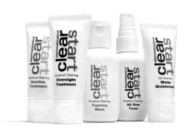

Blemished skincare products

TOP TIP

The need for exfoliation

Exfoliation is recommended for all clients. For example, on younger clients it can ensure the skin is kept clear of excess sebum and dead skin which could lead to blemishes and problematic skin. For the mature client the removal of the surface dead cells has a rejuvenating and brightening effect on the skin's appearance and enables absorption of skincare preparations.

Teenagers regenerate external skin cells every 14 days. This period increases to 30–40 days as a client reaches their forties. This is an important fact to share with your mature clients.

Dry skin may be exfoliated more than oily skin to avoid over-stimulation of the sebaceous gland. However, skin sensitivity and age will affect this and need to be taken in to consideration.

Exfoliation has the following benefits:

◆ Dead skin cells, grease and debris are removed from the surface of the skin.

◆ Fresh new cells are exposed, improving the appearance of the skin.

◆ Skin preparations such as moisturising lotions are more easily absorbed.

◆ The blood circulation in the area is mildly stimulated, bringing more oxygen and nutrients to the skin cells and improving the skin colour.

◆ Hyperpigmentation is improved in appearance by the removal of the pigmented surface skin cells.

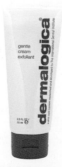

Exfoliation product

TOP TIP

Facial warming

On occasions a skin warming treatment such as steaming may be beneficial before exfoliation to soften the outer skin cells and debris, facilitating removal. This is particularly beneficial when treating a male client.

HEALTH & SAFETY

Body exfoliants

Point out to clients that exfoliants designed for use on the *body* are unsuitable for use on the *face* – their action is not as gentle.

HEALTH & SAFETY

Nut shell exfoliants

Avoid exfoliating products that contain sharp grains of nut shells: these can scrape, split and damage the epidermis. Before purchasing, test the exfoliating product on the back of your own hand to feel its action and assess suitability.

ECO TIP

Micro-beads

There is increasing pressure to stop the use of micro-beads in cosmetics because of their potential to cause environmental damage. They are not filtered from waste water and can enter the food chain, when ingested by fish which we then consume!

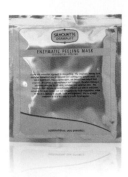

Enzymatic peeling mask

ACTIVITY

Exfoliants

Apply an exfoliant to the back of your own – or a colleague's – hand or arm. Compare the appearance and the feeling of the skin before and after application.

This technique produces a particularly marked effect on black skin, as it reduces the greyish appearance of the skin. (This is due to the skin having a thicker stratum corneum.) This is a great way of visually demonstrating to a client the beneficial effects of using an exfoliant.

TOP TIP

Male skin

A man who shaves, exfoliates every day, as shaving removes the top layer of skin. You can recommend that he also uses a cosmetic exfoliating product on areas such as the nose and forehead where comedones (blackheads) as shown may appear. If a male client suffers from pseudo folliculitis, recommend an electric shave rather than a wet shave, which tends to make this disorder worse.

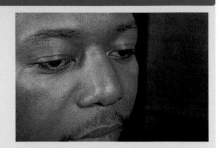

Contra-indications

Exfoliation is beneficial for most skin types; however, avoid application if the client has the following:

◆ highly sensitive skin

◆ a vascular skin disorder such as telangiectases or damaged broken veins in the area of service application

◆ pustular, blemished skin.

Exfoliants Various **exfoliants** are available; they may be of chemical or vegetable origin. Alternatively, mechanical exfoliation may be used using a brush cleanser.

Biochemical skin peel **Natural acids**, alpha-hydroxy acids (AHAs), derived from fruits, sugar cane and milk, or the beta-hydroxy acid (BHA) salicylic acid, may be applied to the skin as a face mask. The natural acids dissolve dead surface cells and stimulate circulation in the underlying skin. These masks are available to suit all skin types.

AHAs may be combined with enzymes derived from fruits such as papaya (papain) and pineapple (bromelain) to help remove surface dead skin to achieve maximum effect. Some of these may require activation using, for example, steam.

When you apply this type of face mask, warn the client that there will be a stinging sensation and then a tightening effect as the mask sets.

Pore grains Pore grains, often referred to as skin scrubs, are the most popular exfoliants: a base of cream or liquid containing tiny, solid spheres of polished plastic called micro-beads or other exfoliant property ingredients such as crushed seeds, fine sea salt, abrasive minerals such as Solum Diatomeae (Diatomaceous Earth), is gently massaged over the skin's surface.

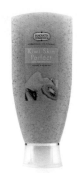

Dual action cleanser and exfoliator

Clay exfoliants Gentler **clay exfoliants** have a clay base, which is applied like a face mask and requires friction applied with the hands to remove it manually. As it dries, the clay absorbs dead skin cells and sebum. The mask is then gently stroked away, using the pads of the fingers. A mask style exfoliant is more suitable for a blemished skin accompanying an oily skin type.

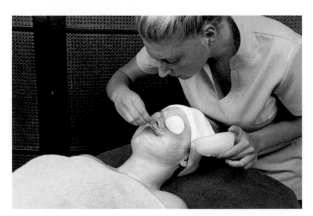

Clay exfoliant application

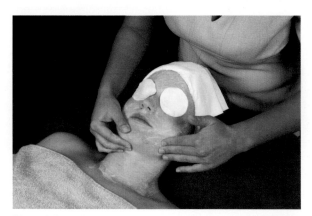

Clay exfoliant removal

Mechanical exfoliation **Mechanical exfoliation**, or 'facial brushing', softens and cleanses the skin. Dead skin cells and excess sebum are removed as the soft hair bristles rotate over the skin's surface. The rotary action also increases the cleansing action of exfoliation.

If the skin is warmed before mechanical exfoliation, this will soften the dead skin cells, and **skin peeling cream** may be applied: together these will maximise the result of exfoliation.

Be careful to avoid over-stimulation and over-exfoliation, resulting in sensitising the skin's surface, or disturbing the skin's natural protective qualities. Permanent sensitisation could result from incorrect exfoliation techniques or over-exfoliation.

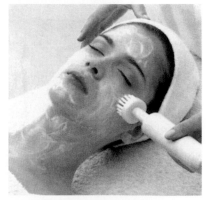

Mechanical exfoliation

EXFOLIATION TREATMENT EXAMPLES

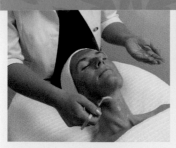 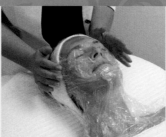 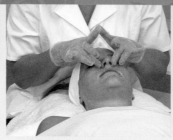 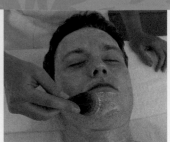

1 Biochemical skin exfoliation - the facial exfoliant is applied to the skin following cleansing and skin warming to heat and soften the skin. The exfoliant containing AHAs removes dead skin cells and stimulates skin renewal. Warn the client a mild stinging sensation may be experienced, but will disappear quickly upon removal.

2 Plastic film is placed over the exfoliant to speed up the action of the exfoliant lotion. Carefully ensure the film does not cover the client's nose and mouth.

3 A facial pore grain scrub is applied to the skin's surface and light circular petrissage movements are applied concentrating on the chin, nose and forehead. Care must be taken over areas of sensitivity, broken capillaries and around the eye area.

4 A soft facial brush may be used in a rotary action to further enhance the effectiveness of some exfoliants, removing areas of dead skin and sebum. This is particularly beneficial when working on a male client to loosen dead skin and debris surrounding coarse terminal facial hair. A client may also purchase the brush to use as part of their home care programme.

Client advice and recommendations

The client can be advised to use exfoliants at home as a specialised cleansing service after normal cleansing and toning. Exfoliants should be applied once a week for all skin types, except oily, for which it may be applied twice a week. Always be guided by manufacturers' instructions.

The application and removal technique will differ according to the exfoliant product type. If a facial scrub, advise the client to massage the recommended product amount gently over the skin using their fingertips. Application should always be in an upwards and outwards direction.

After application, any product residue should be thoroughly rinsed from the face using clean, tepid water. The client may then apply a face mask or tone the skin and apply a nourishing skin moisturiser if performed at night.

A UV sunblock should be used to protect the skin to avoid skin damage following application.

Warming the skin

A **steam treatment** is the ideal means of producing the required warming effect on the skin to achieve both cleansing and skin stimulation. Skin warming is often incorporated into a facial treatment after the manual cleansing, so making it more receptive to subsequent treatments.

The effects of steam treatment are:

◆ The pores are opened.

◆ Locally, the blood circulation and the lymphatic circulation are stimulated.

◆ The surface cells of the epidermis are softened, which helps desquamation.

◆ Sebaceous gland activity is improved, which benefits a dry mature skin.

ACTIVITY

Retail skincare devices

There is an increasing retail opportunity for clients to use equipment at home alongside their skincare products to maintain the health of the skin between salon visits. Research the availability of such devices.

REVISION AID

What does the term 'desquamation' mean?

ALWAYS REMEMBER

Steam equipment is sometimes referred to as a vaporiser.

◆ The facial muscles are relaxed, due to the raise in temperature locally.

◆ Skin colour is improved.

Steam is provided by heating distilled water electrically until it boils to create steam.

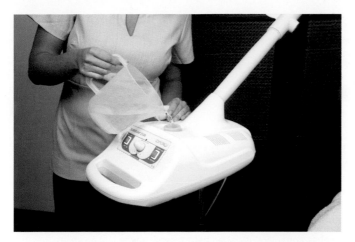

Filling the water reservoir in the steam unit with distilled water

The resulting steam is applied as a fine mist over the facial and neck area. As the steam settles upon the skin it is absorbed by the surface epidermal cells. These cells are softened and can be gently loosened with an exfoliation service.

Some equipment has a feature where essential oils may be added to a basket chamber within the unit. Oils are selected according to the client's physiological/psychological needs.

ACTIVITY

Steam units

Collect literature on different steam units. Compare their efficiencies and features. Which would be the best buy? Consider:

◆ Is the equipment transportable, suitable for promotional activities?

◆ Is it height-adjustable, and is the arm and nozzle of the steamer rotation capacity sufficient to suit the differing needs of clients positioned on the treatment couch?

◆ Is it easy to clean?

◆ If floor-standing; does it move easily?

◆ Does it allow the addition of aromatic oils?

◆ Does it have safety features to prevent overheating or the water reservoir running dry?

Contra-indications
Although the service is suitable for most clients, do not use steam if your client has any of the following:

◆ *Respiratory problems*, such as asthma or a cold.

◆ *Vascular skin disorders* – these would be aggravated by the heating action and increased blood circulation.

◆ *Claustrophobia* – fear of enclosure or confined space.

◆ *Skin with reduced sensitivity*.

◆ *Diabetes*, unless the client's GP has given permission.

◆ *Rosacea* – a vascular skin disorder, where excess sebum production combined with a chronic inflammatory condition is caused by dilation of the blood

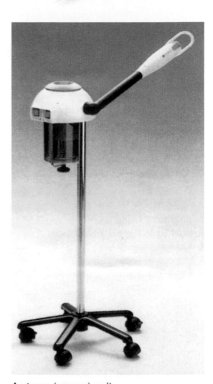

capillaries. The skin becomes coarse, the pores enlarge, and the cheek and nose become inflamed.

◆ *Dilated capillaries*, where there are excessive capillaries near the surface of the skin that are permanently dilated.

Explain to the client:

◆ how long the treatment is to be applied for

◆ that you will not leave them during the steam application

◆ the sensations that will be experienced

◆ the physical effect on the skin.

The duration of the application and the distance differ according to the skin type and related conditions.

The client should be positioned in a semi-reclined position for facial application.

Before applying steam, protect the client's eyes with damp cotton wool. Areas of delicate skin should be protected with damp cotton wool and if necessary a suitable barrier cream.

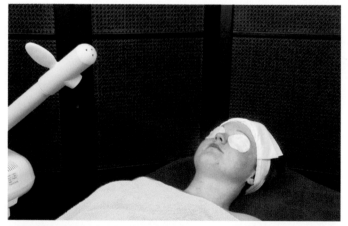

A client positioned for steam treatment

The distance between the steam outlet and the client's skin to be treated should be approximately 30–35 cm. The application time will depend on the treatment effect and the type of skin that is being treated. Generally allow:

◆ 10 minutes for the face.

Ensure that an even flow of steam covers all the area being treated; this will require movement of the steamer arm and nozzle which can usually rotate 180 degrees. Reposition as necessary.

HEALTH & SAFETY

Steam application

Oily skin will tolerate a shorter application distance and a longer application time. For sensitive skin, increase the application distance and reduce the time. If the skin is very sensitive, steam treatment may be omitted due to its stimulation of the blood capillaries. What are the manufacturer's application guidelines for your steam equipment? Remember that these are only *guidelines* – observe the skin's reaction and check that the client is comfortable.

If you are using ozone, this is applied following the steam application for the final few minutes, as directed by the manufacturer. The steam will change in appearance to a bluish-white cloud.

After applying steam, blot the skin dry with a soft facial tissue and proceed to remove any blockages.

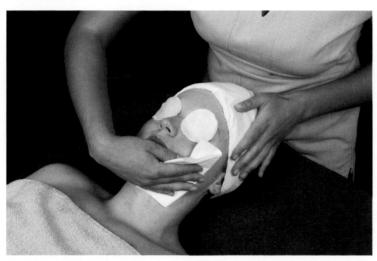

Blotting the skin after steaming

At the end of the treatment, turn off the machine and unplug it, thereby saving energy. Check that you have tidied away the trailing lead so that there is no risk of it causing an accident.

HEALTH & SAFETY

Ozone

Most steam units produce ozone when the oxygen in the steam is passed over a high-intensity quartz mercury arc tube. Ozone is thought to be beneficial in the treatment of blemished skin, as it kills many bacteria, but it may also be carcinogenic (liable to cause cancer) if inhaled. Use the steam unit only in a well-ventilated room, and only for short periods of time.

HEALTH & SAFETY

Safe use and care of the steam unit

◆ Always follow manufacturer's instructions on correct usage. Have the unit tested annually by a qualified electrician to ensure its safety in compliance with the Electricity at Work Regulations (1989).

◆ Always use distilled water to avoid limescale mineral build-up in the heating element, which can lead to damage.

◆ Never fill the water reservoir past the recommended level or 'spitting' could occur, where hot droplets of water are ejected and could burn the client's skin.

◆ Never use the equipment if the water reservoir is below the recommended level or the heating element could be damaged. Most units have a cutout feature so that the equipment switches off if this occurs.

◆ Never leave the lead trailing across an area where somebody could trip and fall.

◆ Never leave the client unattended whilst receiving the treatment. Use the time to talk about their skincare requirements, or update their treatment record.

Contra-actions Contra-actions to steaming include the following:

◆ *over-stimulation of the skin*, caused by incorrect application distance and duration of the steam

◆ *scalding*, caused by spitting from a faulty steam jet or by the vessel being overfilled

◆ *discomfort*, caused by the steam being too near the skin, leading to breathing difficulties, or by the treatment being applied for too long.

Towel steaming Towel steaming or hot towels is an alternative to steaming that can be used to achieve the same beneficial effects if an electrical steam unit is not available. Several clean small towels are required: these are heated in a bowl of clean hot water, or specialised unit, and are then applied to the face. The towels must not be too hot to handle or you could burn the client's skin. Always check the towel temperature before application.

Application Seat the client in a semi-reclined position. Neatly fold a small clean towel and immerse it in very warm water. Wring it out quickly and, standing behind the client, transfer it to the face. With the towel folded in half, place it over the lower half of the face, directly under the client's lower lip; then unfold it to cover the upper face, leaving the mouth and nostrils uncovered.

Press the towel gently against the face for 2 minutes; during this time the towel will begin to cool. Remove the towel and replace it with another heated towel. Continue in this way, heating and replacing the towels, for approximately 10 minutes.

After towel steaming, blot the skin dry with a soft facial tissue and proceed to remove any blockages.

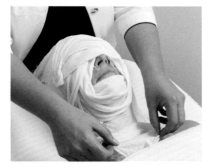

Towel steaming

Removing skin blockages – extraction

After the skin has been cleansed, you may wish to remove minor skin blemishes such as comedones (blackheads). Milia (whiteheads) removal is advanced and may be studied as part of Level 3 beauty therapy qualifications. It is preferable to warm the tissues first as discussed previously: this softens the skin and relaxes the openings of the skin that are blocked.

Comedones are areas of sebum and dead skin cells located in the hair follicle, which turn black when exposed to oxygen in the atmosphere.

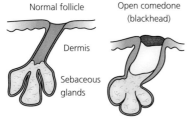

Comedone (blackhead) formation

Products, tools and equipment

You will need all of the basic equipment listed earlier in this chapter, and the following specialist tools and equipment:

Tools and equipment

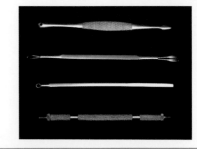

◆ **Single use disposable non-latex (synthetic) powder-free gloves**
◆ **Medical swabs** impregnated with isopropyl alcohol or skin disinfectant lotion.
◆ **Stainless steel comedone extractor** (selection shown in image)

Safety and hygiene

The skin must be cleansed and disinfected with a suitable skin disinfectant/alcohol preparation before skin blockage removal to minimise secondary infection.

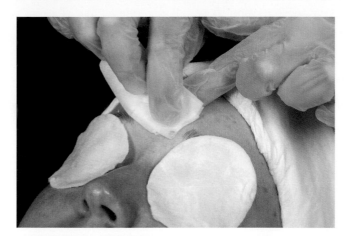

Cleaning the skin before removal of skin blockage/ extraction

All contaminated waste material from this service (such as facial tissues and gloves) should be disposed of in an identified waste container, as directed by your local health authority.

After use, the stainless steel comedone extractor should be cleaned with a disinfectant/ alcohol preparation, whilst wearing disposable gloves before sterilising in an autoclave.

Single use disposable non-latex (synthetic) powder-free gloves must always be worn while carrying out the treatment.

Treatment application

Comedone removal For **comedone removal** using the loop end of the extractor tool, apply gentle pressure around the comedone.

HEALTH & SAFETY

Client comfort

◆ Never obstruct the client's nostrils when removing a comedone from the nose area.
◆ Never apply pressure on the soft cartilage of the nose.

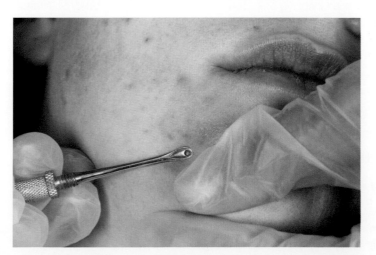

Comedone extraction

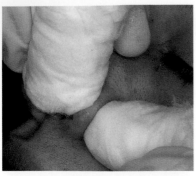

Manual extraction of comedone (blackhead)

The comedone should leave the skin with ease, apparent as a plug, wipe away extraction with damp cotton wool. You may need to use manual extraction too and apply gentle pressure with your fingers at the sides of the comedone to ensure that it is effectively removed; when doing this, wrap a tissue or damp cotton wool around the pads of the index fingers, sometimes using a gentle rocking motion. It is important that all excess sebaceous matter from the comedone is removed to prevent infection.

Contra-actions:

◆ Incomplete extraction could lead to cellular decomposition and secondary infection.

◆ Skin bruising could occur if too much pressure is applied.

◆ Capillary damage could result if too much force is used when squeezing the comedone. The surrounding blood capillaries can rupture, causing permanent skin damage.

◆ If extraction results in tissue damage and blood loss, a medical swab should be applied to the area.

HEALTH & SAFETY

Skin blockages

Never attempt to remove larger skin blockages such as sebaceous cysts – these should be treated by a GP.

HEALTH & SAFETY

Skin blockage removal

If the client suffers from severe congestion, do not attempt to carry out all the removals in one session. This would sensitise the skin, making it appear very red, and would be most uncomfortable for the client. Instead they should visit the salon weekly for you to clear the skin gradually as part of an overall treatment programme including home care recommendations to be followed.

HEALTH & SAFETY

Avoiding contamination

Clay mask-sourced ingredients must always be made from sterilised materials, because of the danger from tetanus spores.

ALWAYS REMEMBER

Face packs

The term *face pack* is sometimes used instead of face mask: a face pack does not set, but remains soft; a face mask sets and becomes firm.

Mask treatment

The **face mask** is usually a skin-cleansing preparation which may contain a variety of different ingredients selected for their deep cleansing, toning, nourishing or refreshing effect on the skin. The mask achieves this through the following actions. If it contains:

◆ *absorbent* materials, dead skin cells, sebum and debris will adhere to it when it is removed

◆ *astringent* ingredients, the pores and the skin will tighten

◆ *emollient* ingredients, the skin will be softened and nourished

◆ *soothing* ingredients, the skin can be desensitised to reduce skin irritation

◆ *skin-lightening* ingredients; these will help to reduce the appearance of areas of pigmentation e.g. hyperpigmentation.

There are basically two types of mask: setting and non-setting. You will need to know when and how to apply each.

Setting masks

Setting masks are applied in a thin layer over the skin and then allowed to dry. The mask need not necessarily set solid – a solid mask can become uncomfortable, and be difficult to remove, especially if the client has a sensitive skin condition.

Setting masks come in these varieties:

◆ clay masks

◆ peel-off masks including – gel, polyvinyl acetate (PVA) and paraffin wax

◆ thermal masks.

Clay masks

The **clay mask** absorbs sebum and debris from the skin surface, leaving it cleansed. It can also stimulate or soothe the skin, according to the ingredients chosen. Various clay powders are available – select from these according to the physiological effects that you require:

◆ **Calamine** A light pink powder that soothes surface blood capillaries. For sensitive or delicate skin.

◆ **Magnesium carbonate** A very light, white powder that creates a temporary astringent and toning effect. For open pores on dry and normal skins.

◆ **Kaolin** A cream-coloured powder that has a very stimulating effect on the skin's surface capillaries, thereby helping the skin to remove impurities and waste products. For congested, oily skin.

◆ **Fuller's earth** A green, heavy clay powder. It has a very stimulating effect, such that the skin will show slight reddening. It also produces a whitening, brightening effect. For oily skin with a sluggish circulation. Due to its strong effect, it is not suitable for a client with sensitive skin.

◆ **Flowers of sulphur** A light, yellow clay powder, which has a drying action on pustules and papules. Applied only to specific blemishes (pustules).

To activate these masks it is necessary to add a liquid – an **active lotion** – that turns the powder to a liquid paste. Active lotions are selected according to the skin type of the client and the mask to be used; they reinforce the action of the mask. Examples are:

◆ **Rose water and orange flower water** These are very popular; they have a very mild stimulating and toning effect.

◆ **Witch hazel** This has a soothing effect on blemished skin; it is also an astringent natural antiseptic and is suitable for use on oily skin.

◆ **Distilled water** This is used on highly sensitive skins.

◆ **Almond oil** This is mildly stimulating. Because it is an oil, it does not allow the mask to dry: it is therefore recommended for highly sensitive skin or dehydrated skin.

◆ **Glycerol** A humectant, which is hydrating, prevents the mask drying and is suitable for dry mature skin.

When treating a black skin, clay masks tend to leave a white residue on removal. Choose a mask that does not have this effect.

The mask should be kept in place for about 10–15 minutes.

ALWAYS REMEMBER

Setting masks

When using a setting mask, ensure that the mask is evenly applied or it will dry unevenly.

REVISION AID

When is extraction included in a facial treatment?

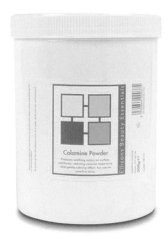
Calamine powder

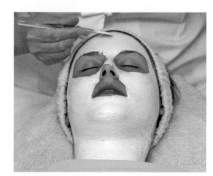
Clay mask

ACTIVITY

Choosing face masks

Which clay powder and which active lotion would you mix for clients with the following skin types and conditions:

1   A mature, sensitive skin type.
2   A young, normal skin type.
3   A combination skin type: cheeks, neck area dry; forehead, nose and chin area oily.

Peel-off masks   **Peel-off masks** may be made from gel, PVA or paraffin wax. Because perspiration cannot escape from the skin's surface, moisture is forced into the stratum corneum. The mask also insulates the skin, causing an increase in temperature.

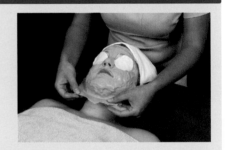

The **gel mask** is either a suspension of biological ingredients, such as starches, gums or gelatine, or a mixture of synthetic non-biological resin ingredients. The mask is applied over the skin; on contact with the skin it begins to dry. When dry it is peeled off the face in one piece. Depending on the biological ingredients added, the gel mask can be used to treat all skin types. (If the client has excessive facial hair, such as at the sides of the face, this mask may cause discomfort on removal. To avoid this, place a lubricant under the mask, or use a different sort of mask.)

Synthetic resin emulsions such as **PVA** resin are used to tighten the skin temporarily, and are suitable for mature skin; they can also be used with dry skin. Algae may be used as an ingredient, which causes rapid setting.

The **paraffin-wax mask** is stimulating in its action. The paraffin wax is blended with petroleum jelly or acetyl alcohol, which improve its spreading properties. The wax is heated to approximately 37°C and is then applied to the skin as a liquid. It sets on contact, so speed is essential if the mask is to be effective. The wax mask is loosened at the sides and removed in one piece after 15–20 minutes. The paraffin-wax mask is suitable for dry skin. Because of its stimulating action, it is unsuitable for oily skin or highly sensitive skin.

Thermal masks The **thermal mask** contains various minerals. The ingredients are mixed and applied to the face and neck, avoiding the mouth and eye tissue. The mask warms on contact with the skin: this causes the pores to enlarge, thereby cleansing the skin. As the mask cools it sets, and the pores constrict slightly. The mask is removed from the face in one piece. Thermal masks have a stimulating, cleansing action, suitable for a normal skin or for a congested, oily skin with open pores.

Non-setting masks

Some **non-setting masks** stay soft on application; others become firm, but they do not tighten like a setting mask. For this reason they do not tone the skin as effectively as setting masks. Non-setting masks include:

- warm oil
- natural masks – fruit, plant and herbal
- cream.

Warm-oil masks A plant oil, typically **olive oil** or **almond oil**, is warmed and then applied to the skin. It softens the skin and helps to restore the skin's natural moisture balance. Warm-oil masks are recommended for mature skin and dry or dehydrated skin. Ideally it can be used with a gauze mask.

Gauze masks A **gauze mask** is cut to cover the face and neck, with holes for the eyes, nostrils and lips. This is then soaked in warm oil. A dampened cotton wool eye pad is placed over each eye. The gauze is then placed over the face and neck. It is usually left in place for 10–20 minutes.

Impregnated sheet masks These are sheets, usually cotton, gauze or silk, placed over the skin, which have been impregnated or saturated in active ingredients to achieve specific treatment results, i.e. collagen to hydrate and rejuvenate the skin.

Natural masks Natural masks are made from natural ingredients rich in vitamins and minerals. Fresh **fruit** and **vegetables** have a mildly astringent and stimulating effect. Usually the fruit is crushed to a pulp and placed between layers of gauze, which are laid over the face.

Honey is used for its toning, tightening, antiseptic and hydrating effect. **Egg white** has a tightening effect and is said to clear impurities from the skin. **Avocados** have a nourishing effect; **bananas** soften the skin, and are used for sensitive skins.

HEALTH & SAFETY

Allergies

When using biological masks, always check first whether the client has any food allergies.

When using a commercial mask, try to find out *exactly* what it contains, so that you don't apply a sensitising ingredient to an allergic skin type.

Cream masks Cream masks are pre-prepared for you. They have a softening and moisturising effect on the skin. Each mask contains various biological extracts or chemical substances to treat different skin types or conditions. Instructions will be provided with the mask, stating how the product is to be used professionally.

These masks are popular in the beauty salon: they often complement a particular facial treatment range used by the salon, and they are available for retail sale to clients.

HEALTH & SAFETY

Contra-indications

Do not use thermal masks on a client with a circulatory disorder or one who has lost tactile sensation.

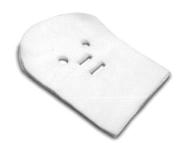

Pre-cut gauze mask

TOP TIP

Sheet masks

Sheet fabric masks made from materials such as cotton and silk are similar in appearance to moist facial tissues. They are often coated in foil to maximise their effectiveness. They are a great way of retailing masks and are available in all shapes and sizes.

Mini masks or micro masks are available to apply to targeted areas such as the skin under the eyes.

HEALTH & SAFETY

Client comfort

If a client is particularly nervous, choose an effective non-setting mask. Some clients feel claustrophobic when wearing a setting mask.

TOP TIP

Gauze masks

Ensure that you position the gauze correctly so that the nose and eye holes are properly placed.

HEALTH & SAFETY

Natural masks

Because natural masks are prepared from natural foods, they must be prepared *immediately* before use – they very quickly deteriorate.

HEALTH & SAFETY

Acidic fruit

Lemon and grapefruit are generally considered too acidic for use on the face.

ACTIVITY

Creating natural masks

Create some masks, listing the ingredients to suit each of the following skin types:

◆ dry

◆ oily

◆ mature, with superficial wrinkling

◆ sensitive.

If possible, arrange to carry out one of the masks on a suitable client in the workplace. Evaluate the natural face mask. Consider: cost, preparation, application, removal and effectiveness. Remember to ask your client for *their opinion*!

Contra-indications

The **contra-indications** to general skincare apply also to face mask application. In addition, observe the following:

◆ **Allergies** *Check* whether your client knows if they have allergies. If so, avoid all contact with known allergens.

◆ **Claustrophobia** Do not use a setting mask on a particularly nervous client. Some clients feel claustrophobic under its tightening effect.

◆ **Sensitive skins** Do not use stimulating masks on clients with highly sensitive skin.

ALWAYS REMEMBER

Cotton wool

Ensure that you have plenty of dampened cotton wool – it is used to apply toner to the skin before mask application, to remove the mask or mask residue left on the skin, and to apply toner to the skin after mask removal.

Ideally, buy cotton wool discs to use for the eye pads during a face mask. They will ensure an evenly shaped protective shield for the eye area. Alternatively apply a specialist eye treatment mask.

Products, tools and equipment

When applying masks you will need all of the basic equipment listed earlier in this chapter, and the following specialist products, tools and equipment.

Products, tools and equipment

◆ **Cotton wool (2)** Pre-shaped, round and dampened **or specialist eye treatment pads**

◆ **Scissors** To cut cotton wool eye pads (if cotton wool discs are not used) or other associated mask resources

◆ **Face-mask ingredients**

◆ **Gauze** Used in applying certain masks

◆ **Flat mask brushes (3)** Disinfected brushes to apply the mask. Disposable may also be used

◆ **Facial toning lotions (a selection)** To suit various types of skin

◆ **Sterilised mask-removal sponges (2) or facial mitts/ towels** For use when removing the mask using clean warm water

◆ **Lukewarm water** If required for mask removal

◆ **Moisturisers (a range)** To suit different skin types for use after mask removal

Safety and hygiene After applying the mask, clean the mask brush thoroughly in warm water and detergent. Next, place it in a chemical disinfecting agent, rinse it in clean water, allow it to dry, and then store it in the UV cabinet.

When you use a paraffin-wax mask, remove as much mask residue as possible from the brush, then place the brush in boiling water to remove excess wax. Disinfect the brush as usual before use.

If you use sponges to remove the mask, place them in warm water and detergent. After rinsing them, place them ready for disinfection in an autoclave. (With repeated disinfection, sponges will begin to break up so will need to be replaced.) Thermal mitts and towels should be washed at a temperature of 60°C. A large, high-quality, disposable cotton wool disc may be purchased, and disposable towels may also be used in mask removal.

Clean and wipe non-single use non-biodegradable plastic spatulas with disinfectant and then place in the UV cabinet.

Preparing the work area Check that you have all the products, tools and equipment you need to carry out the treatment. You may like to place a paper roll at the head of the treatment couch, underneath the client's head, to collect any mask residue on mask removal.

The head of the treatment couch should be flat or slightly elevated. Don't have it in a semi-reclined position during mask application; often masks are liquid in consistency and may run into the client's eyes or behind their neck.

Mask treatment

Preparing the client For maximum effect the mask must be applied on a clean skin. If the mask application follows a **facial massage**, ensure that the **massage medium** has been thoroughly removed.

Select the appropriate mask ingredients to treat the skin type and the facial conditions that require attention.

HEALTH & SAFETY

Maintaining hygiene

You need several mask brushes and mask sponges to allow effective disinfection of the tools, and so that you can provide freshly disinfected tools for each client.

ALWAYS REMEMBER

Brushes

When purchasing mask brushes, note that a plastic-handled brush is preferable to one with a painted wooden handle – the painted one would be likely to peel on immersion in water and disinfectant, which spoils the professional image!

Disposable mask brushes are ideal and may be recommended as a retail item for a client's personal home use.

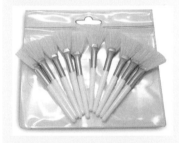

REVISION AID

Which mask is most suitable for cleansing and absorbing dead skin cells and surface debris?

ALWAYS REMEMBER

Preparation

◆ Place a clean facial tissue under the edge of the headband if worn at the forehead, so that it overlaps the headband. This will protect the headband from staining.

◆ Don't mix a clay mask with the mask brush – if you do, the solid contents will tend to collect in the bristles, the mask won't be mixed effectively, and the brush won't spread the mask evenly.

How to apply and remove the mask The mask is usually applied as the *final* facial treatment, because of its cleansing, refining and soothing effects upon the skin. The methods of preparation, application and removal are different for the various face mask types, so the guidelines below are a general outline of effective treatment technique.

1 Having determined the client's treatment requirements, select the appropriate mask ingredients. If you use a commercial mask, always read the manufacturer's instructions first and follow their guidance.

2   Discuss the treatment procedure with the client. Explain:

◆ what the mask will feel like on application

◆ what sensation, if any, they will experience

◆ how long the mask will be left on the skin.

Generally the mask will be left in place for 10–20 minutes, but the exact time depends on the client's skin type, the type of mask and effect required.

3   Prepare the mask ingredients for application. Commercial non-setting cream mask shown.

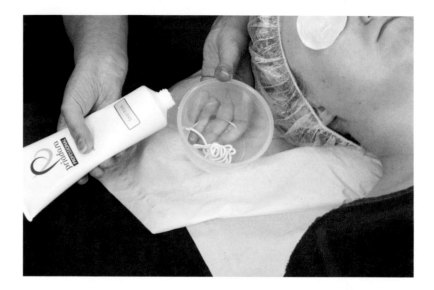

4   Using a disposable or disinfected mask brush or spatula, begin to apply the mask. The usual sequence of mask application is neck, chin, cheeks, nose and forehead.

If you are using more than one mask to treat different **skin conditions**, apply first the one that will need to be on longest. This is a popular trend and is known as multi-masking, where different products are layered on the skin.

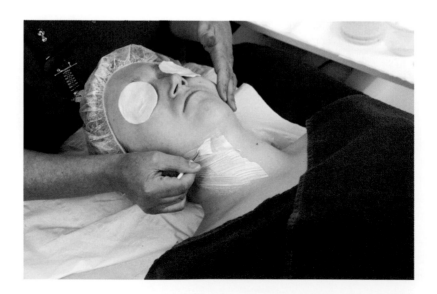

Apply the mask quickly and evenly so that it has maximum effect on the whole face. Don't apply it too thickly; as well as making mask removal difficult, this is wasteful as only the part that is in contact with the skin has any effect.

Keep the mask clear of the nostrils, the lips, the eyebrows and the hairline.

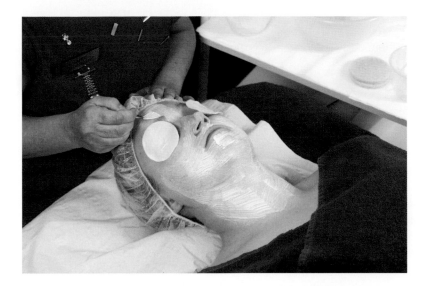

ALWAYS REMEMBER

Efficient working

While the mask is on the face you can tidy the working area and collect together the materials required for mask removal. Do not disturb the client, who will be relaxing at this time. A hand massage may also be offered.

5 To relax the client, apply cotton wool eye pads dampened with clean water.

6 Leave the mask for the recommended time or according to the effect required. Take account also of the sensitivity of the skin and your client's comfort.

7 Wash your hands.

8 When the mask is ready for removal, remove the eye pads.

Explain to the client that you are going to remove the mask. Briefly describe the process, according to whether this is a setting or a non-setting mask.

Remove the mask using an appropriate technique, i.e. mask sponges or warm towel method. Mask sponges, if used, should be damp, not wet, so that water doesn't run into the client's eyes, nose or mouth.

HEALTH & SAFETY

Client comfort

It is important to check that your client is comfortable while the mask is on their face. They will suffer discomfort if their skin is intolerant to a particular mask or ingredient.

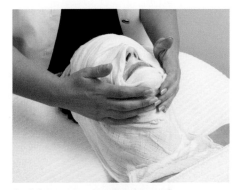

Applying a warm towel to the mask

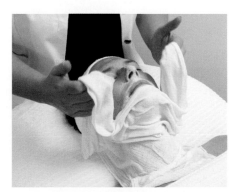

Removing the mask with a warm towel

9 When the mask has been completely removed, apply the appropriate toning lotion using dampened cotton wool. Blot the skin dry with a facial tissue.

10 If this is the final treatment, apply an appropriate moisturiser and other specialised products to the skin, explaining their purpose.

ECO TIP

Mask removal

When using water to remove a mask you may need to renew the water as you work to ensure effective removal.

Do not leave the water running unnecessarily during this time.

11 Remove the headband, and tidy the client's hair.

12 With a mirror, show the client their skin. Evaluate the treatment.

13 Record the results on their treatment plan record.

Contra-actions Before you apply the mask, explain to the client what the action of the mask will feel like on the skin. This will enable them to identify any undesirable skin reaction, evident to them as skin irritation – a burning sensation.

Ask the client initially whether they are comfortable: this will give them the opportunity to tell you if they are experiencing any discomfort. Should there be a contra-action to the mask, remove the mask immediately and apply a soothing skincare product.

If on removal of the mask you can see that there has been an unwanted skin reaction (that is, if you see inflammation), apply a soothing skincare product. In either case, note the skin reaction on the treatment record for future guidance and choose a different mask next time.

Client advice and recommendations The client may be given a sample of the face mask for use at home. Explain to them the procedure for application and removal, so that they achieve maximum benefit from the mask. Encourage them to purchase a suitable mask for their skin type and condition and apply a mask once or twice a week, depending on manufacturer's instructions and their skin type and condition, to dislodge dead skin cells and to cleanse, nourish and stimulate the skin. Following a mask application, inform the client of what a contra-action may look like and if it occurs what action to take.

Advise the client not to apply the mask directly before a special occasion, in case it causes blemishes, as sometimes happens. The skin should be toned and moisturised after removing the mask.

The suitability of the mask must be reviewed periodically dependent upon the client's skin needs and environmental and lifestyle factors.

Facial massage

Manual massage is the external manipulation, using the hands, of the soft tissues of the face, neck and upper chest. Massage can improve the appearance of the skin and promote a sensation of stimulation or relaxation.

Each massage performed is adapted to the client's physiological and psychological needs. The skin's physiological needs are observed during the skin analysis; the client's psychological needs are usually discovered during the consultation.

The benefits of the facial massage include the following:

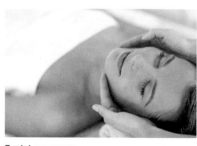

Facial massage

◆ Dead epidermal cells are loosened and shed. This improves the appearance of the skin, exposing fresh, younger cells.

◆ The muscles receive an improved supply of oxygenated blood, essential for cell growth. The tone and strength of the muscles are improved, firming the facial contours.

◆ The increased blood circulation in the area warms the tissues. This induces a feeling of relaxation, which is particularly beneficial when treating tense muscles.

◆ As the blood capillaries dilate and bring blood to the skin's surface, the skin colour improves.

◆ The lymphatic circulation and the venous blood circulation increase. These changes speed up the removal of waste products and toxins, and tend therefore to purify the skin. The removal of excess lymph improves the appearance of a puffy skin (provided that this does not require medical treatment).

◆ The increased temperature of the skin relaxes the pores and follicles. This aids the absorption of the massage product, which in turn softens the skin.

◆ Sensory nerves can be soothed or stimulated, depending on the massage manipulations selected.

◆ Massage stimulates the sebaceous and sudoriferous glands and increases the production of sebum and sweat. This increase helps to maintain the skin's natural oil and moisture balance.

Treatment information to provide at the initial point of interest

Facial massage is carried out as required, usually once every 4 to 6 weeks. Before the facial massage is given, the skin is cleansed; afterwards it is usual to apply a face mask, which may absorb any excess massage medium from the skin or can enhance further the skin nourishing effect of the treatment.

When booking a client for this treatment, allow 1 hour. The facial massage itself should take approximately 20 minutes, but this may vary according to the client's skin type and condition.

Warn the client that the skin may appear slightly red and blotchy after the treatment, due to the increase in blood circulation to the area: this reaction will normally subside after 4 to 6 hours. If it doesn't, the client should be advised to contact the salon for further guidance.

Because of the stimulating effect on the skin, recommend to the client that they receive this treatment when they do not have to apply any cosmetic products directly afterwards.

Sometimes the skin develops small blemishes after facial massage; this is due to its cleansing action. Therefore, if the client is preparing for a special occasion, such as a wedding, make the appointment for at least 5 days in advance.

Massage manipulations

The facial massage is based on a series of classic massage movements, each with different effects. There are five basic groups of massage movements:

◆ effleurage

◆ petrissage

◆ percussion (also known as tapotement)

◆ frictions

◆ vibrations.

You can adapt the way each of these movements is applied, according to the needs of the client. Either the *speed of application* or the *depth of pressure* can be altered.

ALWAYS REMEMBER

Client care

The headband can spoil the hair, and the massage medium may enter the hairline. Recommend that the client does not style their hair directly before the facial treatment. Often male clients may prefer not to wear a head band.

TOP TIP

Practice your massage techniques

When learning facial massage you need to practice. Practice the movements to perfect the manipulations. Practice each manipulation – this will increase the agility and strength of your fingers and wrists.

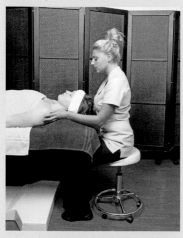

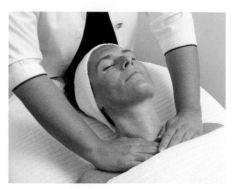

Speed of massage application can be altered

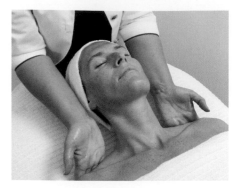

Depth of massage pressure may be altered as well

Effleurage Effleurage is a stroking movement, used to begin the massage, as a link manipulation, and to complete the massage sequence. This manipulation is light, has an even pressure, and is applied in a rhythmical, continuous manner to induce relaxation.

The pressure of application varies according to the underlying structures and the tissue type, but it must *never* be unduly heavy.

Effleurage has these effects:

◆ Desquamation is increased.

◆ Arterial blood circulation is increased, bringing fresh nutrients to the area.

◆ Venous circulation is improved, aiding the removal of congestion from the veins.

◆ Lymphatic circulation is increased, improving the absorption of waste products.

◆ The underlying muscle fibres are relaxed.

Uses in treatment: to relax tight, contracted muscles.

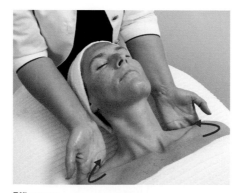

Effleurage

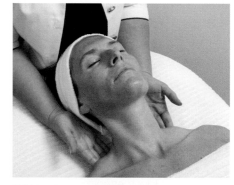

Petrissage

Petrissage Petrissage involves a series of movements in which the tissues are lifted away from the underlying structures and compressed. Pressure is intermittent, and should be light yet firm.

Petrissage has these effects:

◆ improvement of muscle tone, through the compression and relaxation of muscle fibres

◆ improvement in blood and lymph circulation, as the application of pressure causes the vessels to empty and fill

◆ increased activity of the sebaceous gland, due to the stimulation.

Movements include picking up, kneading, knuckling, pinching, rolling, frictions and scissoring.

Uses in treatment: to stimulate a sluggish circulation; to increase sebaceous gland and sudoriferous gland activity when treating a dry skin condition.

Percussion

Percussion, also known as **tapotement**, is performed in a brisk, stimulating manner. Rhythm is important as the fingers are continually breaking contact with the skin; irritation could occur if the movement were performed incorrectly.

Percussion has these effects:

◆ a fast vascular reaction because of the skin's nervous response to the stimulus – this reaction, **erythema**, has a stimulating effect

◆ increased blood supply, which nourishes the tissues

◆ improvement in muscle and skin tone in the area.

Movements include clapping and tapping. In facial massage, only light tapping should be used.

Uses in treatment: to tone areas of loose, crepey skin around the jaw or eyes. Particularly beneficial for a mature skin type.

TOP TIP

Stimulation

When a stimulating massage is required, incorporate more petrissage and tapotement into the massage sequence.

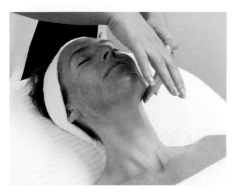

Percussion (tapotement)

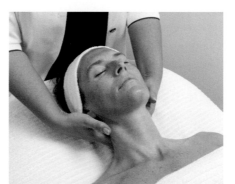

Vibrations

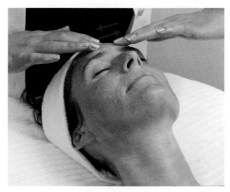

Frictions

Frictions

Frictions cause the skin and superficial structures to move together over the underlying structures. These movements are performed with either the fingers or the thumbs and concentrated in particular areas, applied with regulated pressure. Used in treatment to relieve stress and relax tension in the forehead muscle. The movements include scissor movement to the forehead.

Frictions has these effects:

◆ increased desquamation (surface skin removal)

◆ gentle stimulation and improved function of the superficial tissues

◆ improvement in scar tissue by breaking down the tissue adhesions

◆ improved blood and lymph circulation

◆ breaking down tight nodules (tension in muscle fibres).

Vibrations

Vibrations are applied on the nerve centre. They are produced by a rapid contraction and relaxation of the muscles of the therapist's arm, resulting in a fine trembling movement.

Vibration has these effects:

◆ stimulation of the nerves, inducing a feeling of wellbeing

◆ gentle stimulation of the skin.

Movements include *static* vibrations, in which the pads of the fingers are placed on the nerve, and the vibratory effect created by the therapist's arms and hands is applied in one position; and *running* vibrations, in which the vibratory effect is applied along a nerve path.

Uses in treatment: to stimulate a sensitive skin in order to improve the skin's functioning without irritating the skin's surface.

ACTIVITY

Planning a massage

How will observations from the skin analysis and the client consultation influence the facial massage service?

TOP TIP

Pressure used at the neck and shoulders

Pressure may be increased when working on larger muscles in the neck or shoulders such as the trapezius muscle, especially if the client has tension in this area.

Products, tools and equipment

The massage is carried out using a **massage medium** that acts as a lubricant. A massage balm, cream or oil may be used; these are slightly penetrating, and soften the skin. Choose a product that contains ingredients to suit the client's skin type, condition and the age of the skin.

Massage balm Typically a mixture of oils and waxes which, when warmed in the hands, melts and softens into the skin, creating an ideal medium for massage which is readily absorbed. Active ingredients include essential oils such as rose and geranium. The client will benefit from the inhalation of the essential oils.

Massage cream This is ideal for those clients who require a richer, creamier texture. Also ideal for those who dislike the sensation of oil on their skin. This is more readily removed from the skin than oil. Creams are more rapidly absorbed than massage oils so may require further applications during the massage.

Massage oil Traditionally plant sourced, examples include jojoba, apricot kernal oil and sweet almond oil. These are readily absorbed by the skin whilst providing adequate slip and control to apply the massage techniques.

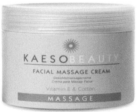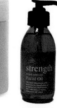

Massage cream   Facial oil

ACTIVITY

Choosing a massage medium

Compare two professional skincare ranges. Look at:

◆ the choice of facial massage preparations available and their suitability for different skin types
◆ the ingredients used in their formulation, and the effects claimed.

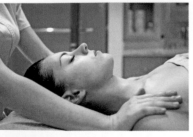

Applying petrissage massage technique to the trapezius muscle, using the heel of the hand

Whichever product you choose, it should provide sufficient slip while still allowing you to control the massage movements.

REVISION AID

What is the anatomical name for the jawbone?

STEP-BY-STEP: FACIAL MASSAGE TREATMENT

There are many different massage sequences, but each uses one or all of the massage techniques discussed above. What follows is a basic sequence for facial massage.

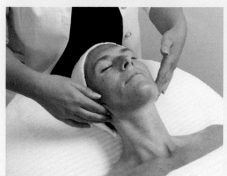 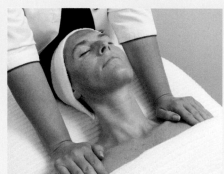 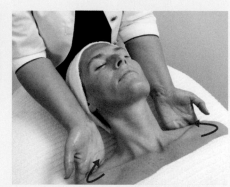

1 Effleurage to the neck and shoulders Slide the hands down the neck, across the pectoral muscles around the deltoid muscle, and across the trapezius muscle. Slide the hands up the back of the neck to the occipital bone at the base of the skull.

Repeat step 1 a further five times.

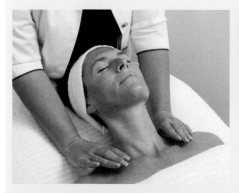 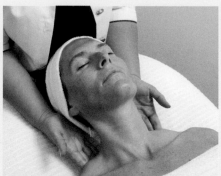 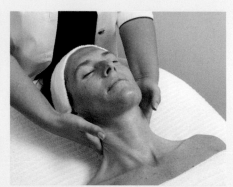

2 Thumb kneading to the shoulders Using the pad of both thumbs, make small circles (frictions) along the trapezius muscle, working towards the spinal vertebrae.

Apply each movement three times; then repeat the sequence (step 2) a further two times.

3 Finger kneading to the shoulders Position the fingers of each hand behind the deltoid, and make large rotary movements along the trapezius.

Apply each rotary movement three times; repeat the sequence (step 3) a further two times.

4 Vibrations Place the hands, cupped, at the base of the neck: perform running vibrations up the neck to the occipital bone.

Repeat step 4 a further six times.

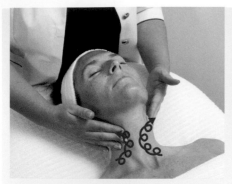

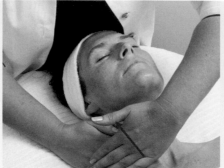

5 **Circular massage to the neck** Perform small circular movements over the platysma and the sternocleidomastoid muscle at the neck.

6 **Hands cupped to the neck** Cup your hands together. Place the hands at the left side of the neck, above the clavicle. Slide the hands up the side of the neck, across the jawline (mandible), and down the right side of the neck; then reverse.

Repeat step 6 a further two times.

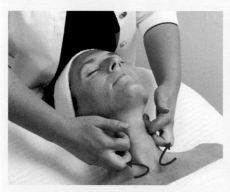

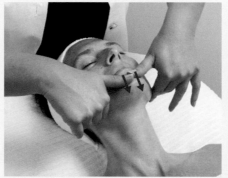

7 **Knuckling to the neck** Make a loose fist: rotate the knuckles up and down the neck area, over the platysma and sternocleidomastoid muscle.

Repeat step 7 to cover, a further two times.

8 **Up and under** Place the thumbs on the centre of the chin, over the mentalis muscle, and the index and middle fingers under the mandible. Slide the thumbs firmly up over the chin. Bring the index finger onto the chin, and place the middle finger under the mandible forming a V shape. Slide along the jawline to the ear. Replace the index finger with the thumb, and return along the jaw line to the chin, sliding the thumbs over the chin. Repeat the sequence.

Repeat step 8 a further five times.

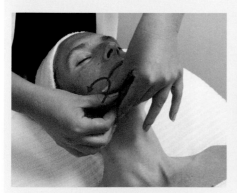

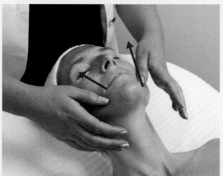

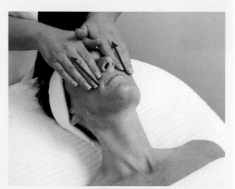

9 **Circling to the mandible** Place the thumbs one above the other on the chin, and proceed with circular kneading along the jawline towards the ear. Reverse and repeat.

Repeat step 9 a further two times.

10 **Flick-ups** Place the thumbs at the corners of the mouth. Lift the orbicularis oris muscle with a flicking action of the thumbs. Do not flick the lips – position the thumbs 5 mm from the corner of the mouth to avoid this.

Repeat step 10 a further five times.

11 **Half face brace** Clasp the fingers under the chin; turn the hands so that the fingers point towards the sternum. Unclasp, and slide the hands up the face towards and over the frontal bone of the forehead.

Repeat step 11 a further two times.

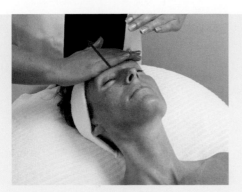
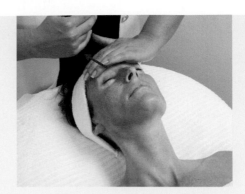

12 **Lifting the eyebrows** Place the right hand on the frontal bone of the forehead at the left temple, and stroke upwards from the eyebrow to the hairline. Repeat the movement with the left hand. Alternate each hand; repeat the movement across the forehead.

Repeat step 12 a further two times.

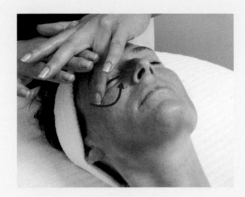
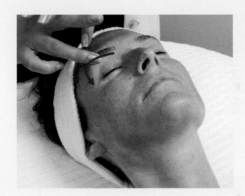

13 **Inner and outer eye circles** Using the ring finger, of each hand, *gently* draw three outer circles and three inner circles on each eye, following the fibre direction of the orbicularis oculi muscle.

Repeat step 13 a further two times.

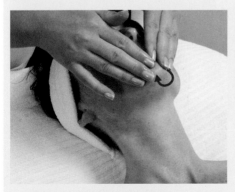
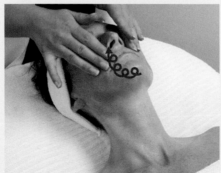
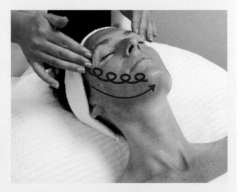

14 **Circling to the chin, the nose and the temples** Apply circular kneading to the chin, the nose and the temples. Return to the starting position.

Repeat step 14 a further two times.

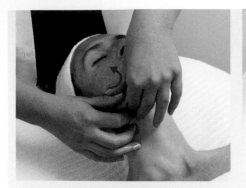

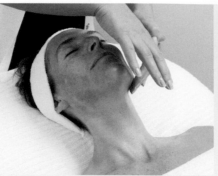

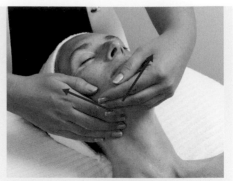

15 **Thumb kneading under the cheeks** Place the thumbs under the zygomatic bones. Carry out a circular kneading over the muscles in the cheek area.

Repeat step 15 a further five times.

16 **Tapping under the mandible** Tap the tissue under the mandible, using the fingers of both hands. Work from the left side of the jaw to the right; then reverse.

Repeat step 16 a further five times.

17 **Lifting the masseter** Cup the hands. Using the hands alternately, lift the masseter muscle, sweeping diagonally upwards over the muscle starting from the chin

Repeat step 17 a further five times.

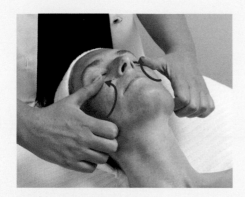

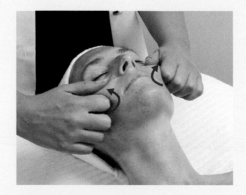

18 **Rolling and pinching** Using a deep rolling movement, draw the muscles of the cheek area towards the thumb which is placed, without moving, on the zygomatic bone in a rolling and pinching movement.

Repeat step 18 a further five times.

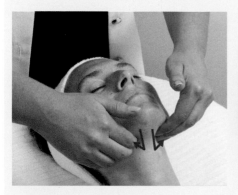

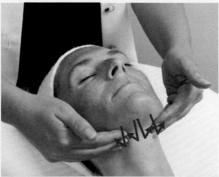

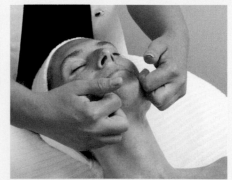

19 **Lifting the mandible** Place the pads of the fingers underneath the mandible and pivot diagonally. Lifting the tissues, work towards the ear.

Repeat step 19 a further two times.

20 **Knuckling along the jawline** Knuckle along the jawline and over the cheek area.

Repeat step 20 a further two times.

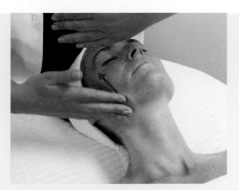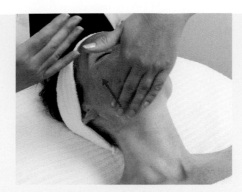

21 **Upwards tapping on the face** Using both hands, gently slap upwards along the jawline from ear to ear, lifting the muscles.

Repeat step 21 a further five times.

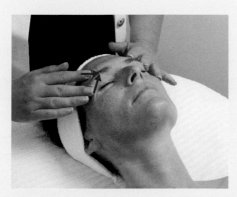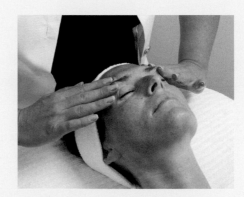

22 **Scissor movement to the forehead** Open the index and middle fingers to make a V shape at the outer corner of each eyebrow. Open and close the fingers in a scissor action moving inwards towards the inner point of the eyebrow. Slide back to starting point and repeat.

Repeat step 22 a further two times.

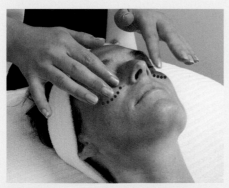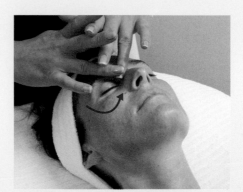

23 **Tapotement movement around the eyes** Using the pads of the fingers, tap gently over the orbicularis oculi surrounding the eye area.

Repeat step 23 a further two times.

24 **Eye circling** Repeat sequence described in step number 13.

Repeat step 24 three times.

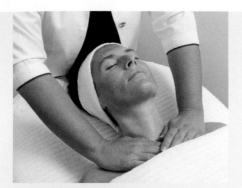
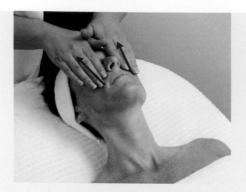

25 Apply effleurage to conclude the massage sequence.
Starting at the base of the neck, open the hands and cover the upper chest, shoulders, trapezius, front and sides of the neck then clasp the jaw and perform a half face brace towards the forehead.

Separate the hands and move the hands over the frontal bone, concluding the massage by applying light pressure at the temples

---

TOP TIP

Client comfort

Read your client's body language. During the facial massage, the client's face should relax. If there are evident signs of tension, such as vertical furrows between the eyebrows, check that the client is warm and comfortable.

After the massage

After the facial massage, remove the massage medium thoroughly using clean, damp sponges, cotton wool, facial mitts or towels. Check thoroughly that all product has been removed.

Apply toner to remove traces of oil, leaving the skin grease-free. Finally, blot the skin dry.

You may then proceed with further skin treatments, such as a face mask, or simply apply an appropriate moisturiser to conclude the treatment.

TOP TIP

Massage medium can easily be overlooked during removal in the following areas: the eyebrows; the base of the nostrils; under the chin; in the creases of the neck; behind the ear and on the shoulders. Ensure all massage medium is thoroughly removed.

ACTIVITY

Massage at home

Design a simple massage routine that a client could be taught to use at home. Moisturising balms and oils are available for retail that the client could use within their home skincare programme.

Which type of manipulation is involved in each movement in your sequence? What effect do you wish to achieve by incorporating it?

A facial chart is provided which you can copy to insert your massage instructions.

An example is provided for you.

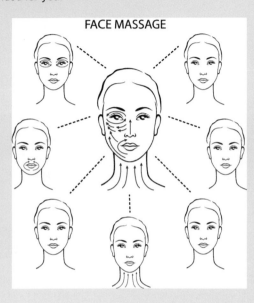

FACE MASSAGE

Client advice and recommendations

Encourage your client to use massage movements when applying emollient skincare products. Show them how to perform such movements correctly. This is great for reducing stress and areas of tension, and improving blood and lymphatic circulation. and getting maximum benefit form the properties of the ingredients such as inhalation of essential oils.

Facial exercises may be given to the client to practise at home. These should be carried out at least four times per week.

ACTIVITY

Hand and wrist mobility exercises

Devise ten exercises to increase the strength and mobility of your hands and wrists.

REVISION AID

Name the massage movement where the skin tissue is lifted away from the underlying structure and compressed.

Specialist facial treatment

Specialist treatments should be offered to your client when there is a specific need or if they feel they would like to benefit from such a service. Specialist training in these advanced techniques is usually offered by the product suppliers.

STEP-BY-STEP: SPECIALIST FACIAL

The model for this specialist facial service is a white, young female client with a combination skin with areas of sensitivity. One hour and 15 minutes was allowed for this facial.

The following facial treatment will:

◆ stimulate the blood circulation

◆ aid with the removal of toxins and waste products through improved lymphatic circulation

◆ have a skin cleansing action

◆ remove dead skin cells (desquamation)

◆ improve the moisture content of the skin

◆ reduce areas of sensivity.

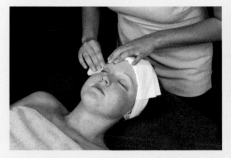

1 Cleansing the eye area. Lip cleansing follows.

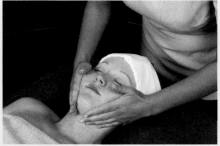

2 Application of facial cleansing lotion. The cleanser selected has ingredients to cleanse the skin, removing excess sebum whilst including anti-bacterial ingredients to promote skin healing. This superficial cleanse is followed by a deeper cleanse. The skin is inspected following the superficial cleanse to ensure that the correct treatment products are selected and applied, modified as necessary to suit the skin type and condition.

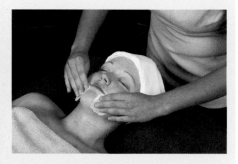

3 Removal of facial cleanser using dampened cotton wool in an upwards and outwards direction.

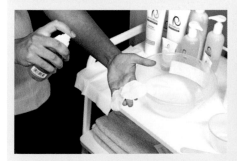

4 This is followed by the application of toning lotion. The appropriate toning lotion is selected and applied to damp cotton wool. This is applied to the skin in an upwards and outwards movement. Alternatively it can be sprayed over the skin from behind the client to cover the skin of the face and neck.

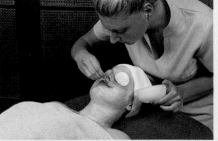

5 A clay exfoliant is applied to the face and neck to absorb excess sebum, gently removing dead skin cells and debris without sensitising the skin further. When it starts to dry, becoming matt in appearance this is removed using an upwards rolling finger action whilst supporting the tissues to avoid stretching the skin.

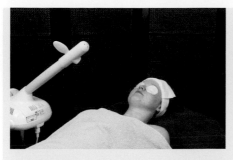

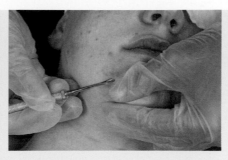

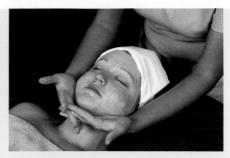

6 Application of a facial steamer. This will have a skin-cleansing action causing the pores to relax and open. It also has additional therapeutic relaxation properties, as the client inhales an aromatic lavender oil which has been added to the filter basket within the unit. The skin is then blotted dry. Comedone extraction may be provided at this stage, only if required, either manually or using a comedone extractor.

7 Facial massage movements are applied to the shoulders and face. An oil is used incorporating essential essences to control the overactivity of the sebaceous gland. Massage techniques are adapted to avoid over stimulation of the sebaceous glands and to psychologically relax the client.

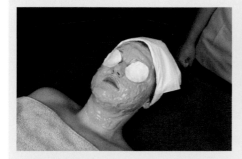

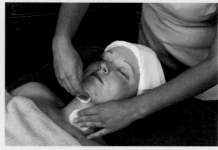

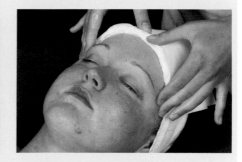

8 A personalised serum is applied to regulate sebaceous secretions and this is placed below a setting (occlusive) type mask. The mask provides a waterproof covering which will aid the absorption of the serum as the skin warms.

9 Skin toning lotion is applied following mask removal.

10 The service concludes with the skin being moisturised. This may include SPF which is recommended to avoid UVL photodamage. The service will provide both psychological and physiological benefits.

Express facial

An express facial may be provided to maintain the health and functioning of the skin, to cleanse refresh and hydrate the skin, or to target a specific area for improvement.

The name 'express' explains its purpose. It is provided quickly and usually lasts for 30 minutes.

Its purpose and benefit is varied.

◆ It can introduce a new client to the facial service, especially if they have never experienced a facial before, such as a teenage or male client.

◆ It is ideal as an interim facial for those clients with busy lifestyles or hectic schedules.

◆ It allows clients to experience the application and effects of products that will benefit their skin type and condition. Typically, it may include the face, neck, décolletage (upper chest) and shoulder areas.

◆ You can target areas of concern, such as treatment for sensitivity or anti-ageing e.g. for the eye area or problematic skin.

◆ You can assess suitability of products on a client who has a sensitive skin type. However, always remember to perform a skin sensitivity patch test 24-48 hours before for anybody who has a history of known sensitivity /skin allergies.

◆ It can be provided as a client reward, for example as part of a loyalty scheme or acknowledgment of special occasion such as a birthday.

◆ You can demonstrate a new product, explaining its application and allowing the client to experience firsthand the benefits such as facial oil, serum, micro mask etc.

◆ If it is part of a skincare promotion, a prescription of priority products can be identified to meet the client's needs.

◆ The client should feel relaxed and revived following the service.

Preparation for express facial

The express facial may not always be delivered in the normal treatment room especially if it is part of a promotional event. However, the facial will need to be delivered either on a facial chair or treatment couch. It will be more comfortable for the client to remove upper outer clothing and perhaps wear a robe. This will also avoid contact between the client's clothing and skincare products. Apply facial preparation requirements in line with removal of jewellery, contact lenses and protection of client's hair.

Following the consultation and skin analysis, the express facial will typically include the following stages.

◆ Cleansing sequence to thoroughly cleanse the area treated.

◆ Tone to remove traces of skin cleanser and skin debris.

◆ Exfoliation to remove surface cells.

◆ Mask, to cleanse, calm or nourish the skin.

◆ Tone followed by serum or moisturiser application to protect and hydrate the skin.

When delivering an express service, use this opportunity to explain the name and purpose of techniques or products used. For example, you may say "I am now applying a gentle exfoliator for the skin. This uses a clay base rather than less- environmentally friendly options. Its role is to remove or polish off dead skin cells from the skin's surface leaving a brighter, clearer, softer and more youthful appearing skin."

Following the express treatment, aftercare advice should be provided including possible contra-actions, post-treatment restrictions and the use of additional retail products and services.

Update the client's records following treatment, noting samples provided, areas that may need attention or follow up at the next treatment.

Client advice and recommendations

Aftercare and advice is discussed throughout the chapter in relation to each of the facial treatment procedures.

On completion of your facial treatment ensure that you have covered the following in your **advice and recommendations**:

◆ provided the client with a glass of water to hydrate and assist the removal of toxins, reminding them of the great health benefits of water to the skin

◆ shared information recorded on their treatment plan and explained its relevance to this service and future treatments

◆ explained what products have been used in the facial treatment and why

◆ taken time to demonstrate the products and explain their benefits, specific to the client's needs

◆ simplified ingredients and technologies used in the products' formulation so that they can be clearly understood

◆ presented a display of these products, which will personalise the service

◆ allowed the client to handle and touch the product

◆ advised what products are a priority for the client to use at home; a basic skincare routine is essential to maintain the maximum benefit from the facial treatment

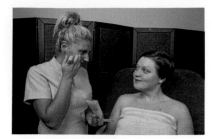

After the treatment provide your client with suitable aftercare advice.

"Great skin therapists know their stuff! Giving clients advice about how to improve a skin condition starts with knowing how your skin works and what happens when it does not function as it should. Effective skin treatments and helping clients select the right home care for real skin results must be based on solid science."

Daniella Norman

◆ advised on product quantity, application and removal, again in order to gain maximum benefit from their use

◆ provided contra-action advice and recommendations, action to be taken in the event of an unwanted skin reaction

◆ discussed the use of make-up following treatment (only eye and lip make-up should be worn directly after a facial treatment; allow up to 8 hours before make-up application to avoid congestion of the stimulated, cleansed skin)

◆ avoid excessive heat or further facial treatments for 24 hours

◆ explained the recommended time intervals between treatments

◆ provided guidance on what further treatments you would recommend to maintain or improve further the facial skin condition

◆ reminded the client tactfully of lifestyle improvements that they could make, which would benefit their skin health and wellbeing, reinforce the importance of wearing SPF to protect the skin from UV damage including premature ageing and pigmentation.

◆ discussed if product samples are to be provided, when and how they are to be used

◆ provided the opportunity for the client to ask any further questions.

"Consumers can be more motivated by how you communicate, not necessarily what you are saying. Speak with passion and authenticity. Know your product and have a thorough understanding of how the skin works."

Daniella Norman

Update and record all details on the client treatment record, including products purchased. You can discuss their effectiveness at the next facial treatment.

Take the client to the reception to book their next appointment if required, or if you have the technology, book the appointment in the treatment area.

Prepare the area for the next treatment:

◆ clean product tops and containers, and store appropriately to maintain their quality

◆ remove items for laundry and dispose of waste associated with the treatment

◆ clean and disinfect work surfaces

◆ prepare the couch following the requirements of your workplace policy.

ASSESSMENT OF KNOWLEDGE AND UNDERSTANDING

Having covered the learning objectives for this chapter test what you need to know and understand by answering the following short questions below.

Anatomy and physiology questions required for this subject are found in Chapter 2.

Organisational and legal requirements

1. What health and safety legislation is relevant to the delivery of a facial treatment? List these and explain briefly their purpose and your responsibility in relation to each.

2. What actions must be taken before a client under 16 years of age receives a facial?

3. Provide three examples to demonstrate how you comply with the legislation of the Equality Act when carrying out facial treatments?

4. What is the significance and why must a client's signature be obtained before commencing facial treatment?

5. Taking into account health and safety hygiene requirements, provide examples of how you would prepare your personal presentation and hygiene for facial treatment?

6. How should all client records be stored to comply with the Data Protection Act (1998)?

7. How long would you allow to complete a full, non-express facial treatment?

8. Why is it important for all staff to be familiar with the different facial pricing structures?

9. What details should be recorded on the client's treatment record and why is it important to keep accurate records regularly updated?

How to work safely and effectively when providing facial treatments

1. What environmental conditions should be considered when setting up for a facial treatment? Why are these important to both you and the client?

2. What do you understand by the terms disinfection and sterilisation? State two methods used in a facial treatment and when these are used.

3. How can you ensure that skincare products and equipment are used hygienically, avoiding cross-contamination?

4. How can you ensure that you and the client are correctly positioned for the facial treatment? What are the consequences (short and long-term effects) that could result from not considering this?

5. It may be necessary when preparing for the facial treatment to dispense products for use in the service. What should be considered when dispensing products?

6. When should electrical equipment, such as the facial steamer, be checked for good repair? Give three examples that would be checked in terms of this piece of equipment.

7. Give five examples of how the work area should be prepared ready for the next treatment following a facial treatment. When should this be carried out?

Consultation, treatment planning and preparation

1. What information may a client request when enquiring about a facial treatment?

2. How will the treatment application differ for a new facial treatment client to ensure they feel confident and will relax during the treatment?

3. Why is the client consultation essential before a treatment is provided?

4. Describe the different types of communication skills that you use when performing a client consultation.

5. At the consultation you notice that the client has what you consider to be herpes simplex. What action would you take? How would you explain the actions to be taken by the client?

6. At the consultation a client asks your advice about a small lump on their skin that occasionally bleeds. What advice do you give them?

7. What is the legal relevance of client-questioning and recording the client's responses?

8. How can you ensure that the client will be relaxed and confident during their facial treatment?

9. What assessment techniques are used to identify a client's skin type and conditions to inform their treatment requirements?

10. How can the client's skincare routine and lifestyle factors relate to their appearance, condition and treatment requirements?

Contra-indications

1. Name three contra-indications that would prevent facial treatment being carried out.

2. Name three contra-indications that would restrict treatment being provided.

3. Provide an example of how a treatment may be modified when a non-preventable contra-indication is present.

4. How would you select and apply skin products for a client with an allergic skin type?

Facial treatments

1. How may facial treatment be adapted when treating a male client?

2. Design a facial treatment lasting 1 hour for each of the different skin types; oily, dry and combination. You may decide the age of the client and identify any accompanying conditions that may be present, related to each skin type. Describe:

   a. the aim of the facial treatment linked to skin type
   b. the facial treatment products, tools and equipment you are going to use
   c. when and how you will apply them
   d. the different stages of the facial and how long each stage will last
   e. any information you may need to gain from the client to assist you in your facial treatment plan.

3. Describe how you would recognise the following skin conditions: sensitive, mature, young and dehydrated skin

4. List the internal and external lifestyle factors that may affect the skin?

5. What influences the regularity of clients receiving facial treatments?

6. When and why would you use a skin warming treatment?

7. What is the purpose of the following skincare products:

   a. cleanser
   b. toning lotion
   c. exfoliant
   d. moisturiser
   e. face masks?

8. What are the names of the different massage techniques? Explain how you would possibly adapt facial massage for a client with mature skin considering the change in facial skin and muscle tone.

9. What is a specialist skin product?

10. How would you select the massage medium to perform a facial massage?

11. What is the name given to excessive redness that can occur during a facial? What could be the cause of this?

12. What is a contra-action? Describe three contra-actions that could occur during or following a facial treatment and how you would deal with each.

Advice and recommendations

1. What skincare products would you recommend that are essential for a new client who has previously used soap and water, to use as part of their home care routine?

2. Why is it important to provide the client with a home care routine?

3. How would you explain the correct application and where relevant, removal of the following products for home use:

   a. cleansing milk
   b. facial scrub
   c. toning lotion
   d. non-setting face mask
   e. eye cream
   f. night cream?

4. Why is it important to tell the client about contra-actions that may occur? What advice would you give to a client in relation to this?

5. A client may visit the salon for a mini, express type-facial. What would this consist of, and when would you recommend this additional treatment?

NOTES

5 Eyelash and Eyebrow Treatments

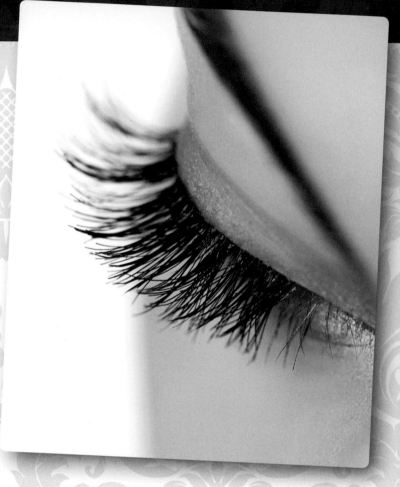

LEARNING OBJECTIVES

This chapter covers how to provide products and treatments that will enhance the client's natural eyelashes and eyebrows.

You will learn more about:

◆ Maintaining safe effective methods when working.

◆ The information that must be obtained at the consultation including the outcomes of the skin analysis and any skin sensitivity patch tests to ensure the client's suitability for treatment and welfare.

◆ Consultation and assessment techniques needed to draw up a treatment plan that meets the client's treatment objectives according to their requirements, including:
   – eyebrow shaping including threading
   – colouring the eyebrows and eyelashes, using temporary cosmetic products and permanent colour tint
   – eyelash enhancement systems, including temporary and semi-permanent techniques.

◆ The key elements of each eye treatment service.

◆ The different tools, products and equipment that may be used within the treatment to meet the client's treatment objectives.

◆ What must be considered following the client consultation, including any treatment modifications.

◆ How to advise the client on any additional products or treatments that will be of benefit to them.

◆ How to provide advice and recommendations to your client following treatment to maintain or further enhance the appearance of the eye area.

KEY TERMS

adhesive

anagen

catagen

consultation

erythema

eyebrow artistry

eyelash attachment

eyebrow and eyelash tinting

eyelash extension adhesive

eyebrow pencil

eyebrow powder

eyebrow shaping

eyebrow template

eyebrow threading

eyelash extensions

eyelash extension solvent

flare lashes

folliculitis

hair colour characteristics

hair cuticle

hair growth cycle

hydrogen peroxide (H_2O_2)

oxidisation

skin sensitivity patch test

single (or individual) lashes

strip lashes

telogen

terminal hair

threading

threading technique (hand, mouth and neck)

toluenediamine

tweezers

vellus hair

WHEN PROVIDING EYE TREATMENTS YOU WILL BE REQUIRED TO

◆ apply environmental and sustainable working practices

◆ follow relevant laws and manufacturers' instructions

◆ use different consultation and assessment techniques to correctly identify your client's needs

◆ use products, tools and equipment that will enhance the required results

◆ adapt the treatment to meet the client's physiological and psychological requirements (where required)

◆ take the necessary actions where a contra-action, contra-indication or treatment modification is required

◆ provide relevant advice and recommendations to support your client's treatment objectives.

INTRODUCTION

The technical skills required to enhance the eye area include a variety of techniques and effects that are continuously evolving. Eye treatments are popular with immediate results that both change and enhance the client's facial appearance. To achieve this, each eye treatment should be modified to suit the client's eye shape, face shape, natural hair growth and colouring, age, gender and the treatment plan agreed at consultation.

Health and safety is always an important part of every treatment, but because of the sensitivity of the eye area a skin sensitivity patch test must be performed before tinting and eyelash extension systems, as the chemicals used have the potential to cause allergic reactions.

Dealing with people in a polite, efficient manner and using good communication and questioning skills to find out exactly what they require from the eye treatment service forms an important part of this treatment.

INDUSTRY ROLE MODEL

SHAVATA SINGH Founder of Shavata Brow Studios

What do you find rewarding about your job? I love being able to make such a difference to someone's look in just a few minutes and seeing how happy they are! This is particularly true for people who have never had a professional shape. The results really can be transformative and instantly make them look younger, fresher and generally look the best they possibly can. I also enjoy meeting new people and find this very rewarding.

What makes a good beauty therapist? Someone who is discreet, attentive, a good listener but also advises the client with an expert eye on how to best accentuate each of their features. Above all a beauty therapist must be honest and must not sell the customer something they do not need.

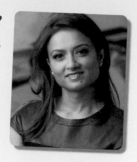

Essential anatomy and physiology knowledge requirements for eyebrow and eyelash treatments are identified in the checklist 'Anatomy and physiology knowledge and understanding requirements for each technical skill' in Chapter 2. In addition it is necessary to have an understanding of the basic structure and function of the eye. This is also discussed in Chapter 2, The Science of Beauty Therapy.

ALWAYS REMEMBER

Transferable knowledge, understanding and skills

When providing eyebrow and lash treatments it is important to use the skills and knowledge you have learnt in the following chapters:

◆ The Business of Beauty Therapy (Chapter 1)
◆ The Science of Beauty Therapy (Chapter 2)
◆ Consultation Practice and Techniques (Chapter 3)
◆ Wax Depilation (Chapter 8).

The eyebrows and eyelashes protect the eye from moisture and dust as well as defining the appearance of the eyes and enhancing the facial features.

The eyebrows can be shaped and coloured. The eyelashes can be coloured and permed, or artificial eye lashes may be attached to the natural eye lashes to both thicken and lengthen.

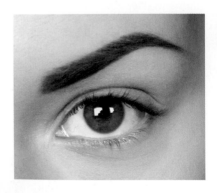

Eyebrow shaping

The eyebrows, situated above the bony eye orbits of the face, help to protect the eyes from moisture and dust, and to cushion the skin from physical injury. Misshapen eyebrows give an untidy appearance to the face but when correctly shaped they give balance to the facial features and enhance the eyes – the most expressive feature of the face.

Eyebrow hair removal can be carried out with temporary or permanent hair-removal techniques. Permanent methods include the advanced treatments of electrolysis and intense pulsed light (IPL). This section covers the temporary removal of eyebrow hair using tweezers and threading.

Shaping the eyebrows can be performed as a reshape, which involves removing eyebrow hair to create a new shape or eyebrow maintenance, which involves removing only a few stray hairs to maintain an existing shape. The period of time between treatments determines whether it is an eyebrow reshape or eyebrow maintenance.

Preparing the work area for eyebrow shaping

Each eye treatment work area should have the following basic products, tools and **equipment** listed below, further equipment relevant to each eye treatment service is discussed in the chapter, starting with eyebrow shaping. The work area should always be prepared and maintained throughout the day, ready for further treatments.

Eye treatment products, tools and equipment

Products, tools and equipment

- **Treatment couch or beauty chair** With an adjustable **back rest** and height, these may offer neck and foot support for the comfort of both the client and the beauty therapist when working. This should be in an easy to clean surface, such as PU vinyl upholstery.

- **Equipment trolley or work surface** Large enough to accommodate all the necessary products, tools and equipment. This should have an easy-to-clean surface; porous surfaces such as wood will stain if in contact with chemicals such as permanent tint, creating an unprofessional appearance.

- **Beauty stool** With adjustable height, back support and covered in a fabric similar to that covering the couch.

- **Step-up stool** To assist clients as necessary to position themselves on the couch.

- **Magnifying lamp** This magnifies the area when assessing client suitability for treatment and treatment requirements. The magnifying lamp is also essential when performing an eyebrow shape to ensure a clean result free from superfluous, unwanted hair.

- **Covered waste bin** Should have an easy-to-clean surface in a colour that will not show stains. The best choice is a stainless steel, foot operated bin.

- **Hand mirror** Must be maintained in a clean condition and is used when consulting with the client before and after their treatment, as well as during for some treatments.

- **Headband** A clean headband or headband bonnet should be provided for each client to secure hair away from the area and prevent you from coming into contact with the hair. You may alternatively use a hair clip to avoid spoiling the hair.

- **Hand disinfectant** Usually containing chlorhexidine, to cleanse and disinfect the hands as required following hand washing.

- **Skin-cleansing preparations** The trolley should carry a display of facial and eye skin-cleansing preparations to suit all skin types and conditions, used for removal of facial make-up and skin debris from the area.

- **Non-oily eye make-up remover** To cleanse the eye area.

- **Spatulas and orange woodsticks** Several clean spatulas in a range of sizes should be provided for each client. One should be used in tucking any stray hair beneath the headband. Others including orange wood sticks, will be used when removing products from their containers and for applying products to the skin.

- **Cotton wool** There should be a plentiful supply of both damp and dry cotton wool, sufficient for the treatment to be carried out.

- **Disinfectant** For cleaning and disinfecting equipment before use and storage following sterilisation.

- **Disposable paper tissue roll** To hygienically protect work surfaces.

- **Tissues** These should be stored in a covered container. These are used for blotting the area dry and occasionally the client's eyes may water so a tissue may be placed at the corner of the eyes.

- **Towel drapes** A small hand towel may be draped across the client's chest and shoulders. Alternatively disposable paper tissue may be used, replaced for each client.

- **Towel** A clean towel should be available for you to wipe your hands on as necessary. A dark coloured towel is most practical for tinting treatments so accidental spillages do not spoil the appearance of the towel.

- **Bowls** To store dry and damp cotton wool.

- **Client treatment record** Confidential record with details of each client, including personal details, products used, retail purchases made and details of each treatment.

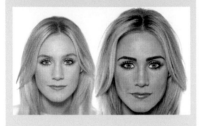

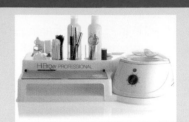

Eyebrow shaping treatments

Specialist products, tools and equipment

Before beginning the **eyebrow shaping** treatment, check that you have the necessary products, tools and equipment to hand and that they meet the legal hygiene and industry requirements for eye treatments.

There are two sorts of **tweezers** used to shape the eyebrows:

◆ automatic, and

◆ manual.

Automatic tweezers have a spring-loaded action and are designed to remove the bulk of excess, unwanted hair.

Manual tweezers are used to remove stray hairs, and to accentuate the brow shape where more accurate care is required. They are available with various ends including slant, claw or pointed; which you use is a matter of personal preference, but slanted ends are generally the most popular choice for eyebrow shaping.

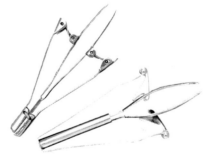

Automatic tweezers

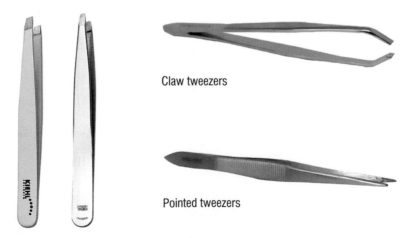

Claw tweezers

Pointed tweezers

Manual slant tweezers

HEALTH & SAFETY

Tweezers

A number of pairs of tweezers must be purchased (perhaps five), due to the length of time required for sterilisation. A freshly sterilised pair should be used for each client.

Buy good quality stainless steel tweezers: cheaper metals rust after repeated sterilisation.

Disposable mascara brushes are ideal for brushing the hairs during brow shaping.

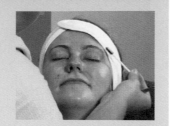

TOP TIP

Purchasing tweezers

When purchasing tweezers, make sure that the ends meet accurately so they will grasp the hair effectively. If the points are too sharp, they can cause the hair to break.

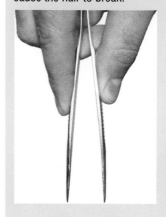

Although many beauty therapists may complete an eyebrow shaping treatment using only one of these – automatic or manual tweezers – it is important to be skilled in the use of both types. The following specialist products, tools and equipment must also be available.

◆ **Orange sticks** to measure the length and arch of eyebrow when planning hair removal.

◆ **Dry and damp cotton wool** to apply skin and eye cleansing and soothing products – and to collect hair removed during treatment.

◆ **Eyebrow brush** or disposable brushes to comb through the eyebrow hair before, during and after shaping to groom the hairs into the final shape. These may be available for the client to purchase too.

◆ **Scissors (stainless steel)** with short, thin points for trimming long hairs, or coarse **terminal hairs** that are unsuitable for removal and require shortening.

◆ **Disposable non-latex (synthetic), powder-free gloves** may be worn to prevent cross-infection and possible contamination with bodily fluids during hair removal treatment.

◆ **Glass jar** to store small stainless steel sterilised tools in a recommended chemical disinfecting fluid suitable for the beauty therapy industry.

◆ **Eyebrow pencil** may be used to mark the skin when measuring brow length, demonstrating the hairs for removal.

◆ **Pencil sharpener (stainless steel)** Suitable for use in the autoclave, used to sharpen the **eyebrow pencil** before contact with the client's skin. The client will then observe good hygiene practice.

◆ **Skin disinfectant** To cleanse the client's skin before treatment, reducing the possibility of secondary infection following the treatment.

◆ **Soothing lotion or gel** With healing and antiseptic properties including ingredients such as witch hazel or tea tree, suitable for application to the skin of the face. Remember, the skin is especially sensitive around the eyes and can easily become irritated and inflamed.

◆ **Client record** To record the client's personal details, products used and details of the treatment.

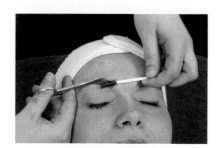

Scissors used to trim hair length

Preparation of the work area

Before the client is shown through to the work area, it should be checked to ensure that the required products, tools and equipment are available for eyebrow shaping and the area is hygienically clean and tidy.

The treatment couch or beauty chair should be clean, having been thoroughly washed with hot soapy water, or wiped thoroughly with a professional disinfectant cleaner. The surface should be protected with a long strip of disposable paper bedroll placed to cover a freshly laundered or disposable covering. A small towel should be placed neatly at the head of the couch – for hygiene and protection during treatment. This will be draped for protection across the client's chest. The tissue will need changing and towels freshly laundered for each client.

The couch or beauty chair should be positioned flat or slightly elevated when performing the treatment.

The work area should be adequately lit to ensure that the treatment can be provided safely, but avoid bright lighting that could cause eye irritation and lead to watery eyes.

Always follow your workplace policy for preparation of the work area.

Safety and hygiene

Sterilise tweezers at an appropriate time during the working day. Ensure that you always have sterile tweezers available for each client. After they have been sterilised in the autoclave, the tweezers should be stored in the UV cabinet or in a disinfected, clean covered container, ideally labelled. After 24 hours the tweezers will be clean but not disinfected. This length of time is extended in a procedure that places the object in a vacuum sealed bag.

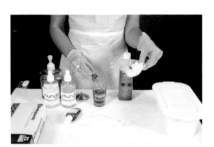

Chemical disinfection of eyebrow shaping tools

A fresh chemical disinfectant solution may be used to store a spare pair of tweezers while carrying out an eyebrow treatment. This solution is usually dispensed into a small jar or container stored on the trolley.

Spare tweezers are necessary in case you should accidentally drop the other tweezers during the treatment. After the eyebrow shaping treatment, tweezers must be replaced, cleaned and re-sterilised.

Sharpen the brow pencil before use on each client when used to measure the eyebrow length.

"For each appointment, use clean, disinfected tweezers, new disposable brushes and keep pencils sharpened."

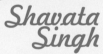

Single use disposable non-latex (synthetic) powder-free gloves may be worn for protection, avoiding cross-infection during the eyebrow shaping treatment – you may come into contact with tissue fluids from the client's skin.

As the waste from the treatment may contain body fluids and pose a health threat, it must be collected and disposed of carefully, in accordance with the Local Authority Environmental Health Department.

Client care, consultation and communication

Treatment information to provide to the client at the initial point of interest

The following points are important for the receptionist to consider when booking a client for an eyebrow shaping treatment.

◆ Eyebrow shaping may be carried out as an independent treatment or combined with other treatments, such as eyebrow artistry, temporary cosmetic and permanent tinting use of colour. Where permanent colour tint is used, the eyebrows should be tinted before shaping to avoid the tint coming into contact with the open follicle and perhaps causing skin irritation or an allergic reaction. Remember to advise the client a skin sensitivity patch test is required before the use of permanent tint.

◆ When a new client makes an appointment for a treatment, always allocate extra time for the consultation beforehand. Inform the client of this requirement and its purpose.

◆ Explain to the client how long they should allow for the appointment. When making an appointment for eyebrow shaping it is usual to allow 15–20 minutes, dependent upon the treatment requirements of reshape or maintenance. For a maintenance treatment usually allow 15 minutes.

It is wise to have a designated time that identifies the difference between the two treatments. For example, for clarity and to avoid confusion, less than two weeks could be regarded as maintenance and over two weeks as a reshape.

◆ If the client has thick, heavy brows, or if they do not have their brows shaped regularly, they should be advised to have them shaped gradually over a period of weeks, until the desired shape is achieved. This will allow the client to become accustomed to the new shape and will minimise any discomfort.

Client arrival

Clients should never be kept waiting on arrival for their appointment unless there is an unavoidable reason.

ALWAYS REMEMBER

Professional treatment timing

Eyebrow shaping treatment: allow 15–20 minutes. If there is insufficient time available, do not book the treatment. Always deliver a quality service.

◆ Eyebrow shaping may be carried out as an independent service, or combined with permanent tinting of the brows. In the latter case, the brows should be tinted before shaping, to avoid the tint coming into contact with the open follicle and perhaps causing an allergic reaction. For a combined treatment allow 30 minutes.

◆ If the client informs you of poor health, or is taking medication that may affect their skin or hair condition, it may not be possible to treat them until the medical condition has been treated by their GP. Tactfully check client suitability, this may involve seeking guidance from others.

ALWAYS REMEMBER

Consultation

Accurately record your client's answers to necessary questions to be asked at the consultation.

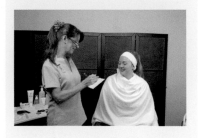

ALWAYS REMEMBER

Compliance with the Data Protection Act (1998)

Ensure all client records are stored securely and only the staff that have permission to are able to access them.

On arrival the client **treatment record** may start to be completed; this may be completed by the salon receptionist if competent to do so. Record the client's personal details, such as their name and address.

The beauty therapist will add further information to the treatment record at the consultation and during treatment in relation to information provided by the client, any modifications required and in relation to the results obtained. Sometimes, You may decide that it is preferable to complete hair removal using threading or waxing methods.

The combination of techniques and products at your disposal allows you to be very creative where colour is applied to define and emphasise the final shape. This is called **eyebrow artistry**.

If a client is a **minor**, under the age of 16 years of age, it is necessary to obtain signed written consent before service is carried out. It is also necessary that the parent, carer or guardian is present when the service is given.

mybrows
BEAUTIFUL EYES

Eyebrow record card

Name	Date of birth
Address	
Telephone (home)	Telephone (mobile)
Email address	
Patch test date	Patch test results

Identifying treatment restrictions at consultation

At the consultation, identify any peculiarities such as bald patches or scarring in the brow area. You may initially feel uncomfortable discussing this, but this will avoid any confusion over what can be achieved, or concern later that the area is devoid of hair!

TOP TIP

Developing your skills

To achieve a quick result (if you are qualified to do so) you may airbrush the eyebrows using specialist make-up. This is an example of how there are always opportunities to update your professional skills.

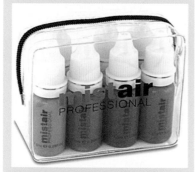

Professional airbrush eyebrow make-up is silicone based, providing a quick, professional, durable finish used in conjunction with an **eyebrow template**

TOP TIP

Up-selling

While the client is having their eyebrows shaped, this provides an ideal opportunity to discuss further suitable related services, such as an eyebrow tint, and use of additional eyebrow products, such as pencils, waxes and powders.

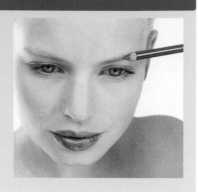

Consultation

Before eyebrow-shaping treatment commences, carry out a **consultation**. Here you will discuss the shape and effect to be achieved. You will use your professional judgment to consider the most appropriate shaping treatment based upon the client's age, hair growth and colour, natural brow shape, facial features, face shape and fashion style.

Before shaping the brows you must consider the following factors:

The natural shape of the brow The eyebrows are situated above the eyes and the natural brow follows the line of the eye socket. This varies greatly between clients, and will affect what is achievable, which is where additional techniques such as tinting, eyebrow artistry and, if qualified, advanced techniques such as the addition of artificial hair may be discussed.

"For me, every client is my most important client, so all my staff are trained to the highest standard and customer service is one of the most important components of my business. We also use a combination of techniques to ensure each customer gets the brow shape that suits them best."

Shavata Singh

If the client has been shaping their own brows, it may be necessary to let them grow for a short period before shaping them professionally. If the brows are very thin or very thick, it may take several sessions before the desired shape is achieved.

If the brows have been tweezed over a long period of time, they may not grow back successfully; this should be discussed with the client. In such instances, temporary eyebrow pencil and brow powder may be used to achieve the required effect. Temporary brow colour is useful to apply when growing hairs into a new brow shape, to create a defined brow shape.

Fashion Each season sees new fashion trends, which also affect eye make-up colours and application techniques and eyebrow shapes.

ALWAYS REMEMBER

Eyebrow hair removal and fashion

Remember, fashions come and go. This should be considered when removing hair using both temporary and permanent hair-removal methods. Even with temporary eyebrow hair removal methods the hair regrowth following regular removal may be patchy and less dense. Permanent methods destroy the cells of the germinal matrix in the hair follicle that create the hair. This should be considered before using any form of permanent hair removal to shape the brows.

Often, to achieve these eyebrow shapes either the removal of hair or the addition of colour and eyebrow product is required. In addition, as different eyebrow styles suit different eye and face shapes, it may be necessary to modify the look to suit the client.

Look at these stylised brow shapes that define an era:

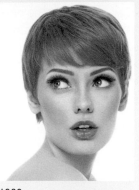
1960s

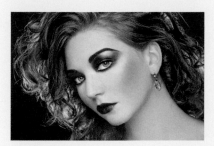
1980s

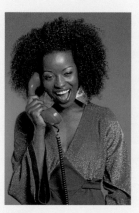
1970s

ALWAYS REMEMBER

Brow tinting

By tinting brow hair before shaping you will colour any finer lighter hairs, which will then form part of the brow. This may improve what is achievable with the brow shape.

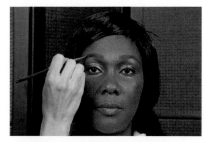

Applying temporary brow colour to define the brow shape

TOP TIP

Male eyebrow shaping

Male clients may require a result that emphasises their natural brow shape and removes stray, untidy hairs. This generally requires removing hair from the area between the brows where the brow hairs may meet, as shown. If not removed this brow hair can give the client a stern look.

Male clients will also often need hair removed from underneath the lower outer brow, which will open up the eye area. If this brow hair is not removed it can create a hooded effect to the eyelid.

Do not define the brow shape unless this is specifically requested.

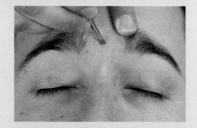
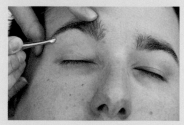

TOP TIP

Temporary brow colour

A sharpened eyebrow pencil may be used to simulate brow hairs – select the correct colour and apply feathery strokes using the pencil point. To create a natural effect, two different pencil colours may be used, for example brown and grey chosen to complement the client's hair and skin colouring.

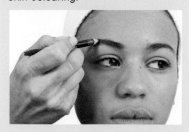

The age of the client The brow hair of older clients may include a few coarse, long, discoloured white or grey hairs. These may be removed provided that this does not alter the brow line or leave bald patches. In general, thick untidy eyebrows make the client look older, by creating a hooded appearance; and thin eyebrows will make the client look severe. Ideally the brows should therefore be shaped to a medium thickness. Remember, as female clients age the eyebrow hair often becomes more sparse due to reduced oestrogen hormone levels and blood circulation to the cells.

The natural growth pattern The shape and effect that the client requests may be made impossible by the pattern of the natural growth of the hair, which is genetically determined. When shaping the brows of an Oriental client, for example, you will notice that the eyebrow hair grows in a downward direction. To create an arch it may be necessary to trim the hairs, using a small, sterile pair of sharp small scissors. Alternatively, you may remove the outer eyebrow length and use an eyebrow pencil to create a new brow line. Use your professional judgement to advise the client.

ACTIVITY

Age of the client

Look at the eyebrows of clients that you treat. Recognise characteristics that you are likely to observe in relation to the skin in the area and hair colour, type and growth.

How does this influence:

◆ what can be achieved?
◆ what other eyebrow artistry techniques you may use?

Provide examples gained from your knowledge and experience at consultation.

"Consultations should determine lifestyle and preference; aftercare should offer advice on maintaining the client's most natural shape, so they are able to comfortably shape their brows."

Shavata Singh

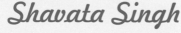

REVISION AID

In which stage of growth are hairs actively growing?

ALWAYS REMEMBER

Eyebrow shape modification

Always consider how you will modify your treatment to meet the client's needs.

◆ Avoid removing hair that conceals a bald area, e.g. a skin scar in the area.
◆ Trim long hair that spoils the brow line.
◆ Consider gender, requirements and suitability of hair removal when shaping a male client's eyebrows.
◆ If applying colour, select what is appropriate to complement the client's natural hair colouring.

Choosing an eyebrow shape

The eyebrows should be in balance with the rest of the facial features: the right brow shape for each client will depend on the client's facial proportions and natural brow shape.

There is no single ideal brow shape; different brow shapes are shown below.

What is achievable? Obviously not all of these brow shapes are achievable for every client, but the skilful application to the eyebrows of temporary cosmetic colour can create the illusion of the desired brow shape. This is referred to as eyebrow artistry.

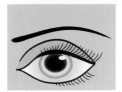
Thin eyebrows: straight shape

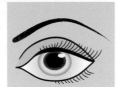
Thin eyebrows: rounded shape

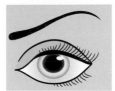
Thin eyebrows: oblique shape

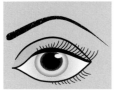
Thin eyebrows: arched shape

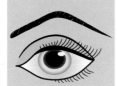
Thin eyebrows: angular shape

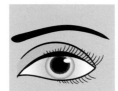
Medium eyebrows: straight shape

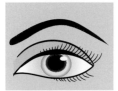
Medium eyebrows: rounded shape

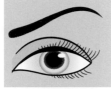
Medium eyebrows: oblique shape

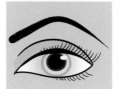
Medium eyebrows: arched shape

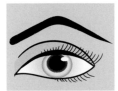
Medium eyebrows: angular shape

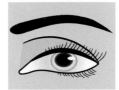
Thick eyebrows: straight shape

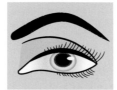
Thick eyebrows: rounded shape

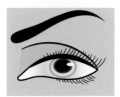
Thick eyebrows: oblique shape

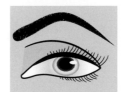
Thick eyebrows: arched shape

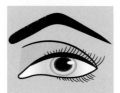
Thick eyebrows: angular shape

The quantity of brow hair removed during shaping produces a thin, medium or thick final shape, as illustrated. Shape and thickness should create balance in the face. The shape can be changed using semi-permanent and temporary techniques. Semi-permanent techniques and eyebrow enhancement are advanced skills but may be offered by your salon. You may offer temporary techniques such as eyebrow artistry.

◆ *Semi-permanent make-up*, is an advanced technique, also referred to as micro-pigmentation. It, can be used to add colour semi-permanently to the brows, for example to disguise a bald patch, thicken and define the shape. A popular technique called microblading applies pigment through a series of needles, allowing you to achieve a more natural look where individual hairs are created to suit the client, rather than a block of colour.

ALWAYS REMEMBER

Eyebrow enhancement

Artificial individual brow hairs are ideal for temporarily disguising any bald areas in the natural eyebrow hair. These are an increasingly popular technique that requires advanced training.

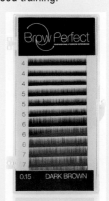

ACTIVITY

Correcting eye shapes through brow-shaping treatment and brow artistry

How would you correct/improve the eye shapes below:

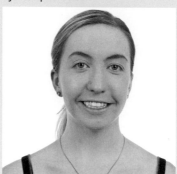

Wide-set eyes

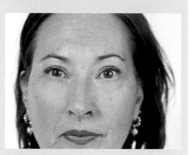

Close-set eyes

◆ *Cosmetic surgery hair transplants* are available for the client with sparse eyebrows.

◆ *Artificial individual eyebrow hairs* are applied in the same way as individual single eyelash extension systems, but differ in positioning and longevity.

ALWAYS REMEMBER

Semi-permanent make-up

Although advanced techniques, it is useful to have a professional awareness of techniques that the client may have read about. An example is semi-permanent make-up where suspended pigment particles in a liquid base are inserted into the outer skin using a disposable needle. Many of the popular dyes are based on plant extracts.

The immediate effect gradually fades, lasting up to 3 years.

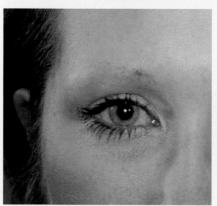

Before

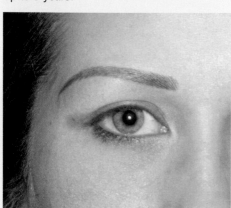

After

Ideally, the distance between the two eyebrows should be the width of one eye. If this is not the case, the illusion may be created by removing hairs or by applying temporary brow colour to create this effect.

Wide-set eyes can be made to appear closer together by extending the brow line beyond the inside corner of the eye; close-set eyes can be made to look further apart by widening the distance between them.

ACTIVITY

Correcting brow shapes

Collect pictures of faces showing different eyebrow shapes. Discuss which you think are correct and which incorrect for each face, explaining why.

How to measure the eyebrows to decide length and arch placement

In order to determine the correct length of the client's eyebrows, there are three main guidelines. Initially these guidelines will be applied to ensure that the correct length and brow shape are achieved, but the experienced beauty therapist will recognise the corrective work to be carried out without the need for measuring.

STEP-BY-STEP: MEASURING THE EYEBROWS

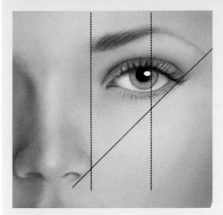

Guidelines to measure the eyebrow to determine arch placement and length

1 Place an orange stick or spatula vertically beside the nose and the inner corner of the eye. This is usually in line with the tear duct. Any hairs that grow between the eyes and beyond this point should be removed. If the client has a very broad nose, however, this guide is inappropriate: tweezing would commence near the middle of the brow. In this instance, use the tear duct at the inside corner of the eye as a guide.

2 Place an orange stick or spatula in a vertical line from the centre of the eyelid, or outside edge of the pupil if the eyes are open. This is where the highest point of the arch should commence.

3 Place an orange stick or spatula in a line from the base of the nose (the side of the nostril) to the outer corner of the eye. Any hairs that grow beyond this point should be removed.

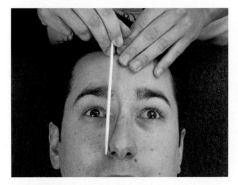

Male client; measuring the eyebrow: the inner corner of the eye, the tear duct is shown here

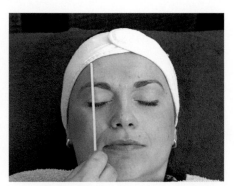

Female client; measuring the eyebrow: the centre of the eyelid, usually in line with the outside edge of the pupil

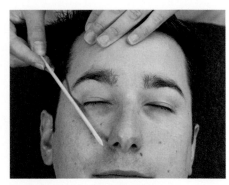

Male client; measuring the eyebrow: the outer eye

ACTIVITY

Correcting brow shapes

You cannot change the bone structure of the facial features without cosmetic surgery, but brow shaping can create the illusion of improved facial balance and proportion. Discuss why each of the brow shapes below would complement the accompanying face shape.

Face shape

Correct brow shape

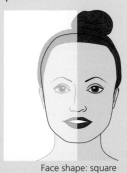

Square

Face shape: square

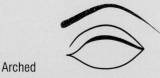

Arched

Correct brow shape: arched or softly rounded

TOP TIP

Measuring tool

A tool may be used to assist you in measuring where the client's brows should start and finish. The arch should be placed using the client's features as a guide when the tool is opened and its arms positioned and placed flat against the face.

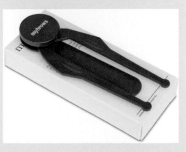

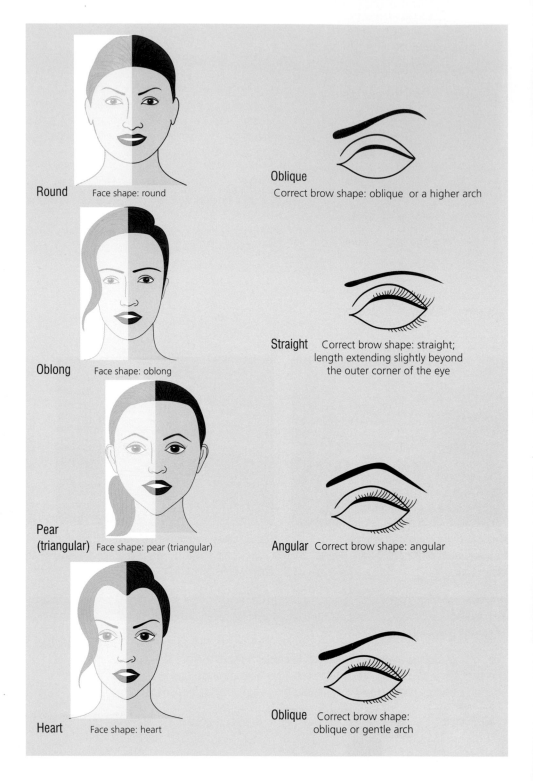

Round — Face shape: round

Oblong — Face shape: oblong

Pear (triangular) — Face shape: pear (triangular)

Heart — Face shape: heart

Oblique — Correct brow shape: oblique or a higher arch

Straight — Correct brow shape: straight; length extending slightly beyond the outer corner of the eye

Angular — Correct brow shape: angular

Oblique — Correct brow shape: oblique or gentle arch

Contra-indications

When a client attends for an eyebrow shaping treatment, you should always check that there are no **contra-indications** that might restrict or prevent the treatment.

If while completing the consultation or on visual inspection of the skin the client is found to have any of the following in the eye area, eyebrow shaping treatment must not be carried out:

◆ *contact lenses* unless removed

◆ *hypersensitive skin* – the skin could become excessively red and swollen

◆ **trichotillomania** – this is a repetitive disorder where the client pulls out their hair voluntarily

◆ **any eye disorder**, such as those listed in the chart following this text

◆ **glaucoma** is an eye disorder where the optic nerve is damaged at the point where it leaves the eye. This damage can be caused by raised eye pressure or because there is a weakness in the optic nerve. This can lead to loss of sight. GP permission should be sought before treatment proceeds

◆ severe **inflammation or swelling** the cause may be medical

◆ **skin disease,** such as impetigo

◆ **skin disorder**, such as psoriasis or eczema

◆ **severe bruising** – client discomfort could be caused and the condition made worse

◆ open **cuts or abrasions** – secondary infection could occur

◆ **chemotherapy** – medical treatment commonly used to treat cancer. A side-effect can be hair loss because all cells of the body are affected by the treatment, not just cancer cells

◆ recent **facial piercing**

◆ recent **semi-permanent make-up**, the area will be sensitive

◆ recent **eye surgery**

◆ **scar tissue under 6 months old** – the skin lacks elasticity.

Contra-indications that would restrict treatment include old bruising, mild eczema or psoriasis, avoid the area. For more information on diseases affecting the eye see Chapter 3, Consultation practice and techniques.

The following eye disorders contra-indicate eyebrow-shaping treatments (including threading and waxing also further eye services including), tinting to the brows and lashes and eyelash enhancement systems.

Name	Description	Name	Description
Conjunctivitis or pink eye 	Bacterial infection causing inflammation of the mucous membrane (conjunctiva) that covers the eye and lines the eyelid. Symptoms include redness, itching, soreness and pus exudate.	**Watery eye** or epiphora 	The eye over-secretes tears, which would normally drain into the nasal cavity.
Stye or hordeola 	Bacterial infection of the sebaceous glands of the eyelash hair follicles. Appears as a small, inflamed (red) and sore lump on the eyelid, containing pus.	**Blepharitis** 	Inflammation of the eyelid caused by infection or an allergic reaction.

(Continued)

Name	Description	Name	Description
Cyst	A localised pocket of sebum, which forms in the hair follicle or under the sebaceous gland in the skin. Semi-globular in shape, either raised or flat and either hard or soft. Cysts are the same colour as the surrounding skin unless an infection occurs which results in redness. A cyst on the eyelid is also known as a chalazion or meibomian cyst.	Benign (non-malignant) tumour	Benign (non-malignant) tumour. Harmless skin-coloured growths. They may appear as a 'thread' of skin on the eyelids growing between the eyelashes. Chemical services such as tinting and perming should be avoided to avoid skin irritation. Refer the client to their GP.

If you are unsure about the safety of proceeding with treatment – for example, if there is an undiagnosed lump in the area – ask your client to seek medical approval first. Remember you are not qualified to diagnose a contra-indication. Refer the client to their GP without giving unnecessary cause for concern.

Discuss possible contra-actions that may occur during or after the eyebrow shaping service with your client at consultation and the action to take. These are discussed below.

Contra-actions

Erythema is considered to be a **contra-action** to the treatment: it is recognised as a marked reddening of the skin seen over the whole area or specifically around one damaged follicle. It is usually accompanied by minor swelling of the area. If this occurs you must try to reduce the redness by applying a cool compress and soothing antiseptic lotion or cream to the area. In extreme cases it may be necessary to apply ice if available.

REVISION AID

What other methods of temporary brow hair removal are often used in the salon?

HEALTH & SAFETY

Contra-action: using ice

To maintain hygiene, place the ice cube in a new small freezer food bag. Dispose of the bag hygienically after use.

Discuss possible contra-actions that may occur during or after the eyebrow shaping treatment with your client at consultation.

Record details of any contra-action on the client's record.

If the reddening reduces in response to your corrective action, you may decide in future to remove only a few stray hairs at each eyebrow-shaping treatment, to minimise the risk of this reaction recurring.

If you accidentally pinch the skin with the tweezers and break the skin, apply a suitable soothing, antiseptic lotion for the skin, whilst wearing gloves. Inform the client not to touch the area and recommend the further application of a suitable antiseptic lotion. The main aim is to avoid secondary infection. All details of action taken must be recorded on the client record.

Following the consultation, record all client details accurately on the client treatment plan record.

The client should be shown through to the prepared work area after the treatment plan record has been completed.

The client record should be signed and dated by the client and yourself following the consultation to confirm the suitability and consent with the agreed treatment.

Keep and store client treatment records in compliance with the Data Protection Act for future reference.

TOP TIP

Relaxing the hair follicles

It is often stated that before beginning shaping, the brows should be prepared with warm, damp cotton wool pads, to relax the hair follicles and soften the eyebrow tissue, making hair removal easier. During treatment, however, you will be wiping over the area with an antiseptic lotion, which has a cooling, soothing and tightening effect on the skin, so this preparation is probably ineffectual unless repeated during the treatment.

STEP-BY-STEP: SHAPING THE EYEBROWS

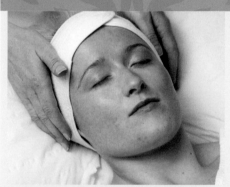

1 Position the magnifying lamp to give maximum visibility of the area. Ensure the client is comfortably positioned on the couch. Clean your hands. Secure a clean headband in place, to keep client's hair away from treatment area.

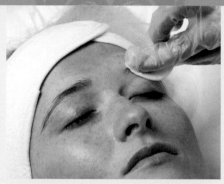

2 Working from behind or to the side of the client, cleanse the eyebrow area, using a lightweight cleansing lotion or non-oily, eye make-up remover.

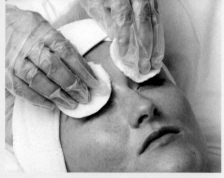

3 Apply a mild antiseptic lotion to two damp cotton wool pads, then gently wipe each eyebrow. This removes all grease from the area, so that the tweezers will not slip. The brow area should then be blotted dry, using a clean, folded facial tissue.

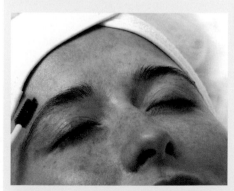

4 Brush the brow hair with the disposable brush, first *against* the natural hair growth, then with it. This enables you to define the brow shape and to observe the natural line.

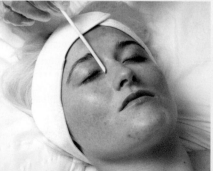

5 Measure the brows (using the guidelines described earlier). Best practice is to wear disposable gloves, as you may come into contact with body tissue fluid.

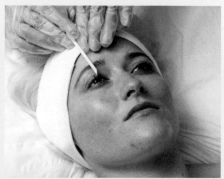

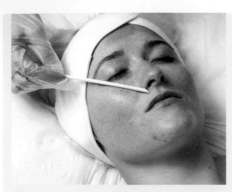

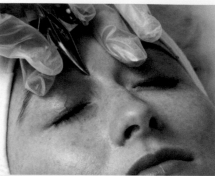

5 continued.

6 Place a clean piece of cotton wool in a convenient position for collecting the removed hairs, for instance at the top of the couch next to the client's head, some therapists wrap tissue or damp cotton wool around their finger to collect hairs. Begin tweezing, using a sterilised pair of automatic tweezers. These are designed to remove hairs quickly and efficiently, and are therefore used for the bulk of the hair identified for removal. It is usual to start at the bridge of the nose: the skin here is less sensitive than under the brow line.

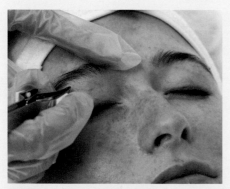

7 Gently stretch the skin between the index and middle fingers, pressing lightly onto the skin. This will help you to avoid accidentally nipping the skin; it will also open the mouth of the **hair follicle** and minimise discomfort to the client.

Hairs should be removed individually, and the tweezers should be wiped regularly on the pad of clean cotton wool used to collect the removed hairs.

Remove the hairs from underneath the outer edge of the brow, working inwards towards the nose. It is advisable to work on each brow alternately. This ensures that the brows are evenly shaped; it also reduces prolonged discomfort in any one area during shaping. Hairs should ideally be removed only from *below* the brow, otherwise the natural line may be lost. It is sometimes necessary, however, to remove the odd stray hair growing *above* the natural line.

During shaping, show the client their brows in a mirror, to confirm the shape and so that you can avoid removing too much hair.

8 Remove the hairs quickly, in the direction of growth. This prevents the hairs from breaking off at the skin's surface. Hair breakage can be seen to have occurred if a stubbly regrowth appears 1 or 2 days after shaping. Incorrect removal may also cause distortion of the hair follicle, or result in the hair becoming trapped under the skin as it starts to regrow (see section on ingrowing hair in Chapter 8 Wax depilation).

9 Long hairs may be trimmed with scissors if necessary. Using an eyebrow brush, brush the brow hair, hold the hair in place and then trim the hairs that you wish to shorten.

Any discoloured, coarse, long, curly or wavy hairs may be removed, as long as this does not alter the line or leave a bald patch.

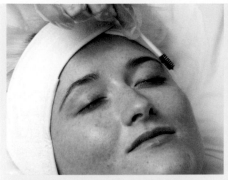
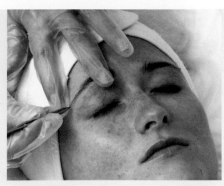
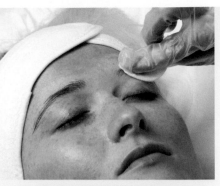

10 At regular intervals during shaping, brush the brows to check their shape. Apply antiseptic lotion or gel to a clean, dampened cotton wool pad, and wipe this gently over the eyebrow tissue to reduce sensitivity and to clean the area.

11 When the bulk of excess hair has been removed, manual tweezers may be used to take away any stray hairs and to define the line.

12 On completion of brow shaping, wipe the eyebrows with the antiseptic soothing lotion or gel, applied with clean, damp cotton wool. Apply a mild antiseptic lotion or cream to the area, using clean, dry cotton wool, to reduce the possibility of secondary infection.

13 The hairs that have been removed should be disposed of hygienically.

14 Brush the brows into shape and show the client the finished effect. The client may wish further hairs to be removed. Ask them to identify these. If you think this would be unsuitable explain why.

15 Record details of the service on the client's record. Advise the client on skincare preparations, procedures and techniques to enhance the brows to follow at home.

TOP TIP

Hair root!

Hairs removed in the anagen stage of hair growth will exhibit a root and inner root sheath on removal. A hair correctly tweezed from the hair follicle is shown here.

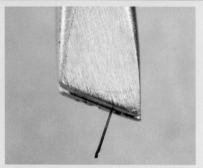

Hair correctly tweezed from the hair follicle

TOP TIP

Atchoo!

Occasionally clients start sneezing when you tweeze hairs at the bridge of the nose. If this happens, leave this area till last.

TOP TIP

Manual pointed tweezers

Manual pointed tweezers are effective at removing those difficult to remove short, coarse hairs.

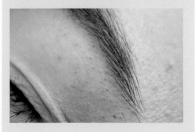

HEALTH & SAFETY

Soothing lotion

Care should be taken when applying soothing lotion. If too much is applied it may run and enter the eye, causing further discomfort. It is often best to apply a small amount of soothing lotion to a clean cotton wool pad, remembering to use a separate one for each eye to avoid cross-infection.

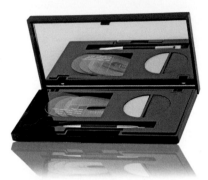

Retail Brow cosmetic kit

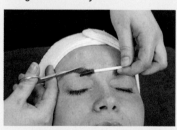

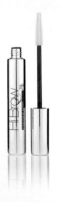

Eyebrow growth and conditioning serum

Client advice and recommendations

Advise the client to receive the treatment as follows:

◆ eyebrow maintenance every one to two weeks

◆ eyebrow reshaping every three to four weeks.

While a client receives an eyebrow shape it is an ideal opportunity to promote other eye treatment services. These include tuition in brow artistry and selling templates and brow colours to achieve the required look; eyebrow waxing; **threading**; tinting; and **eyelash enhancement attachment systems.** Remember a skin sensitivity patch test will be required before certain services.

Retail products can be recommended such as specialist skincare, non-oily eye make-up remover and eye gel.

An eyebrow pencil, which is usually a blend of waxes with a non-oily formula, or brow powder cosmetic can be recommended to emphasise the new eyebrow shape or disguise bald patches in the brows, e.g. scars. Sparse eyebrows can be made to appear thicker. It can also be used to stimulate hairs, or when the length of the brow needs to be increased. Colour choice should always complement natural hair colour. Darker colour may be selected to create a dramatic effect appropriate for evening make-up looks.

> "Always be honest with clients; I never recommend a product or treatment they don't need. However, if they do need it, I will explain the benefits and impact it can have. Relevant link selling when a client is in the chair exposes them to new products/ treatments they had previously not considered."
>
> *Shavata Singh*

A colourless wax is available to shape and fix brow shapes. An invisible layer of wax remains on the eyebrows, maintaining the desired shape all day long. Eyebrow wax may contain argan oil, a popular hair conditioner ingredient, vitamin E and aloe vera to moisturise dry brow hair. Clear brow gels can be applied to keep the hair in shape when brushed.

An oil-based cleansing product may be required to effectively remove pencil and brow powder, especially if waterproof products are used.

A brow enhancing serum may be recommended to condition the brow hair.

Eyebrow make-up tools, such as a brush with comb to blend colour and shape the brow and angled brushes to create the brow shape may be recommended.

Explain to the client that they should only remove hairs every two to three weeks to establish a removal routine in line with the **hair growth cycle**. You may recommend retail tweezers for this purpose.

Explain how to care for the area following the eyebrow shaping treatment to avoid an unwanted reaction – a contra-action. Advise the client not to wear eye make-up for at least six hours following the eyebrow-shaping treatment. The hair follicle has been damaged where the hair has been removed, effectively torn out from the skin: it will be at risk of infection unless the area is cared for while it heals. It should not be necessary for the client to continue using antiseptic preparations at home, but they should be advised to carry out these instructions if discomfort or continued reddening occurs:

1 Explain to the client the action to take in the event of a contra-action.

2 Cleanse the eyebrow area using a mild antiseptic lotion or witch hazel, applied with a small piece of clean, dampened cotton wool.

3 Apply an antiseptic soothing lotion, cream or gel with clean, dry cotton wool.

4 Gently remove excess antiseptic lotion, cream or gel using a clean, soft facial tissue or clean damp cotton wool.

5 Repeat as necessary, approximately every 4 hours. *If the reddening does not subside in the next 24 hours, contact the salon*.

6 Although brow make-up can be applied to brow hair where hair has not been removed, advise client that further eye make-up on the upper lid should only be worn when the redness has gone – usually after 8 hours.

"Practice excellent customer service:

◆ Promote great grooming.

◆ Be passionate about eyebrows.

◆ A successful beauty therapist will have a natural talent with people.

◆ Stay level-headed.

◆ Be precise."

Shavata Singh

Eyebrow artistry

This should be selected to suit the client's colouring, characteristics and the eyebrow appearance agreed at consultation. Eyebrow artistry techniques will both colour and define the overall shape. This will be achieved using the following tools, equipment and products:

◆ Permanent tint mixed with hydrogen peroxide. Permanent tint is applied before hair removal as it colours the hairs (and stains the skin temporarily) in the area.

◆ Temporary colour, available in a range of colours, applied with a cosmetic brow pencil; brow powder, which may be mixed and used in conjunction with translucent wax (when applied, this fixes the brow powder and grooms the brow hair into shape). Some products have waterproof properties to improve durability.

◆ Brow templates may be placed over the natural brows, used to outline, or create a silhouette to fill in the new brow colour and shape temporarily. A block colour is not necessarily required; it may be texture that is to be achieved by simulating hairs with additional colour and tones.

◆ Brow brush used to groom and define the brow hairs and blend the colour.

◆ Small angled brush to apply brow powder to outline the brow shape and add colour to the skin within the brow using feathery strokes.

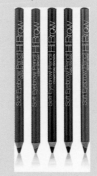

A mirror is required for instructional purposes and when demonstrating how the client is to achieve the new shape.

Temporary brow colour is applied after shaping.

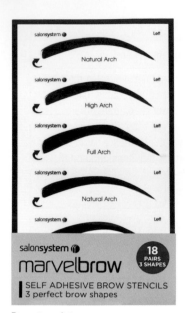

Brow templates

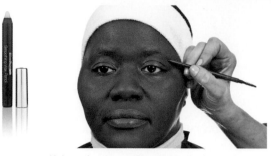

Waterproof brow fix

Using a brow pencil to create the brow shape on sparse brow growth

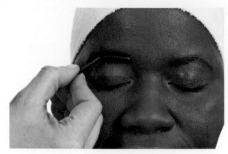

Using a brush to soften and blend the brow pencil

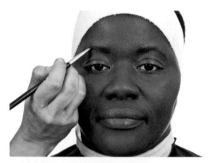

Applying a brow powder with angled brush to colour and set the look

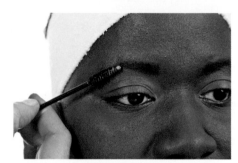

Clear brow gel applied with waterproof properties and to extend durability

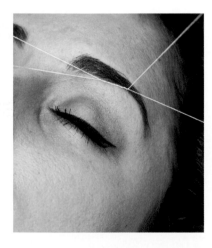

Threading

Hair can also be removed from the eyebrows using a popular technique called **threading**.

During a threading treatment a loop of twisted cotton thread is passed across the skin to trap the hairs and so 'pluck' them from the hair follicles. There are three main techniques of threading: the mouth, neck and hand techniques.

INDUSTRY ROLE MODEL

LORRAINE ONORATO Founder and Principal of The National School of Threading

What do you find rewarding about your job? I find it rewarding to observe learners at the beginning of their journey into the industry and then seeing them flourish.

What do you find challenging about your job? I don't find anything a challenge as long as I am prepared and willing to adapt and adjust, so flexibility is important in order to deal with new situations as they arise.

What makes a good beauty therapist? Compassion, confidence, knowledge and excellent skills combined with a willingness to continue learning throughout your career.

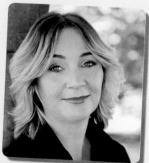

ALWAYS REMEMBER

Transferable knowledge understanding and skills

When providing threading services it is important to use the skills you have learnt in the following units:

◆ The Business of Beauty Therapy (Chapter 1)

◆ The Science of Beauty Therapy (Chapter 2)

◆ Consultation, Practice and Techniques (Chapter 3).

Threading is a relatively inexpensive and effective method of hair removal. Unwanted hair is removed with minimal pain and skin irritation. Neat results are achieved with hair regrowth usually seen in approximately two to six weeks dependent upon the rate of hair growth. Threading effectively removes very short hair with little irritation to the skin as the thread only removes the hair – not the skin surface as in the wax depilation technique. This advantage also makes it possible to go over the treatment area more than once. Hair can be removed individually or in 'lines', creating a precise, defined shape with hair removed from both above and below the eyebrow, giving the threaded eyebrow its characteristic defined shape and appearance. Threading is also beneficial to those individuals that have undergone strong acne treatments, e.g. roaccutane, retin-A, where the skin becomes very delicate, or those that have other contra-indications to waxing, i.e. allergies to ingredients contained in the wax, such as resin.

TOP TIP

Gentle on the skin

Threading creates less trauma on the skin than other hair removal treatments, e.g. waxing, which can cause irritation from heat, allergic reactions and possible skin removal.

Threading advantages	Threading disadvantages
◆ Only removes hair not skin.	◆ Some clients may experience side-effects following the treatment, these include excessive skin reddening (erythema) and short-term puffiness of the skin tissue treated.
◆ Good for removal of short hairs.	
◆ Can isolate one hair at a time.	
◆ Can go over an area more than once without causing skin irritation.	
◆ Sharp, defined shape can be achieved.	◆ The area may be uncomfortable for a short while.
◆ Inexpensive to perform as minimal resources required.	◆ Itching may occur following hair removal.
◆ Fast results.	◆ Ingrowing hair may occur when the hair regrows or as a result of poor technique.
◆ Good for eyebrows and facial hair.	◆ Infections may occur (e.g. **folliculitis**), if homecare advice is not followed as the follicle will remain open for up to 24 hours following the service.
◆ Minimal skin irritation – good for delicate, sensitive skin types.	

Thread

A specialist 100 per cent cotton thread is used for threading. This thread allows strength but resilience during the treatment, which is important in order to perform threading to a high standard.

ALWAYS REMEMBER

History of threading

Threading is an ancient manual method of temporary hair removal, similar to tweezing. Threading has been used for many centuries. Its origin is a little uncertain but it is believed that it was originally used in Arabia, Turkey and India.

HEALTH & SAFETY

Extra protection

Ensure you use a specialist cotton that has an anti-bacterial coating as conventional 'sewing' thread can cause injury to the skin.

Specialist threading thread has an anti-bacterial coating added to it during the manufacture process, giving further protection to the skin while performing the treatment and so reducing the risk of infection.

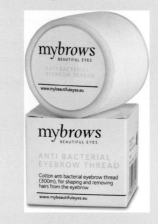

REVISION AID

What is the indention in the skin that a hair grows from?

"Be on time and prepared for your treatment, after all we expect our clients to be on time!"

Lorraine Onorato

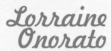

Like tweezing, threading can be combined with other eye treatments to enhance the overall result that can be achieved. A good example would be to apply eyebrow artistry, using tint, cosmetic powder and pencils to colour and define the brow shape.

For male grooming, an **eyebrow threading** treatment can be combined with a barbering treatment. Hair can also be removed from the tops of the cheeks, nose and ears.

Preparing the work area for threading

Before beginning threading, check that you have the necessary products, tools and equipment to hand and that they meet the legal hygiene and industry requirements for threading service. Check the suitability of the environmental conditions. Good ventilation and lighting are important.

Products, tools and equipment

Each threading work area should have the following **basic equipment** listed below, plus the further supplementary products, tools and equipment relevant to the threading treatment.

Products, tools and equipment

- **Client chair or service couch with neck and foot support** A the correct working height for the beauty therapist to carry out the treatment.

- **Equipment trolley or work surface** On which to place products, tools and related equipment.

- **Beauty stool** Adjustable height, back support and covered in a fabric similar to that covering the couch.

- **Step-up stool** To assist clients as necessary to position themselves on the couch.

- **Disposable tissue roll** To protect the clean, disinfected work surfaces and client clothing at the neck area.

- **Headband** A clean headband should be provided for each client to secure hair away from the area. You may alternatively use a hair clip to avoid spoiling the hair.

- **Towel drapes** A small hand towel may be draped across the client's chest and shoulders. Alternatively paper tissue may be used, replaced for each client.

- **Hand disinfectant** Usually containing chlorhexidine, to cleanse and disinfect the hands as required following hand washing.

- **Single use disposable non-latex (synthetic) powder-free gloves** such as nitrile or PVC formulation may be worn to ensure a high standard of hygiene and to reduce the possibility of contamination during service application.

- **Towel** A clean towel should be available for you to wipe your hands on as necessary.

- **Spatulas** Several clean spatulas (preferably disposable) in a range of sizes, should be provided for each client. One should be used for tucking any stray hair beneath the headband. Others will be used in removing products from their containers and for applying products to the skin.

- **Cotton wool** There should be a plentiful supply of both damp and dry cotton wool, used to apply cleansing and soothing skincare preparations.

- **Tissues** These should be stored in a covered container. They are used for blotting the area dry and occasionally the client's eyes may water so a tissue may be placed at the corner of the eyes.

- **Disinfectant** For storing **sterile tweezers and scissors** that may be used in the service.

- **Covered waste bin** It should have an easy-to-clean surface. The best choice is a stainless steel, foot-operated bin.

- **Hand mirror** Maintained in a clean condition and used in consulting with the client before, during and after their service.

- **Bowls** To store dry and damp cotton wool.

- **Client treatment record** Confidential record with details of each client, including personal details, products used, retail purchases made and details of each treatment.

Specialist threading equipment and materials Before beginning the service, check that you have the necessary equipment and materials to hand and that they meet legal hygiene and industry requirements for threading services.

◆ **Bright lighting** and **magnifying lamp** A magnifying lamp enlarges visibility of the area when assessing client suitability for treatment and their service requirements. The magnifying lamp is also essential when performing an eyebrow threading to ensure a clean result free from superfluous, unwanted hair is achieved.

◆ **Specialist threading thread** To remove hair with threading technique.

◆ **Powder** Purified talc or other specialist powder supplied by the manufacturer for threading.

◆ **Specialist stainless steel eyebrow trimming scissors** For trimming long hairs.

◆ **Disinfected or disposable brow brush** To brush the eyebrows into shape before, during and after treatment.

◆ **Client treatment record** For recording confidential details of each client registered at the salon, including the client's personal details, products used and details of the service including any modifications to how the service was performed and why.

The work area should always be prepared and maintained throughout the day, ready for further treatments.

Safety and hygiene

◆ Client hair and clothing should be protected and any clothing and accessories removed where necessary from the area. If the client has brow piercings these should be removed. However, as part of the consultation, check when the piercing was completed. Eyebrow piercing can take between two to four months to heal so the area should not be treated during this period as there is a risk of infection.

◆ Always wash hands before treatment. Wear disposable gloves to avoid cross-infection when possible. However, gloves may hinder technique.

◆ Ensure the skin is clean and grease free. Apply a mild alcohol skin disinfectant to the area.

◆ Ensure that the client's hands do not come into contact with the area being treated whilst stretching the skin, to avoid the possibility of contamination, which could lead to infection.

◆ Prepare a new piece of thread for each treatment area.

◆ Metal tools such as scissors and tweezers must be sterilised before each use on a client.

◆ Maintain accepted industry hygiene and safety practices throughout the treatment.

> "To avoid cross-infection change your thread between each facial area that you are treating and always between clients."
>
> *Lorraine Onorato*

TOP TIP

Powder

Cornflour is traditionally used as an alternative to talc, to dry the skin, absorbing any moisture and lift the hair from the skin before the treatment. Some threading specialists use the powder to ensure the smooth gliding of the thread on the skin's surface.

HEALTH & SAFETY

Hand cleanliness

Before beginning treatment for a new client always wash your hands with an antibacterial cleanser or apply a disinfectant hand gel to clean hands, preferably in front of the client.

HEALTH & SAFETY

Hygiene

Disposable mascara brushes can be used to brush the eyebrows as an alternative to a brow brush, which can then be hygienically disposed of immediately after use.

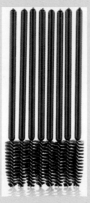

HEALTH & SAFETY

Waste

Contaminated waste must be disposed of in accordance with the environmental health department of your local council.

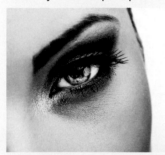
Client care, consultation and communication skills

Discuss the client's requirements, identifying and agreeing shape, thickness and area for hair removal. Also discuss what is realistically achievable with the threading treatment, both short- and long-term. Always be realistic in your recommendations and take the opportunity to discuss other eyebrow services that may enhance the look achieved. Take into consideration the client's eye and face shape.

Treatment information to provide to clients at initial point of interest When a client makes an appointment for a threading treatment, the receptionist will need to check whether the client has received the treatment before. This is to allow for the consultation time, which is usually 10–15 minutes. They must also check which area the client requires threading to book sufficient time.

As contact lenses should be removed when performing eyebrow threading, inform the client of this in order that they can store them safely on removal.

The client will often ask 'is it painful?' The answer is that threading is like tweezing but is much quicker, therefore overall, the client should experience less pain than when tweezing.

All staff, especially staff communicating with clients at reception, should be familiar with the different pricing structures for the range of threading treatments and products available for retail.

Commercially, 20 minutes is allowed for threading for an **eyebrow reshape**.

Consultation Explain to the client that they will be required to support the skin to assist hair removal as instructed. You may wish to demonstrate this to confirm understanding at consultation. Encourage clients to ask questions to clarify any points.

Check client suitability, certain contra-indications will prevent or restrict threading.

If the client is a **minor** under the age of 16, it is necessary to obtain parent/guardian permission for the threading treatment. The parent, carer or guardian will also have to be present when the treatment is received.

Discuss with the client the preferred shape they would like to achieve. Refer to the earlier section in this chapter 'Choosing an eyebrow shape' for detailed information on how to measure a client's eyebrows for eyebrow shaping services and how to decide on a shape to suit the client's face shape and features.

"Always greet clients with a friendly smile and consult with your client at eye level and with adequate eye contact."

Lorraine Onorato

Contra-indications

Although threading is considered to be more suitable for individuals with skin sensitivities resulting from conditions like psoriasis, eczema, dermatitis and diabetes, as with all hair removal techniques **contra-indications** will apply and will be the same as other hair removal techniques (e.g. waxing and tweezing, refer to the section entitled *Contra-indications* earlier in this Chapter, and Chapter 8 Wax Depilation).

Contra-actions

There is also the possibility that **contra-actions** to treatments may arise. This can be avoided by ensuring a thorough consultation prior to the treatment to assess a client's suitability for the treatment and giving clear aftercare advice and instructions on completion of the treatment.

Examples of possible contra-actions:

◆ **folliculitis**

◆ **erythema**

◆ ingrowing hairs

◆ blood spots

◆ broken hair

◆ histamine (allergic reaction)

◆ severe swelling

◆ excessive erythema.

The treatment record should be signed and dated following the **consultation** to confirm client suitability and consent with the agreed threading treatment. Existing clients will need to indicate whether there have been any changes since their last treatment, including their health and any medication taken, which must also be noted down on their record.

Preparation of the client

Preparation of the client for treatment is as important as the preparation of the beauty therapist and must be carried out thoroughly and professionally.

Escort the client to the treatment area and assist with removal of clothing/accessories, e.g. jewellery, scarves, etc. and help the client onto the treatment couch/chair where necessary. Ensure that they are comfortable and positioned at the correct height for you to work.

Confirm the required hair removal discussed at consultation and advise further, where necessary.

Disinfect your hands and, if worn, put on disposable gloves.

Threading techniques

There are three techniques that are commonly used mouth, neck and hand.

1 **Mouth technique** Hair removal using thread where one part of the thread is anchored in the mouth, held between the teeth and lips and the other part is looped in the hands. The loop is created by twisting the middle section of the thread four times; this loop will be used to remove hairs. Using the index and middle fingers of the working hand, the loop is widened and drawn over the skin's surface. The thread is then opened by widening the fingers and thumb of one hand, this action removes the hair. This is the most commonly used technique, originating from the Far East and is also known as the Asian or single loop method.

HEALTH & SAFETY

Contra-action

A contra-action is what may occur as a result of the treatment. This must be discussed at consultation and must be indicated on the client's record where appropriate, with action taken recorded.

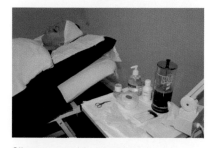

Client prepared for treatment

HEALTH & SAFETY

Personal protective equipment

PPE is recommended to be worn to prevent cross- and secondary infection.

REVISION AID

What should be the qualities of the thread used for hair removal?

TOP TIP

Client sensitivity

If the client is particularly sensitive, warm water cotton pads may be applied to the area before removal to open the hair follicles, facilitating hair removal and reducing discomfort.

ALWAYS REMEMBER

Mouth technique can also be termed Asian or 'single loop method'.

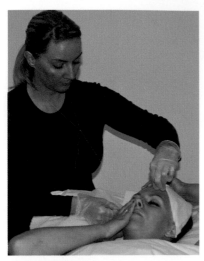

The neck technique

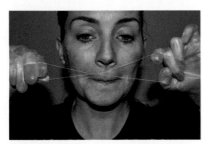

The hand technique (self-threading)

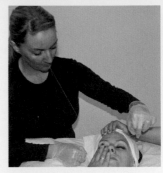

The mouth technique

2 **Neck technique** A substitute for the mouth technique where one part of the thread is anchored around the neck and the other part is looped in the hands as described above. This technique originates from the Middle East and is also known as the Arabian or single loop method.

3 **Hand technique** Hair removal using thread which is held between the index and middle finger of one hand and then the other hand twists the looped thread. The action of widening the thread with the index finger and thumb of one hand traps and removes the hairs as it is moved over the area. Commonly used by practitioners on themselves. This technique is also known as cat's cradle, doubled loop method or self technique.

STEP-BY-STEP: EYEBROW THREADING TREATMENT

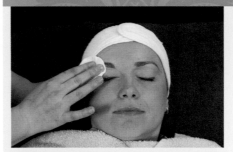

Cleansing the area

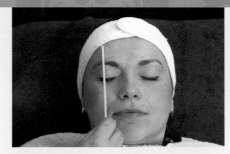

Identifying placement of the eyebrow arch

1 First remove any skin debris, facial creams or cosmetic products, if worn, from the area to be treated using damp clean cotton wool. Then use a professional skin cleanser followed by a skin disinfecting product, e.g. a mild formulation of ethanol, to ensure the area is grease free; blot dry with a clean tissue, disposing of both in a lined metal waste bin. Moisture left on the area will reduce the effectiveness of the thread gripping the hair.

2 Brush the eyebrows in an upwards and then downwards direction to ensure the hairs are laying flat, and trim any long hairs that may spoil the finished result. Brush eyebrows back into place.

You may decide to measure the eyebrows in order to decide the correct length and where the arch should commence to complement both eye and face shape. Brow measurement is discussed earlier in this chapter under the section 'How to measure the eyebrows to decide length'.

3 With a clean piece of cotton wool, apply a light dusting of recommended threading powder (optional) to the area – this will enable the thread to glide over the skin and is particularly good when the skin is warm and moist.

4 Decide on the technique of threading to be used and prepare the cotton. Shorter lengths of thread are easier to handle whilst developing your skills or if you have small hands.

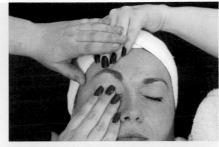

Positioning the client's hands to support the eye area during eyebrow threading

5 The client must now support the area to be treated – for eyebrows one hand should be over the eye and one over the top of the eyebrow. Support the client's hand when positioning it into place, explaining the purpose – to prevent the skin being pinched or cut by the thread.

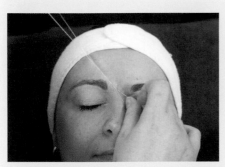

Thread against hair growth, hair removal above the brow

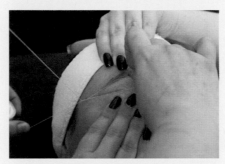

Hair removal below the brow

6 The hairs are removed against the direction of hair growth as the loop closes, in the 'V' shape area of the thread. The thread is firmly placed onto the skin ensuring even tension throughout the treatment. This will enable effective and accurate removal of the hair from the root, avoiding snapping while reducing any discomfort to the client.

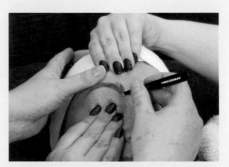

Threading performed between the eyebrows

Tweezers used to define the finished look

6 Remove all hairs as necessary, using the thread to brush away any loose ones dropping onto the skin during the treatment. Keep checking the threaded area to ensure symmetry of both eyebrows. If completing a reshape show the client the eyebrow shape as the treatment progresses to ensure client satisfaction.

7 Tweezers may be used to create the precise, defined look to complete the service.

HEALTH & SAFETY

Checking area for modification requirements

When preparing the eyebrows for threading, whilst brushing through the hair check for further treatment considerations, such as scarring in the eyebrows. Inform the client if identified.

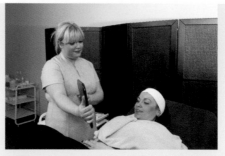

Confirm satisfaction with the finished look

8 Brush the eyebrows into shape and show your client the finished result.

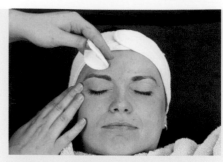

Application of aftercare skincare product

9 On completion of the treatment and when the outcome is to the client's satisfaction apply a soothing, antiseptic aftercare product to the area using clean cotton wool to remove loose hairs, reduce any redness and soothe the skin. This consumable waste is immediately disposed of into a lined, covered bin.

10 Assist client from the treatment chair/couch and provide appropriate aftercare advice and recommendations.

TOP TIP

Threading direction

Ensure that you are always removing hair against the direction of hair growth. This will avoid client discomfort and best results following the treatment.

TOP TIP

Trimming hairs

Eyebrow hairs may be trimmed (especially if long) by first brushing the hair in an upwards direction. The point of the scissors should be angled towards the bridge of the nose with the shank laying flat to the skin's surface. The long hair is then trimmed to match the length of the other eyebrow hair. This process is then repeated underneath the eyebrow by brushing the hair in a downwards direction.

TOP TIP

Managing different hair types

Different hair densities will require an adjustment of tension in the thread, e.g. coarser hair (terminal hair type) requires more tension to remove from the root without snapping it.

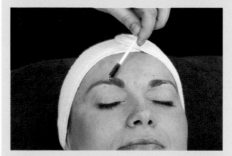

Brushing brow hair

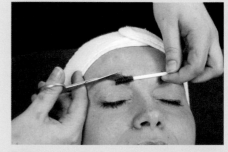

Trimming brow hair

ALWAYS REMEMBER

Although tweezers can be used to help create the finished look, do remember that threading alone should be all that is needed to create the perfect definition.

ALWAYS REMEMBER

Poor technique

Poor technique may result in hair breakage. This results in hair that will reappear quickly in the area with an appearance as if it has been shaved, and will feel bristly as it will have a blunt, rather than a tapered end.

TOP TIP

Client satisfaction

To ensure client satisfaction, especially when re-shaping a thick eyebrow shape, it is advisable to show the client the shape as it is developing.

TOP TIP

Retail opportunities

On completion of the treatment you could recommend a retail product or further eye service, e.g. a soothing massage to the eye area with a suitable aftercare cream to enhance the treatment.

Client Advice and recommendations

For the next 12–24 hours it is important to avoid activities or actions that could lead to skin irritation or infection.

Follow aftercare advice and recommendations as given for eyebrow shaping earlier in this chapter under the section 'Client advice and recommendations.'

To avoid ingrowing hairs it is important to keep the area moisturised and **gently exfoliate** the area after three days and twice weekly thereafter. These products must be suitable for facial use.

"Following an eyebrow threading treatment spend a few minutes with the client discussing and demonstrating how the eyebrows can be enhanced and defined. Use this opportunity to retail your eyebrow kits, gels, pencils and specialist products and further services."

Lorraine Onorato

If needed, the area can be soothed with either a recommended product or a soothing and calming product, e.g. aloe vera gel.

Recommend the application of cosmetic colour to define the brows, especially if the brow hair is sparse or a different shape is to be achieved requiring additional hair growth. This may be a brow pencil or brow powder of a suitable colour.

Recommend other services that will further enhance the eye area such as tinting to the eyebrow/eyelashes and eyelash enhancement. Remember a skin sensitivity patch test will be required before certain services.

If there is a contra-action following treatment, advise the client what appropriate action should be taken. Advise the client to receive the treatment in the specified time according to their hair growth cycle. Repeat bookings vary according to the natural hair regrowth and client requirements.

Ensure that the client's records are up-to-date, accurate and complete following the threading treatment. Provide written instructions in an aftercare leaflet.

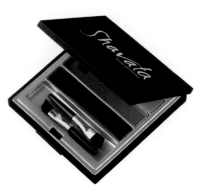

Retail cosmetic colour to define the brows

"Where possible give added value to the client during a treatment. Performing just a 3-minute eyebrow massage makes all the difference and will keep them returning and recommending."

Lorraine Onorato

ALWAYS REMEMBER

Appointments

Schedule the client's next appointment as part of the aftercare advice.

REVISION AID

Why is gentle exfoliation beneficial to the treated area between threading treatments?

HEALTH & SAFETY

Cross-contamination

To avoid cross-contamination, ensure all disposables and waste are put immediately into the bin and not left exposed on the surface of the work area.

REVISION AID

What other services complement eyebrow shaping?

Eyebrow and eyelash tinting

The hair of the eyelashes and eyebrows protects the eyes from moisture and dust, but the lashes and brows also give definition to the eye. Many clients, especially those with fair lashes and brows, feel that without the use of eye enhancement their eyes lack this definition.

Further definition of the brow and lash hair can be created if a permanent dye is applied to them. Most clients, apart from those with very dark hair, will benefit from **eyebrow and eyelash tinting** because the tips and the bases of these hairs are usually lighter than the body of the hairs, causing the hairs to appear shorter than they actually are. Tinting the length of the lash or brow hair makes it appear longer and bolder, yet the effect created if required can look natural.

Because the eye tissue around the eye area is very thin and sensitive, dyes designed for permanently tinting the hair in this area have been specially formulated to avoid any eye or tissue reactions. *The application of any other dye materials in this area is dangerous, and may even lead to blindness*.

Permanent tints are available in different forms, including jelly, liquid and cream tints. The most popular and acceptable permanent tinting product is the cream tint: this formulation is thicker, so that it does not run into the eye and it is easy to control during mixing, application and removal.

Several colours of tint are available, including brown, grey, blue and black.

If the shade you want is not available, you can vary the shade of available tints by leaving the dye on the hair for different lengths of time, or by mixing different colours together. For example mix blue with black, to produce a navy blue colour, leave the tint to process for three to five minutes; if left to process for ten minutes, the same tint will produce a raven blue-black colour.

TOP TIP

Blue tint

When a client requests a blue eyelash tint, make clear that this will not produce an 'electric blue' fashion colour.

HEALTH & SAFETY

Using safe permanent tinting products

Always use a tint that is permitted for use under EU regulations and complies with the Cosmetic Products (Enforcement) Regulations 2013. If you use any other tint your insurance may be invalid.

The development of colour

Two products are essential for the permanent tinting treatment:

◆ professional **eyebrow** or **eyelash tint**

◆ **hydrogen peroxide (H_2O_2).**

The tint usually contains small molecules of permanent dye called **toluenediamine**. These need to be 'activated' before their colouring effect becomes permanent: this is achieved by the addition of hydrogen peroxide. The peroxide is said to **develop** the colour of the tint.

Chemically, hydrogen peroxide is an **oxidant**, a chemical that contains available oxygen atoms and encourages certain chemical reactions – in this case, tinting.

The hydrogen peroxide container will state either its volume or its percentage strength. To activate the tint and for safe use around the eye area, a 3% or 10-volume strength peroxide is used.

When you add the hydrogen peroxide to the tint, the small dye molecules together form large molecules, which remain trapped in the **cortex** of the hair. The hair is thus permanently coloured, but in time, as it continues to grow, the new hair will show the natural colour.

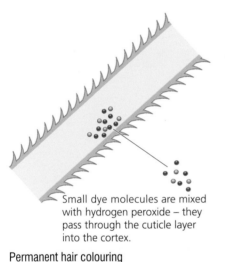

Small dye molecules are mixed with hydrogen peroxide – they pass through the cuticle layer into the cortex.

Small dye molecules swell and join together, becoming permanently trapped in the cortex of the hair.

Permanent hair colouring

HEALTH & SAFETY

Hydrogen peroxide strength

Do not use a higher strength than 10-volume or 3% hydrogen peroxide. If you do, skin irritation or minor skin burning may occur.

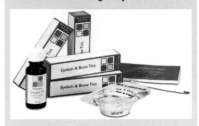

ALWAYS REMEMBER

Hydrogen peroxide

Replace the cap of the hydrogen peroxide container *immediately* after use, or the peroxide will lose its strength.

Preparing the work area for permanent tinting

Specialist products, tools and equipment

Before beginning the permanent tinting treatment, check that you have the necessary products, tools and equipment to hand and that they meet legal hygiene and industry requirements for eye treatments. You will need all of the basic products, tools and equipment listed for eyebrow and lash treatments earlier in the chapter as well as the following specialist equipment:

◆ **Coloured tints (a selection)** Usually in black, blue, brown and grey.

◆ **Disposable cosmetic lip and mascara brushes** To aid application of eyebrow and eyelash tint and to comb through the brow/lash hair before and following treatment.

◆ **Cotton buds** To remove make-up and excess tint from around the eye. They may also be used to apply products such as petroleum jelly.

◆ **Headband (clean)** To protect long hair or bleached hair from accidental contact with the tint.

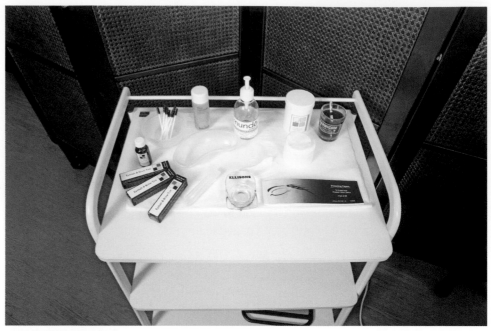

Work surface prepared for tinting of eyebrows and/or eyelashes

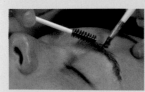
◆ **Eye make-up remover (non-oily)** To cleanse the eye area before treatment application removing make-up if worn, skin debris and natural oils.

◆ **Hydrogen peroxide** (10-volume/3%).

◆ **Petroleum jelly** To protect the skin and prevent skin staining.

◆ **Eye shields (commercial) or cotton wool pads** To prevent skin staining during eyelash tinting.

◆ **Disposable non-latex (synthetic), powder-free gloves** To provide protection from skin staining and to be worn if allergic to permanent tint products.

◆ **Non-metallic bowl** For mixing the permanent tint (note that some metals cause immediate release of the oxygen from the hydrogen peroxide, causing ineffective processing of the tint).

◆ **Skin stain remover** To remove any accidental staining to the skin.

Preparation of the work area

Before the client is shown through to the work area, it should be checked to ensure that the required products, tools and equipment for tinting are available and the area is clean and tidy.

Clean and protect the treatment couch or beauty chair as for the eyebrow-shaping treatment. The treatment couch or chair should be flat or slightly elevated.

The work area should be adequately lit to ensure that service can be given safely, but avoid bright lighting that could cause eye irritation leading to eye watering.

Always follow your workplace policy for preparation of the work area.

Safety and hygiene

◆ It is necessary to use disposable applicators for the application of the petroleum jelly and the tint because it is impossible to disinfect brushes effectively. Disposable make-up lip brushes are ideal for the application of petroleum jelly and disposable make-up lip brushes are ideal for tint application.

◆ Disposable gloves may be worn for protection to avoid skin staining and if you are allergic to the tint.

◆ Dispense products hygienically from containers, e.g. use a clean disposable or plastic disinfected spatula to remove skin barrier product petroleum jelly before use.

◆ Clean the tint bowl immediately following use with hot, soapy water, dry and disinfect.

◆ A negative skin sensitivity patch test result must be obtained before this treatment is carried out.

Treatment information to provide to clients at initial point of interest

The following points are important for the receptionist to consider when booking a client for permanent tinting treatment.

◆ When making an appointment for this service, allow five minutes for a skin sensitivity patch test.

Ask the client to visit the workplace 24 hours before the appointment for a skin sensitivity patch test. How to carry out a skin test is discussed in the Health & Safety box and below.

◆ When a new client makes an appointment for a treatment, always allocate extra time for the consultation beforehand.

◆ Explain to the client how long they should allow for the appointment. When making an appointment for brow tinting allow 10 minutes, and 20 minutes for an eyelash tint.

◆ Brow and lash tinting may be carried out as independent or combined treatments. For a combined treatment allow 30 minutes.

◆ If brow shaping is to be included, this is completed following tinting. Allow a further 15 minutes for this.

◆ If the client informs you of poor health, or is taking medication that may affect their skin or hair condition, it may not be possible to treat them until the medical condition has been treated by their GP. Tactfully check client suitability, this may involve seeking guidance from others.

◆ If they wear contact lenses, ask the client to bring their lens container so that they can safely store the lenses in it during the tinting service.

◆ On average, a client will need their lashes tinted every six weeks, or sooner if, for example, they take a holiday in a climate where sun bleaches them. Eyebrow tinting, on the other hand, should be repeated when the client feels it to be necessary, perhaps every four weeks, as eyebrows seem to lose colour intensity more quickly than lash hair.

ACTIVITY

Choosing brow and lash colours

Which colour do you think would be most suitable for the eyelashes and eyebrows of the following clients:

◆ dark hair
◆ fair hair
◆ red hair
◆ white/grey hair
◆ elderly client?

HEALTH & SAFETY

Skin sensitivity patch test

Each manufacturer will recommend how far in advance a skin sensitivity patch test must be received. You must comply with this requirement or your insurance will be invalidated. Check your manufacturer's instructions.

REVISION AID

What are the names of two active ingredients used when tinting the lashes/brows?

Skin sensitivity patch test

Some clients are sensitive to the tint, and produce an allergic reaction immediately on contact with it; others may become allergic later. For this reason you therefore need to carry out a **skin sensitivity patch test** 24–48 hours before each lash or brow tinting treatment. The National Occupational Standards state the guidance for sensitivity testing as per manufacturers' instructions.

A mixture of the hydrogen peroxide and tint colour to be used should be applied as recommended by the manufacturer to skin, which has been previously cleaned, on the inside of the elbow or behind the ear. Here the skin is thinner and is more likely to show an allergic response, if there is intolerance to the product used.

Two responses to the skin sensitivity patch test are possible – positive and negative:

◆ a **positive skin sensitivity patch test** result is recognised by irritation, swelling or inflammation of the skin – if this occurs, do not proceed with the treatment. The client should be advised to contact the salon in the instance of a positive skin sensitivity patch test result and the product should be removed immediately from the skin.

◆ a **negative skin sensitivity patch test** result produces no skin reaction – in this case you may proceed with the treatment.

In the instance of a positive skin sensitivity patch test, you could try an alternative product as the client may not be allergic to all tinting product ingredients.

Always record the date the skin sensitivity test is given, the result and products used.

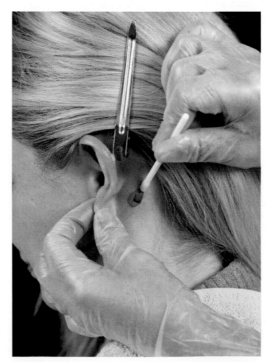

A skin sensitivity patch test for brow/lash tinting carried out behind the ear

Client care, consultation and communication skills

At the consultation, discuss the effect and appearance that the client would like to achieve. For the eyelashes and eyebrows, ideally aim to select a colour that complements the client's hair and skin colour, their age, and usual eye cosmetics if worn. Always discuss the choice of colour carefully with the client to discover their preference. You may ask certain questions in order to help in your selection:

◆ 'What colour mascara do you normally wear?'

◆ 'How dark would you like your eyelashes/eyebrows?'

◆ 'Do you normally wear eyebrow pencil? If so, what colour?'

◆ 'Have you had your eyebrows/lashes tinted before? Were you satisfied with the result? If not, why?'

Explain the treatment procedure and what sensations it is normal to experience and how the finished result should look.

Ask open questions to confirm client understanding about the treatment. For more information on asking open questions see Chapter 3.

Offer the opportunity and invite the client to ask you any questions.

Inform the client at consultation of any relevant contra-indications and contra-actions that may occur during or after the tinting treatment and the action to take. These are discussed next.

Contra-indications

When a client attends for an eyebrow or lash tinting treatment, you should always check that there are no contra-indications that might restrict or prevent treatment. Refer to the chart illustrating contra-indications to eye treatments earlier in this chapter. After completing the treatment plan record visually, inspect the eye area to confirm there are no contra-indications present.

Remember, you are not qualified to diagnose a contra-indication. Refer the client to their GP without creating unnecessary cause for concern.

In addition you must also check the following:

◆ **Results** of the skin sensitivity patch test – *a positive (allergic) reaction* to the skin sensitivity patch test, would contra-indicate treatment.

◆ *Contact lenses when carrying out eyelash tinting* (unless removed) The tint would cause irritation between the lens and the eye or dependent on the type, could tint the lens!

◆ A particularly nervous client would also be contra-indicated for the following reasons, which should be tactfully explained:

   ◆ it would be difficult for them to keep their eyes closed for 10 minutes

   ◆ they might become anxious as the tint was applied, creating the possibility of tint entering the eye

◆ they might blink frequently, making preparation of the eye area and application of the tint both difficult and hazardous.

Inform the client at consultation of any relevant contra-actions that may occur and the action to take.

Contra-actions

TOP TIP

Contra-action to eyelash tinting product resulting in a positive skin reaction

Source an alternative manufacturer. The client may not be allergic to all products if the cause of the contra-action is allergy.

If the client complains of discomfort during the treatment, tint may have entered the eye. Take the following action:

1 Remove the tint immediately from the eye area using clean, damp cotton wool pads in an outward sweep.

2 When you are satisfied that all excess tint has been removed (that is, when the cotton wool shows clean), carefully flush the eye with clean water. Repeat the rinsing process until discomfort has been relieved.

3 Apply a cool compress to cool and soothe the eye area.

If there is a noticeable sensitivity of the eye tissue after eyebrow or eyelash tinting it may be recommended that the client does not receive the treatment again. Alternatively, source an alternative tinting product to test compatibility. Record this on their treatment record so that the offending product may be avoided in the future.

In the event of an allergic contra-action following treatment the client should be advised to apply a cool compress and soothing agent to the skin to reduce redness and irritation. If symptoms persist they should seek medical advice.

Record details of any contra-action on the client's treatment record.

The treatment plan should be signed and dated by the client and yourself following the consultation to confirm the suitability and consent with the agreed treatment.

Keep and store client records in compliance with the Data Protection Act and have them available for future reference.

Clean, sterile water used to flush the eye

Tinting the eyebrows and lashes

1 Position the client comfortably, in a flat or slightly elevated position. If they are wearing contact lenses and receiving an eyelash tint, these must be removed.

2 Place a clean, protective towel across the client's chest and shoulders, and protect their hair with a clean headband.

3 Wash your hands after preparing the client, which assures the client that the treatment is beginning in a hygienic and professional manner.

4 Cleanse the area to be treated with a non-oily cleansing lotion to dissolve facial make-up (if worn). Apply this with clean, damp cotton wool.

5 To ensure that the area is thoroughly clean and grease-free, apply a non-oily eye make-up remover or a mild toning lotion, stroked over the lash or brow hair, with clean damp cotton wool.

Blot the brows or eyelashes dry with a clean facial tissue. This ensures that the tint will not be diluted, and also prevents the tint from being carried into the eye, if an eyelash tint is being carried out. Brush through the brows to separate the hair using a disposable brush. Note if the hair is fair at the lash base.

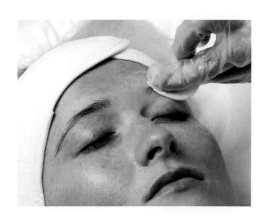

6 Prepare pre-shaped eye shields or cotton wool by applying petroleum jelly to the inner surface (the surface that comes into contact with the skin).

7 Ensure that light is not shining directly into the client's eyes during eyelash tinting. If it were, the eyes might water, carrying the tint into the eye or down the face (possibly causing skin staining).

8 Finally, check that the client is comfortable before beginning tint application.

9 Best practice is to wear disposable gloves to avoid contact with the tint that could lead to skin staining and possibly **contact dermatitis**. If worn, put on at this stage.

ALWAYS REMEMBER

Tone and blot

The brows or lash hair to be tinted must be grease-free – the grease would be come a resistant barrier to the tint. Blotting the hair dry avoids any moisture present weakening the effectiveness of the tinting product.

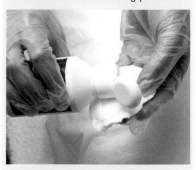

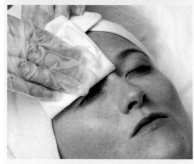

REVISION AID

How can you determine the correct colour choice for an eyebrow tint?

HEALTH & SAFETY

Maintaining hygiene

Do not use the same spatula in the container again when dispensing petroleum jelly, or you might contaminate the product.

TOP TIP

Client communication

Speak to your clients as you apply the eyelash tint. Check that they are comfortable and understand what you are doing at each stage of the treatment. Remember: the eyes are very sensitive and will water readily.

TOP TIP

Tint removal

Use a cotton bud to remove any excess tint from along the lash line on removal. If left, this can often cause eye irritation.

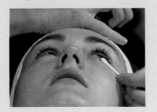

STEP-BY-STEP: TINTING THE EYELASHES

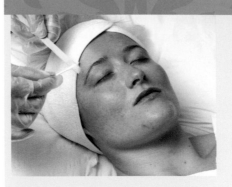

1 Remove some petroleum jelly from its container, using a disposable, or hygienically prepared alternative spatula.

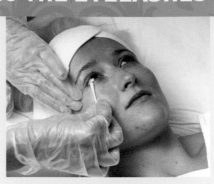

2 Working from behind the client, ask the client to open their eyes and to look upwards towards you. Using a disposable brush or cotton bud, apply petroleum jelly underneath the lower lashes of one eye, ensuring that it extends at the outer corner of the eye. (This is in case the client's eyes water slightly during treatment, which might otherwise lead to skin staining.) The petroleum jelly must not come into contact with the lash hair, where it would create a barrier to the tint.

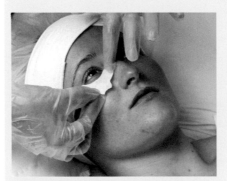

3 Place the prepared eye shield or cotton wool on the skin under the lower lashes, ensuring that it adheres to the skin and fits 'snugly' to the base of the lower lashes.

4 Repeat the above process for the other eye.

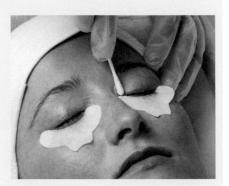

5 Ask the client to close their eyes gently. Instruct them not to open them again until you advise them to do so, in about 10 minutes' time.

6 Apply petroleum jelly to the upper eyelid, in a line on the skin at the base of the lashes avoiding contact with the lash hair.

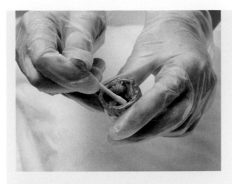

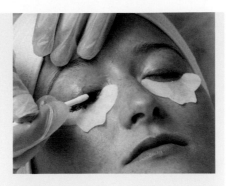

HEALTH & SAFETY

Using eye tints

Always read the manufacturer's instructions carefully before application of your permanent tint.

7 Considering the length and density of the client's eyelashes, mix the required amount of tint with 10-volume (3%) hydrogen peroxide. As a guide, a 5 mm length of tint from the tube, mixed with two or three drops of hydrogen peroxide, is usually sufficient. Mix the products to a smooth cream in the tinting bowl, using the disposable brush. Always recap bottles and tubes tightly after use, to avoid deterioration of products.

8 Wipe excess tint off the brush onto the inside of the bowl. Apply the tint thinly to each hair. Work from the base of the lash to the tip, ensuring that each hair is evenly covered. Press down gently with the applicator to ensure that the lower lashes also are covered. The few inner and outer lashes should also be covered, down to the base.

ALWAYS REMEMBER

Eyelash tint

Allow further processing time to an area where the hair is more resistant to colour, typically red and white hair.

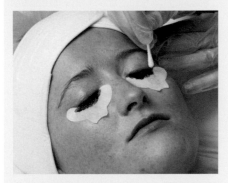

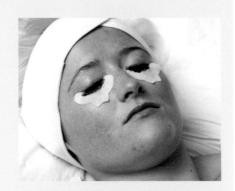

9 Remove any excess tint from the skin with a clean cotton bud immediately following application to avoid skin staining.

10 Allow the tint to process for approximately 5 to 10 minutes from the completion of application, guided by the manufacturers' instructions. A circular cotton wool pad may be placed over each eye which will create additional warmth to speed the tinting process. Discard any unused tint mixture as soon as the tint has been applied.

(Continued over page)

HEALTH & SAFETY

Client comfort

The client should not be left during the lash-tinting treatment. You must be available both to offer reassurance and to take the necessary action if the eyes water and in the instance of a contra-action.

If the eyes do water during an eyelash tint, whilst the eyes are closed, hold a tissue at the corner of the eye to soak up the moisture. Take further action if watering persists and the eyes begin to sting. See contra-action, previously covered in this chapter.

ACTIVITY

Eyebrow and eyelash tinting

List reasons why clients would benefit from this treatment. Such knowledge is essential when promoting eye services.

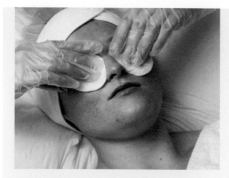

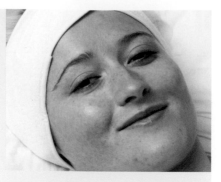

11 On completion of processing, remove the eyelash tint by applying clean, damp cotton wool pads over each eye, wiping away most of the tint and removing the protective eye shield in one movement, an outward sweep. Using fresh dampened cotton wool pads, gently stroke down the lashes from base to tips, until all excess tint has been removed. With a sweeping action on each eye and using one cotton wool pad, wipe from the side to the middle against the lash growth, while the other hand supports the eye tissue. ***All tint must be thoroughly removed before the client opens their eyes***.

12 Ask the client to open their eyes. If removal has been correctly carried out, the lashes and their bases will be free from tint. (While training, if any tint remains at the base of the lashes after the eyes have been opened, ask the client to close their eyes again and finish the removal process using clean, damp cotton wool.) Check that every lash has been tinted, especially the base of each lash and the inner and outer corner lashes. Show the client the result, ensuring the colour is dark enough and that they are satisfied with the final effect.

13 Once you are satisfied that all tint has been removed, place a cool, damp cotton wool pad over each eye for 2 to 3 minutes to soothe the eye tissue.

14 Record details of the treatment on the client's treatment record.

STEP-BY-STEP: TINTING THE EYEBROWS

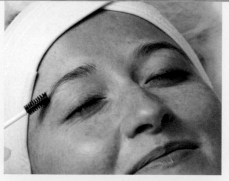

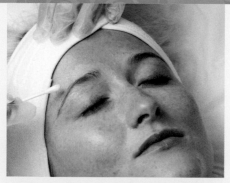

ACTIVITY

Explaining poor results

What reasons can you think of to explain why tint applied to the eyelashes or eyebrows has not coloured the hair successfully? Discuss your answers.

1 Brush the brow hair away from the skin, using a disposable brow brush.

2 Remove some petroleum jelly from its container, using a hygienic disposable spatula.

3 Using a disposable brush or cotton bud, surround each eyebrow with petroleum jelly, as close as possible to the brow hair (to avoid skin staining).

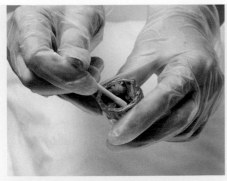

4 Mix approximately 5 mm of the chosen tint colour with two or three drops of 10-volume (3%) hydrogen peroxide in a tinting bowl. Ensure that the tint is mixed thoroughly to a creamy consistency, according to the manufacturer's instructions.

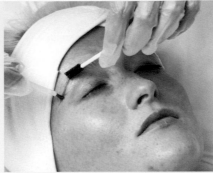

5 Wipe excess tint off the brush onto the inside of the tinting bowl. Apply the tint neatly and economically to the brow hair of the first eyebrow, ensuring that the brow hairs, from the base to the tips, are evenly covered (as shown in the picture).

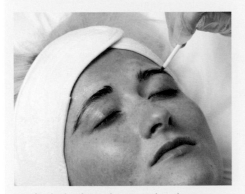

6 Apply the tint to the second eyebrow; following the same procedure.

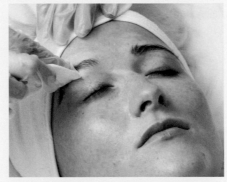

7 Immediately after application of the tint to the second eyebrow, remove the tint from the first eyebrow. Use a clean dampened cotton wool pad. Place it on the eyebrow, then wipe it across the eyebrow in an outward sweep, removing the excess tint. Ensure that all traces of excess tint have been removed, to prevent skin staining.

Never leave tint on the eyebrows for longer than 2 minutes. Eyebrow hair colour develops much more quickly than lash hair.

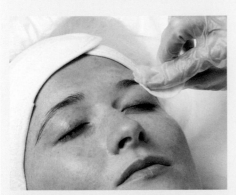

8 Remove the tint from the second eyebrow in the same way.

Show the client the effect of the tinted eyebrows. If the brow hair is not dark enough, reapply the tint to the eyebrow hair, following the same application and removal procedure. Note this on the client's treatment record.

When you are both satisfied with the colour of the tinted eyebrows, complete the client's treatment record, recording all related details of the treatment.

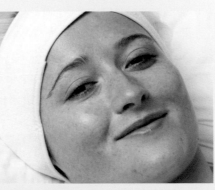

9 The completed effect, showing both eyebrow and eyelash tint.

ALWAYS REMEMBER

White hair

When selecting and using tint for a white-haired client, note that the hair is very often resistant to colour. The processing time may need to be increased. Note any modification on the treatment record for future reference.

TOP TIP

Tint application to brow hair

To ensure even coverage of brow hair, use a brush to lift the hair to enable application at the base of the hair to mid-length of the hair shaft.

REVISION AID

When a client tests positively to a tint skin sensitivity patch test, what eye service could you provide as an alternative to enhance brow appearance?

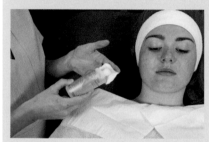
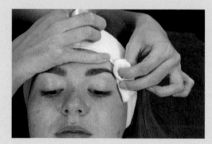

Client advice and recommendations

If an unwanted reaction occurs, a contra-action, e.g. irritation or redness, apply cool water or a damp cotton wool pad to the area.

If reddening continues after 24 hours contact the salon.

Advise the client to receive the treatment as follows:

◆ eyelash tinting every four to six weeks

◆ eyebrow tinting every three to four weeks.

Inform the client that exposure to UV will lighten the tint, such as a holiday in the sun.

Promote cosmetic products where extra definition would be of benefit.

Cosmetic products can be retailed that maintain the condition of the lashes and brows, such as a balm for the brows to keep the colour at optimum appearance.

Recommend brow shaping to enhance the natural brow following tinting.

Eyelash attachment systems

Eyelash attachments are made from small threads of nylon fibre or real hair, referred to as artificial eyelashes. They are attached to the client's natural lash hair imitating the natural eyelashes and making the lashes appear longer and thicker, and thereby drawing attention to the eye. There are several eyelash attachment systems available to be worn temporarily, for a day or special occasion, and if semi-permanently for up to 8 weeks. The design, look and effects differ greatly depending on the choice of lash and application technique.

Artificial lashes are applied for the following reasons:

◆ to create shape and depth in the eye area when completing corrective eye make-up application techniques

◆ simply to add definition to the eye area

◆ to enhance evening or special occasion make-up

◆ to provide thick long lashes for photographic make-up

◆ to provide an alternative eyelash-enhancing effect for a client who is allergic to mascara.

Three eyelash attachment systems will be discussed below: strip, flare and single or individual lashes.

Strip lashes
Strip lashes are designed to be worn for a short period, either for a day or an evening. They are attached to the base of the client's natural eyelashes with a soft, weak adhesive. After removal the strip must be cleaned before reapplication.

Strips designed for use on the lower lashes are called **partial lashes**: small groups of hairs are placed intermittently along the length of the artificial-lash base. These may be applied to the upper lashes also to thicken finer lashes, whilst achieving a natural look. Alternatively, shorter length lashes are available which may be applied to the outer lashes only.

Commercially, the most popular colours are usually black and brown. For special effects, however, strip lashes are available in fantasy colours, complete with feathers, glitter and jewels!

Flare lashes
flare lashes are attached to the natural lashes with a stronger adhesive. They may be worn for up to four weeks, and are sometimes referred to as **semi-permanent lashes**.

Lash length may be short, medium or long; their texture may be fine, medium or thick, with differing lash curls and shapes.

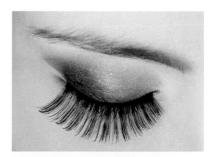

Strip lashes

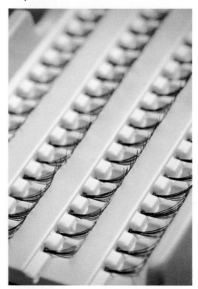

Flare lashes

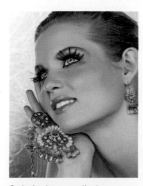

Strip lashes applied to enhance a photographic make-up

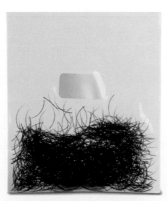

Single or individual lashes

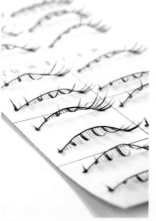

Partial strip lashes

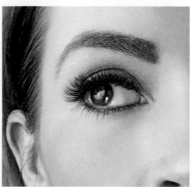

Coloured eyelash extensions to enhance a make-up look

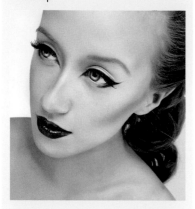

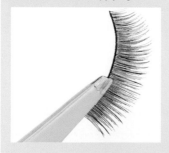

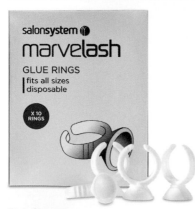

salonsystem
marvelash
GLUE RINGS
fits all sizes
disposable

X 10 RINGS

Glue ring cup

Single or individual lashes Single (or individual) lashes are attached to a single, natural eyelash. They may be worn for six to eight weeks, but maintenance treatments may be received every two to three weeks to replace those lost through the natural growth cycle.

We will discuss strip and flare systems next, which are more temporary than the single or individual lash system.

Preparing the work area for eyelash extensions

Specialist products, tools and equipment

Before beginning the eyelash extension application, check that you have the necessary products, tools and equipment to hand to meet legal, hygiene and industry requirements for eye treatment services. You will need all of the basic tools and equipment listed for eyebrow and lash treatments earlier in the chapter, as well as the following specialist equipment:

◆ **Disposable mascara brush** To brush the natural lashes before application, separating them, which will assist attachment of the artificial lash, creating a professional final result.

◆ **Manual tweezers (two pairs) (sterilised)** Special tweezers are available, designed specifically to assist in attaching individual eyelashes.

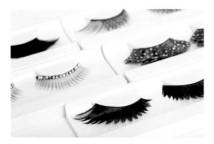

Strip eyelash

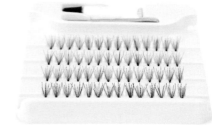

Flare eyelash

◆ **Strip eyelash** A selection of differing lengths, thickness, colours and appearance.

◆ **Flare eyelash** A selection, in a choice of different lengths, thicknesses and colours.

◆ **Eyelash adhesive** The adhesive differs for the eyelash extension type which affects its permanency. The correct adhesive must be used to suit the lash type.

◆ **Eyelash solvent** to dissolve flare lash adhesive when removal is required.

◆ **Sterilised scissors (one pair)** Used for trimming the length of strip lashes.

◆ **Cotton wool buds** To apply solvent when removing flare lashes.

◆ **Surgical spirit** For wiping the points of the tweezers to remove adhesive ensuring efficient application.

◆ **Plastic palette or vinyl pad (disinfected)** On which to place the eyelash extensions prior to application, if not working directly from the tray they are supplied in.

◆ **Disinfected dish (small)** Lined with foil, in which to place the eyelash adhesive during lash extension application, or **glue ring cup**, which you can wear when applying the flare lash and individual lash system.

Preparing the work area

Before the client is shown through to the work area, check it to ensure that the required products, tools and equipment are available for eyelash extensions and the area is clean and tidy.

Clean and protect the couch or beauty chair as for previous eye treatment.

The couch or beauty chair should be in a slightly elevated position, to give the optimum position for the beauty therapist when applying the eyelash extensions. In this position, too, the client will not be staring into an overhead light (which might cause the eyes to water).

Always follow your workplace policy for preparation of the work area.

Safety and hygiene

◆ Disposable gloves may be worn if you are allergic to the eyelash adhesive.

◆ When preparing to apply *strip* lashes, clean the surface of the palette onto which you will stick the lashes once you have removed them from their packet. Use disinfectant, applied with clean cotton wool. The palette may be stored in the UV light cabinet until ready for use.

◆ Flare lashes come in a special 'contoured' package; you can hold this securely while removing individual flare lashes, so the lashes can be kept hygienically until required.

◆ Clean or dispose of the container dependant on type used to hold the individual eyelash adhesive immediately following use.

◆ Always have a spare pair of tweezers available during application of the eyelash extensions. Should you accidentally drop the tweezers with which you are working, you will need a clean, sterile pair available.

◆ Scissors, used to trim strip lashes, should be sterilised before use.

◆ Dispense products from containers, e.g. eyelash adhesive.

◆ A negative skin sensitivity patch test result must be obtained before this treatment is carried out.

Treatment information to provide to clients at initial point of interest

The following points are important for the receptionist to consider when booking a client for eyelash extension treatment:

◆ When making an appointment for eyelash extensions, find out why the client wants eyelash extensions to determine which type would be most appropriate.

◆ Allow 20 minutes for the application of flare and strip lashes; and again allow a further 45 minutes if applying them in conjunction with a make-up.

◆ Although flare lashes can be worn for up to four weeks they look effective only for approximately two to three weeks. After this time, the appearance of the flare lashes begins to deteriorate, the lash **adhesive** becomes brittle, and the eyelash area may become irritated.

◆ Due to the cyclic nature of hair replacement some flare lashes will be lost when the natural lash falls out. These lashes may be replaced every one to two weeks,

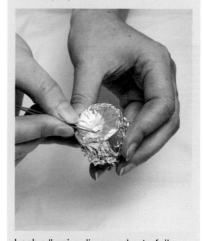

Lash adhesive dispensed onto foil

as necessary; the client is usually charged a price for each individual flare lash replacement – usually referred to as an 'infill service'. The client must be told of this service as part of the aftercare advice and instruction.

When a client makes an appointment for an eyelash extension treatment, they should be asked the following questions:

◆ *Have they had the treatment before?* If they have not, they will need to be advised to visit the workplace to receive a skin sensitivity patch test, in order to assess sensitivity to the adhesive and confirm suitability for treatment. Skin sensitivity patch test results should be recorded on the client record.

◆ *Are they wearing the eyelash extensions for a particular reason, such as a holiday or a special occasion?* In deciding which type of eyelash extension would be most appropriate, take into consideration the effect required and for how long the lashes are to be worn.

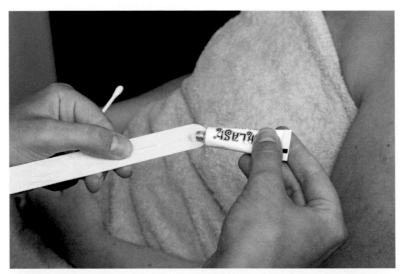

Adhesive is prepared for skin sensitivity patch test

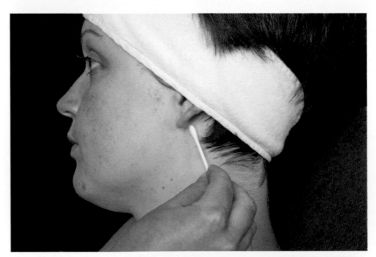

The eyelash adhesive is placed behind the ear for the skin sensitivity patch test as the skin is thinner here, similar to the skin around the eyes

◆ If the client wears glasses, the eyelash extensions must not be so long as to touch the lenses. Also, if the lens magnifies the eye, this must be taken into account. Ask the client to bring their glasses with them to the appointment.

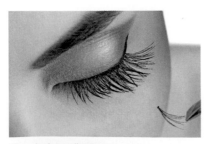

Flare lash application

Remember, if a client is under the age of 16 it is necessary to obtain parent, carer or guardian permission for all eye services. They will also have to be present when the treatment is received.

Client care, consultation and communication skills

Factors when choosing eyelash extensions
Before applying eyelash extensions you should consider the following points, and advise the client accordingly.

Purpose and any limiting factors
Considerations should include if the lashes are to be worn for an occasion or for longer duration. This will affect the time required to apply the eyelash extensions and the maintenance requirements to be followed if worn on a more permanent basis. Also, the overall effect required.

The client's age
Eyelash extensions create a very bold, dramatic effect, which can make an older client look too hard. Remember that the skin colour and the natural hair colour change with age: the lash chosen must enhance the client's appearance.

Fashion
Often clients in their twenties will follow catwalk and social media trends, so it is important you are aware of the latest looks, products and techniques to achieve this.

The client's natural lashes
Does the client have short or long, sparse or thick, very curly or straight lashes? Choose an artificial eyelash to complement the natural lash. Here are some guidelines:

◆ *Short and stubby lashes* These are commonly seen on older clients who have overhanging eyelids. Choose a medium lash length in a medium thickness at the outer corner of the eyelid; the lashes should become gradually shorter from the centre of the eyelid to the inner corner. Brush the artificial and natural lashes together after application to ensure that they blend.

◆ *Sparse lashes* Place individual short lashes along the natural lash line; or, to give a more natural appearance, you may wish to apply partial strip lashes to the upper eyelid.

◆ *Curly eyelashes* These are very common on clients of African descent. Choose a longer, sweeping strip or individual artificial eyelashes, in black. The chosen lashes and colour should give emphasis and depth to the eye.

The client's eye condition
Some clients have oily eyes, which is where a fluid called meibum is secreted from the meibomian gland; a sebaceous gland found in the eye rim. This will affect the durability of the lashes and must be considered when discussing choice of lash with your client.

The natural eyelash colour
Select artificial eyelashes that complement the hair and skin colour. Natural hair artificial eyelashes offer the greatest choice of colour, but these are expensive and may be difficult to purchase. An eyelash tint may be recommended before lash extension application to create a more natural, realistic result. This is especially so if the client has fair or red hair colouring and black lashes are selected.

Using eyelash extensions for corrective purposes
Here are some outlines of corrective techniques for various eye shapes.

TOP TIP

Images of 'before and after' lash extensions

At consultation it is a good idea to share 'before and after' images of different effects that can be achieved with eyelash extensions.

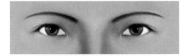
Short and stubby lashes

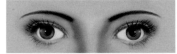
Sparse lashes

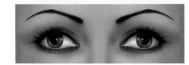
Curly eyelashes

TOP TIP

Streaked lashes

Streaked lashes are available, to give a more subtle effect for the mature client.

Eye shape	Corrective steps
Small eyes	Place eyelash extensions at the outer corners of the upper eyelid. These should be longer than the natural lashes.
Close-set eyes	Place fine, long, flare or partial strip lashes at the outer third of the eye. They may be applied to the lower lashes as well as to the upper.
Wide-set eyes	Apply medium-length lashes at the inner corner of the eye and to the centre, becoming slightly shorter towards the outer corner of the upper eyelid. This may be repeated on the lower lash also.
Downward-slanting eyes	Apply longer lashes (flare or partial strip lashes) to the outer corners of the upper eyelid.
Round eyes	Flare or strip lashes should be used to lengthen the lash line. Apply the eyelash extensions from the centre of the upper eyelid outwards.
Deep-set eyes	Apply fine lashes to the upper and lower lashes. The upper-lid eyelash extensions should be longer, to draw attention to the eye.
Overhanging lids	Apply longer lashes to the upper eyelid, from the outer corner and tapering to a shorter length at the centre of the lid and towards the inner corner.

On completion the eyelash extensions should achieve a balanced and well-proportioned look complementing the client's eye shape, producing the agreed desired effect.

Explain the treatment procedure and what sensations it is normal to experience and how the finished result should look. This is important especially when treating a nervous or new client to provide reassurance.

Ask open questions to confirm client understanding about the treatment.

Invite the client to ask you any questions.

Inform the client at consultation of any relevant contra-actions that may occur during or after the service and the action to take. These are discussed below.

The treatment record should be signed and dated by the client and beauty therapist following the consultation to confirm the suitability and consent with the agreed treatment.

Keep and store client records in compliance with the Data Protection Act and for future reference.

"Never be tempted to cut corners, always strive to be the best you possibly can. Always listen to what your client wants and never be afraid to ask questions. Always be discreet with other staff and clients."

Shavata Singh

Contra-indications

When a client attends for eyelash extension treatment, you should always check that there are no contra-indications that might restrict or prevent eye treatment as listed previously in this chapter in the Contra-indications section. After completing the treatment record visually inspect the eye area to confirm there are no contra-indications present.

Remember, you are not qualified to diagnose a contra-indication. Refer the client to their GP without creating unnecessary cause for concern.

In addition you must also check the following:

◆ **Results of the skin sensitivity patch test** – *a positive (allergic) reaction* to the skin sensitivity patch test, would contra-indicate treatment.

◆ *Contact lenses* (unless removed) The adhesive would cause irritation between the lens and the eye.

◆ A particularly nervous client would also be contra-indicated:

　◆ They might blink frequently, making preparation of the eye area and application of lash extensions both difficult and hazardous.

Use your discretion in deciding on the suitability of a client for treatment.

For more information on asking open questions refer to CHAPTER 3.

For more information on disorders affecting the eye see CHAPTER 3, Consultation Practice and Techniques.

Contra-actions

If during application of eyelash extensions the client's eye starts to water, blot the tears with the corner of a clean tissue. The tears can cause the adhesive to become ineffective or if a stronger glue is used as with flare lashes, this will take on an unsightly white crystallised appearance. Any possible irritation of the eyes should therefore be avoided, during both preparation of the eye area and application itself.

Never place individual flare eyelashes at the base of the natural eyelashes in contact with the skin – eye irritation will occur.

While practising flare eyelash application you may find at some point that you have accidentally glued a couple of the lower and upper natural lashes together. Apply adhesive **solvent** to a cotton wool-tipped orange stick, and gently roll this over the lash length to dissolve the adhesive.

If solvent or adhesive should accidentally enter the eye, remove excess product, rinse the eye thoroughly and immediately, using clean water. Repeat this until discomfort is no longer experienced.

Preparing the client

Show the client through to the prepared work area after the treatment record has been completed. Consult the treatment record and check the area for any contra-indications to treatment.

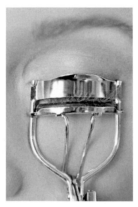

Brushing natural lashes before eyelash extension application

Curling the natural lash to assist contour and contact with artificial lash

1 Position the client comfortably on the treatment couch or beauty chair (which should be slightly elevated). If the client wears contact lenses, these must be removed before the treatment begins.

2 Drape a clean towel across the client's chest and shoulders. Protect their hair with a clean headband or secure hair out of the way with a hair clip.

3 Wash your hands, which indicates to the client that treatment is beginning and in a hygienic and professional manner.

4 It is usual to carry out a full facial cleanse (rather than cleansing only the eye area), as make-up is usually applied to complement the eyelash extensions. Use a professional cleanser to dissolve facial make-up, followed by a non-oily eye make-up remover to cleanse the eye area. Both products should be removed with clean, damp cotton wool.

5 To ensure that the eye tissue and eyelashes are thoroughly clean and grease-free, apply a mild oil-free toning lotion; stroke this over the skin using clean, damp cotton wool.

6 Blot the lashes dry, using a fresh facial tissue for each eye. (Any moisture left on the natural lashes will reduce the effectiveness of the eyelash adhesive.)

7 The natural lashes may be curled before lash extension application, as the natural lash will contour more effectively and bond with the false lash.

8 Brush the natural lashes to separate them before application.

STEP-BY-STEP: APPLYING FLARE LASHES

1 Check that everything you need is available, on a work surface adjacent to where you will be working.

2 Check that the back of the couch or beauty chair is slightly raised, at a height that is comfortable for you.

3 Discuss the treatment procedure with the client. Explain that she will be required to keep her eyes slightly open during the treatment. Reassure her that she may blink during application. Very often clients feel that they shouldn't, and their eyes begin to water.

4 Ask her to tilt her head downwards very slightly. This tends to lower the upper eyelids, making application easier.

5 Depending on the effect required, you may start application of the flare lashes at different positions along the natural lash line. In general, apply shorter lashes to the inner corners of the eyelid, and longer lashes to the outer corners; this creates a realistic effect and ensures client comfort. If you are applying individual flare lashes to the entire upper lid, it is practical to start application at the inner corner of the eyelid and work outwards: this follows the natural contour of the eye.

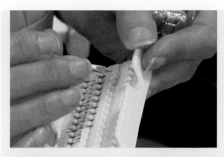

6 With the sterile tweezers, select a lash from the package, holding it near its centre. Brush the underside of the individual flare lash, at the root, through the adhesive. The adhesive should extend slightly beyond the root. You need sufficient adhesive, but not too much – excess adhesive should be removed by wiping the lash against the inside of the adhesive container.

8 Apply the lashes one at a time, to each eye alternately. This avoids sensitising the eye, and makes it easier for you to create a balanced effect.

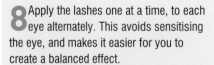

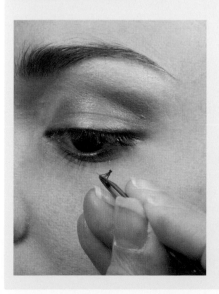

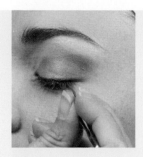

7 Working from behind or the side of the client, hold the tweezers at the angle at which the artificial eyelashes will be applied to the natural lash line. Hold the brow tissue with your other hand to steady the eyelid.

Using a stroking movement, place the underside of the artificial eyelashes on top of the natural lash. Stroke the adhesive along the length of the natural eyelash. Guide the artificial eyelashes towards the base of the natural lash, so that the artificial eyelashes rest along the length of the natural lash. Wait a few seconds to allow the adhesive to dry (to prevent the lashes from sticking together). Continue placing further flare lashes side by side until the desired effect is achieved.

During application, keep checking your work. If a lash is out of line, remove it while the adhesive is still soft. If the adhesive has set, the lash will need to be removed using adhesive solvent.

9 If the client requires eyelashes to be applied to the *lower* lid, the application technique is slightly different.

Work facing the client, with the client looking upwards, her eyes slightly open. Follow the same general procedure for applying the eyelashes to the upper lid; here, however, the lashes curve downwards and the adhesive is applied to the *upper* surface of the lash.

Lashes applied to the lower eyelid are usually shorter than those chosen for the upper lid, and more adhesive is required for the lashes to be secure and have maximum durability.

HEALTH & SAFETY

Applying adhesive

With flare lashes, do not apply adhesive directly from the tube to the eyelash base – you would risk applying too much adhesive and also spoiling the flare lash.

ECO TIP

Preparing lash adhesive

Do not prepare the lash adhesive until you are ready to use it. It tends to dry on contact with air creating product wastage.

ALWAYS REMEMBER

Clean tweezers

To ensure efficient application, don't get adhesive on the points of the tweezers. This would result in wastage of lash extensions and affect the quality of the final result.

TOP TIP

Positioning

When applying the flare lashes to the inner portion of the eyelid, hold the skin taut, stretching the skin slightly. This will enable you to position the eyelash extension more easily.

TOP TIP

Retail opportunity

Mascaras are available, formulated to be worn with individual flare lashes. The product is more easily removed than regular non-waterproof mascaras.

▶

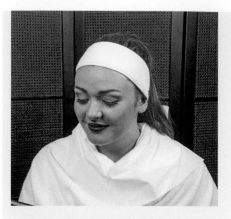

10 When you have completed the flare lash application, ask the client to sit up, and show her the completed effect to confirm suitability.

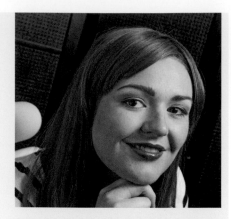

11 If the client is satisfied with the result, you can apply a water- or powder-based eye make-up at this stage if desired. Do not apply mascara, as this will reduce the adhesion to the natural lash. Mascara also clogs the lashes together, and is difficult to remove without affecting the eyelash adhesive. On completion, the natural and flare lashes can be gently brushed – using a disposable brush – to remove particles of eyeshadow.

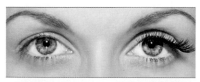
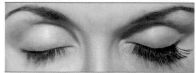

Before and after: strip lashes applied to enhance the natural eyelashes

STEP-BY-STEP: APPLYING STRIP LASHES

Strip lashes may be applied *before* carrying out eye make-up application – this avoids the eye make-up being spoilt if the eyes water slightly during application.

1 Check that everything required for the strip lash application is available on a work surface adjacent to where you will be working.

2 Carefully apply skin preparation products and foundation if being worn in conjunction with make-up, taking care not to get any cosmetic products on the lashes. (If you do, gently wipe over the lashes with non-oily eye make-up remover, and blot the eyelashes dry again with a clean facial tissue.)

3 Brush the lashes to separate them, using a clean disposable mascara brush. This makes strip lash application easier, and removes any fine particles of loose powder.

4 Remove the strip lashes from their container and place them on a clean, disinfected palette. Each strip is designed to fit either the left or the right eye: remember which is which when placing them on the palette.

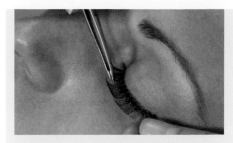

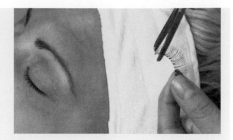

5 Check the length of the strip against the client's eyelid. The strip should never be applied directly from one corner of the eyelid to the other; but should start about 2 mm from the inner corner of the eye, and end 2 mm from the outer corner. This ensures a natural effect and maximises the durability of the artificial eyelashes.

When you remove the strip lash from the package you will find that there is adhesive on the backing strip, which fixes the lash in the container: this adhesive is sufficient to hold the lash onto the client's natural lash while you measure the length.

6 To trim the strip lashes you require a sharp pair of scissors. First, correct the length of the *strip* if necessary. Hold the lashes securely with one hand, and then trim the strip at the outer edge. Then trim the lashes themselves, if necessary. Never reduce the length of the lashes by cutting straight across them: the result would not look natural. Natural eyelashes are of varying lengths, due to the nature of the hair growth cycle; it is this effect that you must simulate. To shorten the lash, 'chip' into the lash. Use the *points* of the scissors to shorten the lash length. Cut the lashes so that the shorter lashes are at the inner corner of the eyelid, gradually increasing toward the outer corner.

7 The couch or beauty chair should be in a slightly raised position. During the treatment you will be working from behind the client: the height must be comfortable for you.

8 Discuss the treatment procedure with the client. Explain to her that she will be required to keep her eyes open during the application. Ask her to tilt her head downwards very slightly – this lowers the upper eyelids, making application easier.

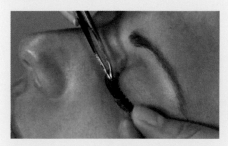

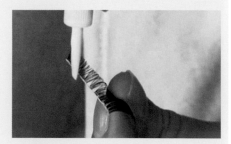

9 Using the sterile tweezers pick up the strip lash, handling it very carefully, as it can easily become misshapen.

Remembering that the strip is designed to fit either the right or the left eye, place it against the appropriate eyelid and check the length (with the client's eyes closed).

10 Once satisfied that the length of the strip lash is correct (see Step 6 for reducing length) place a small quantity of strip lash adhesive onto the disinfected palette. Holding the strip lash with the sterile tweezers at its centre, drag it at its base through the adhesive (the adhesive must be moist). It is usually white, but when it dries it becomes colourless. There should be a generous even application along the length of the strip, especially at each end to ensure it is secured adequately. It is ready to apply when it becomes tacky rather than wet. The glue shown is white, it will become clear as it dries.

Alternatively you may apply the adhesive directly onto the base of the strip lash as shown.

TOP TIP

Dealing with downward growing lashes

If a client has straight eyelashes that grow downwards, curl them slightly using eyelash curlers. If you don't, a gap will be visible between the real lashes and the strip lash.

TOP TIP

Preventing lifting

Extra glue (although not excessive) may be applied to the ends of the lashes to prevent lifting while wearing them.

HEALTH & SAFETY

Lash length

If the lashes are not shorter at the inner corner of the eyelid, they will irritate the client's eye.

▶

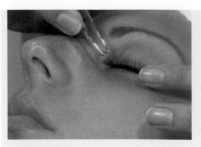

11 Ask the client to look down slightly, with her eyes half open. With one hand lift her brow to steady the upper eyelid.

Position the base of the strip lash as close as possible to the base of the natural eyelash, ensuring that it is about 2 mm in from the inner and outer corners of the eye. *Gently* press the artificial and natural eyelashes together with your fingertips, along the length of the lash and at the outer corners.

12 When you are sure that the first strip lash is secure, apply the second in the same way.

13 If strip lashes are to be applied to the bottom lashes also, apply these now, in the same way as the upper lashes. (Strip lashes for the lower lids are fine, with an extremely thin base. These lashes should be trimmed as before to ensure comfort and durability in wear.)

14 Allow three to five minutes for the adhesive to dry.

15 Gently brush the lashes from underneath the natural lash line, using a clean disposable mascara brush. This will blend the natural eyelashes and strip lashes together. Check that both sets of lashes are correctly positioned, and that a balanced look has been achieved.

16 Strip lashes look more realistic if eyeliner is applied to the client's eyelid: this disguises the base of the strip lash.

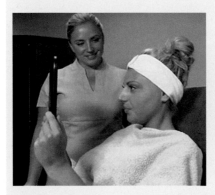

17 Show the client the finished effect to confirm satisfaction.

18 When you are satisfied, update details of the treatment on the client record.

"With lashes take your time. The more precise the application, the better the result."

Shavata Singh

STEP-BY-STEP: HOW TO REMOVE FLARE LASHES

1 Position the client for the removal service.

2 Wash your hands.

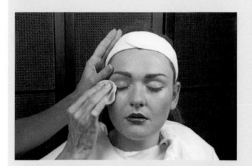 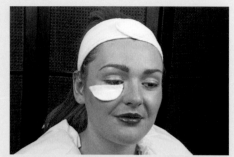

3 Remove make-up and general skin debris from the eye area, cleansing the skin with a suitable eye make-up remover.

4 While the client's eyes are open, place a pre-shaped eye shield underneath the lower lashes of each eye. (This will protect the eye tissue from the solvent.) Position the eye shields so that they fit snugly to the base of the lower lashes.

5 Ask the client to close her eyes gently, and not to open them again until you tell her to do so.

6 Prepare a new disposable orange stick by covering it at the pointed end with clean, dry cotton wool. Alternatively you can use a cotton bud.

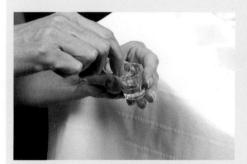 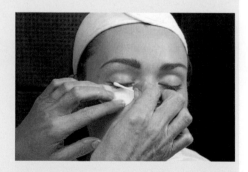

7 Moisten the cotton wool with the flare lash adhesive solvent.

8 Treating one eye at a time, gently stroke down the flare lashes with the adhesive solvent until the adhesive dissolves and the flare lash begins to loosen.

9 When you are satisfied that the lash adhesive has dissolved, the flare lash will start to move away from the natural eyelash, gently attempt to remove the flare lash. Support the upper eyelid with the fingers of one hand, using the other hand to remove the flare lash with a sterile pair of manual tweezers. If the adhesive has been adequately dissolved, the lash extension will lift away easily from the natural eyelash. If there is any resistance, repeat the solvent application until the eyelash comes away readily.

▶

TOP TIP

Continuing professional development

As part of your progression you may develop your skills further in the application of artificial eyelashes by studying the Level 3 Unit, Individual eyelash extensions.

REVISION AID

What type of eye make-up remover is used to cleanse the area before any eyelash service, and why?

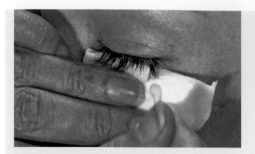

10 As the flare lashes are removed, collect them on a clean white facial tissue or a clean pad of cotton wool.

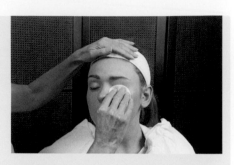

11 Having removed all of the flare lashes from one eye, soothe the area by applying damp cotton wool pads soaked in cool water. (This will also remove any remaining solvent.)

A damp cotton wool pad may be placed over the eye, while you remove the flare lashes from the other eye.

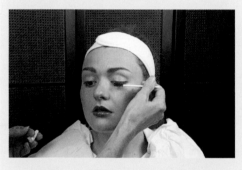

12 Finally, brush through the natural eyelashes to ensure all adhesive has been removed.

HEALTH & SAFETY

Client comfort and safety

Never attempt to remove the flare lash extensions until they have begun to loosen – if you do, the client's natural eyelashes will also be removed, causing them discomfort and noticeable gaps of hair along the lash line.

HEALTH & SAFETY

Eye care

Do not allow eyelash adhesive solvent to come into excessive contact with the eye tissue – it could cause irritation of the skin. Ensure that there is sufficient solvent only on the cotton wool: it should be moist but not dripping wet or the solvent might enter the eye.

How to remove strip lashes

If a client wears strip lashes they will need instructions on how to remove and care for these themselves.

1   Use the fingertips of one hand to support the eyelid at the outer corner. With the other hand, lift the strip lash base at the outer corner of the eye. Gently peel this strip away from the natural lash, from the outer edge towards the centre of the eyelid.

2   **If reusing** peel the adhesive from the backing strip, using a clean pair of manual tweezers. Take care to avoid stretching the strip lash.

3 Clean the strip lash in the appropriate way.

◆ *Strips made from natural hair* Clean with a commercial lash cleaner or 70 per cent alcohol. This removes the remaining adhesive and the eye make-up.

◆ *Synthetic strips* Place in warm, soapy water for a few minutes, to clean the lashes and remove the remaining adhesive. Rinse in tepid water.

4 After cleaning the strip lashes they should be recurled.

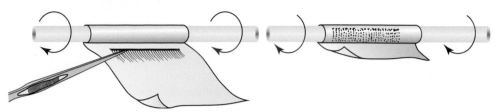

Recurling strip lashes

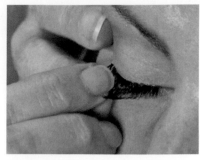

Strip lash removal – support the outer corner of the client's eyelid

How to recurl strip lashes

For reasons of hygiene and because of the time involved, this treatment will not be offered by the salon. The client, however, will need advice on how to recurl the lashes at home.

1 On removal from the water, place the strip lashes side by side, ensuring that the inner edges are together inside a clean facial tissue.

2 Wrap a tissue around an even, round barrel-shaped object such as a felt-tip pen, and secure it with an elastic band.

3 The strip lashes, inside the facial tissue, should then be rolled around this object. Keep the base of the strip lash straight, so that the whole lash length curls around the object.

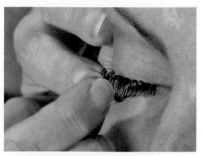

Strip lash removal – carefully peel away the strip lash from the natural lash

Once recurled, the strip lashes can be returned to the contoured shelves in their original container and stored for further use.

HEALTH & SAFETY

Client comfort

When removing the strip lash, avoid pulling the natural lashes with the artificial eyelashes.

Client advice and recommendations

◆ Provide advice on the action to take if an unwanted reaction, a contra-action, occurs.

◆ Avoid rubbing the eyes, or the lashes may become loosened.

◆ Do not use an oil-based eye make-up remover as its cosmetic constituents will dissolve the adhesive.

◆ Use only dry or water-based eye make-up (as these may readily be removed with a non-oily eye make-up remover).

◆ If the lashes are made of a synthetic material, heat will cause them to become frizzy. Advise the client to avoid extremes of temperature, such as a hot sauna.

◆ Do not touch the eyes for one and a half hours after application, while the adhesive dries thoroughly.

If the client has had flare lashes applied, the following advice and instruction should be given on caring for the lashes:

◆ Use a non-oily eye make-up remover daily to cleanse the eyelids and eyelashes. Avoid contact with oil-based skincare and cosmetic preparations in the eye area, such as moisturisers and eyeliners – the oil content will dissolve the adhesive, and the flare lashes would become detached.

◆ Avoid the use of mascara as this cannot be removed effectively without damaging the application of the lash extensions.

◆ Do not attempt to remove the flare lashes – pulling at lash extensions will also pull out the natural eyelashes.

◆ After bathing or swimming, gently *pat* the eye area dry with a clean towel.

◆ A disposable spiral applicator brush may be used to comb through the lashes to separate them.

Clients with flare lashes should have the eyelash extensions maintained by regular visits to the salon. Lost flare lashes can be replaced as necessary; this is often described as an eyelash *infill* service. Schedule this for every 10–14 days.

If the client wishes to have the individual flare lashes removed, recommend that this should always be done professionally.

Single lash extensions

Having learned about flare lash and strip lash systems, there is another choice – single lash extensions – which provide more durability and are referred to as semi-permanent due to the strength of adhesive used with the system. Before you proceed to single lash extensions, you may learn the express system, which involves application of the single lash system hair to create a similar effect to strip lashes and takes approximately 30 minutes, whereas a full application of single lash extensions can take up to two hours.

Formed from synthetic fibre polyester material to resemble natural lash hair, single eyelash extensions are bonded to the natural lashes using a strong adhesive (usually cyanoacrylate), which sets rapidly and can be harmful if in contact with the skin. As the client loses their natural lash after approximately 90 days, they will also lose the artificial lash. From 30–70 **single lashes** are applied to the eyelashes, which can take up to two hours. This requires the client to have their eyes closed continuously during this period. Single lash extensions can be worn for three to eight weeks, depending upon the cyclic nature of the natural hairs; the natural functioning of the eyes – single lashes applied to clients who have oily eyes will not be as durable as the oil weakens the adhesive; and the lifestyle and aftercare procedures followed by the client following application. To keep them looking their best it is necessary to have a maintenance service every three weeks, where lost lashes are replaced.

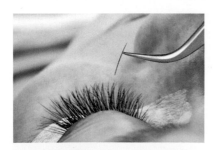

Single lash extension

Hair growth cycle

Single lash extensions are attached to one individual lash, which allows the natural hair to grow normally. When the natural lash is shed, so too will be the artificial extension lash. This must be considered when selecting lash lengths. New short lashes should have a shorter lash length attached to them.

Vision can be affected following single lash extensions. **Thickening of the cornea** can occur as a result of swelling behind the cornea. This is if the eyes are closed for long periods. Once the eyes re-open the cornea reduces its thickness as swelling reduces, restoring normal vision.

Preparing the work area

Before beginning the single lash system application, check that you have the necessary products, tools and equipment to hand to meet legal, hygiene and industry requirements for eye services. You will need all of the basic products, tools and equipment listed earlier in the chapter for eyebrow and eyelash treatments, as well as the following specialist equipment.

Products, tools and equipment

◆ **Eye make-up remover (non-oily formulation)** To remove cosmetics from the eye area and general skin debris and natural oils from the area. Pads are the most convenient for use.

◆ **Single synthetic lash extensions** In a variety of lengths, thicknesses, curvatures and colours (as available from your manufacturer).

◆ **Sterilised tweezers** Of long, pointed design available in a straight, X type and angled as shown. These enable single lash hairs to be isolated during application and precision application. Two pairs are required for each service. Several pairs are required to allow for sterilisation after use.

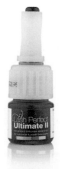

◆ **Single lash system adhesive** To attach the artificial lash to the natural lash. Some glues are odourless, which are more suitable for clients with sensitive eyes.

◆ **Adhesive holder** To hold dispensed adhesive and facilitate application. This may be a disposable ring holder, worn by the beauty therapist, or a jade stone, due to its cooling properties. It helps to keep the adhesive at a constant temperature and optimum consistency.

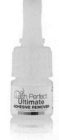

◆ **Single lash system solvent** Used to remove lashes during application if incorrectly applied, in the event of a

contra-action or when performing a maintenance service.

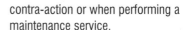

◆ **Small micro-applicators** For the application of adhesive solvent to smooth and even the application of adhesive coating during application.

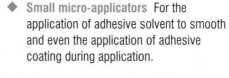

◆ **Eyelash blower** To apply air over the area speeding the lash adhesive drying time.

◆ **Single lash system sealer** To seal the lashes following application. This is a popular retail item.

◆ **Scissors (sterile)** To cut the micropore tape to size.

◆ **Eye shields** Single use, disposable, usually gel pads to cover and prevent the upper and lower lashes from sticking together and also providing a conditioning service for the lower eye tissue if impregnated with therapeutic products.

◆ **Clear surgical tape** Cut to size, used to secure the lower lashes in place following eye shield application and to attach single lashes prior to application, to facilitate application.

◆ **Eyelash combs** Used to brush though the artificial and natural lashes. These are disposable, preventing cross-infection.

◆ **Support cushion** To place under the client's knees when positioned for treatment to avoid discomfort.

A support may be available to place under the client's knees. This helps to to avoid discomfort and strain on pressure points when positioned in one place for for a long period of time.

The couch or beauty chair should be in a slightly elevated position, to give the optimum position for the beauty therapist when applying the single lashes.

Check the lighting, temperature and ventilation is adequate for the treatment. If the temperature is too warm the adhesive will set very quickly, which may cause problems when fixing the lashes in place.

Safety and hygiene

◆ When preparing the single lashes remove from the container and apply to surgical tape when required to reduce contamination.

◆ Always have spare tweezers to ensure if you were to drop a pair you will always have access to a clean, sterile pair. All metal tools, e.g. tweezers and scissors, should be cleaned with disinfectant and then sterilised in the autoclave after use.

◆ Always dispense products into clean containers, e.g. adhesive.

◆ Following the treatment, discard dispensed products that have been exposed to the atmosphere.

◆ Maintain high standards of personal hygiene.

◆ wear the recommended face mask to avoid inhalation of chemicals, i.e. solvents, and to reduce the risk of cross-contamination through airborne viruses, etc. when working in close proximity to the client.

◆ Disinfect work surface after every client and replace consumables.

◆ Protective client coverings, if used, such as towels and headbands, should be freshly laundered for every client.

◆ Dispose of waste into a covered, lined bin at all times.

Provide single eyelash extensions

Treatment information to provide to client at point of interest

When making an appointment for single lash treatment, find out why the client wants to wear the lash extensions and determine which type would be most appropriate. It may be that strip or flare lashes may be most appropriate.

Although single lashes may be worn for up to eight weeks they look effective for up to two to three weeks when through the natural cyclic shedding of the client's natural lash hair, gaps may become evident that will require replacement. The lash extensions may also lift as the adhesive weakens, sometimes twisting from their original placement. This will require a maintenance treatment and the client should be informed of this. The client must be reminded of this requirement as part of the consultation and aftercare advice and recommendations.

When a client makes an appointment for single lash service, they should be asked:

◆ Have they had the service or other artificial lash service before? Further time should be allowed at the initial treatment to discuss the plan and procedure.

◆ All clients, including those who have received the treatment before are required to visit the salon beforehand for a skin sensitivity patch test to assess any skin intolerance to the products used, e.g. adhesive. Results should be recorded on the client record.

◆ Are they having the lashes applied for any particular reason, such as a holiday or special occasion?

Inform the client of the the service time required between 11/2–2 hours, and between 30–60 minutes for a maintenance service.

In deciding which type of lash system would be most appropriate, take into consideration the effect required, how long the lashes are to be worn for. In addition, consider their occupation to see it is compatible to maintaining the lashes, their commitment to the time required for an initial lash application, aftercare maintenance requirements and their agreement to the cost of the treatment.

Also question the client about other chemical services they may have received, e.g. eyelash tinting and eyelash perming. Ask when this was, its success and if there were any comments with regard to the treatment that should be noted, e.g. eye irritation.

"Think on your feet, for example, if a client is running late and there is a way to fit them in, then do it!"

Shavata Singh

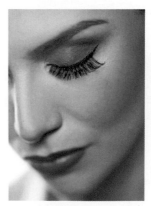

TOP TIP

Confirming client suitability

If the client is unsure about her suitability and commitment to maintaining single lash extensions, a few lashes may be applied initially at the outer corners of the eye.

Check whether the client has had lash services or eyelash extensions before and provide examples so your client can select the required look

Planning the treatment

A variety of lashes are available, these can be applied for corrective purposes as well as to lengthen the natural lash. Lash length may be short, medium or long; their texture may be fine, medium or thick. A Y-shaped lash is also available, which gives the appearance of having applied two lashes, reducing application time to achieve the result. This is ideal when immediate volume is required.

They are also available in a variety of colours, the most popular colours commercially being black and brown. For special occasions and fashion looks lashes are available in fantasy colours including metallic.

Techniques are always advancing, so it is important when you have mastered single lash extensions to look at other techniques, such as Russian layering. This is where lashes are skillfully layered to achieve a strip lash result.

Factors to consider when choosing single eyelash extensions

Before applying single eyelash extensions you should consider the following points and advise the client accordingly.

The client's age The consultation is important to agree the look, which will include the volume and intensity required. As women's hair thins with age, increasing thickness of the

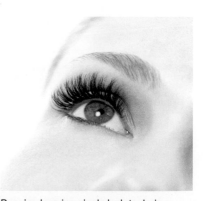

Russian layering single lash technique

lashes is a more subtle change than increasing the length. This is achieved by adding a full set of shorter length single lash extensions.

> "Always take into account the client's age and look: huge false lashes on a client that would suit a more natural look needs to be addressed. Always remain honest."
>
> *Shavata Singh*

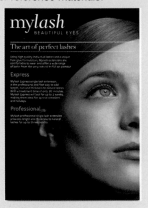
TOP TIP

Lash length

Single lash systems are applied in a variety of lengths to create a natural look simulating the natural cyclic appearance of hair growth.

Longest lashes are usually applied in the centre of the natural lash line. Shorter lashes should be placed on the inner corner of the lash line to avoid eye irritation.

If the length of the single lashes applied is too long for the client's natural lashes, this will result in twisting, where the lashes become crossed over each other.

The client's natural lashes Look at the client's natural lashes: are they short, long, sparse or thick, curly or straight – also their natural curvature? Choice of curvature of the single eyelash extension ranges from natural to dramatic. The single lash should be chosen to complement the natural lash or the result may be unsuitable in terms of appearance and durability. For a natural look, select slightly longer lashes and their application will make the eyelashes look fuller.

For a dramatic look increase the length by half again and select a thickness of 0.2–0.25 T.

The curvature of the lashes affects the curled look. Popular lashes include:

◆ the J shape, which is most natural

◆ the B shape, which is straight with a gentle curl at the end

◆ the C shape, which gives the appearance that you have curled your lashes.

Choose a lash that is one half to one third longer than the client's natural eyelashes. If the single lashes are too long this will affect the durability of the attachment, cause the lashes to become twisted on the natural lash, and may cause stress to the natural lash causing it to weaken.

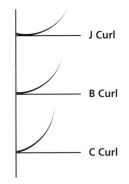

J Curl

B Curl

C Curl

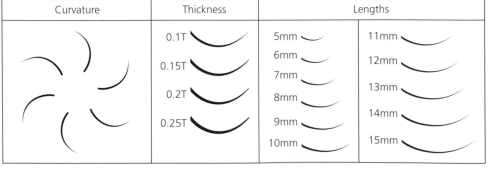

Curvature	Thickness	Lengths	
	0.1T	5mm	11mm
	0.15T	6mm	12mm
		7mm	13mm
	0.2T	8mm	
	0.25T	9mm	14mm
		10mm	15mm

Sample single lash lengths, thicknesses and curvatures

Eyelash and skin colour Select lashes that complement the hair and skin tone. Remember, a client may have their lashes tinted so the lash natural colour should be considered.

Natural eye shape

Using single lash systems for corrective purposes Below are some examples of corrective techniques for various eye shapes.

Eye shape	Corrective steps
Small eyes	Use medium-length lashes at the outside of the eye, longer in the middle and shorter on the insides.
Close-set eyes	Apply differing lengths of medium and longer lashes at the outside corners of the eyes and shorter on the insides.
Wide set	Use medium lashes from the inner portion of the eye with longer in the centre and a mixture of shorter and medium at the outsides.

Contra-indications

Certain contra-indications preclude or restrict single lash extension treatment. If there is any concern over the client's suitability, medical advice should be sought before the treatment proceeds. If following completion of the treatment plan or inspection of the eye area you have found any contra-indications as listed previously in this chapter and identified below, do not apply single eye lash extensions:

◆ a positive (allergic) reaction to the skin sensitivity patch test for adhesive

◆ previous eye service chemical treatments that may have weakened the natural lashes, e.g. eyelash perming.

If the client suffers from allergies such as hay fever there may be occasions when it is impractical for the lashes to be applied as they will be lost more quickly as the eyes become irritated and water.

Because you are working so close to your clients, some may feel uncomfortable or even claustrophobic.

It is a good idea to assess client tolerance to treatment by initially applying several lashes to assess suitability.

"Never agree to conduct a service that you do not feel is correct for the client, for example if the client wants to create something that you simply know will not suit her then be honest, she will appreciate it in the long run."

Shavata Singh

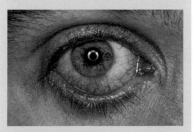

HEALTH & SAFETY

Herpes simplex

If a client suffers from the virus herpes simplex, this in some instances can occur in the eye area affecting the top layer of the cornea. If severe, this can affect the deeper layers of the cornea leading to scarring, resulting in permanent damage to vision. Be aware if your client suffers from this viral condition.

HEALTH & SAFETY

The following disorders restrict treatment

Dry eye syndrome In this condition there is decreased tear production or excessive tear evaporation, which may be caused by age, medical conditions and certain medications such as antihistamines. Its presence may be temporary or permanent. Refer your client to their GP before treatment proceeds.

Glaucoma An eye disorder in which the optic nerve is damaged at the point where it leaves the eye. This can be caused by raised eye pressure or damage occurs because there is a weakness in the optic nerve. This can lead to loss of sight. Refer your client to their GP before treatment proceeds.

HEALTH & SAFETY

Post-chemotherapy treatment

A client may request treatment following chemotherapy. It usually takes three to six months following treatment for hairs to grow back. Hair re-growth may be different from previously, changing texture and becoming curly when previously straight. Seek medical confirmation to treat if the hair growth is new.

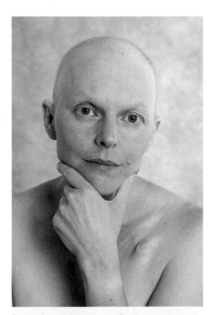

Post chemotherapy, a client may request treatment – seek medical confirmation if hair growth is new

An unduly nervous client with a tendency to blink could prove hard to treat in this way. Use your discretion in deciding the suitability for the treatment.

Those contra-indications requiring GP referral should be tactfully and clearly discussed to ensure client understanding.

Explain to the client what actions to take if a contra-action was to occur.

Contra-actions

If during application of single lashes the eyes start to water, blot the tears with the corner of a clean tissue. The tears can affect the adherence of the adhesive. Any possible irritation of the eyes should therefore be avoided, during the preparation of the eye area and application itself.

If the adhesive has accidentally seeped and glued to the protective eye shield, apply adhesive solvent with an applicator, and gently roll it over the area to dissolve the adhesive. To prevent this you should regularly check during application that the adhesive has not stuck to the shield. This is achieved by lifting the upper eyelid slightly.

If solvent accidentally goes into the client's eye, remove excess product, rinse the eye thoroughly and immediately, using clean water if necessary. Repeat this until discomfort is no longer experienced.

Allergic reaction to the products used – the client will need to have the products removed immediately and a record made of the reaction and action taken. It will be necessary to perform skin sensitivity patch tests with the products used to identify the allergen.

Over-stimulation of the meibomian gland, the sebaceous glands found on the eyelash line, could occur due to incorrect choice of lash length, thickness and wearing of the single lash extensions for long periods.

Skin sensitivity patch test

The adhesive used for single lash extension service should not come into contact with the skin, which means a skin sensitivity patch test should not be necessary. However, accidental contact may be made with the skin and some clients may be sensitive to the lash adhesive, producing an allergic reaction immediately on contact with it; others may become allergic later. For this reason, therefore, it is recommended to carry out a skin sensitivity patch test before each single lash extension treatment.

This test should be given on either the skin on the inside of the elbow or behind the ear. Some manufacturers recommend actually applying several lashes, following the application technique, to assess tolerance of the products used.

Two responses to the skin sensitivity patch test are possible – positive and negative:

◆ A positive skin sensitivity patch test result is recognised by irritation, swelling or inflammation of the skin.

◆ A negative skin sensitivity patch test result produces no skin reaction – in this case you may proceed with the treatment.

Before you proceed with the treatment question your client to confirm their understanding of all aspects of the treatment procedure.

The treatment record should be signed and dated by the client and beauty therapist following the consultation to confirm the suitability and consent of the agreed treatment.

It is important that accurate records are kept and stored in compliance with the Data Protection Act (1998) and for future reference.

Remember, clients classed as minors cannot be treated without signed parental/guardian consent and they must be present throughout the treatment if received.

Preparation of the client

Show the client to the prepared work area after the treatment plan has been completed. Consult the record card and check for any contra-indications to treatment. All accessories must be removed from the eye area including contact lenses. Explain the preparation process for the treatment, describing how the area will be prepared, the sensations to be experienced and how long the eyes will be closed for. It is important that they understand they cannot open their eyes while the treatment is being carried out.

1   Position the client comfortably, and ensure they are relaxed. This is important as the service can take any time between two hours if applying a full set of single lashes or 30–60 minutes if providing a maintenance service. The back of the couch should be slightly elevated without causing unnecessary strain to you while working. Support the client's head or neck with a cushion or pillow. A support cushion may be also placed under the knees to take the strain of the back while lying for a long period.

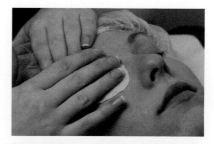

Cleanse the eye using the manufacturer's recommended eye make-up remover

2   Protect the client's hair with a hair headband, preferably disposable. This ideally must cover the whole head, e.g. a head bonnet to avoid beauty therapist contact with the client's scalp hair while working.

3   Protect the client's upper clothing with paper tissue, or small towel according to your workplace policy.

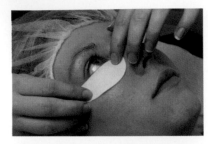

Apply protective eye shield to cover the lower lashes

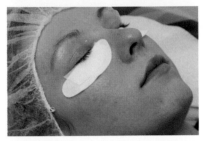

Apply surgical tape to cover any exposed lashes

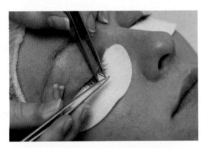

Single eyelash extension application

4   Wash your hands and apply a hand disinfectant after preparing the client. Protective gloves may be worn, especially if the beauty therapist has intolerance to any of the products used in the treatment.

5   Cleanse the eye area using the specialised non-oily eye make-up remover provided by your manufacturer. This will remove natural oils from the lashes that will affect adherence.

6   Comb through the lashes to separate them, allowing them to dry. Check client comfort.

7   Remove the adhesive backing on the reverse of the eye shield. Ask the client to look upwards towards you. Holding the skin around the lower eye taut, usually with the ring finger, apply a protective eye shield to cover the lower lashes of each eye. Ensure that this fits snugly around the eye contour and covers the lower lashes but does not touch the client's inner eye at the corner. Surgical tape is applied to cover any remaining exposed lashes. Apply a primer, recommended by your manufacturer, which prepares the lashes to ensure the lashes are oil free.

Comb through the lashes again as necessary; this straightens the lashes, avoids tangling and loosens any lashes that may be ready to naturally shed.

8   Ask the client to close their eyes. They must now remain closed. The client will only open their eyes when you request this.

9   Finally, check that the client is comfortable before single lash application.

ALWAYS REMEMBER

Avoid eye cosmetics before treatment application

It is best if the client arrives for the treatment wearing no cosmetic products on the eye area. This is because it will take time to remove and the cleansing process may affect the adherence of the lash system and sensitise the eye, causing it to water or create oils, again which will impede adherence.

REVISION AID

How should the client's natural lashes be prepared for treatment?

TOP TIP

Protective shields

The protective shield is usually impregnated with soothing, nourishing ingredients and acts as a service itself for use around the eye.

Products are available for single lash extensions that are designed for sensitive skin types.

HEALTH & SAFETY

Allergy

The adhesive used on the eye shield and surgical dressing to cover the lower lashes may cause irritation/allergy if the client/beauty therapist has an allergy to adhesive. Allergy to plasters must be checked for at consultation. The beauty therapist, if allergic, may have to wear gloves.

TOP TIP

Eyelash blower

If using air to assist drying, blow gentle puffs of air from the top of the lash downwards towards the nose. For some clients this may cause their eyes to water if the cornea becomes dry, so use with caution.

STEP BY STEP: APPLYING SINGLE LASH SYSTEMS

On completion the single lashes should give a balanced, well-proportioned look, complementing the client's eye shape and the agreed desired effect.

1 Select the length of lashes, thickness, colour and curvature to suit your client and agreed in the treatment plan.

2 Place the selected hairs on surgical tape where they are easily visible and accessible.

3 Dispense the adhesive in required amount into a disposable container. Alternatively, it may be applied to a disinfected, taped jade stone.

4 The surgical tape holding the lashes may be applied to the back of the hand.

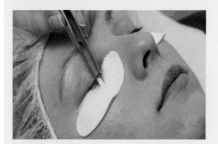
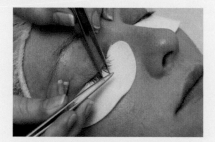
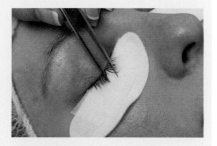

5 Working from behind the client, commence application placing the first lash in the centre, this is usually a longer length of lash. Isolate the natural eyelash by holding the tweezers at a 45° angle in your non-working hand.

Select a hair by its tip, the tapered end and using the pointed tweezers in your working hand, apply adhesive to two-thirds of its length from its base so it appears in small droplets, keeping the adhesive away from the tip.

6 Coat the surface of the isolated natural lash by running the single lash extension in an upward direction, against its length, avoiding contact with the skin.

Secure the lash into position ensuring there are no gaps with the natural hair, approximately 0.5 mm to 1.0 mm from where the base of the lash leaves the skin. Smooth the surface of the small droplets of adhesive using a cocktail stick or micro-applicator so that as it dries a natural appearance is achieved.

7 To create a balanced look and to allow the adhesive to dry, isolate and position the next single lash on the outer portion of the eyelid. You can assist drying using the eyelash blower.

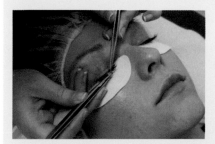
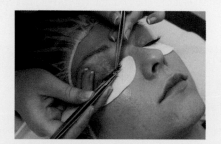
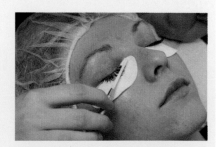

8 Lashes should be positioned at spaced intervals along the lash line in order to achieve a balanced look and to avoid adjacent lashes sticking together during application.

9 On completion of application the lashes may be combed through.

A protective sealer is applied to coat the adhesive and lash and improve the longevity.

10 Remove the adhesive tape and then the protective eye shield from the outside of the eye inwards. This should be easily removed. If excess adhesive has been used or the lower lashes have not been properly covered there can be resistance on removal, which is poor practice. The lashes should feel weightless and totally natural.

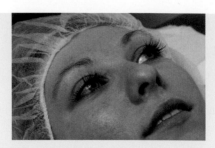

11 Provide the client with a mirror and show the client the finished result.

12 Discuss aftercare advice and recommendations and book a maintenance treatment.

13 Tidy the work area and dispose of any waste.

TOP TIP

Excess adhesive

If there is excess adhesive anywhere following placement, remove immediately while soft, using the professional tool or small applicator provided by manufacturers for this purpose. Also, if the lashes become stuck together, clean and release them immediately.

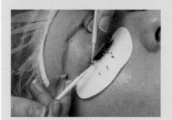

Remove excess adhesive

Once the glue has dried, this task will become more complicated and irritating for the client. A clean small applicator will be required to gently separate them using a small amount of adhesive. Clean tweezer points can also be used to separate the lashes.

TOP TIP

Bonding the single lash securely

If the adhesive has not coated securely the natural lash and single lash extension along its length it will soon be lost as lifting and separation of the lashes occurs.

Too much adhesive can cause lashes to stick together causing a 'clumping' unnatural effect. This may also affect the natural hair growth.

If single lash placement is incorrect when checking, e.g. lifting or crossing other lashes, remove and replace.

ALWAYS REMEMBER

Never apply more than one single lash to a natural lash. this may be too heavy for the natural lashes and may affect their growth and cause lash loss. However, this technique is possible when you have received advanced training and know what will be safe.

TOP TIP

Apply sufficient lashes of a suitable length compared to the natural lash, so that when the natural lash is naturally lost through the hair growth cycle which will mean the loss of the artificial lash also there will be sufficient remaining artificial hairs for the effect to be maintained until the maintenance service two to three weeks after application.

TOP TIP

Application techniques

Outside working inwards

Lash application can commence from the outside working inwards with spaced intervals between each single lash application along the lash line until completed. Each single lash application should be alternated between each eye.

Completing application to one eye, before moving to the other

Commencing lash application in the middle of the lash line, move to the outermost lash then halfway between these two lashes, then halfway again until application to the whole lash line on one eye is completed, before moving to the other.

Maintenance of single eyelash extensions

1 Position the client lying on the couch.

2 Refer to the client's records and check the lashes.

3 Wash your hands.

4 Prepare the lashes as discussed previously for application.

5 It may be necessary to remove some single lashes that require replacement; this is discussed below in removal.

6 Apply replacement lash extensions, required following the chosen application procedure. This will take between 30–45 minutes depending upon the quantity of lash replacement required.

7 Show the client the finished result and review aftercare procedures.

8 Re-book the next maintenance treatment.

9 Tidy the work area and dispose of any waste.

Removal of single eyelash extensions

1 Position the client for removal.

2 Refer to the client's records and check the lashes.

3 Wash your hands.

4 Remove make-up from the eye area, cleansing the skin with a suitable eye make-up remover.

5 Protect the lower lashes and eye by placing a protective eye shield over them. The upper eyelids may also be protected with an eye shield. The eye shields should fit snugly to the contour of the eye lid.

6 Dispense the solvent in the required amount into a container.

7 Apply solvent to an applicator and by treating one eye at a time, gently stroke down the lash extensions with the adhesive solvent until the adhesive dissolves, and the false lash begins to loosen. Use a dry applicator in the other hand to loosen the single eyelash extension.

8 When you are satisfied that the eyelash adhesive has been dissolved, gently attempt to remove the lash extensions. Support the upper eyelid with the fingers of one hand, using the other hand to remove the false lash with a sterile pair of tweezers. If the adhesive has been adequately dissolved, the eyelash will lift away easily from the natural eyelash. If there is any resistance, repeat the solvent application until the eyelash comes away readily.

9 As the lash extensions are removed, collect them on a clean white facial tissue or a clean cotton wool pad.

10 Having removed all the lash extensions lashes from one eye, soothe the area by applying damp cotton wool pads soaked in cool water. (This will remove any remaining solvent.) A damp cotton wool pad may be placed over the eye, while you remove the lash extensions from the other eye.

11 Ask the client to gently open their eyes ensuring that the light is not too bright in the treatment area, as the eyes will be sensitive.

12 Tidy the work area and dispose of any waste.

ALWAYS REMEMBER

Check under lashes

During application gently lift the lashes, lifting the lash line to check underneath that they have not become stuck to the lower lashes/ eye shield below.

Repeat this check several times during application.

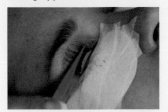

Lift lashes to check underneath

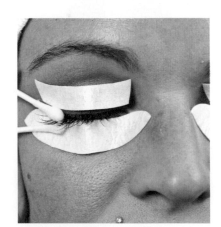

Application of adhesive solvent

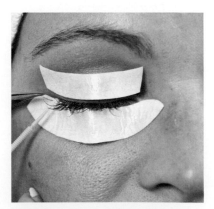

Removal of single eyelash extension using tweezers

HEALTH & SAFETY

Client comfort

Never attempt to remove the lash extensions until they have begun to loosen – if you do, the client's natural eyelashes will also be removed, causing them discomfort.

Avoid excessive use of solvent, which could run and enter the client's eye or cause skin irritation.

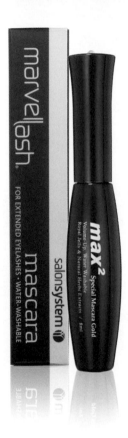

Mascara formulated for removal with water; recommended for use with single eyelash extensions

REVISION AID

When would you recommend a client receives a maintenance treatment and what would this involve?

"Keep yourself updated with the latest celebrity trends, particularly when it comes to lashes. For example, if someone comes into the studio and says that they have seen a certain look on a celebrity, you should always be one step ahead."

Shavata Singh

Aftercare advice and recommendations

◆ Warn the client that when a false lash is lost their natural lashes may appear less noticeable than usual. This does not mean they are weaker in any way. It is simply that the client will be more familiar with the appearance of their eyes with the extensions.

◆ Avoid rubbing the eyes, or the lash extensions may become loosened.

◆ Do not use oil-based eye make-up remover on the area as its cosmetic constituents will dissolve the adhesive.

◆ Use only dry or water-based make-up (as these may readily be removed with a non-oily eye make-up remover).

◆ Avoid extremes of heat, e.g. sauna treatment.

◆ Do not use regular mascara. If necessary to use mascara, this should be especially formulated to wear with single lash extensions, usually water soluble.

◆ Do not use mechanical eyelash curlers, which may loosen the artificial lash and could damage the natural lash, causing loss.

◆ Do not touch the eyes for one and a half hours after application, while the adhesive dries thoroughly. If showering avoid contact with the face. Use a cloth with water to cleanse the face as necessary.

◆ Avoid swimming for 24 hours or other exercise activities that may cause sweating.

◆ Do not attempt to remove the lashes – pulling at the artificial lash will also pull out the natural lashes.

◆ After bathing or swimming, gently pat the eyes dry with a clean towel. As the lashes are synthetic they will not dry like natural lash hair.

◆ An eyelash comb may be used to comb through the lashes to separate them after exposure to moisture, i.e. after showering.

◆ Any contra-action should be reported immediately to the salon.

Clients with single lash extensions should have their lashes maintained by regular visits to the salon. Lost single lashes can be replaced as necessary; this is often described as an infill service. Schedule every two to three weeks, this will enable you to maintain the appearance of the lashes and allow you to assess the health of the natural lashes.

Also recommend the purchase of a mascara formulated for use with the lashes. A sealant is also provided by some manufacturers for use following lash extensions to protect from moisture, helping maintain their appearance.

If the client wishes to have their single lashes removed, this must be done professionally. Recommend other eye services to enhance the eye area.

ASSESSMENT OF KNOWLEDGE AND UNDERSTANDING

Having covered the learning objectives for this chapter, test what you need to know and understand by answering the following short questions. The information covers:

◆ Organisational and legal requirements

◆ Anatomy and physiology

◆ How to work safely and effectively when performing eyebrow and eyelash treatments

◆ Client consultation, treatment planning and preparation

◆ Shaping the eyebrows including threading

◆ Tinting the eyebrows and eyelashes

◆ Applying eyelash attachment enhancement systems

◆ Contra-indications and contra-actions

◆ Client advice and recommendations

Organisational and legal requirements

For full legislation details, see Chapter 1.

1. How should records be stored to comply with the Data Protection Act (1998)?

2. What details should be recorded on the client's treatment record?

3. Why is it important to keep a record of the treatment carried out?

4. How should the client be positioned for eye treatments and why is client positioning important?

5. Why is it important that an eye service is given in the allocated time?

6. How long would you allocate to carry out:

◆ an eyebrow shaping treatment using the threading technique

◆ an eyebrow and eyelash tint

◆ upper lid strip lash application

◆ a full set of single lash extensions?

7. Why is the quantity of tint applied to the area important in relation to both efficiency and the final result?

8. At what age is a person classed as a minor? What would you need to obtain for a minor to receive an eye treatment?

Anatomy and Physiology

1. The small dye molecules used in tinting swell and join together, trapped permanently in the:

a. cuticle of the hair
b. the medulla of the hair
c. the cortex of the hair
d. the papilla

2. What is the hair growth cycle and how does this influence your application of single eyelashes?

3. What types of hair are eyelash hairs? How is this hair type recognised?

4. Draw the structure of the pilosebaceous unit in the skin.

How to work safely and effectively when performing eyebrow and eyelash services

1. What are the acceptable methods of sterilisation for tweezers used within an eye service?

2. What exercises can you perform to prevent repetitive strain injury and fatigue from performing eyebrow threading and regular single eyelash extension services?

3. Name three hygiene and safety precautions to be followed when performing the following eye services:

a. an eyebrow reshape
b. eyelash tinting
c. eyelash enhancement using flare, strip and single lash systems?

4. What should you check on completion of tinting and eyelash extension treatment to maintain products in optimum condition?

5. What personal protective equipment (PPE) may be worn when performing which eye treatments?

6. What environmental conditions should you check are adequate to work safely and effectively when performing eye treatments?

Client consultation, treatment planning and preparation

1. Why is it important to have a thorough consultation before any eye treatment?

Why is it important to confirm the client's understanding of the eye service following the consultation?

2. Why is it important to discuss and agree the treatment plan with the client before treatment commences?

3. If the client is having an eyebrow/lash tint or lash attachment service why is it important to check the results of the skin sensitivity patch test before you proceed?

4. If the client wished to have their fair brows tinted but had a positive reaction to the skin sensitivity patch test, what could you recommend as an alternative?

5. How should the brows be prepared to minimise discomfort and the risk of infection, before shaping commences?

6. What should be considered in the choice of eyelash extension system for a client?

7. How would you prepare the single lashes for application to avoid wastage and tangling?

8. How should the eye area be prepared to ensure that the eyelash extensions adhere securely to the natural lashes?

9. When would you recommend that a client returns to the salon for an eyebrow maintenance, following an eyebrow shape?

10. When would you recommend that a client returns to the salon for tinting treatment to maintain the effect?

   a. to the lashes
   b. to the eyebrows?

11. How long should a client be advised to wear before removal or a maintenance service is required:

   a. strip lashes
   b. flare lashes
   c. single lash extensions?

Shaping the eyebrows

1. What is the difference between eyebrow shaping with threading technique and with tweezers on hair removal in the area?

2. What factors should you consider when deciding the correct eyebrow shape for a client?

3. How can you determine the length of a client's eyebrows that will best suit their facial features?

4. How can you ensure that hairs are removed at their root?

5. What factors should you consider in your approach to eyebrow shaping with the following clients:

   a. a client with excessively thick eyebrows who requests a thin eyebrow shape
   b. a client who has close-set eyes
   c. a client with a round face
   d. a client who has a few stray long, coarse hairs
   e. a client with sensitive skin?

6. Why is antiseptic lotion applied following an eyebrow shaping treatment?

7. It is important to select the correct and most suitable equipment and materials for the treatment. When would you select and in what occasions would you recommend:

   a. automatic tweezers
   b. manual tweezers
   c. permanent tint
   d. temporary brow colour?

Tinting the eyebrows and lashes

1. How should the brow and lash area be prepared to avoid skin staining and to ensure effective tinting?

2. How do you select the colour when carrying out a tinting treatment?

3. a. How would tinting be performed when treating a very nervous client, to ensure a safe, efficient eyelash tinting treatment?
   b In which order would you treat a client who requires an eyebrow shape and an eyebrow tint, and why?

4. What is the difference in processing time between a brow tint and an eyelash tint?

5. How long would you allow the lash tint to process when treating a client with:

   a. blonde hair
   b. white hair
   c. red hair
   d. dark hair?

Applying eyelash extensions

1. Considering each type of lash attachment system, what safety precautions and checks should be taken during the application of each one?

2. When applying eyelash extensions along the length of the eyelid, how can you avoid irritating the corners of the eye?

3. What is the difference between the application of strip and flare lashes?

4. Why should the manufacturer's instructions be referred to when applying eyelash extensions?

5. What may result in poor adhesion of the artificial lash to the natural lash?

6. Which individual single lash type would you select and how would you apply them to suit a client with short, fine lashes and small eyes?

7. Explain the correct removal of:

   a. strip lashes
   b. flare lashes
   c. single lash extensions.

8. Why is it important to check if other chemical eye services have been received before eyelash extension application?

Contra-indications and contra-actions

1. When observing the area for eye treatments, what conditions would contra-indicate service?

2. At consultation you notice that the client has what you think is conjunctivitis. What action should you take?

3. Give two examples of contra-actions that may occur following eyebrow shaping.

4. What action would you take if a skin contra-action occurred following individual single lash application?

5. If a client complained of irritation during an eyelash tinting treatment, what action would you take?

Advice and recommendations

1. What aftercare advice and post treatment restrictions should be given to a client following an eyebrow shaping treatment?

2. What aftercare advice and post treatment restrictions should be given to a client following a tinting service?

3. What aftercare advice and post treatment restrictions should be given to a client following:

   ◆ strip lash application
   ◆ flare lash application
   ◆ single lash application?

4. What product may be recommended for a client following an eyebrow artistry service?

5. What advice would you provide to a client who is concerned that individual single lash extensions may damage their natural lashes?

6. When would you recommend a client received maintenance service? What maintenance procedures are performed at this service to restore the appearance of the lashes?

7. Why and when is it necessary for the client to return to the beauty therapist to have their artificial eyelashes removed?

8. List a range of ideal retail products that could be recommended for each eye service. Explain why they would benefit the client.

6 Make-up

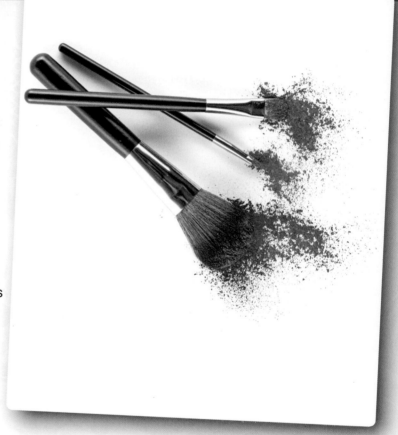

LEARNING OBJECTIVES

This chapter covers how to provide skincare to prepare the skin for make-up application and how to apply make-up products and techniques to suit the client's requirements and occasion.

You will learn more about:

◆ Maintaining safe effective methods when working.

◆ Using consultation and assessment techniques needed to draw up a make-up service plan that meets the client's agreed service plan objectives according to their:

– age group

– skin type and condition (taking into consideration any known allergies or areas requiring disguise or correction)

– facial features

– skin tone

– skin colour

– make-up style – natural, evening and special occasion

– preferences, e.g. colour choice.

◆ How to provide advice and recommendations to your client following the service to maintain and correctly remove the make-up. Also how to advise the client on any additional make-up products or services that will benefit them.

KEY TERMS

age group

consultation

make-up products

make-up style (natural; evening, special occasion)

make-up techniques

make-up tools

primers

skin condition

skin tone

skin type

WHEN PROVIDING MAKE-UP SERVICES YOU WILL BE REQUIRED TO

◆ apply environmental and sustainable working practices

◆ follow relevant laws and manufacturers' instructions

◆ use different consultation and assessment techniques to correctly identify your client's make-up requirements and make-up style

◆ use products, tools and equipment that will achieve the required results

◆ modify application to complement the client's skin condition, tone, face shape and features, and make-up style

◆ incorporate other services to enhance the result, such as eyebrow shaping, eyebrow artistry, lash curling and the application of lash attachments

◆ take the necessary action where a contra-action or contra-indication requires a treatment modification

◆ provide relevant advice and recommendations to support your client's service plan.

INTRODUCTION

This chapter covers the technical skill of make-up application, including how to adequately prepare the skin using appropriate skincare, application and removal techniques to achieve the optimum make-up result. Make-up is applied according to the style required by the client, including natural, evening and special occasion. The choice and application of make-up products and techniques will differ according to the type of light the make-up is to be viewed in. The make-up should also complement the client's skin type, condition, tone, colouring (including their skin, hair and eyes), and their age as well as their clothing and accessories.

Health and safety is an important feature of every service. The suitability of make-up products and any other services to be incorporated must be confirmed at the consultation, therefore avoiding the possibility of an allergic reaction or other service-related contra-action.

Dealing with your clients in a polite, efficient manner, using good communication and questioning skills to find out exactly what they require from the make-up service forms an important part of this technical service.

ROLE MODEL

MARION MAIN Lecturer, Hairdressing and Make-up Artistry, Glasgow Clyde College

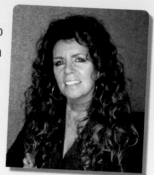

I was lucky enough to start my career working for Irvine Rusk and getting involved in numerous hair shows and photo shoots for magazines. Being part of Salon International also led me into the world of make-up and learning to create a total look was fantastic. Since then, the art of make-up has been my life.

During my career, I have benefited from some great opportunities for development across the make-up industry from applying a basic make-up to working in theatre, TV and film, and everything in-between. I have also been involved in student exchanges in places such as Lithuania and Ireland as well as participating in seminars and training in New York, Barcelona and London.

I am lucky that my career is also my passion. I am able to pass on my experience to students and watch them grow and develop. I am committed to lifelong learning and embrace every new challenge. I am the Chair Elect for the Association of Hairdressers and Therapists which allows students to showcase their work in competitions all over Britain in hair, make-up and beauty therapy. These students are our industry educators of the future and I am very proud to be part of their learning.

ALWAYS REMEMBER

Transferable knowledge, understanding and skills

When providing make-up services it is important to use the skills and knowledge you have learnt in the following chapters:

◆ The Business of Beauty Therapy (Chapter 1)
◆ The Science of Beauty Therapy (Chapter 2)
◆ Consultation Practice and Techniques (Chapter 3)
◆ Facials (Chapter 4)
◆ Eyebrows and Lashes (Chapter 5).

ALWAYS REMEMBER

Uniqueness

Our facial features are unique to us, they are:

◆ our face shape
◆ size and shape of nose
◆ size and shape of eyes
◆ size and shape of the mouth and lips.

Therefore, unique make-up application techniques are required for every client.

Make-up services

Make-up is used to disguise, enhance and accentuate **facial features** to make us appear more attractive – which in turn makes us feel more confident. Make-up is used to create balance in the face, by skilful application of different cosmetic products to reduce or to emphasise facial features.

Each client is unique, so each requires an individual approach for their make-up. The overall effect should enhance the client's appearance and complement their personality, lifestyle and the context for which the make-up is to be worn. Make-up looks and colours change in trend to complement each season's fashions. It is therefore important to keep up-to-date and be aware of how to achieve these different looks. Retail products with instructions should be available for the client to purchase if they wish to achieve the look for themselves.

As well as skin colour (related to the skin pigment melanin) when carrying out make-up, the **skin tone** colour or undertone needs to be considered. This is influenced by our blood

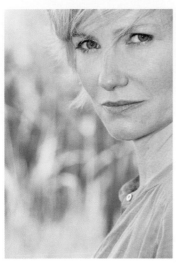
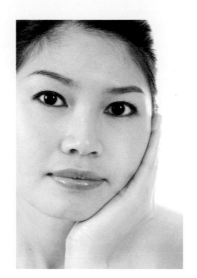

Natural make-up styles

vessels and the blood showing through the skin. The less pigment in the skin, the more undertone will be visible.

Clients may typically have a neutral, warm or cool skin tone. A neutral skin tone is a balance of pink and blue undertones. Warm skin tones usually have yellow and peach undertones. Cool skin tones have blue or pink undertones.

Cool skin tones usually suit cool blue-based colours whilst warmer orange colours suit warmer skin tones.

Make-up products should also improve the appearance and condition of the skin. Products should be selected to suit the client's **skin type**, colouring, condition, gender and age.

The anatomy and physiology knowledge and understanding required is found in the checklist in Chapter 2, and is also discussed within this chapter.

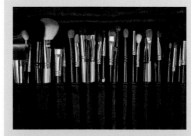

A make-up belt may be worn by the beauty therapist for convenience and efficiency during a make-up service.

Preparing the work area for make-up

The environment where make-up is applied should be decorated in light, neutral colours to avoid the creation of unnecessary shadows. The area should be well lit, ideally with the same kind of light as that in which the make-up will be seen.

Place all the required products, tools and equipment on a trolley, in front of a make-up mirror or other suitable work surface. Make-up brushes may alternatively be placed in a make-up tool belt, in leather, plastic or cloth worn around the waist for convenience during make-up application.

If you are displaying the make-up on a trolley, place the cosmetic products on a lower shelf until required, when they can be moved to the top shelf usually following skin preparation. This avoids cluttering the working area whilst you prepare or 'prep' the skin.

Keeping the work area tidy promotes an organised and professional image, and prevents time being wasted as you try to find products. It also reduces the risk of products dropping on the floor, such as pencils, which would damage the pencil's structure, leading to breakage. The work area should always be in a condition at any time during the working day to provide further make-up services.

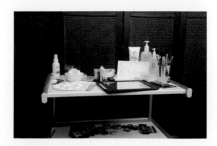

Prepared make-up work surface

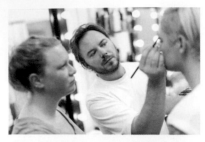

Make-up products may be set out in front of the make-up workstation

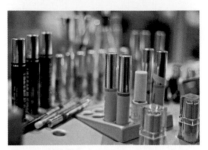

You may work from a retail display with testers, which can be used for make-up applications and demonstrations

HEALTH & SAFETY

Ventilation

Good ventilation is important so that the client's skin does not become too warm. It is easier to apply make-up effectively to cool skin, and the make-up will be more durable.

TOP TIP

Lighting

If working under artificial light, use warm white fluorescent light for day make-up, as this closely resembles natural light.

A diffuser may be used to cover the fluorescent tube. This softens the cool effect on the make-up and reduces the effects of shadows.

REVISION AID

Why is it important to match the make-up style to the lighting of the occasion at which it will be worn?

Lighting   Consider where the make-up is to be seen: in daylight, in a fluorescent-lit office, or a softly lit restaurant? You need to know the *type* of light in which the proposed make-up will be seen: this is important when deciding upon the correct choice of make-up colours, because the appearance of colours may change according to the type of light.

White light (natural daylight) contains all the colours of the rainbow. When white light falls on an object, it absorbs some colours and *reflects* others: it is the reflected colour that we see. Thus, an object that we see as red is an object that absorbs all the colours in white light except red. A *white* object reflects most of the light that falls upon it; a *black* object absorbs most of the light that falls on it.

TOP TIP

Professional lighting

Well positioned, professional make-up bulbs ensure you have enough light that mimics natural daylight to apply a make-up that illuminates the face evenly and indirectly. Often made from special glass they avoid unflattering, harsh shadows as light hits all sides of the face. Lights surrounding a mirror should be placed on the right and left sides of the mirror. Overhead lighting may make dark circles appear worse than they are, encouraging you to unnecessarily over-compensate with concealer!

If the make-up is to be worn in natural light, choose subtle make-up products in neutral colours as daylight intensifies colours. Any imperfection will be clearly seen. Avoid strong contouring techniques, which will appear further exaggerated.

If the make-up is to be worn in the office, it will probably be seen under **fluorescent light**. This contains an excess of blue and green, which have a 'cool' effect on the make-up: the red in the face does not show up and the face can look drained of colour. Reds and yellows should be avoided, as these will not show up; blue-toned colours will. This light also sharpens colours. Don't apply dark colours, as fluorescent light intensifies these. Choose lighter textured products in natural and neutral colours.

In the workplace a warm white fluorescent tube covered with a diffuser is preferable to simulate natural lighting and provides a truer representation of colour.

Evening make-up is usually seen in a darker environment under filament lighting. These create a warm look as they contain the colours red and yellow. Because of this it is necessary to choose the placement of some brighter colour tones and finishes, avoiding shades of brown, which may appear too dark. Emphasise facial features including the eyes using contouring cosmetics and eyeliner. Evening make-up will appear very obvious and dramatic in daylight. Explain to the client the reasons for the effect created, so that if she leaves the salon in daylight she won't feel that the make-up is inappropriate.

Products, tools and equipment

Each make-up work area should have the following **basic products, tools and equipment**. Further products, tools and equipment relevant to the make-up service are described here and discussed in more detail later in this chapter.

Products, tools and equipment

◆ **Couch or make-up chair** With sit-up and lie-down positions and an easy-to-clean surface.

◆ **Trolley** Or make-up work station surface on which to place everything.

◆ **Headband** A clean headband to protect the client's hair when cleansing the skin.

◆ **Hair clips** An alternative to a headband if the client's hair has been styled, is to secure the hair away from the face with a large hair clip.

◆ **Cleansing lotion/make-up remover** Suitable for different skin types and conditions to cleanse and prepare the skin for make-up application.

◆ **Eye make-up remover** To remove eye make-up and prepare the skin in the eye area for make-up application. A non-oily formulation will be required for clients wearing semi-permanent lash attachments.

◆ **Toning lotion** Suitable for different skin types to remove excess **cleanser**, tighten visible pores and restore the skin's pH balance without unnecessary skin stimulation.

◆ **Lightweight moisturiser or primer** Available in different formulations such as serums and gels and for different areas including the face and eyes. Suitable for different skin types to facilitate make-up application, enhance skin appearance and create a barrier between the skin and make-up.

◆ **Bowls** To hold the prepared cotton wool.

◆ **Dry cotton wool** Stored in a covered container, may be used to apply loose face **powder**.

◆ **Damp cotton wool** Prepared for each client and used during skin cleansing facial preparation.

◆ **Cotton buds** To apply make-up products and correct small accidental application mistakes.

◆ **Disposable tissue (such as bedroll)** To cover the work surface and the couch or make-up chair.

◆ **Large white facial tissues** To hygienically place equipment and tools on when preparing the work area, protect the headband from product staining, and to blot the skin after facial toning, absorb perspiration during make-up application and to protect the skin during make-up application.

◆ **Small spatulas (several) preferable disposable** For removing facial skincare make-up products from their containers.

◆ **Pencil sharpener (stainless steel)** Ideally suitable for placement in the autoclave or disinfectant. Used for sharpening cosmetic pencils, to provide a clean hygienic surface for each client and to provide a point for make-up application techniques when required.

◆ **Towels (2)** Freshly laundered for each client – one to be placed over the head of the couch or chair, the other over the client's chest and shoulders to protect their clothing. Alternatively a make-up cape or gown may be worn.

◆ **Bowls and covered, lined metal pedal bin** For waste materials.

◆ **Hand mirror (clean)** To show client the make-up during and after application to ensure satisfaction when a mirrored work station is not used.

◆ **Client treatment record** Confidential record with details of each client including personal details, products used, retail purchases made and details of treatment.

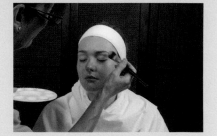
Specialist products, tools and equipment

Before beginning, check that you have the necessary make-up equipment and materials to hand and that they meet legal hygiene and industry requirements for make-up service.

◆ **Make-up (a range)** To suit different skin types, conditions, tones and **age groups**. It is important to choose a range that has retail products which are available for the client to purchase.

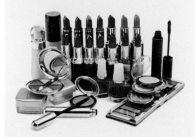

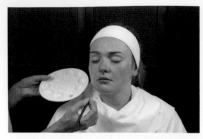

Make-up palette used to hygienically prepare and dispense make-up products

◆ **Bright professional lighting and magnifying lamp** To inspect the skin after cleansing and check for areas requiring special attention, e.g. broken capillaries and dark circles that require **concealer** application.

◆ **Make-up brushes (assorted)** At least three sets are required if this is a popular service you provide, to allow for effective cleaning and disinfection after use.

◆ **Disposable make-up applicators and brushes** Where possible use disposable, for example for **mascara** and the application of **eyeshadow** and **lipstick**.

◆ **Non-latex make-up cosmetic sponge and applicators** For applying **foundation** and other concealing and contouring products.

◆ **Make-up palette** For preparing and dispensing make-up products prior to application.

◆ **Lash extensions and adhesive** Range of lash attachment systems, colours and designs to enhance the eyes and complement the **make-up style** as required.

◆ **Brush cleanser** A proprietary brand cleaner to care for and maintain brushes hygienically.

◆ **Eyelash curlers** Tool used to temporarily curl the eyelashes.

TOP TIP

The benefits of a professional make-up work station

◆ A large mirror is provided, allowing full view of the head and shoulders.

◆ Illumination is provided by specialist make-up bulbs.

◆ The light is reflected from the work shelf and overhead shelf, providing shadow-free light, thus avoiding unnatural shadows.

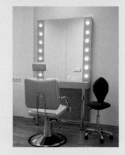

You will need to have to hand a good range of professional make-up in different forms and formulations, suitable for clients with known skin allergies to cosmetics, for contact-lens wearers, for different skin types, conditions, ages and skin colours including:

◆ pre-base products such as **primers**

◆ tinted moisturisers

◆ concealing products

◆ contouring products, including shaders, highlighters and blushers

◆ foundations

◆ translucent powders

◆ eyeshadows

◆ eyeliners

◆ brow pencils and powders

◆ fixing products such as serums and waxes

◆ mascara

◆ lipsticks

◆ lip glosses

◆ lip liners

◆ setting spray.

Other equipment may include:

◆ brow stencils for achieving the silhouette shape of the brows

◆ brow scissors to trim unruly individual brow hairs.

Range of make-up brushes

Name	Description
Large face powder dusting brush	To remove excess face powder or to apply specialised powders such as bronzing and shimmer powders.
Large concealer brush	To apply foundation to specific areas.
Contouring blush brush	To apply facial contouring products to highlight and shade areas of the face. This is achieved as the bristles have a blunt cut or angled end.
Blusher brush (large to medium)	To apply powder colour to the face and for blending.
Small flat angle-edged eyeshadow brush	To apply and blend powder eye make-up products in the socket area of the eye.
Small rounded-edged eyeshadow brush	To apply eyeshadow, blend and shade.
Medium firm eyeshadow blending brush	To blend powder eye colours and soften harsh lines and colour.
Small concealer brush	For exact placement of concealing product in areas such as around the nose and mouth. The brush has a flat surface with a round end; a smaller version of the foundation brush. You may wish to have a medium and large concealer brush as well for application to larger areas.
Lash and brow brush	Brow brush to remove excess make-up from the brow hair and to add colour, blend eyebrow pencil and groom hair into shape. Lash brush to apply mascara, remove excess mascara and to separate the lashes.

(Continued)

Name	Description
Eyeliner brush	A fine brush used to apply make-up eyeliner colour to contour the eyes, creating a precise line. A line and define brush is shown.
Lip brush	To apply lip products and ensure a definite, balanced outline to the lips. These are available in different shapes including angled for coverage, fine-tipped for applying a lip line, flat and diamond-tipped.

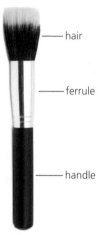

hair

ferrule

handle

The different parts of a make-up brush (fibre optic type)

Make up brushes usually consist of a handle, a piece of metal called a ferrule, which attaches to the handle and holds the brush fibre bristles in place, and bristles themselves.

They are available in different shapes and designs, and are prepared from different fibres, which may be synthetic from fabric and chemical sources or animal including camel, sable, squirrel, pony and goat and contain blends of different animal hairs. Synthetic brushes are non-absorbent and are better for the application of cream or gel textured products as they control the application of the product more.

Powder and blusher brushes may be produced from softer hair, but for the purpose of contouring and blending, brushes must be firmer.

TOP TIP

Fibre optic brushes (as shown on left)

Fibre optic brushes are a mixture of animal hair at the base and synthetic hair at the ends. This combination is great for powder make-up product application as the animal hair holds the powder product and the synthetic end achieves a light final coverage of the make-up product.

Animal hair absorbs products where as synthetic hair will not. Synthetic is ideal to apply liquid foundations, concealer and lip products, for example.

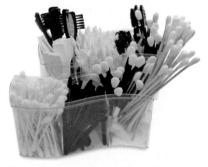

Various types of disposable applicators

ALWAYS REMEMBER

Choosing your make-up brush

Make-up brushes are the tools of your trade!

When buying make-up brushes, make sure that the hairs are secure at the base of the brush – the ferrule. Test the comfort of the bristles; stroke the brush against your skin.

Also if the handle is made of wood, consider if it is a sustainably sourced product e.g. bamboo or recycled resin handles.

Animal hair may be replaced with synthetic hair such as Taklon.

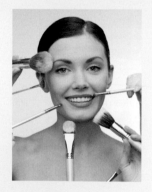

Safety and hygiene

Ensure that **make-up tools** and equipment are sterile or disinfected before use and, where possible, use disposable applicators during make-up application, costing these into the price of the service.

Disinfect non-disposable make-up brushes after each use. An *alcohol-based cleanser* may be used to clean and care for make-up brushes as they contain oils that condition the bristles. The brushes are first cleaned with a solution of warm water and detergent, then thoroughly rinsed in clean water and allowed to dry. They are then briefly immersed or sprayed with the alcohol solution and again allowed to dry. Once dry, place the brushes in a UV light cabinet ready for use.

All cosmetic products should be removed from their containers using a clean spatula or orange stick, and placed on the clean plastic make-up palette before application. This avoids contamination of the make-up with bacteria from unclean make-up applicators. Never 'double-dip' applicators into products.

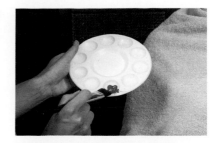

Hygienic removal of make-up product and placement onto a make-up palette

HEALTH & SAFETY

Manufacturer's instructions

Always use brush cleaner following manufacturer's instructions to ensure effective cleaning and care of your brushes.

Application of a professional brush cleaner – always wear PPE to protect your hands; a face mask may sometimes be required in addition when using cleaning agents.

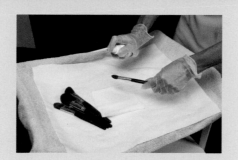

HEALTH & SAFETY

Make-up hygiene

Hygiene is important for clients too. Tom Pellereau, winner of the BBC's Apprentice programme, tested a range of make-up brushes, including some from retail make-up counters. He found that some brushes had 40,000 bacteria on them!

Source: Professional Beauty May 18 2016.

Advise clients to keep their own make-up clean. Dirty brushes spoil effective make-up application, and offer breeding grounds for bacteria.

Make-up generally has a shelf life of 2 years and is then past its best and becomes unhygienic. It is recommended that mascara be replaced every 6 months.

HEALTH & SAFETY

Make-up hygiene advice

To avoid cross-infection, recommend that the client doesn't repeatedly use the applicators supplied with cosmetic products unless they have been cleaned to avoid cross-contamination.

Likewise, applicators provided with cosmetic products should not be used directly on a client, e.g. mascara brush, instead use disposable applicators. Disposable applicators should be discarded after use. This is important information to share with the client too.

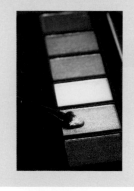

The make-up palette should be cleaned with warm water and detergent, then wiped with a disinfectant solution applied using clean cotton wool. It should be stored in the UV cabinet.

Mascara should be applied using a disposable brush applicator, new for each client.

Sharpen cosmetic pencils with a pencil sharpener before each use. This will ensure contact with the skin is with a clean surface.

Make-up sponges should be disposed of after use, or washed in warm water and detergent where permitted; then placed in a disinfectant solution and rinsed. Allow them to dry, then place them in the UV cabinet, with each side being exposed for at least 20 minutes.

Disinfect work surfaces after every client and always follow hygienic work practices.

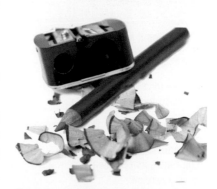

Sharpen cosmetic pencils before each use

"Make-up celebrates diversity: every client and every make-up should be unique.

When performing a service, reassure the client that the make-up is carried out and aims to cater for every situation and client need. Typical examples may be if the client is nervous about having their make-up done, cultural considerations or if there is a specific non-contraindicated health or disability requirement."

Marion Main

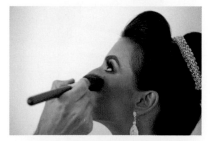

Glamorous bridal make-up style

ALWAYS REMEMBER

Professional service timing

Make-up lesson: allow 1 hour.

Special occasion or evening make-up: allow 45 minutes to 1 hour.

Day natural make-up: allow 45 minutes.

If insufficient time is available, do not book the service. Always deliver a quality service.

Client care, consultation and communication

Information to provide to the client at the initial point of interest

When a client makes an appointment for a make-up service, the receptionist will need to confirm the purpose of the make-up application because this will affect the time that is allocated for the service.

Make-up application is offered for different purposes, called a make-up style.

◆ *A natural make-up* Some clients simply wish to have their make-up professionally applied to enhance their skin and facial features whilst remaining natural, just as they would have their hair professionally styled.

◆ *Evening make-up* will usually be seen under artificial lighting. The effect this has on the appearance of the make-up will depend upon the light source, which must be considered when applying evening make-up. Generally, evening make-up is heavier in application and stronger colours may be applied. Products to emphasise and highlight, such as frosted eyeshadows and **lip glosses** may be introduced.

◆ *Special occasion make-up* is applied to suit the occasion or event for which it is to be worn, such as a party, prom or wedding. If the make-up is for a special occasion it is always recommended to advise the client to visit the salon for a **consultation** and a practice make-up session so that you can decide together on the most appropriate make-up style. Ask the client if possible to bring a swatch of the material with her, so that you can select colours to complement this and to co-ordinate with the accessories.

◆ *Photographic make-up* is applied for many reasons including magazine shoots, portrait work and fashion shows. Make-up application must be skilful to achieve the right end-result as the location may be a photographic studio or outdoors on location. If make-up is to be photographed for a special occasion such as bridal make-up, matt colours may be used to avoid too much light reflection which can be an issue with frosted colours.

◆ *Corrective make-up* may be applied for concealing purposes, and when applying advanced techniques using products that can disguise the appearance of facial disfigurements or birthmarks, and the client may be taught, if you are qualified to do so, how to do this for themselves.

◆ *A make-up lesson* A chance for the client to learn from a professional how to apply make-up that suits them and to learn new techniques.

All staff, especially the staff communicating with clients at reception, should be familiar with the different pricing structures for the range of make-up services and products available for retail. Be aware of market trends – a client may request they only have eye make-up application. If offered this would usually be priced accordingly.

In the workplace, advise the client that if they intend to have their hair washed and styled, this should be done before they have the make-up applied.

If a client requests a deep cleansing facial followed by make-up application, suggest that they have the facial at least five days prior to the make-up. The facial will stimulate the skin, increasing its normal physiological functioning such as localised blood circulation and increased sebaceous gland activity. This will affect how long the make-up lasts; it may even cause the colour of the foundation to change.

Do not recommend an eyebrow reshape at the same service as make-up application – secondary infection could occur; also the skin in the area will be very pink or darker dependent upon skin colouring, altering the colour and thus the effect of eyeshadow. This is because of an increase in blood circulation in the local area. However, it is acceptable to trim hairs or remove stray, or coarse hairs that spoil the appearance of the eye area.

Advise the client to wear something that can be easily removed such as a button-up top, to avoid disturbing their make-up following application.

Client arrival

Clients should never be kept waiting on arrival for their appointment unless there is an unavoidable reason.

On arrival the client **service plan** may start to be completed by the salon receptionist. Record the client's personal details, such as their name and address and if qualified to, check that there are no contra-indications to the make-up service.

Mascara
Black non-waterproof lash-lengthening formula

Eyeliner
Light grey gel liner applied along the outer lash line

Lip liner
Matt red applied to outside of lip line to make the lips appear fuller

Lip product
Cream matt red lipstick and clear lip gloss applied to the centre of the lips

Foundation
Medium beige, liquid foundation with SPF

Powder
Light translucent matt powder

Eyebrow colour
Brown brow powder

Brow bone
Ivory matt eyeshadow

Socket
Matt dark grey eyeshadow

Eyelid
Iridescent light peach eyeshadow

Blusher
Tawny brown applied to cheekbone

Contour
Matt beige powder applied around the jawline and under the cheekbones

Sample record of make-up products applied recorded on a make-up chart

Consultation

The consultation Complete the service plan recording the client's personal details and details of the make-up applied.

If the client is a **minor** under the age of 16, it is necessary to obtain parent, carer or guardian permission for the make-up service. The parent/guardian will also have to be present.

Discuss the make-up style with the client to ensure that the make-up will meet their requirements. You may need to ask questions such as those that follow, but of course the questions depend on the context of the make-up.

Ask the client if she has any images of herself wearing make-up, and to show you which she particularly likes and why.

ACTIVITY

Make-up style book

Just as a hairdresser may refer to hairdressing styles, as a make-up artist you can share make-up styles with the client.

Collect images and build up a make-up style book showing different ages, skin and hair colouring, and make-up contexts and techniques.

"Display make-up in the consultation area to refer to, and to check a client's preferences in relation to colours and textures."

Marion Main

ACTIVITY

Recognising contra-indications

If, on visual inspection, you notice a general contra-indication, the make-up service cannot proceed. What skin disorders can you think of that would contra-indicate, preventing make-up application?

TOP TIP

Seasonality

Analysts at Mintel's Beauty and Personal Care Division have identified that there is a growing trend for seasonality in beauty and facial care products. Seasonal products are growing in popularity and, in 2014 accounted for 11.1% of all beauty launches.

Make-up formulations should be reviewed to see if they meet the client's current skin needs for the different seasons.

- ◆ Do you normally wear make-up?
- ◆ For what occasion is the make-up to be worn?
- ◆ What colour are the clothing and accessories to be worn on this occasion?
- ◆ Are there any colours that you particularly like or dislike?
- ◆ What effect would you like the make-up to create? (This question may be asked in many contexts – the client may wish to achieve a natural or a glamorous effect, or to emphasise or diminish certain facial features.) You may wish to refer to examples of make-up styles to ensure you are accurately interpreting the client's requirements.
- ◆ Are there any products you are allergic to?
- ◆ Do you wear contact lenses?

If the client wears glasses, check the function of the lens, as this can alter the effect of the make-up, for example magnifying the eye area when the glasses are worn.

Provide the opportunity for your client to ask any questions relating to the make-up service.

The service record should be signed and dated following the consultation to confirm the suitability and consent with the agreed make-up service.

It is important that accurate records are kept and stored in compliance with the Data Protection Act and for future reference.

ALWAYS REMEMBER

Each client's make-up requirements will be different

Examples of make-up service modification include:

- ◆ make-up style
- ◆ ethical make-up considerations in choice of products and tools used, for example products not tested on animals
- ◆ choice of make-up products and application techniques for corrective work
- ◆ choice of make-up to suit the client's skin type and condition
- ◆ disguising minor skin imperfections
- ◆ using hypoallergenic products for a client with cosmetic sensitivity
- ◆ age of client, using light-reflecting make-up products for a mature skin or one showing signs of premature ageing.

HEALTH & SAFETY

Allergies

Where possible, before using a new make-up cosmetic, a client with known allergies should first receive a skin sensitivity patch test, or be given a small sample of a product to try on a less sensitive area of the skin, to assess the skin's tolerance. If an allergic reaction occurs, medical attention must be sought immediately.

Inform your client that it is possible to grow out of an allergy to a given product. It is also possible, however, suddenly to become allergic to a product that has not given problems before.

Contra-indications

Certain contra-indications prevent make-up application. These include bacterial, fungal, parasitic and viral infections, which are described in more detail in Chapter 3 Consultation Practice and Techniques, where contra-indications are illustrated and discussed, including those listed below. Check for these at the consultation, and if any of the following are present on further inspection of the skin, do not proceed with make-up application.

Remember that not all contra-indications are visible – a current bone fracture, for example would not be. The following disorders may contra-indicate or restrict make-up service. If you suspect the client has any disorder from the list below, do not attempt a diagnosis but refer the client tactfully to their GP without causing concern.

◆ *pediculosis capitis (head lice)*

◆ *acne vulgaris (active)*

◆ *herpes simplex (cold sore)*

◆ *impetigo*

◆ *styes or hordeola*

◆ *conjuncitivitis (pink eye)*

◆ *watery eye or epiphora*

◆ *blepharitis*

◆ skin disorders such as **hyperkeratosis**, where there is an abnormal thickening of the outer layer of the skin. Psoriasis is an example of this.

In the case of the skin disorder, herpes simplex, the make-up service may be received when the skin is healed and clear.

The following conditions also contra-indicate make-up application:

◆ *skin disorders* including those not listed above, such as bacterial infections (e.g. impetigo), viral infections (herpes zoster) and fungal infections (e.g. tinea corporis)

◆ *psoriasis* and *eczema*, where the skin is broken

◆ *bruising* in the area

◆ *recent haemorrhage*

◆ *swelling and inflammation* in the area

◆ *recent scar tissue*

◆ *sensory nerve disorders*

◆ *cuts or abrasions* in the area

◆ *a recent operation* in the area

◆ *eye disorders* including those not listed in the chart

◆ *parasitic infestation* such as pediculosis and scabies.

Remember – never name a contra-indication, you may be wrong. Refer the client to their GP, it is their role to diagnose the problem.

Ask the client whether they have any known allergies to cosmetic preparations. Note the answer on their record. Care must be taken to avoid contact with an allergen.

REVISION AID

What are the visible facial characteristics of the skin types below that you learned about in Chapter 3?

◆ Oily

◆ Dry

◆ Combination.

REVISION AID

What skin disorders and eye disorders would contra-indicate make-up? List three examples of each.

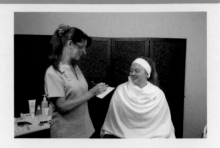

Contra-actions

Certain cosmetic ingredients are known to cause allergic reactions in some people. These ingredients are known as allergens. Allergens may cause irritation, severe redness referred to as erythema, inflammation and swelling, known as a contra-action. This may occur during or following service.

Known cosmetic allergens include the following:

◆ *Lanolin* This is similar to sebum, and is obtained from sheep's wool. It is added to many cosmetics as an emollient.

◆ *Mineral oils* Examples are oleic acid and butyl stearate.

◆ *Eosin (bromo-acid dye)* A staining **pigment**, used in some lip cosmetics and perfumes.

◆ *Paraben* An antiseptic ingredient used as a preservative in facial cosmetics.

◆ *Certain colourants* One example is carmine.

◆ *Perfume* This is added to most cosmetics and is a common sensitiser.

Products should be selected without the allergen where identified.

External contact with an allergen may cause urticaria (hives or nettle rash), eczema or dermatitis. If an allergy occurs, the product should be removed from the skin and a soothing substance applied. The client should be advised not to use the product again. Always record any allergies on the client's record so that the offending product may be avoided in the future.

Other contra-actions include:

◆ *Watery eyes* If the client has minor watery eyes a tissue may be placed at the corners until the irritation has ceased. If the client's eyes water excessively, remove eye make-up and discontinue service.

◆ *Excessive perspiration* Some clients may perspire, which will affect adherence of the make-up and its finished result. Blot the skin with soft facial tissue and apply more loose face powder to absorb perspiration. If the client continues to perspire, and you have exhausted all methods of cooling or ventilating the environment, discontinue treatment.

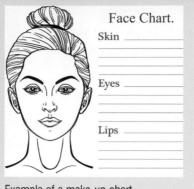
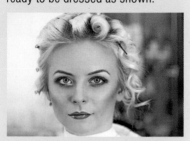
Preparing the client

Take the client through to the make-up work area. Before you start the make-up, you should have discussed and planned the make-up with the client, recording significant details on their service record.

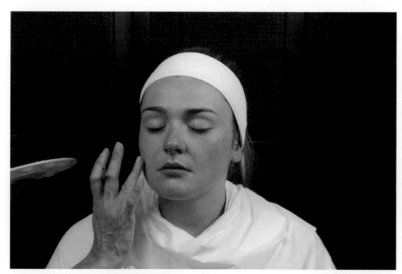

Client prepared for a day make-up style

Before preparing the client for the service, clean your hands using an approved hand cleansing technique in front of your client who will observe hygienic procedures being carried out.

Offer the client a gown, cape or a clean towel according to your work policy, which is placed across their chest and shoulders. Place a headband or hairclip around the hairline, to protect the hair, prevent it from spoiling if previously styled and keep it away from the face.

Any jewellery in the area should be removed. Refer to the service record to check for any known allergies to cosmetic products.

Ensure that the client is comfortable at all times.

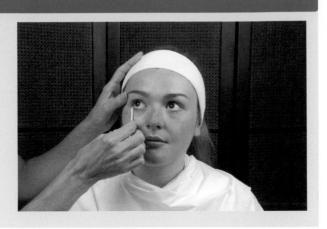

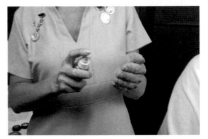

Hands may be disinfected before make-up application where water is not available

After preparing the client, and before touching the skin, clean your hands again. Now cleanse and tone the skin, using products appropriate to their skin type. Just as skincare products vary in their formulation to suit the various skin types, so make-up products are designed for different skins. Record all relevant details on the service record.

Inspect the skin, if necessary using a magnifying lamp. Identify any areas that require specific attention, i.e. broken capillaries, pustules, papules, dark circles, hyper-pigmentation, hypo-pigmentation and scarring. Touch the skin to assess tone and levels of hydration.

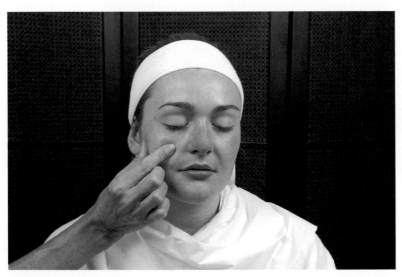

Apply a light-textured **moisturiser** before make-up application. This has the following benefits.

◆ It prevents the natural secretions of the skin changing the colour of the foundation.

◆ It seals the surface of the skin, and prevents absorption of the foundation into the skin.

◆ It contains ingredients to protect, such as SPF, and also to improve skin appearance and performance of the skin type.

◆ It facilitates make-up application by providing a smooth base.

◆ It may be tinted to provide colour when a natural look is required.

Remove excess moisturiser by blotting the skin with a facial tissue.

Special lotions may be applied to improve the skin texture and increase make-up durability, these include skin **primers** and oil control lotions.

Skin primers are silicone-based, creating a film on the skin surface that is hydrating and reflects light. They refine the skin's appearance, minimising open pores and the appearance of fine lines. The formulations can vary to suit the client's skin type and may contain pigments to correct skin tone. The primer provides a base and acts as a barrier, preventing absorption of the make-up products into the skin. Primers are applied as moisturiser but less is required.

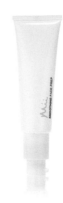

Skin primer

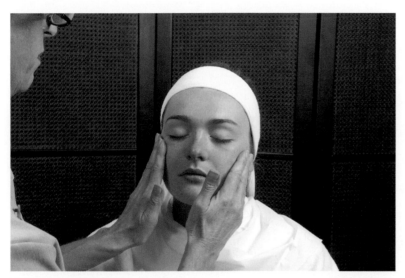

Moisturiser application

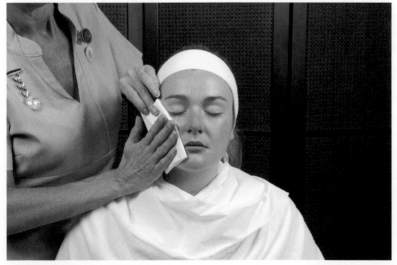

Blotting the skin to remove excess moisturer

REVISION AID

How should the skin be prepared before a make-up application?

ALWAYS REMEMBER

Erythema (skin redness)

Avoid excessive pressure and stimulation of the skin while cleansing and preparing the skin for make-up application.

The skin will become too warm, affecting durability and erythema of the skin will occur – skin reddening requires correction.

Oil control lotions contain powder ingredients that absorb the skin's natural oil, reducing shine and producing a matt finish. They are ideal for preparing an oily or combination skin before make-up application.

Applying make-up products

The make-up sequence

Sequence for applying make-up:

1   Prepare the skin.

2   Conceal any blemishes. This can be checked again following foundation application.

3   Apply foundation.

4   Contour the face (with cream liquid products). Remember: cream on cream, powder on powder. So, if powder products are to be used, this will follow the application of powder in sequence number 5.

5   Apply powder.

6   Contour the face (with powder products).

7   Apply blusher.

8   Apply eyeshadow.

9   Make up the eyebrows.

10   Apply mascara.

11   Make up the lips.

NB. Contour products, used to shade and highlight the face and features, can be applied in powder or cream formulation. Application sequence for contouring will depend upon product formulation chosen.

> **REVISION AID**
>
> Why is it important that make-up is applied in a sequence?

> **TOP TIP**
>
> **Product promotion**
>
> Where possible, use make-up that you also retail in the workplace so that the client can purchase the products if they wish. Use attractive posters and displays in the workplace to raise awareness and interest in the products. Raise awareness on your website if you have one, with professional tips on product use on social media too.
>
>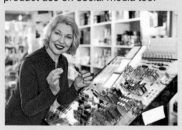

> **ALWAYS REMEMBER**
>
> **Order of application**
>
> Make-up is applied in a specific sequence to ensure:
>
> ◆ a balanced look is achieved
>
> ◆ products are applied effectively, i.e. cream on cream, powder on powder, which allows products to be blended and set appropriately
>
> ◆ the client's understanding, e.g. when carrying out a make-up lesson or demonstrating how to achieve a certain look
>
> ◆ durability and the optimum look of the make-up is maintained.

Age of the client

When applying make-up remember how skin changes with age. This will influence the imperfections and **skin conditions** that may be present and require correction, and the suitability of make-up colour, type and effect.

Age and appearance table

Age	Appearance
<15	Nearly perfect skin. Smooth texture, pores small.
15–25	Acne key factor in surface texture. Fine lines start to appear, pore size increasing.
25–45	More fine lines and appearance of first wrinkles (photo damage). Early signs of sagging near the eye. Some loss of elasticity. Adult acne.
45–55	More wrinkles, rough texture. Sallow yellow colour begins to appear. Pores and age spots enlarge and define. Sagging near eye and cheek.
55+	Wrinkles and fine lines in abundance. Uneven colour, pigmentation. Sagging worsens. Dark circles under eye.

ACTIVITY

Age and corrective techniques required

Depending upon your client's age, there will be corrective techniques that you may anticipate using.

Looking at the *Age and appearance table* on this page, which products and techniques might you select?

How would you modify the application according to skin age?

Concealer

Concealing blemishes

Before you begin to apply make-up to the face, inspect the skin and identify any areas that require concealing, such as blemishes, uneven skin colour, dark circles under the eyes or shadows.

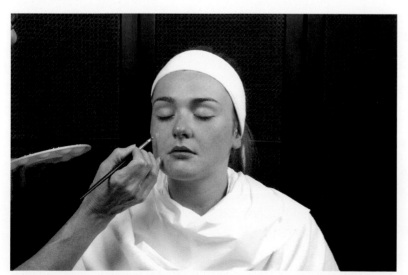

Applying concealer before foundation application to minimise the appearance of a skin papule

ALWAYS REMEMBER

Concealing

Concealing may be completed before or after foundation application.

Foundation may be used to disguise minor skin imperfections, but where extra coverage is required it is necessary to apply a special concealer, a cosmetic designed to provide

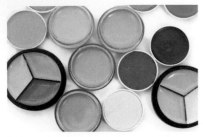

Colour corrector concealing products

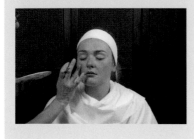
maximum skin coverage. The concealer may be applied directly to the skin after skin moisturising, or following application of the foundation.

Choose a concealer that is one to two shades lighter than the client's skin tone. In the case of pigmentation, however, this may vary according to the colour difference between the area being concealed and the skin's natural colour.

Concealers designed for use around the eye area are often in the form of a pen containing liquid, and are light in texture, lighter in colour than the foundation with a yellow tone to minimise the appearance of dark circles. Concealers designed for covering blemishes are unsuitable for application around the eyes.

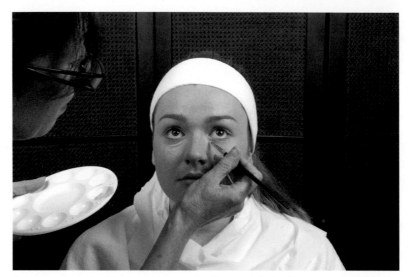

Applying concealer after foundation application to minimise the appearance of dark circles under the eye

Concealer can contain pigment to help correct skin tone.

◆ **Green** helps to counteract high colouring where the skin appears red, and to conceal dilated capillaries. Yellow may also be selected.

◆ **Lilac or pink** counteract a sallow skin colour.

◆ **Peach and pink** counteract dark circles around the eyes and are suitable for darker skin tones.

◆ **White or cream** help to correct unevenness in the skin pigmentation.

◆ **Yellow** helps to counteract the appearance of dark circles around the eyes.

Concealers come in a range of colours and consistencies including liquid, cream, stick, pencil and tube, to suit all skins and differences in skin texture. Mix different colours together to obtain the required colour.

Colour correctors target problem areas and contain pigments that balance skin tone. Select lighter shades, e.g. light pink for lighter skins; if the skin is darker select shades of peach. Peach is particularly effective to counteract bluish under-eyeshadows. Green correctors counteract areas of redness. Yellow counteracts pink tones.

Correctors are applied like concealer and may be followed with concealer or foundation dependent upon the coverage they provide.

Applying concealer to blemishes

Use concealer sparingly. Remove a small quantity of the concealer from its container, using a clean disposable spatula. If it has a brush applicator attached to the product, for reasons of hygieneu this cannot be used.

Apply the concealer to the area to be disguised, using either a clean make-up sponge or a soft concealer make-up brush. Blend the concealer to achieve a realistic effect. Reapply concealer as necessary until correction is achieved.

ALWAYS REMEMBER

Concealing products

Zinc oxide and titanium dioxide are examples of ingredients that increase the coverage of concealer-type make-up preparations and are white in colour. Several colours are required in order to obtain the correct shade to blend into the area. Orange colour corrector is useful to help reduce the appearance of hyperpigmentation on a darkly pigmented skin.

ALWAYS REMEMBER

Common ethnic skin problems:

◆ White skin – easily damaged by exposure to high temperatures and UV light, leading to broken veins and pigmentation disorders.

◆ Oriental – prone to uneven pigmentation on UV light exposure.

◆ Asian – often has uneven pigmentation skin tones; darker skin is often found around the eyes.

◆ Black – melanin is present in all layers of the epidermis; this can cause scarring following skin damage, possibly leading to uneven pigmentation, vitiligo and keloids.

How to apply concealer to disguise minor skin pigmentation disorders

Concealer is useful to disguise minor pigmenation disorders such as hypopigmentation (reduced melanin production, lighter areas of skin) and hyperpigmentation (increased melanin production, e.g. darker areas of skin). Advanced training is required to achieve the requirements for a camouflage make-up. Always check the manufacturer's instructions on how best to apply the concealing product for different coverage requirements.

1 Select the chosen colour or colour mixture that best matches the skin tone surrounding the area to be treated. Select tools that make application easier, such as a small non-absorbent concealer brush.

2 Blend the make-up thinly over the problem area, extending it past the edge. If disguising minor scarring, a brush may be used to feather the make-up at the edges to create a natural effect.

HEALTH & SAFETY

Medicated concealers

Advise clients to avoid medicated 'lipstick'-type concealers – these are too thick for general concealing. They are also unhygienic, as they are designed to be directly applied to a blemish: this means that the product becomes a breeding ground for bacteria.

TOP TIP

Concealer application

It is preferable to build up several layers of product to achieve the desired effect, rather than applying a thick layer.

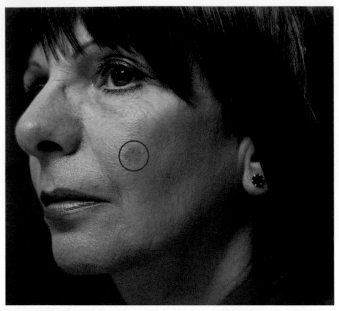

Hyper-pigmentation – Chloasmata to the face (area circled)

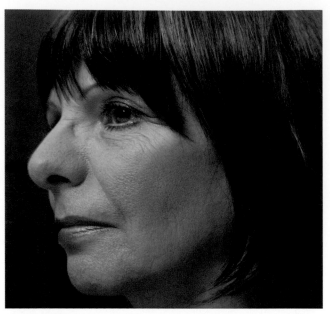

The area of hyperpigmentation chloasmata is disguised

3 Build up the colour depth to ensure the blemish is completely covered, thinning the colour at the edge to blend in. A small concealer brush can be used to blend in the edges of the make-up.

4 Once the required result has been achieved, apply a fixing powder generously with a large powder puff.

5 Brush off any excess powder with a large, soft make-up brush, e.g. powder brush. The area to be disguised should not be obviously detectable.

6 If concealing is completed first the full make-up may now be applied.

7 Apply foundation up to the area of concealing make-up and blend so that an invisible finish is created. Putting an oily cream foundation over the make-up will move or remove the concealer make-up; it is best to use a non-oily, foundation.

8 Record on the client make-up record the make-up products selected and application technique used.

REVISION AID

When might you apply a concealer product?

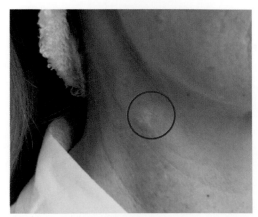

Hypopigmentation in the neck area (area circled)

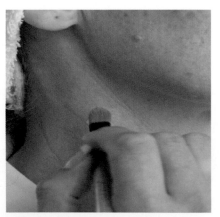

Make-up applied using a synthetic non-absorbent brush to cover the hypopigmenation

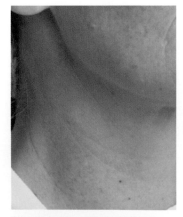

The area of hypopigmentation is disguised

Foundation

Foundation is applied to provide a base for further make-up products, produce an even skin tone, to disguise minor skin blemishes, and as a contour cosmetic.

Foundation is available as cream, liquid, compact stick, gel, cake, mousse, powder, mineral-based and tinted moisturiser.

Foundations can contain different formulations including **'anti-ageing' ingredients** such as vitamins A, C and E. These are to neutralise **free radicals**, natural chemicals thought to be responsible for damaging the skin and producing the signs of ageing – the lines and wrinkles! Sunscreens and moisturisers are commonly included in foundations to protect the skin from the environment.

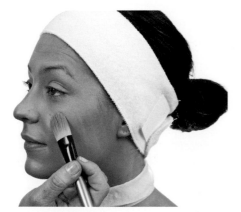
Applying foundation

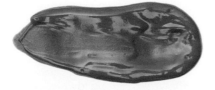
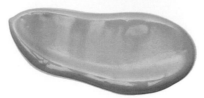
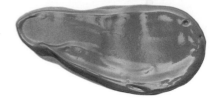
Colour swatches of foundation creams

Silica beads can be included in the formulations, especially for combination/oily skin, to absorb the skin's natural sweat and oil.

Foundations can create different finishes to the skin including:

◆ Matt: popular with an oily skin type, creating a powder finished appearance.

◆ Semi-matt: popular with mature and combination skin types. A smooth moist sheen is created, which may require the addition of translucent powder.

◆ High shine: an oil-based foundation suitable for a mature skin type and one requiring heavier coverage.

◆ Luminous: a shimmery effect is created, which achieves a radiant, healthy skin appearance. Ideal for creating a radiant, healthy appearance to the skin, especially in drier facial areas.

TOP TIP

Coverage to create a natural appearance

To achieve a sheer, healthy, natural appearance quickly, the client may like to apply a tinted moisturiser instead of a foundation. Blemish or beauty balm which is also known as BB cream, and colour corrector or CC cream, provide the consistency of tinted moisturiser. Both treat the skin with additional skincare ingredients and CC cream provides a slightly heavier coverage to even out skin colour, e.g. for disguising areas of redness.

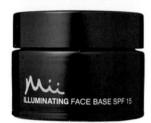

Cream foundation

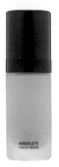

Liquid foundation

Foundations provide different coverage including:

Sheer: a light, natural coverage to enhance balanced skin requiring little correction.

Medium: a heavier coverage that can correct the appearance of uneven skin tone and blemishes.

High: used when maximum coverage is required, usually to conceal a scar or birthmark. You may wish to use the foundation just in the area requiring concealment.

Types of foundation

Each foundation differs in its formulation to suit a particular skin type. The correct choice will guarantee that the foundation lasts throughout the day.

Cream foundations Cream foundations are usually oil-based and blend easily on application. They provide a heavy coverage, and have these specific service uses:

◆ dry skin

◆ normal skin

◆ mature skin.

Liquid foundations Liquid foundations are oil-, water- or mineral-based, providing light to medium coverage.

Oil-based liquid foundations have these specific uses:

◆ dry skin

◆ normal skin

◆ mature skin

◆ combination skin (apply the foundation to the *dry* areas).

Water-based liquid foundations have the following uses:

◆ normal skin

◆ oily skin

◆ combination skin (apply the foundation to the *oily* areas)

◆ dehydrated skin.

Liquid foundations are composed of water, powder, oil, humectant (such as glycerol), pigments and additives.

Water-based foundations do not spread very easily because the water content rapidly evaporates, so these foundations must be applied quickly.

Mineral make-up is created from finely ground minerals, a process called micronisation. Pure mineral powders feel weightless, reduce cosmetic congestion as they do not contain synthetic powders and filler ingredients such as talc.

The make-up may contain a selection of the following minerals, which all contribute an effect to the finished look of the make-up:

◆ Titanium dioxide, a natural white mineral powder providing opacity – titanium is also an ingredient used in cosmetics for its SPF effect.

◆ Zinc oxide, a natural white mineral powder that enhances the appearance of the crystallised minerals provides bacterial protection; mica, a natural mineral that has light-reflecting properties showing a range of colours. (It also affects the finished formulation providing slip to facilitate make-up application.)

◆ Bismuth oxychloride, a synthetic white mineral with a silvery metallic sheen providing coverage to the make-up; iron oxide, a synthetic mineral iron used to add colour.

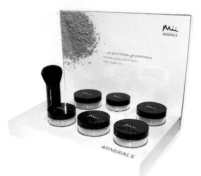

Mineral make-up foundation

TOP TIP

Mineral make-up

Mineral make-up can be applied following a facial as the blend of minerals and pigments form microscopic flat crystals due to their formulation, which will not clog the pores.

Mineral liquid foundation This contains the natural light-reflecting properties of micro-minerals. It provides a low to medium coverage, with a skin enhancing, slightly luminous look.

◆ It helps make the skin appear healthy and fresh.

◆ It is suitable for all skin types, especially normal to dry skin.

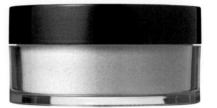

Mineral foundation

Mineral powder foundation Mineral powder foundations contain micro-minerals in a solid powder with a binding ingredient such as algae. Again, suitable for all skin types providing a heavier coverage through layer application.

Gel foundations Gel foundations provide sheer, oil-free, non-greasy coverage and a matt finish. Light-reflective properties are achieved through the addition of pigments. They have these specific uses:

◆ black, unblemished skin

◆ tanned skin

◆ skin on which a natural effect is required.

Compact skin or cake foundation Compact skin or cake foundations may have an oil, wax or powder base. They give a heavy coverage, and have these specific uses:

◆ dry skin

◆ normal skin

◆ badly blemished or scarred skin.

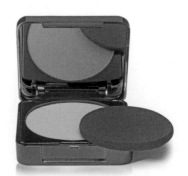

Compact all-in-one or cake foundation

Mousse foundations Mousse foundations provide light to medium coverage depending on application technique. They have a mineral oil base. Their specific uses are:

◆ normal skin

◆ combination skin.

Care must be taken to apply the mousse foundation to an area of the skin and blend quickly or it may start to dry on the face, creating a chalky appearance.

HEALTH & SAFETY

Choosing a foundation

◆ If the skin is oily and blemished, a *medicated* foundation may be used.

◆ If the client suffers from the skin disorder, acne vulgaris, it is preferable not to apply foundation at all – bacterial infections might be aggravated. Mineral foundations may be the most suitable choice.

◆ If the skin is sensitive, select a *hypoallergenic* foundation.

Tinted foundation A tinted foundation is similar to a tinted moisturiser but provides a heavier to medium coverage, although still natural. It offers protection from the environment, especially if containing added sunscreen and skin moisturisers. A disadvantage is it will not cover blemishes.

◆ It helps make the skin appear natural, healthy and fresh.

◆ It may contain light-reflecting ingredients, making mature skin look more radiant.

◆ It is suitable for all skin types available in oil or oil-free formulations.

Tinted moisturiser This provides a very light coverage and finish, ideal for when a natural look is required and the skin is to be seen. As they often contain a sun protection factor (SPF) they are a good choice when make-up is not to be worn as the skin is protected from sun damage. These are a suitable choice for a normal to dry skin type, requiring little correction.

Foundations continuously develop to meet the skin's needs. The serum foundation is an emulsion that provides a sheer natural finish whilst providing colour correction and coverage. The serum contains an SPF, ingredients that firm the skin and have anti-ageing properties.

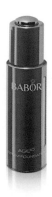

Serum foundation

Foundation colour

The colour or shade of the foundation should match the client's natural skin colour. The skin should ideally be viewed in daylight to choose the best match when testing. Foundation colour may be yellow to orange (warm), red to pink (cool) and both warm and cool (neutral) or olive. Mix colours so that it blends into the surrounding skin, appearing to disappear. Test the foundation for compatibility on the client's jawline or forehead.

If an incorrect colour is selected, or if the foundation is insufficiently blended on application, there will be a noticeable **demarcation line**.

Skin tones may vary on the face with lighter and darker areas, especially on black skin. If the lighter tones are to be emphasised, a lighter coverage foundation product should be selected allowing the skin's natural tone to show. Many skins, especially multi-ethnic skin will require mixing products and shades to create a balanced look. Remember, products can be layered to increase coverage.

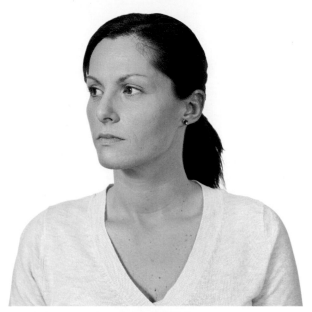

Foundation compatible to the client's skin tone

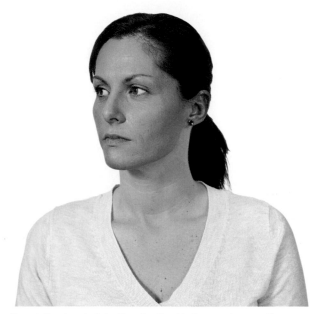

Foundation too dark for the client's skin tone, a demarcation line is visible

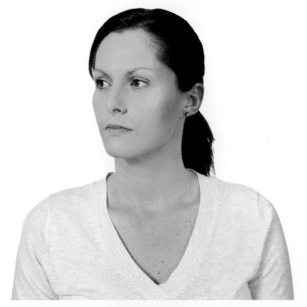

Foundation applied too light for the client's skin tone

TOP TIP

Foundation formulation suitability

On a black skin, avoid powder-based foundations as these will make the skin look grey and dull.

Skin colour	Foundation colour
White	Ivory or light beige, with warm tones of pink or peach.
Olive	Dark beige or bronze.
Suntanned	Bronzer (to suit skin colour).
Florid	Matt beige with a green tint.
Sallow	Beige with a pink tint.
Light brown	Light brown foundation with a warm tone.
Medium brown	Light brown with a yellow/orange tone.
Dark brown	Deep bronze foundation with a yellow/orange tone.
Black	Dark golden bronze.

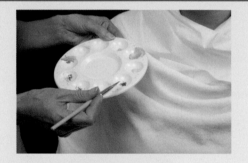

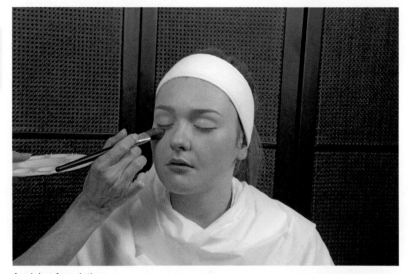

Applying foundation

Applying foundation

If the foundation is in a container with a lid, remove some from the container using a clean disposable spatula, placing it onto a clean make-up palette.

Foundation may be applied using either a foundation brush, which is stroked over the surface of the skin, a large powder brush or a cosmetic sponge. Formulation will dictate the best choice of applicator. Foundation brushes are available in different sizes enabling you to control where you are applying the foundation. It should be applied to one area of the face at a time, with an outward stroking movement.

TOP TIP

Transporting make-up

◆ If you intend to apply make-up at different locations, buy a large make-up case so that you can transport the make-up easily and hygienically.

◆ If you are transporting your make-up in a box, keep the box clean. Clients won't be impressed if they see soiled, dirty make-up containers.

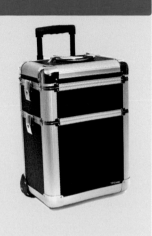
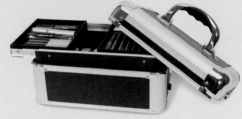

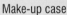
Make-up case

A cosmetic sponge is often also used to blend foundation. Take care that you blend it at the hairline and at the jawline. Avoid clogging the eyebrows with foundation. The **cosmetic make-up wedge** is designed to apply varying amounts of pressure to the different areas of the face, and to ensure even coverage of the foundation.

If applying foundation around the eye area, use a small foundation brush or the angular edge of a cosmetic sponge. This will help you achieve accuracy in application.

The extent of coverage can be controlled by the method of application and where you hold the brush.

Apply foundation to cover the entire face, including the lips and the eyelids. Do not extend the make-up to the neck unless the occasion requires this – for example, if a bride's dress exposes part of the upper chest – because the foundation will mark clothes at the neckline.

Some areas may require to be concealed with a concealing product following foundation application such as dark circles under the eyes.

TOP TIP

Application coverage

If the cosmetic sponge is damp, coverage is light and sheer. To achieve a heavier coverage, use a dry latex-free make-up sponge.

If you hold the foundation brush handle nearer to the ferrule, application will be heavier.

TOP TIP

Professional foundation application

Professionally, avoid applying foundation with the fingers. Apart from being less hygienic, with this method the warmth of your hands may cause streaking. Contact with the fingers and the skin should be minimal. It may also cause disturbance of the placement of concealing product.

ALWAYS REMEMBER

Application of mineral powder foundation

Apply using a large powder brush and tap to remove excess powder before application.

HEALTH & SAFETY

Product formulation MSDS

Legally the manufacturer must produce a list of ingredients used in their product.

Request a MSDS to refer to and ensure safe product selection.

HEALTH & SAFETY

Make-up cosmetic sponges

Keep a store of spare make-up cosmetic sponges – they soon crumble with repeated cleaning.

REVISION AID

How would you select foundation for different skin colours?

HEALTH & SAFETY

Avoiding contamination

Before application, always remove sufficient loose powder from the container and replace the lid. This minimises the chances of bacteria entering the powder.

REVISION AID

Where would shader be applied for a client who has a deep forehead?

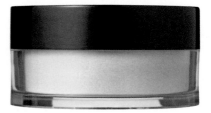

Loose powder

HEALTH & SAFETY

Client advice on hygiene

If the client uses a pressed powder, advise them to wash and replace the powder applicator regularly to minimise the reproduction of bacteria.

Face powder

Face powder is applied to set the foundation, disguising minor blemishes and making the skin appear smooth and oil-free. It protects the skin from the environment by acting as a barrier. It also allows the application and smooth blending of other powder products such as blusher and eyeshadow.

Most powders are based on **talc** as the main ingredient, but talc particles are of uneven size, and substitutes such as the mineral **mica** are now becoming popular. These give a more natural, flattering appearance to the skin.

Powder adheres to the foundation through the addition of **zinc, magnesium stearate** or **fatty esters**. These chemicals set the make-up and remove tackiness. Further powder products can then be applied to the skin.

Face powder contains absorbent materials such as **precipitated chalk, rice powder** or **nylon derivatives**. These absorb sweat and sebum throughout the day, reducing shine and giving the foundation greater durability.

Light-reflecting ingredients such as mica and moisturising ingredients are popular to reduce and soften the signs of ageing such as fine lines.

Shine control ingredients or 'blot powder' is created for use in professional situations and for touch-ups. Blot powder contains crystallised minerals and silica to absorb excess oils and reduce shine on the skin's surface.

Types of face powder

There are two basic products: loose powders and compact powders.

Loose powders Loose powders do not contain any oils or gums to bind the powder together. They are available in a range of shades, with different pastel pigments added to counteract skin imperfections. Colours include pink and lilac, which are flattering when viewed under artificial lights; yellow, which enhances a tanned skin; and green, which counteracts a red skin. Iridescent ingredients may be included to produce shimmering and highlighting effects. Translucent powder has no colour.

Many cosmetic products contain **titanium dioxide**, an opaque white pigment, to provide coverage. When applied to black skin, this can give the skin a chalky appearance. When selecting products for black skin, bear in mind not just the shade but also the ingredients.

Compact powders Compact powders contain a gum, mixed with the ingredients to bind them together. These powders provide a greater coverage, especially if they contain titanium dioxide. Pressed powders should be recommended mainly for a client's personal use, and then only to remove shine from the skin during the day, as required.

How to apply powder

Face powder is applied *after* the foundation, unless a water-based foundation or a combination powder foundation has been selected. Select a matt powder for a daytime make-up, and an iridescent shimmer powder for an evening make-up.

Loose face powder

1 Remove the loose powder from its container, using a clean spatula or, if the powder is in a shaker, by sprinkling it out. Place the powder on a clean facial tissue.

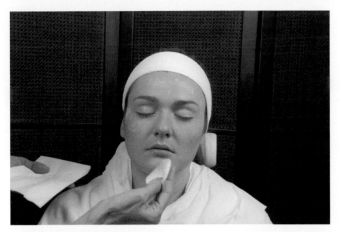

Loose powder application

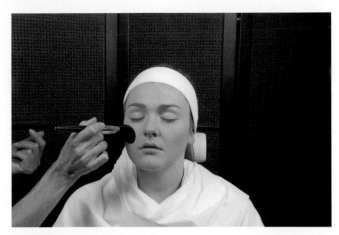

Removal of excess loose powder

2 Ask the client to keep their eyes closed. Using a clean piece of cotton wool or velour sponge, press into the powder and then press the powder all over the face.

3 Remove excess powder using a large, disinfected facial powder brush. Direct the brush strokes first up the face, which dislodges the powder, then down the face, which flattens the facial hair and removes the final residue of excess powder.

Compact powder Apply powder with a brush or velour powder puff.

Facial contouring using powder products may now be carried out.

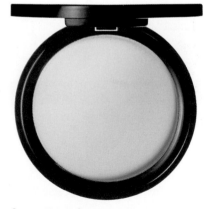

Compact powder

TOP TIP

Applying powder

◆ Don't apply face powder to excessively dry skin, as it would aggravate and emphasise the dry skin condition.

◆ Beware of applying powder if a client has superfluous facial hair, as it may emphasise this.

◆ If the skin appears too pale apply a facial bronzer product to correct.

◆ Oily skin can make the powder darker. If this occurs apply a lighter powder to correct.

TOP TIP

Powders

Some powders reflect light while appearing subtle and non-shiny. These are most flattering for mature skin, as wrinkles appear less obvious.

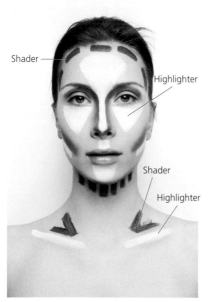

Changing the appearance of the facial shape and features using contouring cosmetics to shade and highlight

Contouring

When applying make-up you will emphasise or diminish the facial shape or features. This is achieved by using corrective contouring techniques.

Contour cosmetics

Changing the shape of the face and the facial features can be achieved with the careful application of **contour cosmetics**. These products draw attention either towards or away from facial features, and can create the optical illusion of perfection.

Each face differs in shape and size, so each requires a different application technique.

Contour cosmetics include **highlighters, shaders** and **blushers**. They are available in powder, liquid and cream forms.

◆ *Highlighters* Draw attention towards – they emphasise. Highlighters must be lighter or the same tone as the skin; formulations will differ, creating either a light matt effect or a pearlescent or shimmery effect. The popular technique, strobing, uses highlighter suited to skin type with the aim to achieve a fresh finish and sheen, whilst also bringing light to facial areas that require emphasis.

◆ *Shaders* Draw attention away – they minimise. When selecting a shader, choose a colour two or three shades darker than the client's natural skin tone. The careful application and blending can be used to sculpt the facial features.

◆ *Blushers* Add warmth to the face and emphasise the facial contours.

Before applying these products, decide on the effect you wish to achieve. Study the client's face from the front and side profiles, and determine what facial corrective work is necessary. Corrective techniques for different face shapes and facial features are discussed below.

Following application of shader and highlighter, contour the cosmetics as shown on the image. Blend and soften the harsh lines, using a sponge or brush, into the surrounding skin colour.

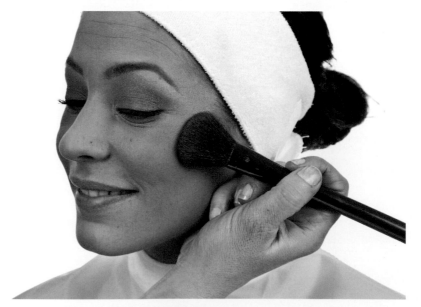

Blusher application to emphasise cheek bones

Blushers The colour should brighten the face. Hold different blusher shades next to the face to identify a suitable colour. Peach, apricot colours suit all skin tones. Reds and berry tones are suited to dark skin tones. Consider the age of the client where natural shades are preferable rather than bright fashion colours. Some blushers appear very vibrant in the container, yet when they are applied to the skin they are subtle.

Blushers are available in powder, cream and liquid formulations.

Powder blushers Mineral powder blusher is formulated using pigments to add colour and warmth to the skin. Alternatively, synthetic or natural pigments are formulated with a face powder with a talc base to add bulk, and zinc stearate to bind the ingredients together with various skin conditioning agents. A softer look is achieved with powder blusher.

Cream blushers A cream or wax base holds the pigment colour. Silicone is added to cream blushers to facilitate application. Cream blushers are highly pigmented so consider this when applying, 'less is more'.

Liquid blusher Pigment providing the tint shade is suspended in a liquid containing water, glycerine, silica and alcohol.

If liquid or cream cosmetics are used, these must be applied on top of a liquid or cream foundation before powder application. (If powder contour products are used, these should be applied after the application of the loose face powder. The rule of contour cosmetic application is: powder on powder; cream on cream.)

Mineral powder blush Minerals are refined to a lightweight, sheer application where colour is achieved by layering. Its ideal usage is for a mature skin.

How to apply powder blushers

Stroke the contour brush over the powder blusher. Tap the brush gently to dislodge excess blusher.

Apply the blusher to the cheek area, carefully placing the product according to the effect you wish to create. The direction of brush strokes should be upwards and

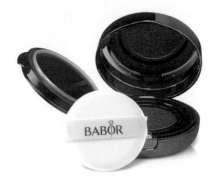
Powder blusher

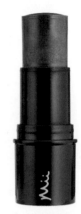
Cream blusher

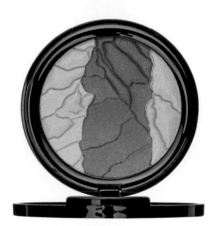
Blusher duo providing colour and highlighting shimmer

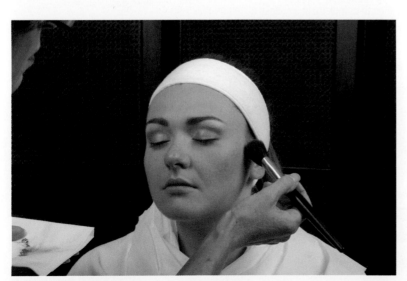
Powder blusher application

TOP TIP

Blusher application

Blusher can be applied to the cheeks and temples to add warmth to the face.

outwards, towards the hairline. Keep the blusher away from the nose, and avoid applying blusher too near the outer eye. Ensure the edges of the blusher application are blended and softened.

Apply more blusher if necessary. The key to successful blusher application is to build up colour slowly until you have achieved the optimum effect.

If too much blusher is applied, tone down with the application of a loose face powder.

How to apply cream blushers

Remove the cream blusher hygienically from its container.

Apply the cream blusher after foundation application. Using the fingertips dot the cream blush colour sparingly onto the fullness of the cheek area and blend towards the hairline. Alternatively a synthetic brush may be used. Cream blusher is suited to all skin types except oily. Place a loose translucent powder over the cream blusher to set if required. Alternatively it can be left unpowdered for a 'dewy' effect.

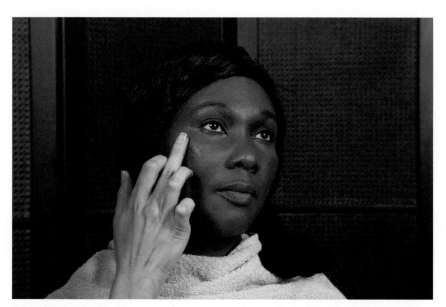

Cream blusher application to complement a special occasion make-up

How to apply liquid blushers

Liquid blusher provides a sheer to strong, stained look, dependent upon product usage. It is best to apply to a normal skin as it is difficult to blend and would be generally unsuitable on a dry skin type.

Dot the liquid blush on the cheek area and blend well. Remember it must be worked with quickly, if left in an area too long it will stain and remain.

Bronzing products

Bronzing products are applied to create a healthy, natural or subtle tanned look. They are formulated to create a matt or shimmer effect and are also suitable as a highlighting contouring product.

When choosing a colour, avoid going more than two shades darker than your client's skin colour, or the look will appear artificial.

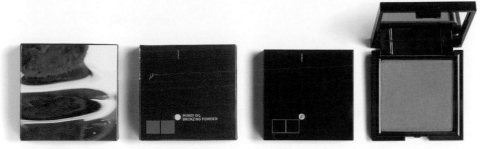
Bronzing products

Types of bronzing product

Bronzing products are available in powder, gel and liquid formulation. Powder bronzers, a tinted powder available in different shades, give skin natural colour effects and highlight and enhance a client's skin tone or tan. Powder bronzers are suitable for all skin types, although they can emphasise a dry or mature skin and can also emphasise blemished and oily skin characteristics, such as open pores. Gel bronzer contains gel and glycerine in which the pigment is suspended. Gel bronzer is preferable for a dry, mature skin and can be applied to the whole face or specific areas. Liquid bronzer is suitable for all skin types and contains a pearlised, light-reflective micro-fine powder with an oil-free formulation. Silicone enhances its application.

Apply bronzing products according to the effect you want to achieve after powder application or in the case of gel and liquid after foundation application. Remember you can use bronzers as a contour product also. It is important that bronzer is applied in daylight-type lighting to avoid excessive application.

Powder Using a large powder brush apply the bronzer powder. Stroke the brush over the cheek area, followed by nose, chin and neck area.

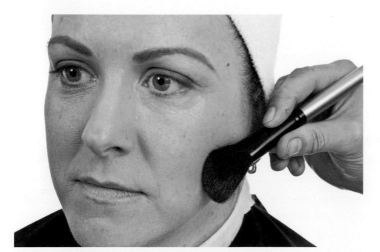
Bronzing powder application: matt powder bronzer applied under the cheekbones

Gel You need to blend the gel bronzer quickly over each area. Apply with the fingers or a damp sponge. Commence at the cheek area, forehead, nose and chin.

Liquid Apply as for gel bronzer.

TOP TIP

Bronzer application

When applying bronzer avoid using a brush that is too large or the bronzer will extend beyond where it is required.

TOP TIP

Bronzers for males

A bronzing powder designed for males is available, which is matt and natural, creating a healthy appearance.

TOP TIP

Cotton buds for accidental mistakes

Have clean cotton buds available so that you can remove the powder from any minor mistakes during application.

Face shapes and features

Face shapes

To guide you on where to contour the face, it is important to assess the client's **face shape**. Take the hair away from the face – hairstyles often disguise the face shape. Study the size and shape of the facial bone structure. Consider any excess fat and the muscle tone.

Oval	**Oval** *Bone structure* This is regarded as the perfect face shape. *Corrective make-up* Corrective make-up application usually attempts to create the *appearance* of an oval face shape. Draw attention to the cheekbones by applying shader beneath the cheekbone, and highlighter above. Blusher should be drawn along the cheekbone and blended up towards the temples.	
Round	**Round** *Bone structure* Broad and short. *Corrective make-up* Apply highlighter in a thin band down the central portion of the face to create the illusion of length. Shader may be applied over the angle of the jaw to the temples. Apply blusher in a triangular shape, with the base of the triangle running parallel to the ear.	
Square	**Square** *Bone structure* A broad forehead and a broad, angular jawline. *Corrective make-up* Shade the angles of the jawbone, up and towards the cheekbone. Apply blusher in a circular pattern on the cheekbones, taking it towards the temples.	
Heart	**Heart** *Bone structure* A wide forehead, with the face tapering to a narrow, pointed chin, like an inverted triangle. *Corrective make-up* Highlight the angles of the jawbone and shade the point of the chin, the temples and the sides of the forehead. Apply blusher under the cheekbones, in an upward and outward direction towards the temples.	
Diamond	**Diamond** *Bone structure* A narrow forehead, with wide cheekbones tapering to a narrow chin. *Corrective make-up* Apply shader to the tip of the chin and the height of the forehead, to reduce length. Highlight the narrow sides of the temples and the lower jaw. Apply blusher to the fullness of the cheekbones to draw attention to the centre of the face.	

Oblong

Bone structure Long and narrow, tapering to a pointed chin.

Corrective make-up Apply shader to the hairline and the point of the chin to reduce the length of the face. Highlight the angle of the jawbone and the temples to create width. Blend blusher along the cheekbones, outwards towards the ears.

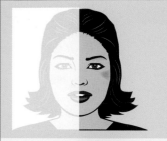

Oblong

Pear

Bone structure A wide jawline, tapering to a narrow forehead.

Corrective make-up Highlight the forehead and shade the sides of the chin and the angle of the jaw. Apply blusher to the fullness of the cheeks, or blend it along the cheekbones, up towards the temples.

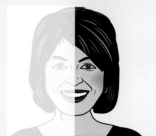

Pear

TOP TIP

Contouring with foundation

Foundation may be suitable as a contour cosmetic. Choose a foundation either two shades lighter (as a highlighter) or two shades darker (as a shader) than the base foundation.

Here shading is applied to emphasise the cheek bones.

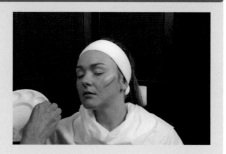

ACTIVITY

Facial bone structure

Draw and label the main facial bones. It is the differing sizes and proportions of these bones that give us our individual features.

To discover the size of each facial feature, feel the bony prominences of your own face with your fingers.

ALWAYS REMEMBER

Accuracy when contouring

Thoroughly clean your brush between shading and highlighting techniques.

Features

Contouring techniques can be applied for corrective purposes to the facial features.

Noses

◆ *If the nose is too broad:* apply shader to the sides of the nose.

◆ *If the nose is too short:* apply highlighter down the length of the nose from the bridge to the tip.

◆ *If the nose is too long:* apply shader to the tip of the nose.

◆ *If there is a bump on the nose:* apply shader over the area.

◆ *If there is a hollow along the bridge of the nose:* apply highlighter over the hollow area.

◆ *If the nose is crooked:* apply shader over the crooked side.

Foreheads

◆ *If the forehead is prominent:* apply shader centrally over the prominent area, blending it outwards toward the temples.

TOP TIP

Foreheads

Foreheads can be improved by a flattering hairstyle:

◆ *Prominent forehead*: choose soft, flat, textured fringes.

◆ *Shallow forehead*: choose a shorter, soft fringe. Height will make the forehead appear longer.

◆ *Deep forehead*: choose a longer, soft fringe.

◆ **If the forehead is shallow:** apply highlighter in a narrow band below the hairline.

◆ **If the forehead is deep:** apply shader in a narrow band below the hairline.

Chins

◆ **If the jaw is too wide:** apply shader from beneath the cheekbones and along the jawline, blending it at the neck.

◆ **If the chin is double:** apply shader to the centre of the chin, blending it outwards along the jawbone and under the chin.

◆ **If the chin is prominent:** apply shader to the tip of the chin.

◆ **If the chin is long:** apply shader over the prominent area.

◆ **If the chin recedes:** apply highlighter along the jawline and at the centre of the chin.

Necks

◆ **If the neck is thin:** apply highlighter down each side of the neck.

◆ **If the neck is thick:** apply shader to both sides of the neck.

The eyes

Make-up is applied to the eye area to complement the natural eye colour, to give definition to the eye area, and to enhance the natural shape of the eye.

Eyeshadow

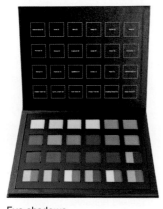

Eye shadows

Eyeshadow adds colour and definition to the eye area. The different types include matt, pearlised, metallic and pastel. They are available in cream, crayon or powder form. Eyeshadows are composed of either oil-and-water emulsions or waxes containing inorganic pigments to give colour.

◆ **Powder eyeshadows** have a talc base, mixed with oils to facilitate application. Lighter shades are produced by the addition of **titanium dioxide** – avoid these on dark skin as they contrast too harshly with the natural skin colour. Pigment shadows are loose powders which provide an intense colour and have light reflective properties.

◆ **Cream eyeshadows** contain wax, oil and silica.

◆ **Liquid eyeshadows** contain water, mica, glycerine and butylene glycol to achieve the correct viscosity.

◆ **Crayon eyeshadows** are composed of wax and oil, and are similar in appearance and application to an eye pencil.

Pearlised mineral eyeshadows are created by the addition of **bismuth oxychloride**, a fine crystalline powder or **mica**, a light-reflecting mineral powder; a *metallic* effect is created by the addition of fine particles of **gold leaf, aluminium** or **bronze**.

ALWAYS REMEMBER

Too much powder

When applying powder colours, always tap the brush before application to remove excess eyeshadow. If too much colour is deposited on the applicator, stroke it over a clean tissue to remove the excess.

Remember, it is better to apply more product in stages until you create the look you want to achieve.

Pigment powders provide a long lasting result but require care and careful placement in their application. It is better to build up the colour gradually as only a small amount is required.

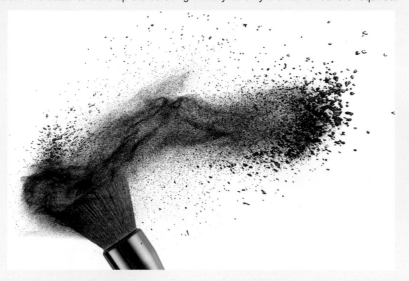

How to apply eyeshadow

Eyeshadow application will differ according to the eye shape of the client and the look to be achieved.

Powder eyeshadow

1 Protect the skin beneath the eye with a clean tissue or loose powder as shown – this is to collect small particles of eyeshadow that may fall during application.

2 Lift the skin at the brow slightly to keep the eye tissue taut, enabling you to reach the skin near to the base of the eyelashes.

3 Apply the selected eyeshadow to the eyelid, using a sponge or an eyeshadow brush applicator.

4 Highlight beneath the brow bone.

5 Using a brush, apply a darker eyeshadow to the socket area, beginning at the outer corner of the eye. Blend the colour evenly, to avoid harsh lines.

6 Ask your client to open her eyes during application so that you can look at the effect created.

Cream eyeshadow
Apply over a base to hold the cream shadow in place. It may be applied with a brush and blended with a sponge or small brush.

Liquid eyeshadow
Apply the liquid shadow colour with a brush, stroking and blending over the eyelid where required.

HEALTH & SAFETY

Eye cosmetics

The eye tissue is particularly sensitive. Eye cosmetic products should be of the highest quality, and be permitted for use according to the Cosmetics Products (Safety) Regulations (2008).

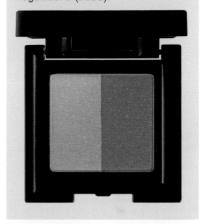

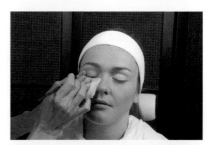

Applying colour shadow to the eyelid at the base of the lashes

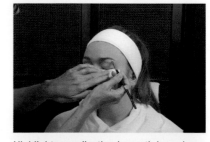

Highlighter application beneath brow bone

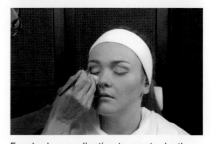

Eyeshadow application to create depth and contour the eye socket

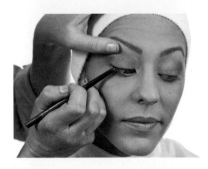

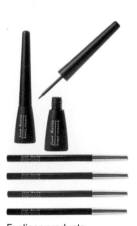

Eyeliner products

Eyeliner

Eyeliner defines and emphasises the eye area. It is available in pencil, liquid or powder form.

◆ *Eye pencil* Made of wax and oil, and contains different pigments that give it its colour.

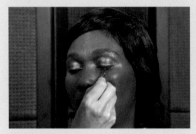
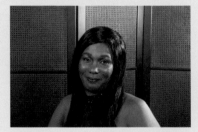
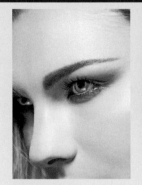
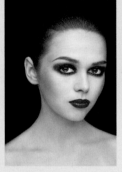
◆ *Liquid and gel eyeliner* A gum solution, in which the pigment is suspended.

◆ *Powder eyeliner* A powder base with the addition of mineral oil.

Powder eyeliner is the most suitable choice for a client who is exposed to a warm environment, as it will not smudge. Sharpen the pencil if used to achieve a sharp point and to provide a clean, uncontaminated cosmetic surface for each client.

How to apply eyeliner If you are using a powder or liquid eyeliner, apply it with a clean eyeliner brush.

1 Lift the skin gently upwards at the eyebrows, to keep the eyelid firm and make application easier.

2 Draw a fine line along the base of the eyelashes (as close to the lashes as possible), as required. Start application at the outer corner of the eye and apply towards the inner corner of the eye. The length of the line applied and angle will differ dependent upon the look to be achieved.

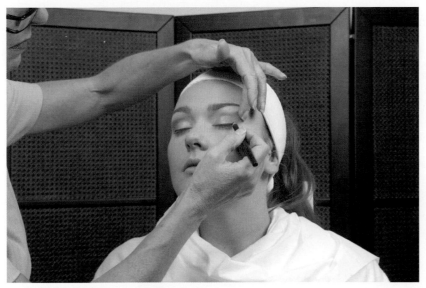

Eye pencil application to the upper eyelid

3 If using an eye pencil or powder line, lightly smudge the eyeliner to soften the effect of the line. (This is not effective with liquid liner.) If required, a further application may be applied for a thicker line. Liquid liner is applied with a fine-tip brush. To help stability when applying, place the base of the hand on a tissue against the client's cheek.

4 Eyeliner may be applied to the inner eye, usually accompanying a 'smoky' eye-shadow look. This technique is unsuitable on small eyes as it would make them appear smaller.

Eyebrow colour

Eyebrow colour emphasises the eyebrow, darkens the hair, alters their shape, disguises bald patches and can make sparse eyebrows look thicker. It is available in pencil, liquid or powder form.

◆ *Eyebrow pencil* Firmer than an eye pencil, and is composed of waxes that hold the inorganic pigments.

◆ *Powder brow colour* Composed of a talc base, mixed with mineral oil and pigments.

◆ *Liquid eyebrow* A fluid, quick-drying eyebrow colour to define the brows.

◆ *Eyebrow mascara* Composed of mineral oil and waxes with pigment suspended in it. The mascara defines the brows and controls and shapes them.

Further guidance on changing the appearance of or enhancing the natural brow shape with temporary colour can be found in Chapter 5.

TOP TIP

Sparse lashes

To provide the illusion of thicker lashes, eyeliner can be applied close to the lashes, making the base of the lash appear thicker.

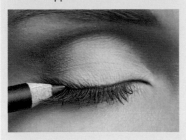

TOP TIP

Lasting liner

Powder eyeshadow may be applied over the eye pencil application to increase its durability, as heat and moisture can disturb the wax/oil content of a pencil. Alternatively the eyeliner can be applied over the powder.

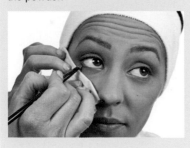

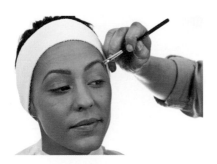

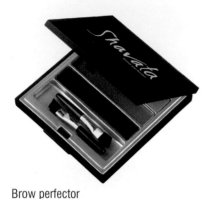

Brow perfector

How to apply eyebrow colour

1 Select an appropriate colour of powder or eyebrow pencil according to your client's colouring characteristics and the effect required. Brush the eyebrows with a clean brow brush to remove excess face powder and eyeshadow. A specialised wax or gel can be applied, which aids adherence of powder brow shadow and separates and defines the brow hair. Here the aim is to emphasise the natural brow shape, outlining the silhouette and filling in gaps with powder colour.

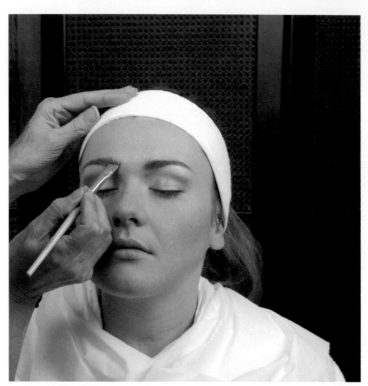

Eyebrow colour application

2 Simulate the appearance of brow hair by using fine strokes of colour, or disguise bald patches with a denser application. Use a pencil or liquid eyebrow to apply feathery strokes or alternatively use a brush apply powder to the prepared brow hair.

3 Brush the eyebrows into shape using an eyebrow brush if necessary without disturbing product application.

Mascara

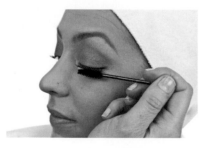

Mascara enhances the natural eyelashes, making them appear longer, changed in colour and thicker. It is available in liquid, cream and block-cake forms. It is composed of waxes or an oil-and-water emulsion, and contains pigments that give it its colour, although clear mascara products are available too. Other ingredients can be added to increase its effect on the appearance of the lashes to thicken or increase length, for example, and durability. If waterproof it will require a special eye make-up remover.

◆ **Liquid mascara** – a mixture of gum in water or alcohol; the pigment is suspended in this. It may also contain short textile filaments that adhere to the lashes and have a thickening, lengthening effect. Water-resistant mascara contains resin instead of gum, so that it will not run or smudge.

◆ **Cream mascara** – an emulsion of oil and water, with the pigment suspended in this.

◆ **Block mascara** – composed of mineral oil, lanolin and waxes, which are melted together to form a block on setting. It must be dampened with water before application.

How to apply mascara Using a disposable mascara brush, put the brush into the mascara and dispense sufficient mascara onto the brush to coat the lashes. Do not 'double dip'. Replace the mascara wand as required. Apply mascara to the eyelashes:

1   Hold the brush horizontally to apply colour to the length of the lashes. Where the lashes are short and curly, or difficult to reach, hold the brush vertically and use the point of the brush.

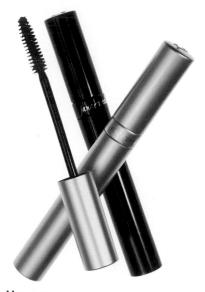

Mascara

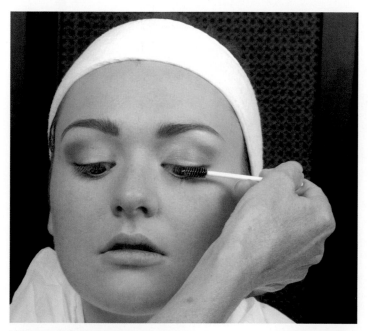

Mascara application to the upper lashes

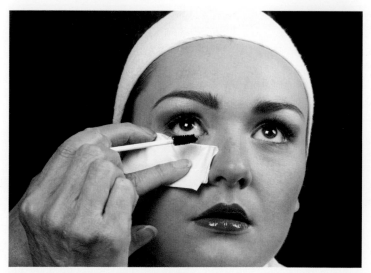

Mascara application to the lower lashes

2   Place a clean tissue underneath the base of the lower eyelashes, and stroke the brush down the length of the lashes from the base to the tips.

3 Lift the eyelid at the brow bone. Ask the client to look down slightly while keeping their eyes open. From above, stroke down the length of the lashes from the base to the tips.

4 Using a zigzag motion draw the brush upwards through the upper and lower surfaces of the lashes, from the base to the tips. Apply several coats to create a dramatic evening look. Ensure the short lashes at the corners of the eyelids are not missed.

5 Finally, separate the eyelashes with a clean brush or lash comb.

TOP TIP

Mascara brushes

There are various designs of mascara brush, each of which are designed to achieve different results according to the individual bristle shape. This unique selling point should be shared with the client as it will also influence their choice of which mascara to choose.

Bristles at the end of the mascara wand apply the mascara product and are made from natural or synthetic fibres, plastic and rubber.

◆ **Short**, **dense** bristles create volume.

◆ **Long**, **sparse** bristles create length.

◆ **Tapered wands** taper to a pointed end from a thicker barrel-shaped body. The pointed end can be used on shorter lashes and to separate the lashes. The barrel distributes the product.

◆ **Spherical wands** are used on short lashes to coat and separate each lash.

◆ **Curved mascara** wands follow the natural shape of the lashes, fanning and separating them. They are ideal to define longer lashes.

◆ **Telescope mascara** wands apply the product just where you want it and are great for hard to reach shorter lashes at the corner of the eyelids.

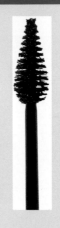

ALWAYS REMEMBER

Curly lashes

Curly lashes will require brushing, using a clean brush, both before mascara application and after each coat, to separate the lashes. A specialised gel may be applied before mascara application which, on drying, separates the lashes.

HEALTH & SAFETY

Mascara hygiene

Mascara when purchased is usually provided with a brush applicator. This applicator cannot be effectively cleaned and disinfected, however, so it should not be used. Instead use a disposable mascara brush for each client.

Recommend to your client that mascaras should be replaced ideally every six months.

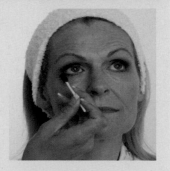

Eye make-up for the client who wears glasses

If the client wears glasses, check the function of the lens, as this can alter the appearance and effect of the eye make-up.

◆ *If the client is short-sighted, the lens makes the eye appear smaller.* Draw attention to the eyes by selecting brighter, lighter colours. When applying eye-shadow and eyeliner, use the corrective techniques for small eyes. Apply mascara to emphasise the eyelashes.

◆ *If the client is long-sighted, the lens will magnify the eye.* Make-up should therefore be subtle, avoiding frosted colours and lash-building mascaras. Careful blending is important, as any mistakes will be magnified!

How to apply corrective eye make-up

Dark circles Minimise the dark circles by applying a concealing, peach coloured corrector product.

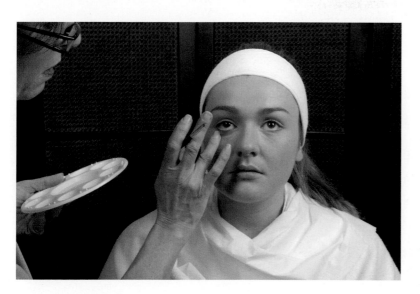

Wide-set eyes

1 Apply a darker eye colour to the inner portion of the upper eyelid.

2 Apply lighter eyeshadow to the outer portion of the eyelid.

3 Apply eyeliner in a darker colour to the inner half of the upper eyelid.

4 Eyebrow pencil may be applied to extend the inner brow line.

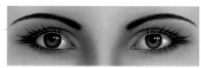
Wide-set eyes

ACTIVITY

Brow colour

What brow colour product would you select for the following and how would you apply it:

◆ fair-haired client, natural daytime make-up style
◆ dark-haired client, evening make-up style
◆ red-haired client, special occasion make-up style
◆ white haired client, sparse brow hair, natural daytime make-up style?

Close-set eyes

1 Lighten the inner portion of the upper eyelid.

2 Use a darker colour at the outer eye.

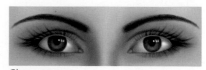
Close-set eyes

HEALTH & SAFETY

Allergies

If the client has hypersensitive eyes or skin, use hypoallergenic cosmetics that contain no known sensitisers.

Contact lenses

If the client wears contact lenses, don't use either lash-building filament mascaras or loose-particled eyeshadows, which have a tendency to flake and may enter the eye.

TOP TIP

Prominent eyes

To make the eyes appear less prominent, select matt eyeshadows applied over the eyelid – pearlised and shimmery eyeshadows will highlight and emphasise the eye.

3 Apply eyeliner to the outer corner of the upper eyelid.

4 Pluck brow hairs at the inner eyebrow – this helps to create the illusion of the eyes being further apart.

Round eyes

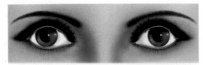
Round eyes

1 Apply a darker colour over the prominent central upper-lid area.

2 Elongate the eyes by applying eyeliner to the outer corners of the upper and lower eyelids.

Prominent eyes

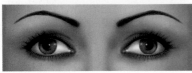
Prominent eyes

1 Apply dark matt eyeshadow over the prominent upper eyelid.

2 Apply a darker shade to the outer portion of the eyelid, and blend it upwards and outwards.

3 Highlight the brow bone, drawing attention to this area.

4 Eyeliner may be applied to the inner lower eyelid.

Overhanging lids

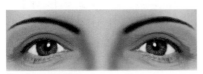
Overhanging lids

1 Apply a pale highlighter to the middle of the eyelid.

2 Apply a darker eyeshadow to contour the socket area, creating a higher crease (which disguises the hooded appearance).

Deep-set eyes

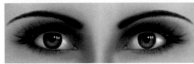
Deep-set eyes

1 Use light-coloured eyeshadows.

2 Eyeshadow may also be applied in a fine line to the inner half of the lower eyelid, beneath the lashes.

3 Apply eyeliner to the outer halves of the upper and lower eyelids, broadening the line as you extend outwards.

Downward-slanting eyes

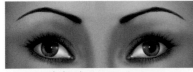
Downward-slanting eyes

1 Create lift by applying the eyeshadow upwards and outwards at the outer corners of the upper eyelid.

2 Apply eyeliner to the upper eyelid, applying it upwards at the outer corner.

3 Confine mascara to the outer lashes.

Small eyes

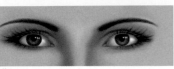
Small eyes

1 Choose a light colour for the upper eyelid.

2 Highlight under the brow, to open up the eye area.

3 Curl the lashes before applying mascara.

4 Apply a light-coloured eyeliner to the outer third of the lower eyelid.

5 A white eyeliner may be applied to the inner lid, to make the eye appear larger.

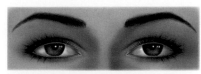

Narrow eyes

1 Apply a lighter colour in the centre of the eyelid, to open up the eye.

2 Apply a shader to the inner and outer portions of the eyelid.

Narrow eyes

TOP TIP

Mascara accidents!

If you accidentally get mascara on the skin, remove with a cotton bud. If waterproof you may need a small amount of eye make-up remover on the bud. Apply any corrective make-up to follow and conceal.

The eyelashes

To emphasise the eyelashes, making them appear longer temporarily, curl them using eyelash curlers. If performing after mascara application, the mascara must be dry.

How to curl the eyelashes

1 Rest the upper lashes between the upper and lower portions of the eyelash curlers.

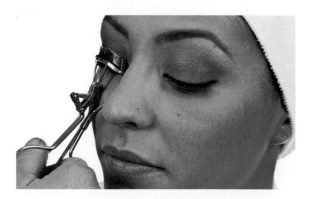

2 Bring the two portions gently together with a squeezing action.

3 Hold the lashes in the curlers for approximately 10 seconds, and then release them.

4 If the lashes are not sufficiently curled, repeat the action.

The lips

Lip cosmetics add colour and draw attention to the lips. As the lips have no protective sebum, the use of lip cosmetics also helps to prevent them from drying and becoming chapped.

It is not uncommon for the lips to be out of proportion in some way. Using lip cosmetics and corrective techniques, symmetrical lips can be created. A careful choice of product and accurate application are required to achieve a professional effect.

The main lip cosmetics are lip liner, lipsticks, lip tints, lib balm and lip glosses. Sometimes the lips may be unevenly pigmented. The application of a lip toner or foundation over the lips corrects this.

TOP TIP

Short straight lashes

Eyelash curling is beneficial for clients who have short lashes that grow downwards. The curled result opens up the eye area.

HEALTH & SAFETY

Eyelash curling

Repeated eyelash curling can lead to breakage. The technique should therefore be used only for special occasions.

ACTIVITY

Choosing mascara

What colour mascara should be applied if the client has the following hair colouring: brown, red, black, white?

TOP TIP

Eyelash curling

The eyelashes may be temporarily curled before mascara application to open up the eye area.

TOP TIP

Natural mascara

Clear mascara defines the lashes and makes them appear thicker, while appearing very natural.

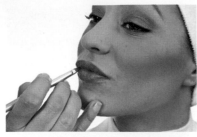

Lipstick application

ALWAYS REMEMBER

Mascara

Never pump the mascara wand when loading it with mascara. This encourages air to enter and makes the mascara dry out.

REVISION AID

What other services could you consider for a client with small eyes?

REVISION AID

What is the purpose of eyelash curlers?

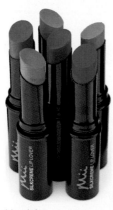

Lipsticks

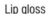

Lip gloss

Lip liner

Lip liner is used to define the lips, creating a perfectly symmetrical outline. This is coloured in with another lip cosmetic, either a lipstick or a lip gloss. The lip liner also helps to prevent the lipstick from 'bleeding' into lines around the lips.

Lip liner has a wax base, which does not melt and can be applied easily. It contains pigments that give the pencil its colour.

When choosing a lip liner, select one that is the same colour as, or slightly darker than, the lipstick to be used with it.

HEALTH & SAFETY

Lip pencils

Always sharpen the lip pencil before use on each client, to provide a clean, uncontaminated cosmetic surface. The point may be softened if required, before use.

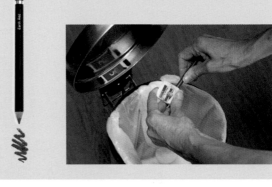

Lip pencil

Lipstick

Lipstick contains a blend of oils and waxes, which give it its firmness, and silicone, essential for easy application. It also contains pigment to add colour, an emollient moisturiser to keep the lips soft and supple, and perfume to improve its appeal. In addition it may include vitamins, to condition the lips, or sunscreens, to protect the lips from UV rays. Some lipsticks contain a relatively large proportion of water – these moisturise the lips and provide a natural look. The coverage provided by a lipstick depends on its formulation.

Lipsticks are available in the following forms: cream, matt, frosted and translucent. Frosted lipstick has good durability, as it is very dry. Some other lipsticks also offer extended durability, and are suitable for clients who are unable to renew their lipstick regularly.

When choosing the colour of lipstick, take into account the natural colour of the client's lips (it is best if it is the same colour tone), the skin and hair colours, and the colours selected for the rest of the make-up.

Lip gloss

Lip gloss provides a moist, shiny look to the lips. It may be worn alone, or applied on top of a lipstick. Its effect is short-lived. Lip gloss is made of mineral oils, with pigment suspended in the oil.

Note that mature clients often have creases on the lips that extend to the surrounding skin. If lip gloss is used it will often bleed into these lines.

HEALTH & SAFETY

Lipstick hygiene

For reasons of hygiene, remove a small quantity of lipstick by scraping the stick with a clean spatula – don't apply the lipstick directly. Use disposable lip brushes to apply lip cosmetics hygienically.

HEALTH & SAFETY

Allergies

Lipsticks often contain ingredients that can cause allergic reactions, such as lanolin and certain pigment dyes. If the client has known allergies, use a hypoallergenic product instead.

TOP TIP

Colour mixing

To obtain the correct colour of lipstick, you may need to mix different lipstick shades together.

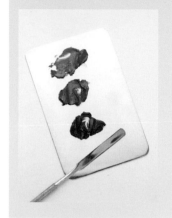

Lip stain

Lip stain adds intense colour to the lips and is made of water, glycerine, skin-conditioning ingredients and mineral pigments. Prepare the lip with lip liner. Apply to lips quickly, using the fingertips or a make-up sponge. Build up the colour to achieve the result required.

Lip balm

Lip balm is a lip moisturiser usually containing oil and beeswax, and sometimes vitamins C and E to help prevent dryness and improve skin texture, to add colour (if the balm contains pigment) and sheen. Following the lip liner, apply to the lips with a brush. A gloss may then be applied to enhance the lips.

Dry lips Sometimes the lips become dry and chapped. A lip balm or conditioner may be applied to the lips before make-up application, allowing it to be absorbed. Recommend that the client keeps them moisturised at all times, especially in extremes of heat, cold or wind. Some facial exfoliants can be professionally applied over the lips to remove dead skin.

If the client does not like to wear make-up during the day, or if the client is male, recommend that the lips be protected with a lip-care product.

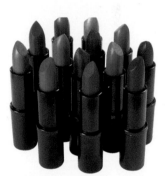

Lip cosmetics

How to apply corrective lip make-up

Thick lips Select natural colours and darker shades, avoiding bright, glossy colours.

1 Blend foundation over the lips to disguise the natural lip line.

2 Apply a darker lip liner inside the natural lip line to create a new line.

Thicker upper or lower lip

1 Use the technique described above to make the larger lip appear smaller.

2 Apply a slightly darker lipstick to the larger lip.

3 If the lips droop at the corners, raise the corners by applying lip liner to the corners of the upper lip, to turn them upwards.

Thin lips Select brighter, pearlised colours. Avoid darker lipsticks, which will make the mouth appear smaller.

1 Apply a neutral lip liner just outside the natural lip line.

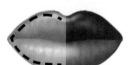

Thick lips

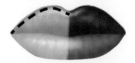

Thick upper lip

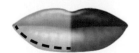

Thick lower lips

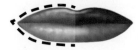

Thin lip

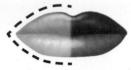

Small mouth

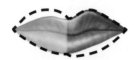

Uneven lips

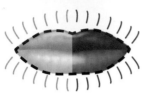

Lines around the mouth

Small mouth

1 Extend the line slightly at the corners of the mouth, with both the upper and the lower lips.

Uneven lips

1 Use a lip liner to draw in a new line.

2 Apply lipstick to the area.

Lines around the mouth

1 Apply lip liner around the natural lip line.

2 Apply a matt cream lipstick to the lips. (Don't use gloss, which might bleed into the lines around the mouth.)

How to apply lip liner, lipstick and lip gloss

1 Select a lip pencil and lipstick to complement the client's colouring and the colour theme of the make-up.

2 Using a pencil sharpener sharpen the lip pencil to expose a clean surface.

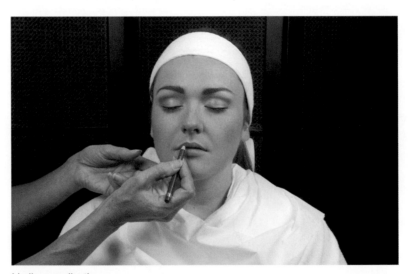

Lip liner application

3 Ask the client to open her mouth slightly.

4 Outline the lips, carrying out lip correction as necessary. Begin the lip line at the outer corner of the mouth, and continue it to the centre of the lips. Repeat the process on the other side of the lip, commencing at the outer corner of the mouth.

5 Remove sufficient lipstick using a clean spatula.

6 Using a disinfected lip brush, apply the lipstick to the lips.

7 Apply a clean facial tissue over the lip area, and gently press it onto the lips. This process, known as blotting, removes excess lipstick and fixes the colour on the lips.

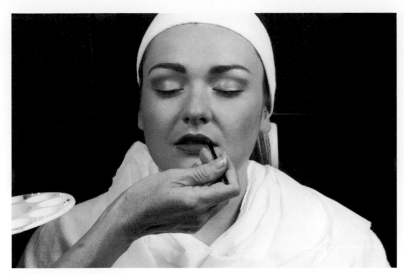

Lipstick application

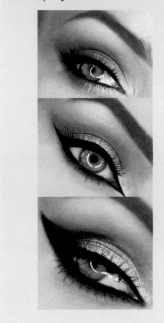

8 The application of powder on the first application of lipstick will make the lipstick longer lasting.

9 A second light application of lipstick may then be applied.

10 If desired, lip gloss may be applied over the lipstick to add sheen, again using a disinfected or disposable lip brush.

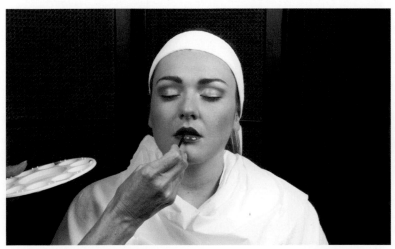

Lip gloss application

Finishing the service

After applying the make-up, confirm that the client is satisfied with the finished result. Then remove the client's headband/clips and fix their hair. You can discuss the finished result in front of the make-up mirror. If the client is satisfied, a fixing spray may be applied to keep the make-up style looking fresh for as long as possible.

Wash your hands. Record details of the service on the client's record.

Provide aftercare advice and recommendations.

"Client make-up records can be completed on laminated cards which can be photographed and uploaded onto their service record. The laminated card can then be cleaned and used for further services, avoiding paper wastage."

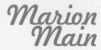

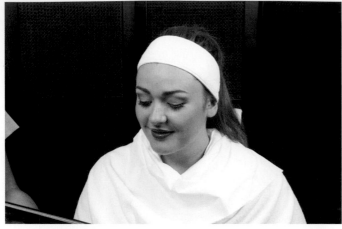

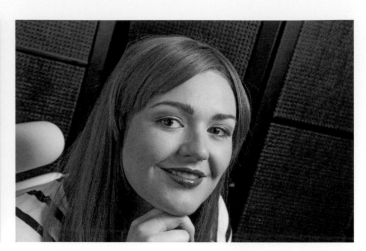

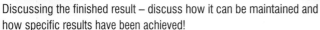
Discussing the finished result – discuss how it can be maintained and how specific results have been achieved!

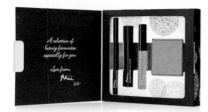

INCLUDES ENCHANT 01

Retail lip products

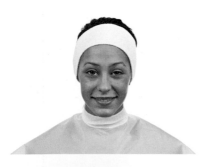

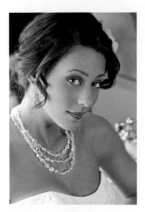
Before and after special occasion make-up application

Advice and recommendations

Following make-up application, recommend the correct skincare products to remove the products you have applied.

Eye cleansing advice

◆ Cleanse the eye area using a suitable eye make-up remover.

◆ Support the eye with one hand and avoid dragging the eye tissue outwards.

◆ Remove waterproof mascara usually using an oily eye make-up remover or one formulated for its removal.

◆ If lash extensions have been applied their removal must also be discussed (see Chapter 5).

Skincare advice

Recommend the correct skincare products to remove the products you have applied.

◆ Apply cleansing preparations to remove facial make-up with an appropriate cleanser in an upwards and outwards direction. Remove with damp cotton wool or clean facial sponges.

◆ Apply a suitable toner to suit skin type and condition to remove excess cleanser and restore the skin's pH balance.

◆ Apply day or night moisturiser, in small dots to the neck, chin, cheeks, nose and forehead. Quickly and evenly spread a thin film over the face, using light upward, outward stroking movements. Additional skincare may be recommended to meet the client's treatment needs.

◆ Blot the skin with a soft facial tissue to remove excess moisture.

Advise the client on re-application techniques to maintain the effect, e.g. removal of facial shine from the face with pressed powder, lip liner to stop 'bleeding', reapplication of blusher to add warmth.

Explain to the client that you can provide make-up instruction in which you would discuss the reason for the selection of make-up products and colours, and the techniques for applying them.

If you have provided make-up instruction, you may provide a before and after picture or a make-up chart showing which products have been used and where.

Have retail products available for the client to purchase. These include the products that you have used during the make-up application and skincare products for preparation and removal of make-up.

Inform the client of eco-friendly advice where available such as refillable product containers.

The client should avoid touching their skin; this will ensure the longevity of the make-up.

Share tips that will ensure that the client gets the best out of any products purchased. Product usage is important when advising the client on retail products. Demonstrate the correct amount of product to dispense to avoid wastage and so that the required look can be recreated.

If a client is colour blind, you can help them by numbering the make-up colours on the products and the make-up style chart for reference and home use.

Explain how to use the product hygienically and when it should be replaced.

Explain what action to take in the event of a contra-action.

Finally, at the end of the make-up service ensure that the client's records are updated, accurate and signed by the client and beauty therapist.

The client's needs

Natural day make-up

The natural day make-up look and any corrective work carried out should be very subtle and kept to a minimum, as if viewed in natural daylight this will make any imperfections appear obvious.

Select a foundation the same colour as the skin – aim to even out the skin tone. Set the foundation with a translucent face powder.

Apply a subtle, warm blusher or bronzing product to add colour to the face. Avoid strong colours of cosmetics, especially on the eyes. The mascara colour should be chosen to complement the client's natural lash and skin colours. Mascara should be used to emphasise, adding colour, texture and separating the lashes without exaggeration of the length and thickness of the eyelashes. Eyeliner may be used, but it should be carefully placed and blended.

Line the lips in a colour that will co-ordinate with the lipstick to be applied, which again should be quite natural.

Evening make-up

This should be applied bearing in mind the type of lighting in which the client will be seen. Artificial light dulls the effect, and changes the colour of the make-up: dark shades lose their brilliance, appearing 'muddy', so you need to use brighter colours. Emphasise the facial features with the careful placement of contouring cosmetics.

Areas where shadows may be created, such as the eyes, should be emphasised using light, bright and highlighting cosmetic products. Add warmth to the face with an intense colour of blusher placed on the cheekbones. A highlighting or shimmer powder in a pearlised or metallic shade may be applied directly on top of or over

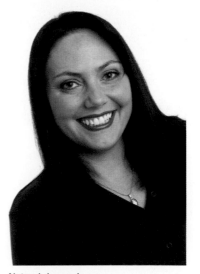

Natural day make-up

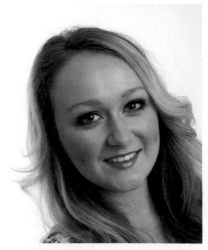

Evening make-up

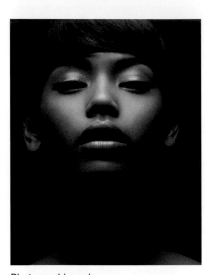

Photographic make-up

the blusher. The client may like to try adventurous cosmetics such as metallics and frosted eye products.

Curl the eyelashes with eyelash curlers or apply false eyelashes to emphasise the eyes. Fashion shades of mascara may be selected, in purples, greens and blues, to complement the make-up and produce the effect required. Light shades of eyeliner may be used to frame the eyes and to 'open' them up.

Add a lip gloss to the lips, or apply a frosted lipstick to emphasise the mouth.

Colour the eyebrows, and carefully groom them to frame the eye area.

Special occasion make-up

A special occasion is usually an important event such as a wedding, day at the races, graduation ceremony or New Year's Eve party.

Whatever the occasion, whether daytime or evening, indoors or outdoors, you will need to consider the type of lighting the make-up will be viewed in – natural or artificial – and any other factors, such as how long it is to be worn for.

The selection of colours should co-ordinate with what the client will be wearing, and finally you need to know the effect they wish the make-up to create – should it be subtle or glamorous? Make-up products can then be selected and appropriately applied to suit the occasion.

Photographic make-up

If applying make-up for photographic purposes, it is important to consider the effect to be created. This should be planned with the photographer in advance of the make-up application.

Consider the brightness of the lighting used. The brighter the lighting, the lighter the make-up pigment will appear. Make-up will therefore need to be applied more strongly. Lighting can be hot and may affect the make-up application making it melt, especially with oil-based make-up. Therefore, avoid oily make-up and regularly apply powder to remove shine.

Generally, matt colours are used, as the lighting will emphasise any shine.

For black and white photography remember dark colours will appear darker when photographed. Therefore, it may be necessary to apply lighter shades in preference to dark – for example, a dark shade of cheek colour would create a dark shadow.

Avoid lip gloss unless you wish the lips to appear full.

It is important to define facial features using shading and highlighting techniques, as photographic make-up removes natural shades and highlights.

Care should be taken to blend all make-up to avoid any demarcation lines, which will be emphasised in the photograph.

Make-up to suit skin and hair colouring

White skin and blonde hair If the client has blonde hair colour, and white skin, keep the skin colour natural. Apply a blusher in rose pink or beige.

Define the eyes with soft tones of browns and pinks. Apply a brown-black mascara.

Colour the lips with a rose-pink or peach lip colour. Avoid lip colours lighter than the natural skin tone.

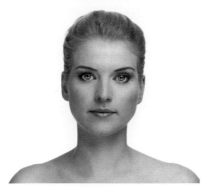

White skin and blonde hair

Oriental skin and black hair For creamy, sallow skin with dark hair, use blusher to add warmth and to brighten the skin, in either pink or brown.

The eyes are dark, with a prominent brow bone. Emphasise the socket of the eye with careful shading; extend this upwards and outwards. Place highlighter along the brow bone.

Pastel colours complement the eye colour. Select black mascara to emphasise the eyes. Deep pinks and orangey-reds suit the lips.

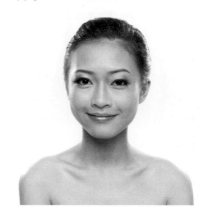

Oriental skin and black hair

White skin and red hair Redheads usually have fair skin with freckles. The skin will flush and colour easily, probably requiring the application of a green-tinted moisturiser, concealer or face powder. Apply blusher in a warm rose or peach colour. Browns, rusts, greens and peach eyeshadow colours suit this skin and complement the eyes. Brown mascara is preferable, to avoid making the eyes appear hard.

For the lips, select a lipstick in peach, golden rust or pink.

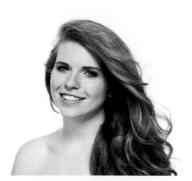

White skin and red hair

Black skin and black hair A yellow-toned foundation is required: it may be necessary to blend foundations to obtain the correct colour. Avoid pink-toned foundations, which make the skin appear chalky.

Women with dark skin tend to have dark brown to brown-black eyes, and can use a wide range of heavily pigmented colours, especially browns and bronzes. Dark shades of blusher in red and plum may be chosen; eyeliner and mascara can be black, or any other dark shade.

Avoid lip colours lighter than the skin tone. A lip liner darker than the lip colour may be used.

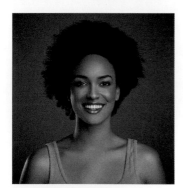

Black skin and black hair

Olive or fair skin and dark hair Select a foundation to suit the basic skin tone. If the skin is fair, choose an ivory base; if it is sallow, select a foundation with a rusty, yellow tone. (With a sallow skin, avoid the use of pinks on the eyes – they make the eyes look sore.)

A beige blusher suits this skin colour, and is complemented by the selection of brown or green shades for the eyes. Black mascara should be used for the eyelashes.

For the lips, choose warm reds or beige.

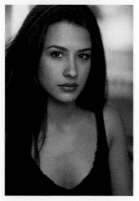

Olive skin and dark hair

Make-up for mature skin

As the skin ages it becomes sallow in colour and appears thinner. Small capillaries can be seen, commonly on the cheek area, and small veins may appear around the eyes. Pigment changes in the skin become obvious, and remain permanently.

At the make-up consultation, discuss your ideas with your client. Sometimes a mature client will have been using the same colours and the same make-up cosmetics for many years, and they may not even be complementary. You will need to advise them tactfully on a fresh approach.

Select a foundation that matches the skin colour yet enhances the skin's appearance. An oil-based foundation is appropriate for use on mature skin: it keeps the skin supple and prevents the foundation from settling into the creases and emphasising the lines and wrinkles. Other alternatives are mineral and serum based foundation.

A concealer may be applied to cover obvious capillaries and small veins, or a foundation may be selected that provides adequate coverage.

A lighter coloured foundation or sheer, lightweight concealer may be applied over wrinkled areas, to make them less obvious.

These areas include:

◆ around the eyes (crow's feet)

◆ between the brows

◆ across the forehead

ACTIVITY

Shading on an ageing skin

Where would you place contouring products in order to correct the appearance of poor muscle tone in the an ageing skin? Copy the following face chart and write in your answers.

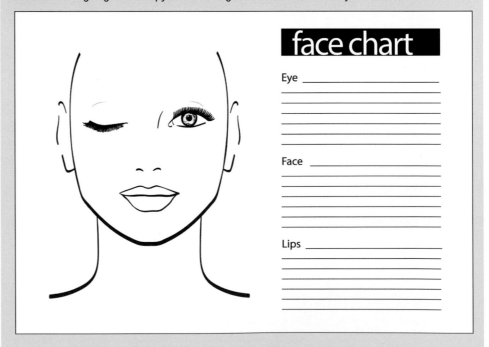

face chart

Eye _____

_____

_____

_____

_____

Face _____

_____

_____

_____

Lips _____

_____

_____

_____

- between the nose and the mouth (nasolabial folds)
- around the mouth (the lip line).

With age, the contours of the face lose their firmness as the fat cells that plump the face reduce, and the facial muscles lose tone and sag. Poor muscle tone can be seen in the following areas:

- the cheek area
- loose skin along the jawline
- loose skin under the brow and overhanging the lid
- loose skin on the neck.

The application of a shader, subtly blended, can improve the appearance of such areas.

Apply translucent powder. It may be preferable to avoid doing so in the eye area as it can emphasise lines around the eyes. To reduce the powdery effect, which may make the skin appear dry, you may direct a fine water spray from a suitable distance to set the make-up.

Apply a blusher with a warm tone – avoid harsh, bright shades. A cream blusher may be applied after the foundation. Place it high on the cheekbone and blend it upwards at the temples, drawing attention upwards rather than downwards.

The lip line becomes less obvious as one grows older, and lines often appear along it. Lip liner should be applied to redefine the lips and to prevent the lipstick from 'bleeding' into the lines. Select a lip liner that is the same colour as, or slightly lighter than, the lip colour. (A darker lip colour would create an unwanted shadow.) A special lip fixative may be recommended, and a durable nourishing cream lipstick applied. Avoid the use of a gloss lipstick, which emphasises lines around the mouth.

The angle of the mouth may droop. Corrective techniques may be used to disguise this.

Powder matt eyeshadows should be selected for use on the eyelid: these soften the appearance of any lines in the area. Choose natural, light shades. Dark colours can make the eyes appear small and tired.

Eyeliner should be used in neutral shades of brown and grey – avoid harsh, bright colours, which will give a hard appearance.

Eyebrows should be perfectly groomed, and arched to give lift to the eye. Bushy eyebrows give the eyes a hooded appearance. If eyebrow colour is required, select a colour that is slightly lighter than the brow colour, or a blend of two colours. If the client has grey hair, use grey and charcoal to provide a natural effect.

Eyelashes should be emphasised with a natural-looking shade of mascara, lightly applied. (If the eyelashes lose their colour, you can recommend that the client has their lashes professionally – and permanently – tinted. Individual short lash extensions may be recommended for corrective purposes to add colour and density.)

"Using photographs of make-up styles previously taken or sourced from the internet is great to share at consultation to start discussions about what the client wants.

Photograph make-up styles for reference later, developing a make-up style portfolio. Use social media to share your make-up looks, following your salon policy and legislative requirements."

Marion Main

STEP-BY-STEP: SPECIAL OCCASION MAKE-UP APPLICATION FOR MATURE CLIENT

The client has dry skin as the sebaceous and sudoriferous glands have become less active as part of the ageing process. Noticeable facial **skin conditions and characteristics** include the following:

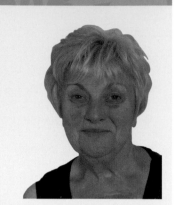

◆ Dark circles appear around the area of the eyes.

◆ Thin, delicate tissue is found around the eyes with small veins and capillaries showing through the skin.

◆ Habitual frown lines occur.

◆ Poor muscle tone has resulted in slack facial contours, e.g. double chin.

◆ Poor skin tone exists because the skin loses its elasticity, resulting in wrinkling and loss of firmness.

◆ Sallow skin colour is due to poor blood circulation.

Make-up is to be applied to a mature client to achieve a glamorous appearance for a social evening. We allowed 45 minutes to achieve this look.

1. The client's skin has been cleansed, toned and moisturised with a product containing a sun protection factor (SPF).

2. A skin primer has then been applied containing silicone to provide a smooth base, fill fine lines and improve skin texture to facilitate make-up application.

3. A yellow-toned concealer has been applied to the skin under the eye and over the eyelid using a concealer brush. This is to disguise dark circles and small veins and capillaries visible in this area.

4. A lightweight liquid foundation with light-reflective properties in medium beige is applied using a foundation brush.

5. A highlighting liquid (lighter than the foundation) is applied using a small concealer brush to the habitual lines located between the eyebrows.

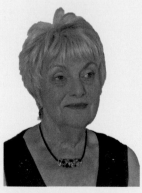

Finished special occasion make-up style

6. Loose mineral powder with illuminating properties is applied to set the foundation. This also counteracts the skin's sallow appearance. A large powder brush is used to remove excess powder.

7. Using a contouring blush brush, a mineral blush powder is applied to the cheekbones in medium pink.

8. Matt beige powder is applied under the cheekbones and along the jaw line to diminish the appearance of slack tissue and provide contour to these areas.

9. A pale pink matt powder mineral eyeshadow is applied to the eyelid and a matt ivory eyeshadow to the brow bone. The socket is defined with a matt grey dark eyeshadow. A medium firm eyeshadow blending brush is used to soften and seamlessly blend application in the socket area.

10. A medium blonde brow powder is applied using a stiff angle brush to add shape and depth to the brows.

11. Dark grey eye liner is applied to the upper and lower outer lash line, approximately halfway along. This is set using a light grey powder applied with an eye liner brush along the length of the lash line.

12. The eyelashes are curled using eyelash curlers and two coats of mascara are applied in black using a lash-lengthening mascara applied with a disposable mascara brush.

13. The lips are outlined slightly beyond the natural lip line using lip pencil in matt pink, providing a fuller appearance.

14. This outline is filled in using a moisturising lipstick in pink, enhanced by a clear gloss in the centre of the lips. Both lip products are applied with a disposable lip brush.

STEP-BY-STEP: NATURAL DAY MAKE-UP APPLICATION FOR ASIAN SKIN

Corrective work completed is subtle, as natural daylight makes any imperfections seem more obvious.

The client's skin has been cleansed, toned, moisturised and blotted to remove excess moisturiser. This look was achieved in 30 minutes.

This is an oily skin type, where overactivity of the sebaceous glands in the skin is creating a shiny, sallow appearance. Darker skin underneath the eye area requires concealer correction.

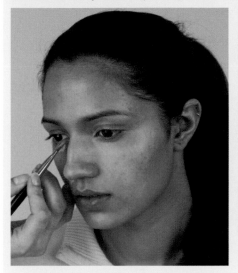

1 A concealer is applied with a brush underneath the eyes to disguise the darker skin tone.

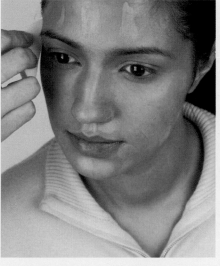

2 A liquid foundation matched to the client's skin tone is applied. Application is over the whole face, including the eyelids and lips, as this gives an even skin tone.

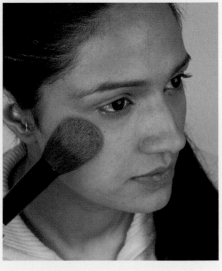

3 Following the application of loose powder, again matched to the client's skin tone, excess powder is removed using a large powder brush. Application is upwards and outwards.

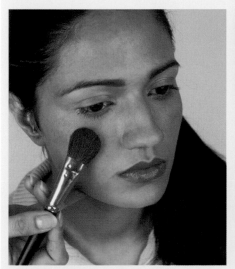

4 Blusher colour is applied to accentuate the cheek area and add colour to the face.

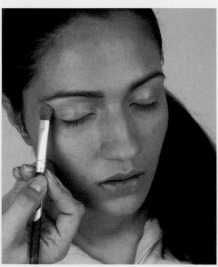

5 Colour applied to the eye emphasises the eye area. We used complementary colours in a purple range. A highlighting colour accentuates the brow bone.

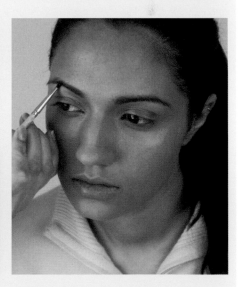

6 The eyebrows are accentuated using a dark matt brown colour applied with a stiff eyebrow brush. This gives definition to the eyebrow, disguising sparse hair and gaps.

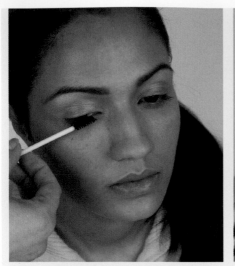
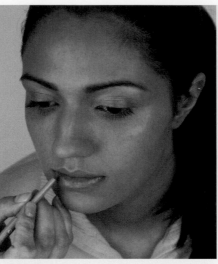
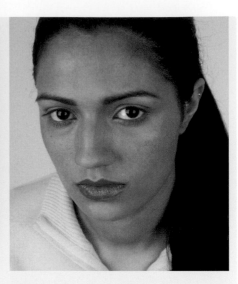

7 The lashes are lengthened using a lash-building mascara in black.

8 Lip liner colour is applied to define the desired lip contour. A co-ordinating lip colour is selected and applied to match the lip liner and complement the eye make-up colour.

9 The final natural day make-up style.

STEP-BY-STEP: EVENING MAKE-UP APPLICATION FOR BLACK SKIN

Make-up that will be seen under artificial lighting is applied. Stronger pigmented make-up colours have been selected, and the make-up effect emphasises facial features through the choice and application of make-up products. Forty-five minutes were allowed to achieve the look.

The client's skin has been cleansed, toned, moisturised and blotted to remove excess moisturiser.

This is a combination skin type and the sebaceous glands are overactive in the T zone – forehead, nose and chin – and the pores appear larger in this area. The sebaceous glands are less active in the cheek, which results in dry skin with tight pores.

Other noticeable facial characteristics include the following:

◆ The skin tone of the face has uneven pigmentation.
◆ The face shape requires balance, which can be achieved using shaded contour colour.

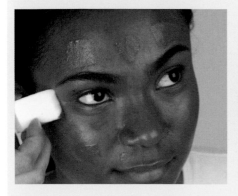
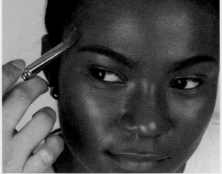
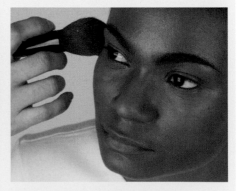

1 Foundation is selected to match the client's skin type and even the skin tone. A mousse foundation has been used to provide a medium coverage and has been blended quickly to avoid a chalky appearance.

2 A cream formulation shading product, in a darker shade than the foundation, is applied underneath the cheekbone and at the temples to accentuate the cheekbones and reduce the width of the face at the temples.

3 Loose powder matching the client's skin tone is applied to set the foundation and facilitate application of further powder products. Powder blusher is applied to the cheekbone.

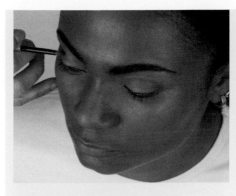

4 Following application of a neutral eye-shadow matt colour, a darker shading product is used to emphasise the eye socket.

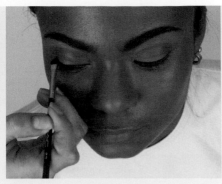

5 The natural lash line is accentuated by eyeliner application. A steady hand is required!

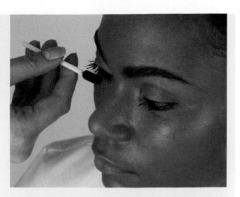

6 Mascara application is applied to lengthen and thicken the lashes, emphasisng the eyes.

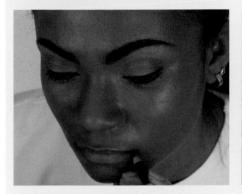

7 Lip liner is applied to define the perfect lip line.

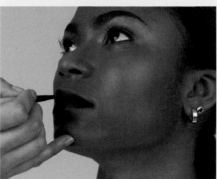

8 The lips are coloured in using a matt lipstick co-ordinated to suit the lip liner. Lip gloss achieves a final touch, which will focus attention and add emphasis in darker lighting.

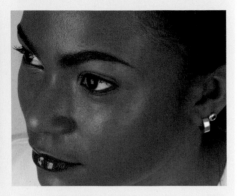

9 The final evening make-up.

Bridal make-up

Bridal make-up requires planning to ensure that you fully understand the client's requirements and can achieve the perfect, unique look for each bride.

In advance of the wedding it is important to trial the look on the client to ensure the make-up style suits the bride and she is confident with the effect achieved.

Remember, this can be a stressful time for the bride, so you need to be able to keep calm and professional throughout the make-up service.

TOP TIP

If possible, make-up should be applied prior to hair being styled. For Asian bridal make-up, the hair will have pieces of hair padding added to it which is used to hold the bride's veil in place as it will be extremely heavy, and this can restrict the bride's head movement.

TOP TIP

If you are right handed, work from the bride's right side to apply the make-up. The same applies if you are left handed, work from the bride's left side. This will stop you straining your wrist and upper body and it will mean that make-up application is easier.

STEP-BY-STEP: ASIAN BRIDAL MAKE-UP APPLICATION

Bridal make-up is personal to every bride suiting their tastes and preferences, be it light and natural, or vibrant and bold. Exotic, beautiful, vibrant, perfection—are some of the words that are often used to describe an Asian bride. The bride wears traditional dress, either the saree or lehenga which varies according to the region, culture and personal preference. Accessories including facial and head adornments, all play a part in the choice of colours selected in the make-up design. The clothing, jewelled accessories and head pieces worn by the bride hold a meaning within the bridal ceremony.

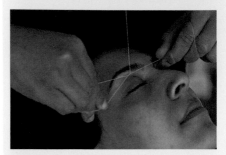

1 Shape eyebrows using threading technique. Eyebrows should be shaped a few days prior to the wedding. The threading method of hair removal is effective for thick strong eyebrow hair.

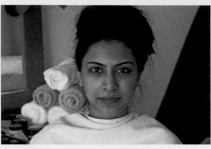

2 Skin has been prepared for the application of make-up.

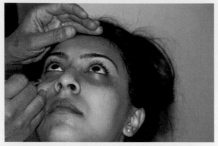

3 Apply primer to the entire face using a small flat tipped brush including the eyelid using a specialist eye primer. Apply orange concealer under the eye area to conceal any dark circles present and also apply to any other blemishes that may need concealing using the correct colour corrector.

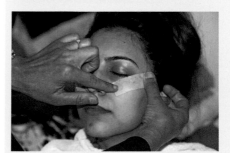

4 Surgical tape may be applied to both eyes as shown and used as a guide line for symmetry of both eyes during eyeshadow application. Also as a guide when applying eyeliner later. Do not use a tape that has strong adhesive. As an alternative to tape, the handle of the make-up brush can be used as a guide line.

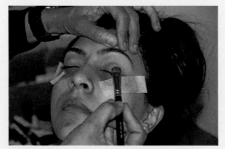

5 Eyeshadow base colour: apply a base beige tone colour to the entire area of the eye to give an even base. Use a medium soft brush and blend well.

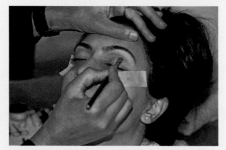

6 Apply eyeshadow on the socket line. Start by applying a darker rust tone eyeshadow to emphasise the socket using a small flat brush, blend in the eyeshadow.

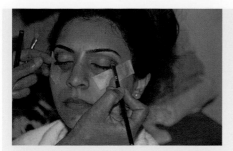

7 Apply a dark grey eyeshadow to the outer edges of the eyes creating a 'C' shape on each eye. Blend using a small soft brush so the end result is a diamond shape at the outer edges of each eye.

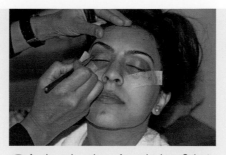

8 Apply main colour of eyeshadow. Select the main eyeshadow colours to match the colour of wedding dress. This colour is placed in front of the diamond shape and blended well towards the centre of the eye using a small soft brush.

9 Apply inner eye colour using a light pearilised colour. This colour will make the eye 'pop' open and contrast well with the other colours. Adding lighter pigment to your eyeshadow will enhance the colour.

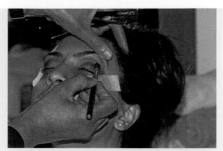

10 Add depth with eyeshadow. At this stage use a small dome shaped soft brush to apply a small amount of black shadow which will provide depth at the outer edges, this must be blended well.

11 Assess the application and effect of the eyeshadow applied. Are your colours blended well? Can you see the gradual change of colour? If the effect is not gradual, you may need to blend the edges of the colours a little more to obtain a soft gradual effect.

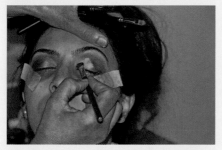

12 Add lighter pigment eyeshadow to the inner eye to achieve a strong look against the eyeliner and lashes when applied. Apply using a soft small flat brush, then blend with a small dome shaped brush as if you are pushing the eyeshadow into the skin.

13 Eyeshadow blending. Use a clean soft flat brush. Blend the pigment over the socket line, merging the colours on the outer eye to achieve a soft shimmer.

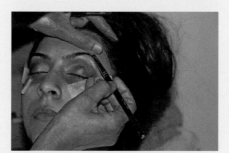

14 Apply highlighter by using a small amount of pearlised eyeshadow pigment placed on the brow bone. Blend well to create a soft effect. Using the same colour keeps the colours flowing, so avoiding harsh lines.

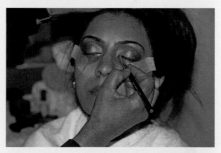

15 Apply definition using a small flat angled brush. Apply eyeshadow pigment to the inner eye and blend towards the lower lash line.

(Continued over page)

TOP TIP

Most Asian brides prefer to have slightly lighter skin colour on their wedding day. Make sure you colour the neck too. The wedding dress will conceal all other skin. This is where airbrushing is a must for all-over even foundation application of face and neck, and will not rub off the neck onto the wedding dress.

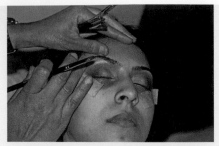

16 Eyebrows: define, colour and shape the eyebrows. Brush the eyebrows to remove any eye shadow residue. Using a slim angled eyebrow brush define the eyebrows using a dark brow powder. An eyebrow stencil can be used to define the shape and colour the eyebrows if preferred.

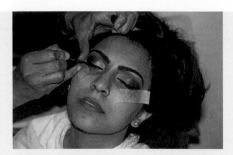

17 Apply eyeliner to the upper lash line. Hold the eye taut from the outer edge and draw the line using liquid or gel liner from the inner eye, outwards. Use the tape on the eyes as a guide. This will ensure that both eyes are symmetrical, ensure that the eyeliner is broad enough so that it will still be seen when artificial strip eye lashes are placed on top. Allow eyeliner to dry on the upper lash line, then gently remove the tape from both eyes. You may need to gently blend the edges of the orange concealer after removal

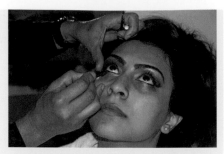

18 Apply eyeliner to the lower lash line. Use a soft eyeliner pencil, line the lower lash line then gently smudge this, ideally using a small rubber smudge brush. Use a sharpened soft black kohl pencil to line the inside of both upper and lower eye lid rims, finishing at the inner eye.

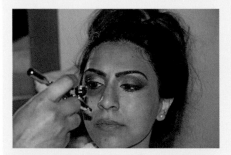

19 Apply a light concealer to cover the orange concealer. This provides an even base on which to apply foundation. The orange conceals the dark circles completely.

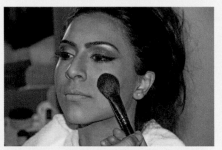

20 Apply foundation using a foundation brush.

21 Contouring can be applied to the face either before or after foundation. In this example, it has been applied on top of the foundation and using a small flat brush, blending lightly. Concealers are an ideal product to use as they are oil based and easy to blend. When choosing your shade to highlight, it should be one or two shades lighter than your chosen foundation. For shading one to two shades darker than chosen foundation, blend so there are no harsh lines as this does not look good in photographs. Where possible take a photograph at this stage to assess the effect of contouring on the final look.

22 Apply blusher to the apple of the cheeks starting in line with the centre of the eye and working out towards the hair line. Bronzer is also a great product to use to achieve a healthy glow. Apply blush or bronzer just above the temples to give the forehead definition.

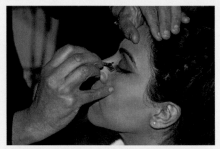

23 Apply strip false lashes.

24 Outline the lip with a lip pencil then using the pencil colour both lips. This will give a good base for the lipstick. Apply the lipstick using a lip brush, blend well. Apply a gloss over the lipstick and tidy the edges with a cotton bud.

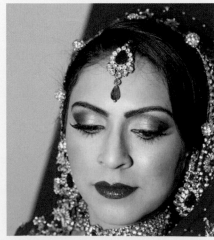

25 Completed make-up with head dress.

ASSESSMENT OF KNOWLEDGE AND UNDERSTANDING

Having covered the learning objectives for this chapter, test what you need to know and understand by answering the following short questions.

The information covers:

◆ Organisational and legal requirements

◆ Anatomy and physiology

◆ How to work safely and effectively when performing make-up services

◆ Client consultation, service planning and preparation

◆ Contra-indications and contra-actions

◆ Make-up application

◆ Client advice and recommendations.

Organisational and legal requirements

See Chapter 1 for details of legislation.

1. What are your responsibilities under the relevant health and safety legislation for make-up services?

   Provide three examples supported by the relevant legislation they relate to.

2. What actions must be taken before a client under 16 years of age receives make-up?

3. How can you ensure you comply with the legislation of the Equality Act 2010 when completing make-up services?

4. Why must a client's signature be obtained before commencing a make-up service? What does this confirm?

5. Taking into account health and safety hygiene requirements, how would you prepare yourself for service?

6. What should you consider when completing make-up services in order to comply with the Data Protection Act (1998)?

7. How long would you allow to complete a make-up style for a client?

8. Why is it important for all staff who will be in contact with clients to be familiar with the make-up pricing structures?

9. What details should be recorded on the client's service record for make-up and why is it important to keep accurate records which are maintained?

10. How can repetitive strain injury be avoided when performing make-up services? Give **three** examples.

Anatomy and physiology

Refer to Chapter 2 The Science of Beauty Therapy and Chapter 3 Consultation Practice and Techniques for further information on the related science and skin diseases and disorders for make-up services.

1. How is the skin affected by the ageing process?

2. How do lifestyle factors affect the skin?

3. a. What happens to the skin if you get an allergic reaction?
   b. How can this be recognised?

4. The skin has both a secretion and excretion function. Describe what occurs with each and the importance of a good skincare routine for these aspects of the skin's function.

How to work safely and effectively when performing make-up services

1. How can you ensure that the make-up environment is suitable for the application of make-up?

2. a. What do you understand by the terms disinfection and sterilisation?
   b. State **two** methods used in a make-up service and when they would be used.

3. How should the make-up brushes be prepared for each client to avoid cross-infection?

4. Why is it important to have a variety of make-up products available?

5. How should the client be positioned when performing make-up?

6. Why is it important to match lighting with the occasion for which the make-up is to be worn?

7. Give **three** examples of how you can be environmentally friendly in your make-up work.

Client consultation, service planning and preparation

1. How can you ensure that you fully understand the effect to be achieved with the make-up style?

2. In order to select the correct skincare and make-up products to complement the client's skin, it is necessary to identify the skin type. What are the facial characteristics of the following skin types that you learnt about in Chapter 4, Facials:

   a. oily
   b. dry
   c. combination?

3. How should the skin be prepared before the application of make-up?

4. What factors should be considered when planning a make-up with a client?

5. Why should you encourage the client to ask questions about the planned make-up?

6. Why is it important to check if the client wears contact lenses or glasses and check the function of the lens?

7. The client should be comfortable and relaxed following the consultation and preparation for the service. How could you tell if the client was relaxed or tense through their body language?

8. What is the legal relevance of client questioning and recording the client's responses?

9. Why is it important that you never diagnose a contra-indication?

10. When would you perform a skin sensitivity patch test before make-up application?

Contra-indications and contra-actions

1. Name **three** skin disorders and **three** eye disorders that would contra-indicate make-up service.

2. What product ingredients are known to cause allergic reactions, and should therefore not be used on a client with a sensitive skin?

3. Name **three** contra-actions that could occur during or after make-up application. What action should be taken?

Make-up application

1. What is the difference in application technique for the following make-up contexts:

   a. natural
   b. evening
   c. special occasion?

2. How is the correct colour of foundation selected for your client?

3. Why is it important that make-up is applied using the appropriate make-up tools?

4. How can you ensure hygienic practice when applying the following products:

   a. foundation
   b. face powder
   c. mascara
   d. lipstick?

5. For what purposes would you apply concealer?

6. Why does the client's age influence make-up product selection and application technique?

7. a. What is a colour corrector?
   b. Why is it pigmented?

8. What is the purpose of:

   a. shader
   b. highlighter?

9. What corrective **make-up techniques** would you apply for each of the following:

   a. square face
   b. mature skin, with slack tissue along the jawline
   c. narrow eyes
   d. small area of hyperpigmentation
   e. small area of hypopigmentation?

10. When would you apply a bronzer product?

Advice and recommendations

1. What aftercare advice and recommendations should be given to a client following make-up application?

2. How can you promote the sale of skincare and make-up products during make-up application?

3. From a magazine, collect a photographic image from the client groups below where make-up has been applied:

   a. Black
   b. Asian
   c. White
   d. Oriental

   Describe how each look has been created, explaining the make-up application and products used.

4. What reapplication make-up tips could you recommend to a client to increase the durability of their make-up?

5. Clients should be advised of suitable make-up removal techniques. Explain the skincare products required and how they should be used.

6. How can clients maintain the hygiene of their make-up products?

7 Hand and Foot Services

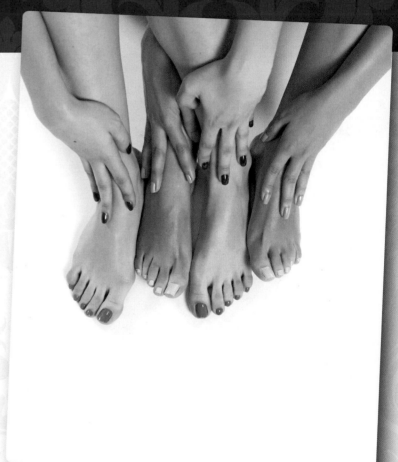

LEARNING OBJECTIVES

This chapter covers how to provide hand and foot services, including specialised treatments. Different techniques and products are applied to improve or maintain the health of the skin and nails, and nail finishes to enhance their appearance. You will learn more about:

◆ Maintaining safe effective methods when working.

◆ The information that must be obtained at the consultation; including the outcomes of the skin and nail assessment and any skin sensitivity patch tests to ensure the client's suitability for service and their welfare.

◆ Preparing the nails to ensure an effective final result and nail finish, including the use of gel polish.

◆ The different tools, products and equipment that might be applied within a nail service to meet the service plan objectives.

◆ How the service can be adapted or personalised for each client, through the selection of appropriate product, tools and equipment to meet their needs identified at the consultation.

◆ How to provide advice and recommendations relating to a client's service, including the use of additional products and further services that may be of benefit to them.

KEY TERMS

Hands and feet
base coat
bevelling
buffer
curing equipment,
    UV and LED
cuticle cream
cuticle nippers
cuticle oil
cuticle remover
exfoliation
gel polish
massage
    technique
nail conditions
nail finish
nail growth

natural nail shapes
nail polish
nail polish drier
nail polish
    remover
nail polish solvent
nail structure
paraffin wax
scissors
service plan
skin structure
top coat
warm-oil service

Hands
anatomy of the hand
    and arm

hand and nail
    treatments
manicure
nail strengthener

Feet
anatomy of the foot
    and leg
foot and nail
    treatments
foot rasp
foot spa
pedicure
toenail clippers

Nail art
blending
dotting technique

dotting tool
embellishment
foiling
freehand technique
glitters
jewellery tool
marbling
marbling tool
nail art
nail art techniques
nail shapes
polish secures
transfers
striping

WHEN PROVIDING NAIL SERVICES YOU WILL BE REQUIRED TO

◆ apply environmental and sustainable working practices

◆ follow relevant laws and manufacturers' instructions

◆ use different consultation and assessment techniques to correctly identify your client's needs

◆ select and use products, tools and equipment that will enhance the required results

◆ adapt the service to meet the client's physiological and psychological* requirements (where needed)

◆ take the necessary actions where a contra-action, contra-indication or treatment modification is required

◆ provide relevant advice and recommendations to support your client's service objectives.

INTRODUCTION

This chapter is about providing nail services to the hands and feet as a beauty therapist. These are referred to as manicures for the hands and pedicures for the feet. However, different parts of these services can be received independently. Manicures will be discussed first, followed by pedicures.

*An example of a psychological requirement is where the client has a habit such as nail biting or picking at the skin surrounding the nails. You need to to provide the client with the support and motivation to help them to stop.

Manicure

The word **manicure** is derived from the Latin words *manus*, meaning 'hand', and *cura*, meaning 'care'.

A manicure aims to improve and maintain your client's hands, nails and surrounding skin. The manicure procedure includes filing the nails to shape, buffing the nail plate surface, using specialised nail products, cuticle products and treatments, massaging the lower arm and hand and providing a complementary **nail finish** to suit the client and their service requirements.

Health and safety is an important feature of every service and delivery of the manicure service must avoid any cross-infection, cross-contamination or harmful chemical exposure. Dealing with your clients in a polite, efficient manner, using good communication and questioning skills to find out exactly what they require from the manicure service, forms an important part of this technical service.

INDUSTRY ROLE MODEL

MARIAN NEWMAN Freelance session nail technician, author and industry consultant

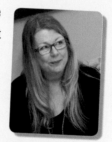

What do you find rewarding about your job? One of the most rewarding aspects is the variety of work I do and the many interesting people I get to meet. I really enjoy seeing the nail industry grow so much and the new developments in technology and products that have taken the industry to even greater levels.

What do you find challenging about your job? My most challenging aspect is remembering which role I am playing each day!

What makes a good beauty therapist? The best nail technicians are those who do not scrimp on their learning, understanding and skills. It really is a 'lifetime of learning' career. It obviously starts in the classroom but continues with additional classes, Internet research, trade magazines, professional forums and trade shows. Practise and practise!

INDUSTRY ROLE MODEL

LAURA DICKEN Managing Director of Podology, Saltburn-by-the-Sea, North Yorkshire

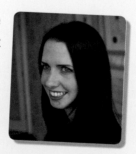

I graduated from New College Durham with a BSc (Hons) degree in Podiatry in 2003. After working for the NHS for two years I realised my dream of setting up my own private podiatry clinic in 2005.

Although I began with a podiatry clinic, it became clear that my clients wanted more. Happy with their traditional chiropody/podiatry treatments they wanted the finishing touches so I trained in manicures and pedicures, and introduced the medical pedicure to my treatment list.

Now after 12 years in business, my chiropody and beauty clinic business—Podology—employs both podiatrists and beauty therapists and has developed an extensive treatment menu. The unique concept of combining the two disciplines means that Podology can offer prescriptive finishing touches to every treatment and meet the client's every need.

Podology has been a finalist in the Professional Beauty awards in London, and in Scratch Magazine's award for Nail Salon of the Year.

Over time, I have developed a special interest in cosmetic podiatry treatments and improving hygiene standards in beauty therapy and speak regularly on these matters at the Professional Beauty shows in London and Manchester.

Anatomy and physiology

The anatomy and physiology knowledge and understanding required is found in the checklist in Chapter 2, and is also discussed within this chapter.

When performing hand and foot nail services you are required to apply your knowledge of the structure and function of the skin, including:

◆ identifying skin type and conditions

◆ the structure of the nail and **natural nail shapes**

◆ identifying nail health and conditions

◆ nail growth

◆ the bones of the hand and lower arm

◆ the bones of the feet and lower leg

◆ the muscles of the hand and lower arm

◆ the muscles of the foot and lower leg

◆ the blood circulation to the hand and lower arm

◆ the blood circulation to the foot and lower leg.

ALWAYS REMEMBER

Nail service products

Hand and nail products that may be used within a manicure include:

cuticle cream/oil; cuticle remover; hand cream/oil; buffing paste; **nail polish** (base coat, top coat and different nail finishes, which may be coloured); nail polish drier; nail polish remover; nail polish solvent; range of specialist nail treatment products, e.g. nail strengthener.

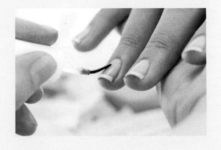

Gel polish is increasingly popular as a finish of choice. It is also more durable.

ALWAYS REMEMBER

Transferable knowledge, understanding and skills

When providing nail services it is important to use the skills you have learnt in the following:

◆ The Business of Beauty Therapy (Chapter 1)

◆ The Science of Beauty Therapy (Chapter 2)

◆ Consultation Practice and Techniques (Chapter 3)

ALWAYS REMEMBER

Hand, foot and nail services

Hand and nail services include different products and specialised treatments applied to improve and maintain the overall appearance and health of the nails and skin.

These include exfoliant products, hand and foot masks and therapeutic ingredients used to hydrate, nourish and care for the skin.

According to a research report by Kline, the international professional nail care market is set to grow at an average rate of 6% a year to reach £1.13bn by 2019.

Products, tools and equipment

Before beginning the manicure, check that you have the necessary products, tools and equipment to hand and that they meet legal hygiene and industry requirements for nail services. Each manicure work area should have the following basic equipment listed below. Additional products, tools and equipment relevant to manicure and pedicure service are also discussed.

Products, tools and equipment

- **Nail bar workstation** On which to place everything.
- **Cotton wool** To remove nail polish and excess nail product preparations. Cotton wool may also be used to tip wooden disposable cuticle sticks. Cotton wool filled gauze pads are also available, which are more absorbent.
- **Tissues** To protect client's clothing in the area, drying the treatment area, removing excess product and for drying tools after removal from the disinfectant solution, etc.
- **Disinfecting solution** To store small plastic and stainless steel sterilised tools.
- **Skin disinfectant** To cleanse and disinfect the client's skin. Specialised sprays and gels are available for this purpose.
- **Medium-sized towels (3)** To dry the skin, nails, etc.
- **Small bowls (3)** For storage and to dispense products into.
- **Disposable paper tissue** To collect waste and should be replaced as necessary during the service.
- **Waste container** This should be a lined bin with a lid to contain vapours from solvents.
- **Client service record** Used to record confidential details of each client registered at the salon, products used and details of the service provided.
- **Cuticle pusher** To gently push back the softened cuticles. This may be plastic or metal; when plastic it is often called a *hoof stick*.
- **Emery boards** Used to shorten and shape the nail free edge.
- **Cuticle nippers** To remove excess cuticle and dead, torn skin surrounding the nail.
- **Nail scissors** To shorten nail length.
- **Wooden cuticle sticks (often called orange sticks)** Tipped at either end with cotton wool. (**Wooden cuticle sticks** should be disposed of after each client, as they cannot be effectively sterilised.) Used to remove products from containers and, when tipped at either end with cotton wool, to ease the cuticle back and clean under the free edge.
- **Hand emollient such as cream, lotion or pre-blended oil** To massage the skin of the hand and lower arm.
- **Cuticle remover** Used to soften the skin cells at the cuticle so excess epidermal skin can be easily removed.

- **Cuticle oil or cream** Used to condition and rehydrate the skin of the nail cuticle; especially beneficial for dry nails and cuticles.
- **Base coat** To prevent nail staining, improve appearance and health of the nail and provide an even surface to improve nail polish application and adherence.
- **Coloured nail polish** (enamel) A selection for the client to choose from in cream or pearlised (also termed crystalline) formulations. Many will have additional ingredients that alter the final nail finish.
- **Top coat** To provide shine and strength to protect the nail polish. Reduces peeling and chipping and increases durability of the nail polish.
- **Nail polish remover** To remove nail polish and excess nail care and skincare preparations from the nail plate.
- **Nail polish drier** An aerosol or oil preparation applied to speed up the drying process of nail polish.
- **Cuticle knife** To remove excess epidermal skin called eponychium and perionychium from the surface of the nail plate.
- **Buffers** Used to improve nail shine, stimulate blood circulation and remove surface cells reducing the appearance of ridges when used with a buffing paste.
- **Four-sided buffer** To remove dead skin cells and provide shine improving the nail plate appearance.
- **Buffing paste** Used to smooth the nail plate and reduce the appearance of ridges in conjunction with a nail buffer tool.
- **A manicure finger bowl** To place the fingers in at different stages of the service. It usually contains a nail cleansing agent to soak, soften and cleanse the skin and nails.
- **Hand and nail service specialised treatment equipment including:**
  - paraffin wax
  - hand masks
  - thermal mitts
  - exfoliators
  - warm oil.

Products used in both manicure and pedicure services

Product	Ingredients	Uses
Nail polish remover	Acetone or ethyl acetate – solvent. Perfume -usually synthetic. Colour. Oil – emollient to reduce drying effect of solvent. Acetone-free nail polish removers are available made from soya and corn-based agricultural chemical compounds called esters with the addition of an ingredient to reduce evaporation of the product such as the emollient glycerine.	To remove nail polish. To remove grease from the nail plate prior to applying polish.
Hand/foot cream/lotion/oil	Vegetable oils (e.g. almond oil) synthetic chemical oils are also available Perfume – synthetic or organic. Emulsifying agents (e.g. beeswax, gum tragacanth, glycerol stearate and cetyl alcohol). Emollients (e.g. glycerine, lanolin and shea butter). Preservatives.	To soften, hydrate and nourish the skin and cuticles. To provide slip during hand/foot massage.
Nail bleach	Citric acid or hydrogen peroxide – bleaches the nail. Glycerine – emollient. Water.	To whiten stained nails and the surrounding skin.
Nail polish	Nitrocellulose resin – film-forming plastic provides a hard, shiny surface. Solvent e.g. butyl and ethyl acetate creates a suitable consistency when applying, and helps polish dry at a controlled rate. Colouring agents and pigments – creating nail polish colour. Pearlised particles - create a pearlised or crystalline effect. Resin e.g. tosylamide resin – improves adhesion of polish to nail plate and flexibility. Solvent such as ethyl alcohol that dissolves ingredients together in nail polish. Plasticisers e.g. triphenyl phosphate – to provide flexibility after the polish has dried, reducing chipping. Pearlised particles – create a pearlised or crystalline effect.	To colour nail plates To provide some protection.
Cuticle cream	Emollients (e.g. lanolin, beeswax or glycerine). Perfume. Colour.	To soften and condition the nails, cuticles and surrounding skin.

(Continued)

HEALTH & SAFETY

Chemical formulations

It is important to keep up to date with the formulations of your products. Nail service technology is advancing all the time, with the aim to reduce toxicity, damage to the client's nails, harm to the beauty therapist through exposure and damage to the environment.

ALWAYS REMEMBER

Pearlised polishes

Pearlised polishes are created by the addition of sparkling, reflective particles such as mica, a synthetic product.

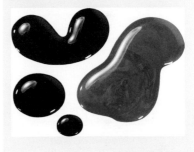

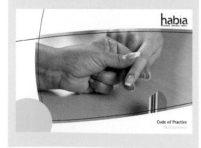

Product	Ingredients	Uses
Cuticle oil	Emollient oils such as lanolin and organic oils such as almond oil.	To soften and condition the nail cuticles and surrounding skin.
Nail strengthener	Nitrocellulose resin – film-forming plastic resin containing ingredients to strengthen nails, e.g. tosylamide/formaldehyde resin.	To strengthen and condition weak, brittle or damaged nails and protect them from breaking, splitting or peeling.
Nail conditioners	Organic oils that are vitamin enriched and provide excellent emollient properties.	Formulation designed to rehydrate, improving the appearance and health of the nail, encouraging **nail growth**.
Cuticle remover	Potassium hydroxide – a caustic alkali. Glycerine – a humectant added to reduce the drying effect on the nail plate.	To soften the skin of the cuticles.
Buffing paste	Perfume. Colour. Abrasive particles (e.g. pumice, talc or silica) to remove surface cells.	To provide a shine to the nail plate (used with a buffer).
Nail polish drier	Mineral oil – assists drying. Oleric acid or silicone – lubricant.	Increases the speed at which the polish hardens.
Nail polish solvent	Ethyl acetate – thins nail polish consistency. Toluene – solvent that dissolves nail polish ingredients.	Thins nail polish that has thickened, restoring consistency.

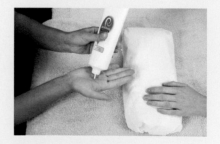

Safety and hygiene

◆ Ensure that your nail workstation is positioned and prepared to avoid unhealthy working positions and posture which could lead to strain and injury of the body.

◆ Ensure that tools and equipment are clean, disinfected and where required, according to legal requirements, sterile before use.

◆ Having sterilised or disinfected tools and equipment store them in a chemical disinfectant, UV cabinet or closed container until ready for use. Remember, they will remain clean but will not be sterile after 24 hours.

◆ Dispense products from containers, e.g. creams and lotions, with a clean, disposable spatula to prevent cross-infection and contamination.

◆ Use, store and dispose of products as recommended by the manufacturer.

◆ Use disposable products and equipment wherever possible.

◆ Refer to your workplace policy, manufacturers' guidelines and related legislative guidelines to ensure safe usage, prevention of cross-infection or contamination, safeguarding the health and welfare of yourself, clients and others.

Manicure and pedicure tools and equipment can be disposable or can be sterilised or disinfected by the following methods:

Tool/Equipment	Method	Term used
Cuticle knife	Autoclave	Sterilisation
Cuticle nippers	Autoclave	Sterilisation
Wooden cuticle stick	Throw away after use	Disposable
Callus file	Autoclave	Sterilisation
Bowl	Chemical (e.g. disinfectant)	Disinfection
Emery board	Throw away after use	Disposable
Buffer	Wipe handle with chemical disinfectant	Disinfection
	Wash buffing cloth in hot (60°C) soapy water	Cleaned
Towel	Wash in hot soapy water (60°C), or if disposable towels, throw away after use	Cleaned
Spatula	Throw away after use	Disposable
Nail clippers	Autoclave	Sterilisation
Scissors	Autoclave	Sterilisation
Hoof stick	Immerse in chemical (e.g. disinfectant)	Disinfection
Trolley	Wipe with chemical (e.g. disinfectant)	Disinfection

HEALTH & SAFETY

Disinfecting sprays

Disinfecting sprays may be used to disinfect the surface of the tools before further disinfection or sterilisation. Any debris must first be removed using a detergent and hot water before its use. Use in a well-ventilated area and avoid contact with flame and excessive heat.

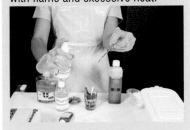

REVISION AID

In what state of hygiene should metal tools be in before use?

HEALTH & SAFETY

Metal in the autoclave

Any metal to be placed in the autoclave should be of a high-quality stainless steel, to prevent rusting. Always dry immediately to prevent damage.

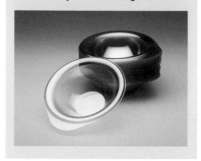

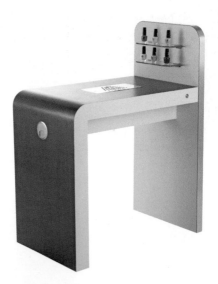

"Nail technicians work every day with products classed as 'hazardous'. Understanding these hazards and working to minimise any potential harm they could cause is essential.

Maintaining and improving the health of the natural nail should be the basis of all nail services. Avoid any damaging techniques but make sure to use the modern products and techniques that are now available."

Marian Newman

Metal tools when ready for use should be placed in a disinfecting solution. After the nail service they must be replaced and re-sterilised.

Environmental and sustainable working practice

Use biodegradable nail polish wherever possible as an alternative to chemical-based acetone nail polish remover. This is naturally derived from agricultural crops and does not contain petroleum ingredients. This also reduces chemical fumes created by acetone-based polish removers created as the volatile (unstable) ingredients evaporate into the air.

The nail plate benefits also from this alternative as acetone can be drying for the nail plate.

Only dispose of chemicals as recommended. Do not pour directly down the sink unless permitted to do so.

Select alternative products with ingredients that are the least hazardous wherever possible. Always read labels and check for environmental kite marks.

Disposable towels and robes may be used to reduce the cost and energy used in laundering items.

Preparation of the service area for manicure

Ensure that all manicure products, tools and **equipment** are clean, sterilised and disinfected, as appropriate, and that all necessary materials are neatly organised at the work station, which should be suitably positioned.

Repetitive strain injury (RSI) is caused by repeated movements of a particular part of the body. This can result in injury to the skeleton and muscle of the upper body and limbs, referred to as musculo-skeletal disorders (MSDs). Consideration should be given to assess the ergonomic design of the workplace equipment and seating to ensure that it promotes the beauty therapist's welfare and productivity by reducing fatigue and discomfort. A height adjustable chair with back support should be used, ensuring it is the correct height for the nail workstation. Foot rests should be used for beauty therapists who cannot place their feet flat on the floor. All equipment, products and tools should be easily accessible between knee and shoulder height. If positioned at the nail workstation for long periods, regular breaks should be taken to avoid fatigue.

ACTIVITY

Stretching exercises to avoid RSI

Perform regular, daily stretching exercises to reduce tension and improve flexibility for the fingers, wrists, hands, arms, shoulder, neck and upper back. These are shown for the fingers, wrists and hands.

Research simple stretching exercises suitable for the shoulder neck and upper back.

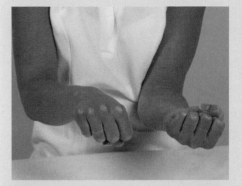
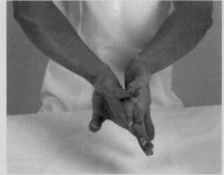
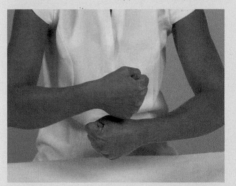
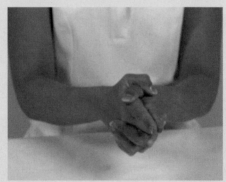
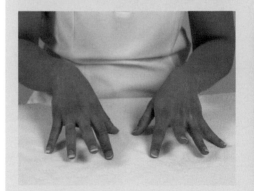
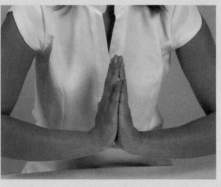

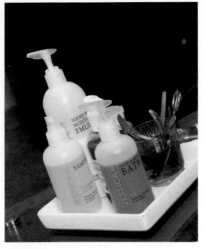

Manicure products, tools and equipment placed in the work area ready for the nail service

ALWAYS REMEMBER

Freelance

When working freelance it is important to consider your welfare and the ergonomics of the area you will be performing your services in.

Look for portable options, such as the portable manicure station and couch, shown below.

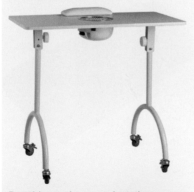

Portable manicure work station

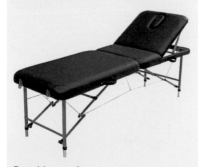

Portable couch

Keeping the work area tidy promotes an organised and professional image, and prevents time being wasted as you try to find products, tools and equipment. Always leave the work area in a condition suitable for further nail services.

The manicure service may be carried out at a purpose-built nail work-station, over a beauty treatment couch as shown or whilst the client receives another service such as a facial. What is important is that your workstation and stool are suitable for your working position.

HEALTH & SAFETY

Preventing injury and fatigue

When you are positioned at the nail workstation, performing repetitive actions, it is important that you are comfortable.

Employers are required to provide seating that is suitable and safe for the needs of the individual within their work role.

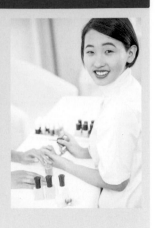

◆ Ensure your seat offers adequate support and is height adjustable.

◆ There should be adequate length between your knee and the back of the seat in order for you to distribute your body weight evenly along your thighs. This also allows satisfactory blood circulation in the area.

◆ The client should be at the correct height, including their hands, to avoid you leaning or stretching unnecessarily.

◆ Adequate breaks should be taken. Consider this when booking your appointments to ensure you carry out a variety of services.

◆ Carry out stretching exercises.

REVISION AID

What actions could lead to RSI when carrying out nail services?

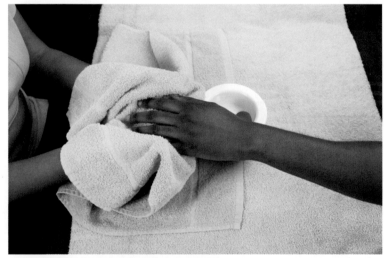

Manicure service performed over a beauty treatment couch

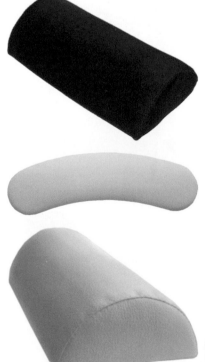

Select your manicure hand rest according to the service being completed

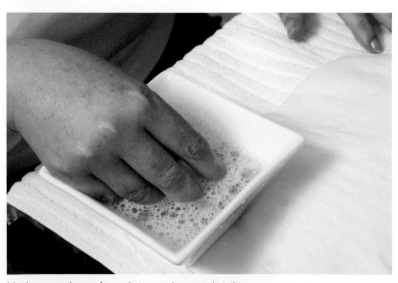

Manicure service performed at a manicure workstation

Prepare your nail workstation according to your workplace policy. The example shown in the image is to place a towel over the work surface, then fold another towel forming a pad and place it in the middle of the work surface. The pad helps to support the client's forearm and wrist during service. Place the third towel over the pad, with more of the towel on the manicurist's side – this is used to dry the client's hands during service.

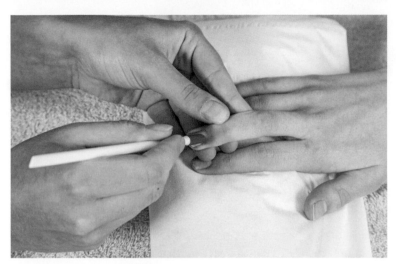

Covered pad placed to provide support

A tissue or disposable manicure mat may then be placed on top of the towels, to catch any nail clippings or filings. This is disposed of later for reasons of hygiene and to avoid irritation to the client's and beauty therapist's skin from filings. All towels should be replaced with freshly laundered or disposable ones according to your workplace policy following each service.

The environmental conditions must be suitable. Lighting must be adequate to avoid eye strain. Additional lighting such as a table lamp may be required to complete tasks competently and safely, such as nail art and cuticle nipping.

The nail workstation must not be positioned in direct sunlight to avoid heat and light discomfort to the client or yourself. Heat can also spoil many manicure products. Ventilation should be adequate to avoid breathing in hazardous dust and chemical vapours from the products used.

Background music, if provided, should be at a sound level that allows effective communication with your client.

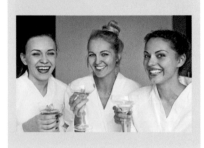
Client care, consultation and communication

Service information to provide to the client at the initial point of interest

When a client makes an appointment for a manicure service, the receptionist should ask a few simple questions that will help guide how long the service will take.

◆ Do they require a nail finish? Time must be allocated for the type of finish required, so the client should be made aware of this.

◆ If the client is new to this service, explain what is involved. Some clients may be embarrassed so providing this information is helpful.

◆ Make clients aware of any promotions or incentives. An example could be that the bride will receive a complimentary nail service if other members of the bridal party are recommended.

ACTIVITY

Making appointments

What questions could the receptionist ask when booking a client for a manicure in order to make the appointments run more efficiently? Write down your questions stating how they will assist with the smooth running of the reception.

ACTIVITY

Communication skills

Positive communication is essential. Give three examples of communication techniques used when carrying out a nail service.

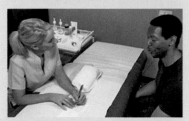

Communication with a male client when performing a hand nail service

TOP TIP

Benefits of manicure service

The beneficial effects of manicure service should be explained to a client at consultation and how regular treatments will help improve and maintain healthy nails and skin.

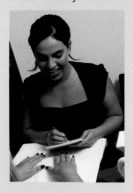

◆ Do they require any **hand and nail treatments** in addition to the manicure, such as **exfoliation** or hand mask? Allow extra time accordingly.

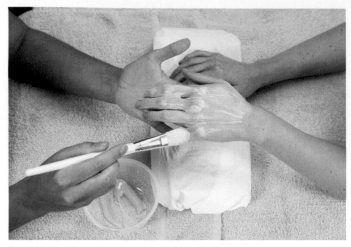

Specialist hand treatment – hand mask application

Has the client had artificial nail enhancements or **gel polish** applied previously which require removal? Allow approximately 20 minutes for this process. Removal must only be carried out if you are qualified to do so.

ALWAYS REMEMBER

Artificial nail enhancements

It is important to discuss the client's previous service history at the consultation. For example, if the client has had several new sets of artificial nail enhancements applied this will create some damage to the natural nail.

The nail plate may be thin, ridges may appear upon the nail plate and the removal technique may cause dehydration. All of these effects will need to be discussed with your client at consultation and an appropriate service plan including treatment products discussed.

Allow 45 minutes for a manicure service.

Allow 20–30 minutes for a file and finish; gel polish takes longer than nail polish.

Allow up to 1 hour for a specialist hand-nail service.

All staff, especially the staff communicating with clients at reception should be familiar with the different pricing structures for the range of manicure services and products available for retail.

The receptionist should also check the age of the client. If the client is a minor under the age of 16, it is necessary to obtain parent, carer or guardian permission for treatment. The parent/guardian will also have to be present when the treatment is received.

"Developing a good style of communication with your clients is essential. This will develop with practice and experience but must start at the beginning of your education. Your clients need to be confident in your professional skills and you need to be able to correctly identify their skin and nail conditions (without diagnosing medically based conditions). Treat every client as an individual and not a series of 'step by steps'. Lead them through your consultation to make sure you understand what they actually want and balance that with what you believe they need."

Marian Newman

Consultation

Before carrying out a manicure service, it is necessary to assess the condition of the client's skin, nails and cuticles. This is important to ensure that the most appropriate hand and nail treatments and products are chosen. Also, by correctly assessing and analysing the client's hand condition and writing this on their client record you will be able to see over a period of time how the condition is improving and progressing.

Assess the condition of the following:

◆ **The cuticles** Are they dry, tight or cracked, or are they soft, intact and pliable?

◆ **The nails** Are they strong or weak, brittle – hard and non-flexible and shatter easily? Or flaking? Are they dry, lacking moisture with visible ridges? Are they discoloured or stained? What natural shape are they – square, round, oval? Are they long or short? Are they bitten?

◆ **The skin** Is the skin dry, rough or chapped, or is it soft and smooth? Is the colour even? Also check the skin in between the fingers.

While assessing the client's hands for service, you should also be looking for any *contra-indications* to the service that may prevent or restrict treatment.

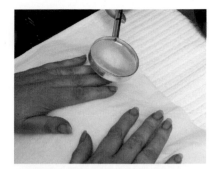

Assessing the nails and skin using a manufacturer's nail magnifier tool or a magnifying lamp may be used.

ALWAYS REMEMBER

Discoloured or stained nails

Discoloured nails may be related to:

◆ a medical condition such as nail fungus, tinea unguium, psoriasis and skin jaundice

◆ medication, for example those containing beta-carotene

◆ trauma to the nail such as bruising

◆ lifestyle, such as contact with nicotine if a smoker

◆ application of dark polish without a protective base coat

◆ not wearing PPE when applying preparations such as self tan, which will stain the skin

◆ contact with hair colourants such as toning lotions and coloured mousses

◆ dark streaks on the nail plate associated with melanin distribution. This is more commonly seen on dark-skinned clients.

At consultation question the client and share advice and recommendations.

ALWAYS REMEMBER

Record keeping

Accurately record your client's answers to necessary questions to be asked at consultation on their treatment record. This is a legal requirement.

ACTIVITY

Assessing the hands' treatment needs

Look closely at your own hands. Assess their condition, considering the skin of the hands surrounding the nail and the nail plate itself, and make notes about everything you see.

Then assess the hands of a colleague. How do they differ from your own?

Complete a treatment record and note the condition of the nails and surrounding skin.
Design a suitable service plan for your client to meet their needs.

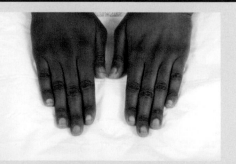

For more information on diseases affecting the skin and recording information related to skin and nail assessment see CHAPTER 3, Consultation Practice and Techniques.

Skin and nail disorders of the hands

When a client attends for a manicure service, as part of the **consultation** and assessment of the client's needs, the beauty therapist should always look at the client's skin and nails to check that no infection or disease is present that might contra-indicate service. Bacterial, fungal, viral and parasitic infections prevent service. These are described in more detail in Chapter 3, where **contra-indications** are illustrated and discussed.

If the client is wearing nail finish that conceals the natural nail plate, this must be removed before inspecting the health of the nail plate.

Contra-indications The following disorders both contra-indicate or restrict services to the hands and also feet. If you suspect the client has any disorder from the chart below, never attempt a diagnosis, but refer the client tactfully to their GP without causing unnecessary concern.

HEALTH & SAFETY

Contact dermatitis

Contact dermatitis is a skin problem caused by intolerance of the skin to a particular substance or a group of substances. On exposure to the substance the skin quickly becomes irritated and an allergic reaction occurs. This may occur when a manicurist's skin is exposed to dust and chemicals on a regular basis. Follow all HSE guidelines to reduce the risk of developing this skin disorder, which could result in the need for a career change!

Always follow workplace policies, procedures and manufacturers' guidelines on the use of products.

Disorder	Description
Broken bones 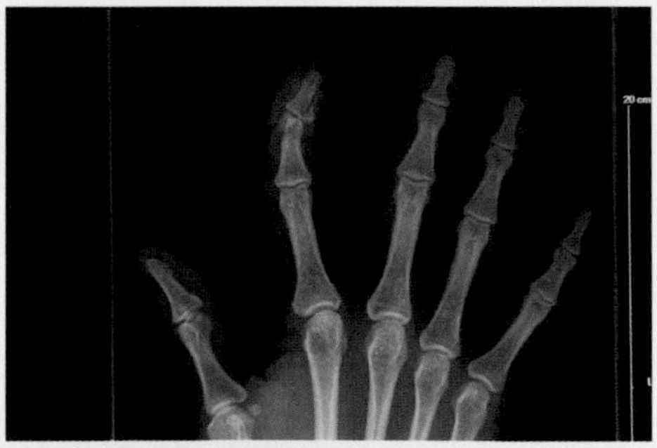 	Injury resulting in a broken bone can often not be seen; confirm at consultation that there is no known injury in the service area. Here a distal phalange bone of the hand is broken. If one bone is affected in the finger of one hand, the service may be modified if the area can be avoided.
Broken skin 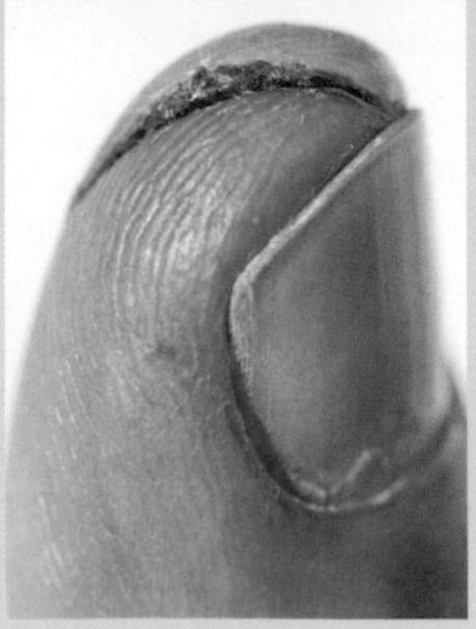 	Any cut or abrasion could lead to secondary infection and the area should not be treated until healed.

(Continued)

Disorder	Description
Diabetes	If a client has a diabetic hand or foot condition, they are vulnerable to infection as they have slow skin healing. Care should be taken also with heat treatments due to impaired circulation. This could be problematic if the skin was accidentally broken during a pedicure service. Permission must be obtained from the client's GP before service can be received.
Paronychia	Infectious bacterial infection. Swelling, redness and pus appears in the cuticle area and skin of the nail wall. Service cannot be provided. Permission must be obtained from the client's GP before service can be received.
Scabies or itch mites	An infestation of the skin by an animal parasite passed on by prolonged direct contact. The animal parasite burrows beneath the skin and invades the hair follicles. Papules and wavy greyish lines appear approximately 1 cm in length, where dirt enters the burrows. Secondary bacterial infection may occur as a result of scratching. Common sites where this is seen include: between fingers or toes, palm of hands, wrists, elbows, soles and sides of the feet. Service cannot be provided. Permission must be obtained from the client's GP before service can be received.
Severe eczema of the skin	Inflammation of the skin caused by contact internally or externally, with an irritant. Reddening of the skin occurs with swelling and blistering; the blisters leak tissue fluid, which later hardens and forms scabs. There is potential for contact with body tissue fluids, cross-contamination and the risk of secondary infection. When severe, service must not be provided due to the risk of discomfort and secondary infection.
Severe eczema of the nail	Differing changes to the nail may occur, including the appearance of ridges, pitting, **onycholysis** or nail thickening (hypertrophy).

(Continued)

Disorder	Description
Severe nail separation (onycholysis) 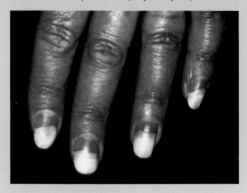	Lifting of the nail plate from the nail bed, may be caused by trauma or infection to the nail or surrounding area; where separation has occurred this appears as a greyish-white area on the nail as the pink undertone of the nail bed does not show. If only one nail is affected and the service can be modified, service can be provided. However, this decision will be based upon the cause of the nail separation.
Severe psoriasis of the nail 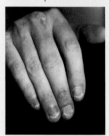	An inflammatory condition where there is an increased production of cells in the upper part of the skin. Pitting occurs on the surface of the nail plate. Separation (onycholysis) may also occur. Service may be modified if there is no risk of discomfort or potential harm to the area.
Severe psoriasis of the skin 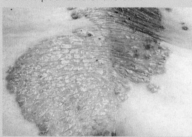	Red patches of skin appear covered in waxy, silvery scales. Bleeding will occur if the area is scratched and the scales are removed. There is potential for contact with body tissue fluids, cross-contamination and the risk of secondary infection. The cause is unknown. When severe, service must not be provided due to the risk of discomfort and secondary infection.
Tinea corporis (body ringworm) 	Fungal infection of the skin, which may occur on the limbs. Small scaly red patches, which spread outwards and then heal from the centre, leaving a ring. Contagious; medically refer the client to their GP.
Tinea unguium 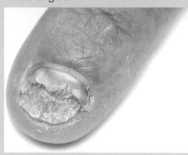	Fungal infection of the nails. The nail plate is yellowish-grey and may thicken. Eventually the nail plate becomes brittle and separates from the nail bed. Contagious; medically refer the client to their GP.

(Continued)

Disorder	Description
warts or verrucae 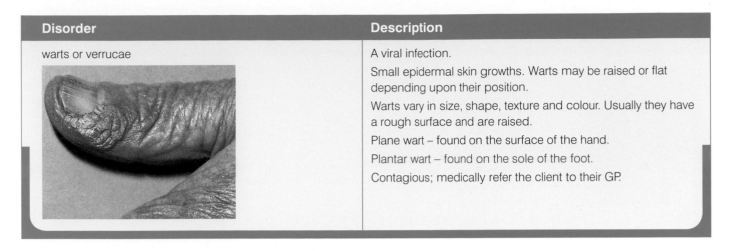	A viral infection. Small epidermal skin growths. Warts may be raised or flat depending upon their position. Warts vary in size, shape, texture and colour. Usually they have a rough surface and are raised. Plane wart – found on the surface of the hand. Plantar wart – found on the sole of the foot. Contagious; medically refer the client to their GP.

Further common disorders that may be seen on the hands. Some may also appear on the feet. Not all of these contra-indicate service.

Disorder	Cause	Appearance	Salon service	Advice and recommendation
Blue nail	Poor blood circulation in the area. Heart disease.	The nail bed does not appear a healthy pink colour but has a blue tinge.	Permission to treat must be received from the client's GP. Regular manicure, including hand treatment service to improve circulation.	General manicure advice. Hand exercises and massage to improve circulation.
Bruised nails	Trauma to the nail (e.g. trapping it in a door); severe damage can result in loss of the nail.	Part of the nail plate may appear blue or black where bleeding has occurred on the nail bed.	Although this disorder does not contra-indicate service, it is advisable to postpone manicuring the nails until the condition is no longer painful. Nail polish may be used to disguise the damaged nail.	Seek medical advice if swelling is present or if pain persists.
Eggshell nail	Linked to Illness, medication and nutritional deficiency.	Thin, fragile, white nail plate, curving under at the free edge.	Permission for treatment must be received from the client's GP. Regular manicure.	General manicure advice. Strengthening base coats incorporating ingredients such as calcium and protective hydrating oils. Seek medical advice regarding health and consider healthy lifestyle factors such as a nutritionally balanced diet.

(Continued)

Disorder	Cause	Appearance	Salon service	Advice and recommendation
Hangnail	Cracking of a dry skin or cuticle condition. Nervous habit of picking or biting the skin around the nail. Associated condition of onychopagy, nail biting. Poor care of the skin surrounding the nails leading to dry skin condition. Link to occupation, regular contact with water such as washing the hands.	Epidermis around the nail plate cracks and a small piece of skin protrudes between the nail plate and the nail wall, sometimes accompanied by redness and swelling: this condition can become extremely painful.	**Warm-oil services**, hand massage and hand masks to moisturise and soften the skin and cuticles. Remove the protrusion of dead skin with cuticle nippers: never cut into live tissue.	Regular use of a rich hand cream/lotion. Regular use of cuticle cream/oil. Wear protective gloves when carrying out domestic or occupational related chores. Wear warm gloves in cold weather. Ensure a balanced diet.
Leuconychia	Trauma to the nail plate or matrix, due to pressure or hitting the nail with a hard object. Air pockets form between the nail plate and nail bed. A deficiency in the mineral zinc in the diet can also lead to the appearance of white spots.	White spots or marks on the nail plate: will grow out with the nail.	General manicure service. Coloured nail polish application will disguise their appearance until the damaged area disappears as it grows towards the free edge. Avoid applying unnecessary pressure at the matrix/lunula area where the nail plate is softer.	Be careful with the hands. Wear protective gloves when carrying out domestic chores or gardening. Do not use the nails as tools! Do not apply unnecessary pressure if pushing back the cuticles. Leave the treatment of the overgrown cuticles to the professionals! Consider healthy lifestyle factors such as a nutritionally balanced diet.
Longitudinal ridges in the nail plate (corrugated nails)	Illness. Damage to the matrix. Age, associated with the ageing process.	Grooves in the nail plate running along the length of the nail from the cuticle to the free edge: may affect one or all nails.	Abrasive buffing paste applied to the nail plate used in conjunction with a buffer helps smooth out the ridges. Use of a **ridge-filling base coat** prior to nail polish application.	General manicure advice. Use of a ridge-filling base coat polish. Ensure a balanced diet.

(Continued)

Disorder	Cause	Appearance	Salon service	Advice and recommendation
Minor **nail separation** (onycholysis)	Lifting of the nail plate from its bed. Can accompany a medical condition such as eczema or psoriasis or a fungal infection in the area.	Where separation has occurred this appears as a greyish-white area as the pink undertone of the nail bed does not show through the nail plate.	It is advisable to postpone manicuring for this nail until the condition is corrected.	Be careful to avoid infection of the nail bed. Protect the nail with a protective dressing. Refer the client to their GP to confirm cause.
Onychophagy (excessive nail biting)	Stress and anxiety can be a trigger that can develop into a permanent nail-biting habit that can permanently damage the nail and surrounding skin.	Very short or little nail plate; bulbous skin appears at the fingertip; nail walls often red and swollen, due to biting of the skin surrounding the nails. Hang nails and peeling skin are often present and broken skin can lead to infection.	Regular weekly manicures. Cuticle service to maximise the visible nail-plate area. Nail conditioning services to prevent dry cuticles and hangnails.	Bitter-tasting nail preparations painted onto the nail plate. Wear gloves to avoid biting in bed. A retail package of products may be provided to gain client motivation in improving the growth and appearance of the nails and surrounding skin. Strategies can be discussed on how to avoid biting nails during periods of stress.
Onychorrhexis	Exposure to water and chemicals causing the nails to become dry. Poor diet. Not wearing gloves in cold weather.	Split, flaking nails.	Warm-oil manicures on a weekly basis.	Regular use of a rich hand cream/lotion. Always wear protective gloves when carrying out domestic tasks and if your work requires contact with chemicals. Always wear warm gloves in cold weather. Ensure a balanced diet. Prescribe nail base coat to protect split, flaking nails.
Pitting	Eczema. Psoriasis.	Pitting resembling small irregular pin pricks appear on the nail plate. The number varies.	Regular manicure with gentle buffing to the nail plate surface.	General manicure advice. Ridge-filling base coat polish. Refer the client to their GP for permission to treat if required.

(Continued)

Disorder	Cause	Appearance	Salon service	Advice and recommendation
Pterygium	Neglect of the nails. Associated with other medical conditions and skin disorders. Hereditary. Injury to the matrix.	Overgrown thickened triangular, wing-shaped skin located at the cuticle and adheres to the nail plate as it grows forward: if left untreated, this may lead to splitting of the cuticle and subsequent infection.	If overgrown cuticle is excessive, refer client to their GP. Warm oil or paraffin wax services weekly. Use of specialist cuticle oils and removers. Once softened, remove excess skin with cuticle nippers. It is important that treatment is gradual to avoid sensitivity and inflammation, which could lead to possible infection.	Regular application of a specialist cuticle oil/cream, in line with manufacturer's instructions. Wear protective gloves when carrying out domestic chores. Gently push back the cuticles with a soft towel when softened, e.g. after bathing.
Transverse furrows in the nail plate (Beau's lines)	Temporary slower development of the nail in the matrix, due to illness or trauma of the nail. Horizontal Grooves occur when nail growth is interrupted, becoming visible later as the nail grows.	Horizontal Groove in the nail plate, often on all nails simultaneously, running from side to side: this will grow out as the nail grows.	Regular, e.g. weekly manicure until normal cells replace the damaged cells.	General manicure advice to care for the nail. Ensure a nutritionally balanced diet.
Koilonychia (spoon-shaped nails)	Hereditary. Iron deficiency due to diet or anaemia, a condition where there are reduced red blood cells. Softened nail plates through immersion in water and detergent or oils leading to lifting of the sides of the nail plate.	Nail plate surface is flat and concave, spoon-like in appearance.	Nails to be kept short and file to achieve a balanced look.	Wear PPE if the nails are regularly exposed to detergent and water. Ensure a nutritionally balanced diet.

(Continued)

Disorder	Cause	Appearance	Salon service	Advice and recommendation
Loss of skin sensation – numbness in the extremities of the hands and feet	Nerves in the extremities, hands and feet are damaged, irritated or compressed impairing sensation. This can lead to loss of sensation numbness, termed sensory neuropathy. Carpal tunnel syndrome is an example related to a medical condition where compression of nerves that control sensation in the hands can lead to loss of sensation. Other factors include medication and injury.	N/A	Without GP consent to treat, service must not be carried out as the client could not indicate discomfort or pain during the service application. If loss of sensation is temporary then service can proceed with caution. However, medical approval should be sought.	Refer the client to their GP for diagnosis and treatment.
Onychauxis (hypertrophy)	Advanced age – nails thicken with age. Psoriasis. Nail trauma. Pressure to the nail, such as ill-fitting shoes.	Excessively thickened nail plate. Can affect the nails of the hands or feet.	Buff the nail plate to reduce thickness.	Regular professional nail service to keep the nail plate smooth and thinned. If on the toenails it may be preferable for the nails to be treated by a chiropodist who can use appropriate tools.
Onychotrophia (atrophy)	Injury to matrix. Poor blood circulation. Diabetes.	Thin fragile nail plate. May lift from the nail bed, resulting in loss of colour.	With permission to treat, take care when filing the nail plate. Avoid any service that may thin the nail plate. Apply nail strengthening products.	Initially refer the client to their GP for diagnosis and treatment. Regular professional nail service. Application of nail strengthening products. Protect the nails, e.g. wear gloves when carrying out domestic tasks.

(Continued)

Disorder	Cause	Appearance	Salon service	Advice and recommendation
Onychocryptosis Ingrowing nail	Incorrect cutting and filing of the nail. Incorrect, ill-fitting foot wear.	Can affect the nails of both the hands and feet. The edges of the free edge part of the nail plate grow into the lateral walls of the nail leading to redness, swelling and inflammation. Bacterial infection may also be associated with this disorder.	If not present, but has been previously identified. Always file the nails correctly according to location – hands/feet. Do not cut/file toenails at the free edge into the corners.	If an ingrowing nail is present, refer the client to a chiropodist. Advise the client on how to correctly cut and shape the nails applicable to the hands/feet.
Onychomycosis (ringworm)	Fungal infection of the nail plate. Regular exposure to water and chemicals, leading to nail softening.	Yellow, brown, white areas on the nail plate.	Can treat again when the area is visibly clear.	Contagious, therefore refer the client to their GP for diagnosis and treatment. Wear PPE if the nails are regularly exposed to detergent and water.
Sepsis	Life-threatening condition whereby the body's immune system responds to infection.	High temperature. Cold, clammy skin which is mottled in appearance.	N/A	Refer the client to their GP for diagnosis and treatment.
Black streaks (linear melanonychia)	Melanin – hyperpigmentation. Form of skin cancer – subungual melanoma.	Dark streaks appearing along the nail length.	Treat as normal with GP permission.	Refer the client to their GP for diagnosis and treatment. Coloured nail polish will disguise the discolouration appearance affecting the nail/s.
Onychogryphosis (rams horn nails)	Nail neglect. Congenital. Psoriasis. Trauma. Poor blood circulation. Ill-fitting footwear. Advanced age – nails thicken with age.	Claw like, thickened nails. These may curve forwards or sideways. More common in toenails.	File the nails short.	Receive regular nail service dependent upon nail growth rate to keep the nails short and even in length. This will reduce the curvature appearance. Advise the client to see a chiropodist if the nails are thickened and too difficult to cut.

(Continued)

Disorder	Cause	Appearance	Salon service	Advice and recommendation
Onychoptosis (shedding of the nail plate)	Trauma. Medically related symptom. Medication. Pressure on the nails, may be caused by ill-fitting footwear.	Shedding of the nail plate in parts or whole.	Can be treated when the nail regrows.	Refer the client to their GP for diagnosis and permission to treat. Avoid reason for initial shedding of the nail plate.

Contra-actions Contra-actions should be discussed with the client at consultation. Certain cosmetic ingredients are known to cause allergic reactions in some people.

The client – or the beauty therapist – may at some time develop an allergy to a manicure product that has been successfully used previously. This could be for a number of reasons, including new medication being taken or illness.

The symptoms of an allergic reaction could be:

◆ redness of the skin (erythema)

◆ swelling

◆ itching

◆ raised blisters.

The symptoms do not necessarily appear on the hands. In the case of nail polish allergy, the symptoms often show up on the face, which the hands are continually touching.

In the case of an allergic reaction:

◆ Remove the offending product immediately, using water or, in the case of polish, nail polish solvent.

◆ Apply a cool compress and soothing agent to the skin to reduce redness and irritation.

◆ If symptoms persist, seek medical advice. If the client receives medical advice, ask them to inform you of the advice and/or service received so you can include this in your records.

Always carry out a skin sensitivity patch test if a client has known sensitivity to product ingredients identified at consultation. The patch test should be performed 24–48 hours before using any new or known ingredient within the nail service or treatment that may cause sensitisation. A negative patch test result is required.

Always record any allergies on the client's treatment record, so that the offending product may be avoided in future.

Further contra-actions may occur as a result of poor manicure techniques, e.g. failing to check the temperature of **paraffin wax** before application, which if too hot could cause skin sensitivity, even burning! Always perform a thermal skin sensitivity test before heat treatments. Tissue damage could result in blood loss, e.g. incorrect nipping removal technique when using cuticle nippers may result in pulling and tearing the skin. Incorrect positioning and use of the cuticle knife may lead to piercing the cuticle with the knife blade.

Avoid cutting the nails too short as again this can result in possible damage to the hyponychium, the part of the epidermis under the free edge of the nail. This may affect its protective function leading to possible infection.

REVISION AID

Where are contra-indications checked for during a nail service?

HEALTH & SAFETY

Diagnosis

You are not qualified to diagnose; this is the job of a medical practitioner.

Therefore if you are unsure about any nail or skin condition present refer the client to their GP.

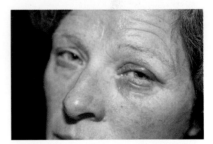

Client with an allergic reaction that has affected the eyes, causing redness and swelling

"Beauty therapists should never work on any client presenting with something they cannot recognise. When in doubt send it out."

Laura Dicken

"You must continue learning and improving. Do this by taking as many short courses as you can. Read the trade press and visit trade shows to keep up with latest products and developments. Have a basic understanding of all the most popular brands, products and technology even if you don't use them. Clients need to know that your knowledge is current and your advice comes from an educated viewpoint."

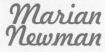
Marian Newman

Service plan

After analysing the client's nails and adjacent skin, a **service plan** should be considered and agreed with the client to meet their needs. In order to correct skin and nail problems, the client should attend the salon regularly, this is weekly or every two weeks. They should also be advised of the appropriate nail and hand products to use, so as to support the salon service. The type of specialist nail services to use, including products, will depend upon the nail and skin condition and the client's time and financial commitment.

- *Nail strengthener* This is used on brittle, damaged nails to strengthen, condition and protect them against breaking, splitting or peeling.
- *Ridge filler* This is used on nails with ridges to provide a more even surface, creating a bond between the **base coat** and polish, allowing a smoother application of polish.
- *Nail oil* This contains ingredients to rehydrate the nail and soften the cuticle.
- *Cuticle creams* These nourish the skin and restore the condition of the cuticle.
- *Hand cream/lotions or oil* Used to protect the skin, maintaining skin hydration and reducing the negative signs of dryness and neglect. In the foot area dry, cracked skin and on the hands rough, dry skin. Some hand creams contain UV filters to protect against UV damage and premature ageing.
- *Specialist hand and nail services* These may also be recommended within the manicure service to improve the appearance of the skin texture, nail and cuticle condition and provide a number of physiological benefits. These may be offered each time the client has a manicure service to maintain the condition of the nails and hands. Their use may be recommended as part of a homecare routine e.g. a hand exfoliant and mask.

Explain to the client how long the service will take, stages of the service and sensations to be experienced.

Provide the opportunity for your client to ask any questions relating to the manicure service or service plan.

The treatment record should be signed and dated by the beauty therapist and client following the consultation to confirm the suitability and their consent with the agreed nail service.

It is important that accurate records are kept and stored in compliance with the Data Protection Act for future reference.

ALWAYS REMEMBER

GP referral

A client referred from their GP will usually have a letter. This would be the case when confirmation of suitability for service has been requested and should be retained with the client's service plan.

ALWAYS REMEMBER

Modifying your treatment to meet your client's needs

Following your consultation, you may need to adjust your manicure to meet your client's needs by modifying:

- the depth of massage pressure when applying hand and arm massage and choice of massage movements applied; e.g. an elderly client's skin is thinner, has less elasticity and they may have reduced joint mobility. Pressure will be reduced; techniques will avoid stretching the skin further and joint mobilisation may be avoided. Explain the benefits of the massage. A deeper hand and arm massage may be applied for a male client as their skin is thicker, and arms tend to be more muscular.
- the choice of massage medium when client has excessively hairy arms; the product must avoid sufficient slip without dragging the hairs, causing discomfort
- the choice of nail polish product and ingredients including base, colour and top coat to improve the nail condition and enhance appearance.

Preparing the client

Consider the client's comfort with the location of the manicure treatment area. Some clients may require a more private area than a busy area with lots of traffic (people walking past). Check suitability of location with your client.

A lightweight protective gown may be offered to the client to cover their clothing. This will prevent damage to their clothes from accidental contact with products during service. Ask them to remove any jewellery from the area to be treated, to prevent the jewellery being soiled or damaged by creams and to avoid obstructing massage movements.

Place the jewellery where the client can see it. Alternatively, ask the client to take possession of it for safe-keeping – follow your workplace security policy. Ensure that the client is seated at the correct height, and close enough to you to avoid having to lean forward. There should be adequate support of the client's arm and wrist throughout.

When the client is comfortably seated, clean your hands using an approved hand cleaning technique – preferably in view of the client, who can then observe hygienic procedures being carried out.

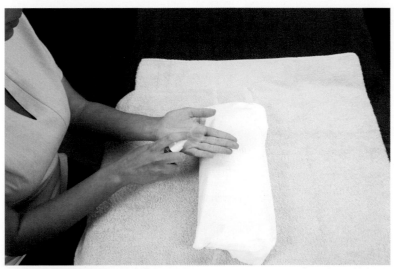

Hand disinfection for manicurist

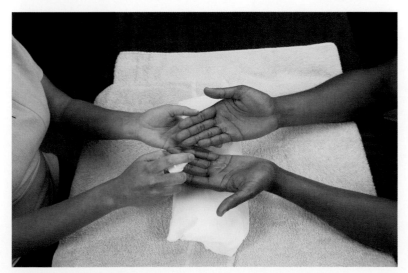

Hand disinfection for client

ALWAYS REMEMBER

Removal of existing finish

If the client is wearing a gel polish finish, refer to later in this chapter where removal of this popular nail finish is discussed.

REVISION AID

What should be considered when positioning the client for nail service?

ALWAYS REMEMBER

Security

Keep the client's jewellery in full view throughout the service, so that they don't forget it when they leave.

Alternatively they may take possession of it. Follow your workplace policy, which will ensure compliance with your insurance requirements.

This will assure them that they are receiving a professional service. The client should also wash their hands before the service commences. The client's skin can also be cleaned with a disinfectant gel or spray. Continue to check for any contra-indications.

Consult the client's treatment record, and begin the service.

STEP-BY-STEP: MANICURE PROCEDURE

This procedure briefly shows the stages in the manicure. Each step is discussed in detail later in the chapter. The procedure may start with the right or left hand.

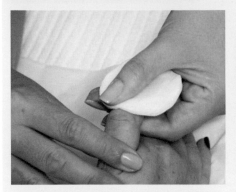

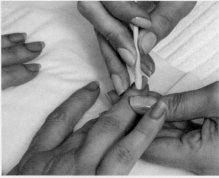

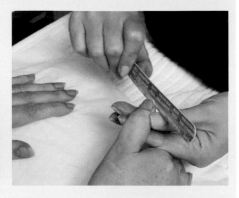

1 Remove any existing nail polish from each nail with nail polish remover. Hold the cotton wool in contact with the nail plate for two to three seconds, then wipe towards you from cuticle to free edge in three strokes – left side, centre and right side of the nail plate. Work methodically from the little finger to the thumb. Then repeat on the other hand. Check for contra-indications and take the necessary action if present. Replace cotton wool regularly to maintain its effectiveness.

2 Use a cotton wool-tipped cuticle stick to apply nail polish remover around the cuticle area as necessary to remove any excess nail polish that may be present. Avoid unnecessary contact with the skin to avoid drying out.

3 File the nails of the right hand to the agreed length and shape. Scissors or nail clippers may be used to reduce length if long. Hold the emery board at a 45 degree angle to the free edge, and apply strokes in one direction. Ensure the free edge is smooth with rough edges removed by performing upward strokes with the file often referred to as **bevelling**.

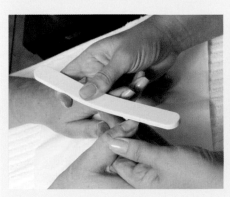

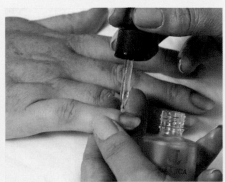

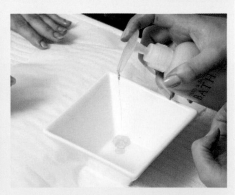

4 Buff the nail plate of the right hand. Apply from cuticle to free edge in one direction only. When used with buffing paste this will remove surface cells providing a smooth finish. If buffing is to be provided as a nail finish this will be carried out towards the end of the manicure.

5 Apply cuticle cream or oil to the cuticle area.

6 Place a small amount of liquid soap formulated for use in nail services and add warm water when ready to use. Place the right hand in the manicure bowl containing warm water and liquid soap. Repeat steps **2–6** for the left hand.

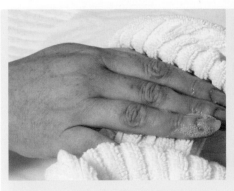

7 Remove the right hand from the manicure bowl and dry with a towel whilst gently pushing back the cuticles. Place the left hand into the manicure bowl.

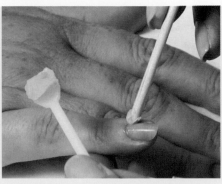

8 Apply cuticle remover to the right hand. Avoid unnecessary contact with the product and the skin of the finger.

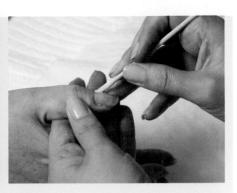

9 Push back the cuticle with a cotton wool-tipped cuticle stick or hoof stick.

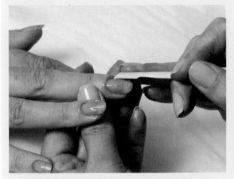

10 Remove excess eponychium with a cuticle knife. The blade should be kept flat and slightly wet to avoid scratching the nail plate.

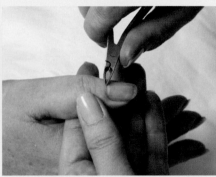

11 Remove excess dead cuticle with nippers.

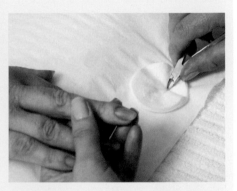

12 Collect excess cuticle and skin tissue on a clean piece of cotton wool or nail wipe and dispose of it hygienically, immediately following completion of this stage of the service. Wipe the nails with damp cotton wool to remove excess cuticle remover. This product could cause skin dryness and irritation.

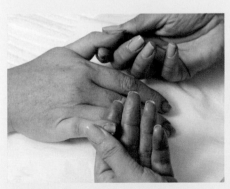

13 Apply cuticle oil and massage it in with your thumbs to hydrate the area. Repeat steps 7–13 for the left hand. Apply massage routine to both hands and forearms.

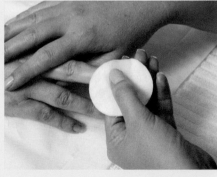

14 Remove grease from the nail plate with a cotton wool pad soaked in nail polish remover.

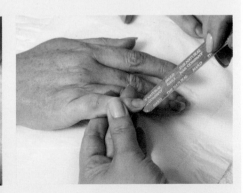

15 Refile and bevel the nails as necessary to ensure they are smooth and even. The client may find it convenient to pay for her service at this stage, to avoid smudging her polish later. Also, if jewellery has been removed ask her to replace it to avoid damage to the polish after application.

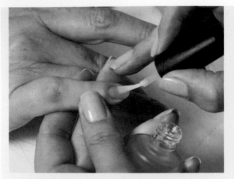

16 Confirm and apply the nail finish. If applying the polish, apply: base coat (once); polish (twice); and top coat (once). If a pearlised polish is used, a top coat is not required and a third coat of polish may be applied. If the client doesn't want polish, buff to a shine with buffing paste or use a four-sided buffer.

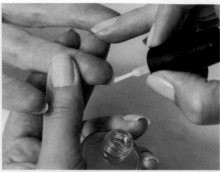

17 Base coat may be applied under the free edge of the nail to create a protective seal.

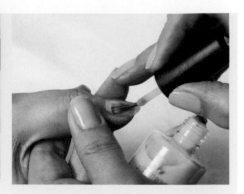

18 French manicure polish application finish: neutral coloured nail polish is applied in soft beige to evenly cover the nail plate surface. Apply one or two coats.

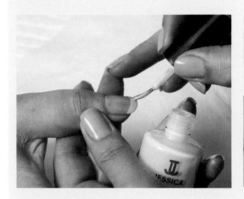

19 The free edge is painted white ensuring that the line is even. Apply one coat. If the nails are particularly stained the reverse of the free edge may be painted also.

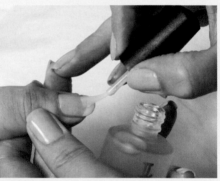

20 Apply a top coat to seal and protect the nail polish. A quick-drying spray or oil may be applied to speed the hardening process.

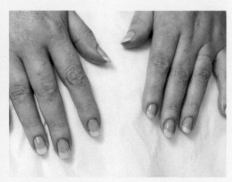

21 The completed manicure with French finish.

"Practise and practise. Don't shy away from the French manicure because it's a bit tricky! Don't spend valuable practice time playing with nail art until you have honed your polishing skills. Beautifully polished nails will bring your clients back again and again."

Marian Newman

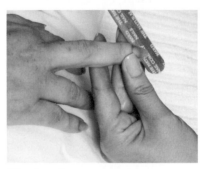

Filing the nails

Filing

The part of the nail that is filed is the free edge. This should be filed to complement the nail shape and condition. When filing the natural nail, use a fine grit **emery board**. Very often emery boards have different degrees of coarseness on either side, indicated by different colours. Use the darker, rougher side to remove excess length, and the lighter, smoother side for shaping and bevelling to remove rough edges. A flexible emery board is preferable to a stiff one as it generates less friction.

When shaping the nail always file the nails from the side to the centre, with the emery board sloping at a 45 degree angle to the nail, slightly under the free edge. If a square shape is required, file straight across the free edge in one direction to create a uniform square shape and then smooth the outside edges to remove roughness, which may lead to accidental damage and breakage.

Use swift, rhythmical strokes. Avoid a sawing action – this would generate friction and might cause the free edge to split.

Never file completely down the sides of the nail, as strength is required here to balance the free edge. Always allow about 4 mm of nail growth to remain at the sides of the nail.

ALWAYS REMEMBER

Nail shapes

When filing the nails ensure that the finished appearance complements the client's nail/hand.

Be guided by the cuticle; use the shape as a guide when shaping the free edge.

If the fingers are long and thin, select a rounded/square shape and keep the nail length short.

If the fingers are short and fat, the nails should be filed into an oval shape and the nail length should be longer to elongate the fingers.

ALWAYS REMEMBER

Emery boards

Cost the emery board into the manicure service as it is a consumable and cannot be used again. The client can keep the emery board for personal use. Instruct the client on how the nails should be filed to avoid nail damage.

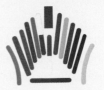

Cutting the nails
Where it is necessary to reduce nail length, it is more efficient to do so by cutting the nail free edge. This is performed using nail scissors or sometimes nail clippers, which have been sterilised before use on each client. Support the nail wall with one hand on the free edge being cut. This minimises client discomfort. Dispose of the trimmed nail plate hygienically in the metal lined waste bin.

Deciding nail shape
The nail shape should complement the client's fingers, nail condition and hand length and size. The shape of the free edge that will most complement a client's nails is one that is similar to the shape of the nail at the base of the nail plate.

Nail shape trends change but both natural and popular **nail shapes** are shown below.

Oval The classic nail shape is oval. This is the shape that offers the most strength to the free edge.

Square A fashionable shape chosen by many clients. The client should be informed, however, that if they have severe corners on the nails they will be more likely to catch and break them.

Pointed This shape is suitable only for longer nails and leaves the nail tip very weak and likely to break. Stiletto nails are an extreme example where the nail is sharply tapered.

TOP TIP

Nail filing

Some nail product suppliers consider the nails best filed after specialised oil application. It is considered less damaging than filing the natural nail when dry.

HEALTH & SAFETY

Personal protective equipment (PPE)

When cutting the nail length you may wish to wear safety glasses, which protect the eyes from flying debris reducing potential injury.

REVISION AID

How do you decide on the shape of the free edge for your client?

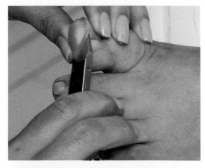
Cutting nails

REVISION AID

What is the name of the bacterial infection that could result from piercing the skin accidentally when performing cuticle work?

Squoval A combination of oval and square nail shape. The nail is filed to a square finish at the free edge and is then gently curved at the corners.

Round The free edge is rounded and is an ideal shape for short nails. This style is popular with male clients.

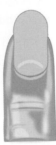 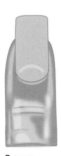 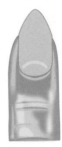 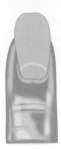 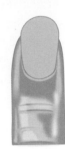

Oval   Square   Pointed   Squoval   Round

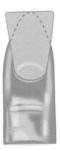 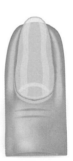 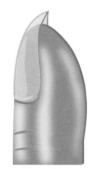

Fan   Tapered nail   Claw nail

Correcting natural nail shapes Sometimes the natural nail shape will require filing into a suitable shape to maintain nail strength, improve the look of the nail and create overall balance.

Fan The nail becomes broader as it grows towards the free edge, appearing as a fan shape. The wider sides of the nail at the free edge should be shaped to achieve an oval shape.

Tapered nail The free edge part of the nail plate is slimmer than that at the cuticle area, which makes it weaker in strength. The free edge should be filed to a squoval shape to maintain strength.

Claw nail Also referred to as hook or convex nail. The nail is excessively curved at the free edge. The nail should be kept short and filed to a round shape. Often this shape can occur as a result of nail injury.

Spoon shape Also referred to as ski jump or concave. The nail plate curves upwards as it grows from the free edge. File into an oval or squoval nail shape.

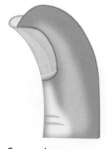

Spoon shape

Buffing

In manicure, **buffing** is used for these reasons:

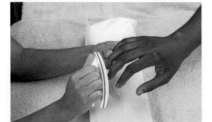

◆ to give the nail plate a sheen

◆ to stimulate the blood supply in the nail bed, increasing nourishment and encouraging strong, healthy nail growth

◆ to smooth any nail plate surface irregularities.

Buffing manicure tools vary. A traditional chamois leather **buffer** may have a handle made of plastic and a replaceable convex pad covered with chamois or soft leather. **Buffing paste** is the cream used to help smooth out surface irregularities, and thereby giving the nail plate a shine. It contains abrasive particles such as pumice, talc or kaolin.

The two-, three- or **four-sided buffer:** this is shaped like a thick emery board and has up to four types of surface, ranging from slightly abrasive to very smooth. It can be used to bring the nail to a shine without the need for buffing paste. It cannot be effectively sterilised, however, and must therefore be discarded after use on one client.

Buffing is carried out after filing to stimulate healthy nail growth and before the nails are soaked in the finger bowl. It could also be used instead of polish at the end of the manicure, or as a nail finish. It is popular when performing a male manicure service as an alternative finish to nail polish, usually followed by a nail conditioning treatment oil application.

If it is being used, **buffing paste** is applied by taking a small amount out of the pot with a clean cuticle stick and applying this to each nail plate. With the fingertip, use downward strokes from the cuticle to the free edge to spread the paste without getting it under the cuticle (which would cause irritation). With the buffer held loosely in the hand, buff in one direction only from the base of the nail to the free edge, using smooth, firm, regular strokes. Use approximately six strokes per nail. Avoid excessive strokes which would cause friction and heat to the nail plate, resulting in drying.

Cuticle work

Cuticle work is carried out to keep the cuticle area attractive and also to prevent cuticles from becoming overgrown and sticking to the nail plate, which could lead to splitting of the cuticle as the nail grows forward, and subsequently to infection of the area.

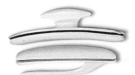

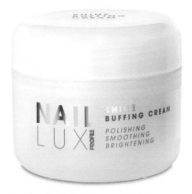
Chamois nail buffer

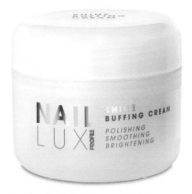
Buffing paste

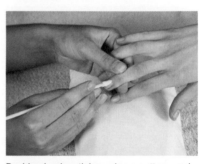
Pushing back cuticles using a cotton wool-tipped cuticle stick

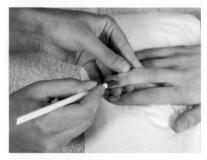
Pushing back cuticles using a hoof stick

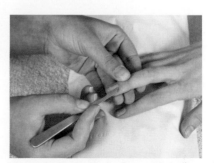
Using a cuticle knife

The work is carried out after soaking the nails in warm soapy water. This step loosens dirt and debris from under the nail free edge and softens the skin in the cuticle area, keeping it pliable and supple.

STEP-BY-STEP: HOW TO PROVIDE CUTICLE WORK

1   Take the fingers from the soapy water and pat them dry with a soft towel, gently pushing back the cuticles. Ensure all cuticle oil/cream is removed.

2   Apply cuticle remover to the cuticle and nail walls, using the applicator or a cotton wool tipped cuticle stick. (Cuticle remover is a slightly caustic solution that helps soften and loosen the cuticles and the eponychium and perionychium from the nail plate.)

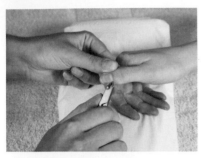

Using cuticle nippers

3 Gently push back the cuticle with a cotton wool-tipped cuticle stick or **hoof stick**. (The cotton wool is to avoid contact with splinters from the wood, and also may be easily replaced if necessary.) Use a gentle, circular motion to push back the cuticle, holding the cuticle tool like a pen.

4 Hold the cuticle knife flat to the nail plate and stroke it in one direction only, gently loosening any eponychium and perionychium that has adhered to the nail plate: do not scratch it backwards and forwards. The **cuticle knife** should have a fine-ground flat blade, which can be re-sharpened when necessary. Dampen the blade with water regularly in the manicure bowl to prevent scratches occurring on the nail plate.

5 Hold the nippers comfortably in the palm of the hand, with the thumb resting just above the blades – this gives firm control over what can be a dangerous tool.

6 With the nippers applied point down, use them to remove any loose or torn, dead pieces of cuticle, and to trim excess dead cuticle. Never pull the tissue as this can lead to skin tearing.

HEALTH & SAFETY

Hygiene

Use a fresh cuticle stick for each stage of the manicure service, and when working on different hands, to prevent contamination of products and cross-infection. The cuticle stick is disposed of after use.

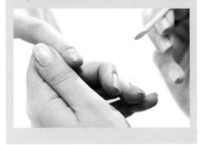

HEALTH & SAFETY

Cuticle care

Do not cut into live cuticle: if you do, it will bleed profusely and will be very uncomfortable for the client. Not every client will require the use of **cuticle nippers** – use them only when needed. Cuticle nippers should have finely ground cutting blades to give a clean cut and to avoid tearing the cuticle. Avoid over-trimming the cuticle, which can lead to overgrown, thickened cuticle.

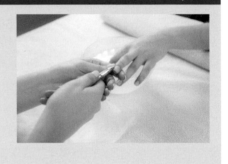

"In my experience, manicurists need to put a lot of emphasis on the importance of cuticle work and preparation of the nail. Sometimes this should take up the main part of the treatment. Good cuticle work is something that clients can rarely do for themselves. It is about thorough removal of the non-living cuticle from the nail plate and NOT about cutting the living skin at the base of the nail (nail fold)."

Marian Newman

Hand and nail treatments

In addition to a manicure service, further hand and nail treatments may be included as appropriate to achieve the treatment plan aims.

Hand, foot and nail treatments include:

Warm-oil treatment

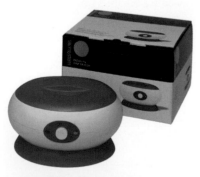

A warm oil /paraffin wax heater

◆ Warm-oil treatment involves gently heating a small amount of organic oil (such as almond, apricot kernel, grape seed or jojoba) and soaking the cuticles in it for

10 minutes. This nourishes the nail plate, softens the cuticles and the surrounding skin, and is an excellent service for clients with dry, cracked cuticles.

◆ Warm oil may also be applied with massage to the skin of the hand and forearm to improve skin texture, colour and blood circulation in the area.

Exfoliating treatment

Exfoliating treatment is carried out as part of the massage routine. The massage is performed as usual, using an **exfoliant** – a mildly abrasive cosmetic product. It may also be applied prior to hand and arm massage to expose new cells and aid the absorption of the massage oil/cream. This treatment offers the following benefits:

◆ the removal of dead skin cells

◆ improvement of the skin texture

◆ improvement of the skin colour

◆ increased blood circulation

◆ increased lymph circulation.

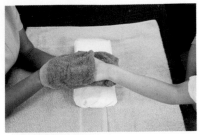

The hands are cleansed before nail and hand treatment

HEALTH & SAFETY

PPE and exfoliation

If performing regular exfoliation treatments, wear PPE to protect the skin on the hands.

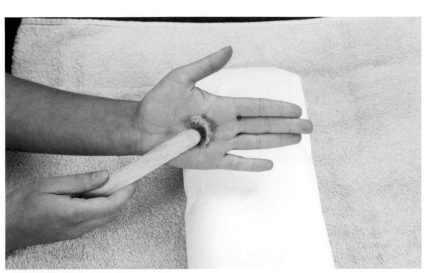

Dispensing exfoliant product for application to the hand and forearm

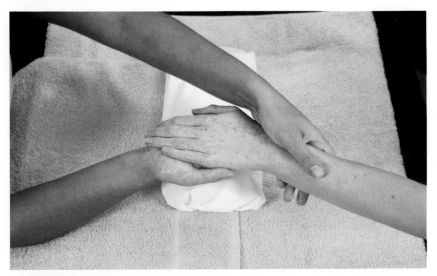

Exfoliant product massaged over the skins, surface, which removes dead skin cells and improves superficial blood and lymphatic circulation

ECO TIP

Microbead exfoliants

Microbeads are solid plastic particles less than five millimetres in diameter. These have been a popular addition to exfoliation products due to their spherical shape, which effectively contours the skin's surface. However, microbeads have been found to enter the water system, endangering marine life, and when ingested they can then enter the food chain. Manufacturers are sourcing ethically preferable alternatives.

The abrasive particles must be thoroughly removed with warm, damp towels before continuing with the rest of the manicure.

Hand treatment mask

An appropriate treatment **mask** may be applied, according to the client's service requirements. This may be either stimulating and rejuvenating, or moisturising. The hands may be placed inside warm thermal mittens or hand gloves for 10 minutes to aid absorption, enabling the mask to penetrate the skin's epidermis. Alternatively a protective film can be placed over the mask. The mask is then removed, and followed with massage medium. Some products may also be used as the massage medium, so are massaged into the skin before removal.

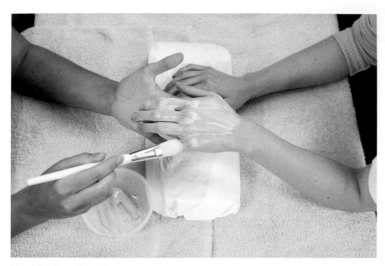

Hand treatment mask

Paraffin wax treatment

The paraffin wax is heated in a special bath to a temperature of 50–55°C. It is then applied to the hands and usually over the wrists too with a brush. It is then covered with a plastic protective covering and left to set for 10–15 minutes before removal. Several layers are applied. This offers the following benefits:

◆ the heating effect stimulates the blood circulation

◆ eases discomfort of arthritic and rheumatic conditions

◆ softens the skin; improving the appearance and condition of the nails and dry skin

◆ soothes sensory nerve endings.

After use the wax is disposed of.

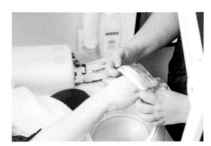

Paraffin wax has been applied with a brush and is being wrapped with a plastic protective covering.

Paraffin wax resources

ACTIVITY

Researching hand and nail treatments

Research other types of hand and nail treatments. Write down the details of your research, including resources, application techniques, benefits and costs.

Thermal mitts

These are electrically heated gloves in which the hands are placed for approximately 10–15 minutes.

They are usually used following the application of a treatment within the manicure routine, e.g. a hand treatment mask. The hands are prepared by wrapping them in a plastic protective covering before placement in the mitts.

The treatment has the following benefits:

◆ decreases joint stiffness in the case of a client suffering from arthritis

◆ improves the condition of dry skin of the cuticles and hands by increasing the absorption of moisturising products

◆ improves skin colour and blood and lymph circulation.

Always follow manufacturer's guidelines in the application procedure for hand and nail treatment services.

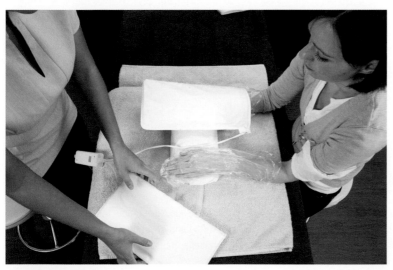

Thermal mitts

REVISION AID

What is the purpose of a nail treatment?

HEALTH & SAFETY

Check the temperature of the paraffin wax and thermal mitts before application.

STEP-BY-STEP: SPECIALIST HAND AND ARM TREATMENT

Specialist hand and nail treatments should be offered to your client when there is a specific service need or if they feel they would like to benefit from such a service. These treatments can be offered independently.

Specialist training in these advanced techniques is usually offered by major product companies.

The following hand and arm treatment service will:

◆ stimulate the blood circulation

◆ have a skin cleansing action

◆ remove dead skin cells (desquamation)

◆ improve the moisture content of the skin

◆ improve joint mobility.

Your services should be adapted the meet the service objectives for the client.

Allow 30 minutes for this specialist hand and arm treatment service.

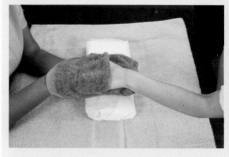

1 The hands and arms are cleansed using warm water with towelling mitts infused with lime oil for its therapeutic, refreshing and energising properties.

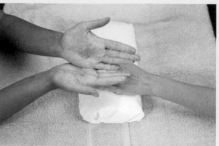

2 The hands are exfoliated to remove all dead skin cells and brighten the skin. A salt-based preparation with emollient, skin-softening ingredients is applied to the skin of each hand and is massaged gently over the skin's surface.

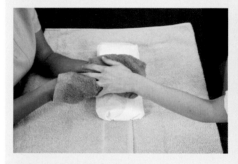

3 Towelling mitts are used to remove the exfoliating product. These have been steamed in a warm towel heater and are warm when used.

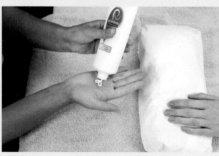

4 A skin-nourishing lotion is applied to each hand and arm. The lotion is particularly beneficial for dry, sensitive skin.

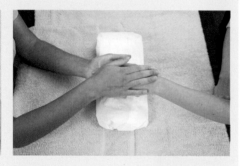

5 Massage movements are applied to the hand and lower arm using effleurage and petrissage massage manipulations.

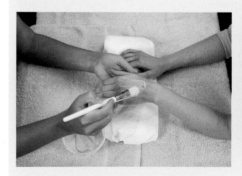

6 A further skin treatment hand mask is applied. The hands are then placed in plastic bags to aid the absorption of the product.

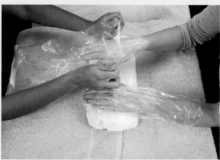

7 The hands are then placed in electrically heated thermal mitts for 10–15 minutes. Remove thermal mitts and plastic bags and remove the product. Continue with a nail finish, if required, after thorough preparation of the nail plate.

Hand and lower arm massage

A **hand massage** sequence is generally carried out near the end of the manicure service, prior to nail finish. It can also be carried out on its own if the client wants the effects of the massage but does not need or request a further nail service.

The massage incorporates classic massage techniques, each with different effects:

◆ Effleurage – gentle stroking movements, which introduce the therapist's hands to the area and are used to start, link massage movements and conclude the massage routine.

◆ Petrissage – kneading, picking up, movements that increase blood circulation locally to the skin and underlying structures.

◆ Tapotement – a light hacking or tapping movement may be used to stimulate the circulation locally. Application technique must be modified in relation to the area treated and the density of the underlying skin and structure to avoid discomfort and a contra-action, e.g. bruising.

◆ Passive movements – gentle manipulation of the joints, which stretch and mobilise the joints, helping to keep them supple whilst maintaining the elasticity of the muscles and removing tension, which could lead to adhesions in the muscles.

◆ Frictions – localised kneading, which stimulates the skin and reduces muscular adhesions and tension in the muscles.

You can adapt the massage application according to the needs of the client. Either the **speed of application** or **depth of pressure** and choice of **massage technique** can be altered.

The reasons for offering a hand and lower arm massage during a manicure are as follows:

◆ to moisturise the skin with massage medium, improving skin hydration

◆ to increase blood circulation, transporting oxygen and nutrients to the lower arm and hand

◆ to increase lymph circulation, transporting waste products in the lymph from the lower arm and hand

◆ to help maintain joint mobility

◆ to ease discomfort from arthritis or rheumatism

◆ to relax the client

◆ to help remove any dead skin cells (desquamation), exposing new cells.

REVISION AID

How long would you allow for a manicure service including hand massage and polish finish?

For detailed information on the different types of massage movement and their benefits refer to **CHAPTER 4**.

REVISION AID

What difference should you consider when performing a hand and arm massage on a male and female client?

TOP TIP

Positive promotion-link selling

Hand massage can be included during a facial while the mask is applied, maximising service benefits and client relaxation. It also gives you the opportunity to promote another product or service to the client.

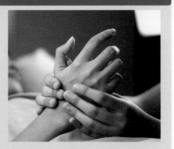

HEALTH & SAFETY

Joint mobility

If the client has any joint mobility restrictions, e.g. arthritis, you will need to modify your massage technique avoiding joint manipulations.

STEP-BY-STEP: HAND AND LOWER ARM MASSAGE

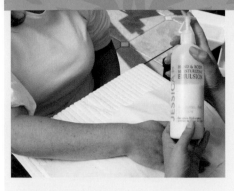

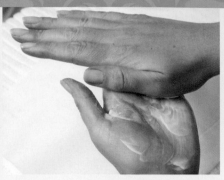

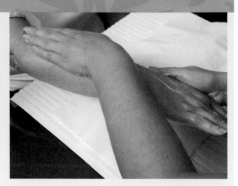

1 Select an appropriate massage medium for the service and for the client's skin. Dispense the massage medium into the hands.

2 Warm the product over the palms and apply to the client's skin using effleurage technique.

3 **Effleurage to the whole hand and forearm** Use long sweeping strokes (using alternate hands) from the hand to the elbow, stroking over the outer and the inner sides of each forearm.

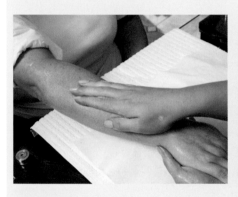

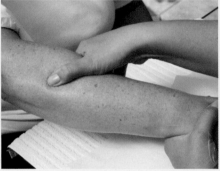

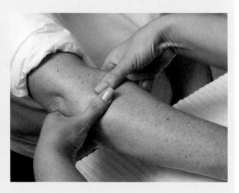

3 **Continued**

4 Using a **petrissage movement** pick up the flexor and extensor muscles of the lower arm.

5 Move from the hand towards the elbow applying frictions over the interosseous membrane located between the radius and ulna bone, then slide the thumbs back down to the hands.

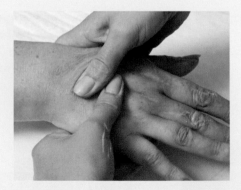

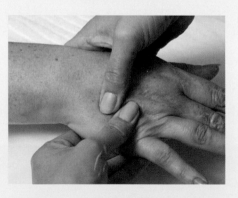

6 **Thumb kneading to the back of the hand and the forearm** Use the thumbs, one in front of the other, and rotate each thumb one in a clockwise direction, the other anti-clockwise, in a gently kneading action between each metacarpal bone.

Repeat step 6 a further two times.

7 **Perform a scissoring, friction movement** using both thumbs between each metacarpal bone in the hands.

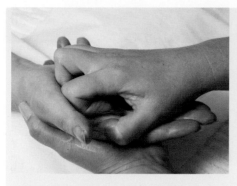
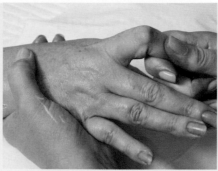
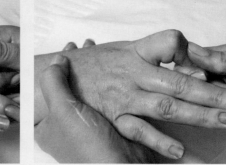

8 Perform a 'knuckling' petrissage movement rotating the fingers in a small fist shape against the muscles in the palms of the hand.

9 Perform passive joint manipulations on the fingers, moving the phalangeal bones of each finger individually.

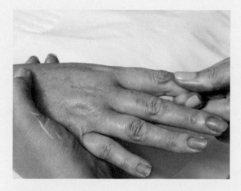
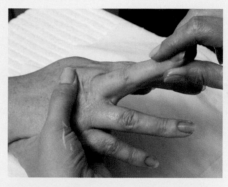

9 Continued. Bend the finger at each joint and then straighten in a resistance movement.

10 Finger circulations, supporting the joints Supporting the knuckles with one hand, hold the fingers individually and gently take each through its full range of movements, first clockwise and then anticlockwise. Move from the little finger to the thumb.

Repeat step 10 a further two times.

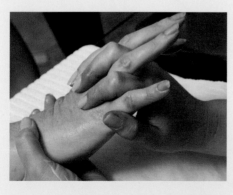
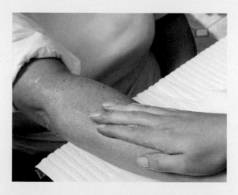

11 Passive wrist circulations, supporting the joints Support the wrist with one hand and put your fingers between the client's fingers, gently grasping their hand. Move the wrist through its full range of movement, first clockwise and then anticlockwise.

Repeat step 11 a further two times.

12 Effleurage to the whole hand and forearm Use the same movement as in step 3.

Repeat step 12 a further five times.

TOP TIP

Special occasions

Many clients will have the nail polish applied for a special occasion, such as a holiday or wedding and it is important to practice to ensure you are consistent in your quality of application as it needs to be right first time.

Pop-up salons at airports are now an option for the client to have a pre-holiday nail service – remember, the client has a plane to catch!

Nail polish application

Nail polish is used to coat the nail plate for a number of reasons:

◆ to decorate the nail plate

◆ to disguise stained nails

◆ to add temporary strength to weak nails

◆ to improve the condition or appearance of the natural nail

◆ to co-ordinate with clothes or make-up

◆ to create designs and effects, called 'nail art'.

As the nail finish is what the client will be looking at following the service it is important that a high-quality finish is achieved that has durability.

Before nail polish is applied, the client's hand jewellery may be replaced, to avoid smudging afterwards.

Styles of polish application

◆ *Traditional application* This style is the one most commonly requested by clients: the entire nail plate is covered with polish in block colour.

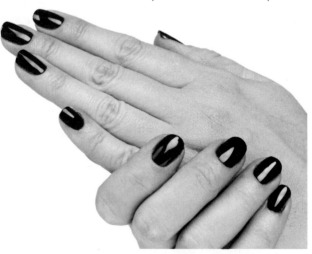

◆ *French polish application* This style involves painting the nail plate of the nail bed pink or pale beige, and the free edge white. This can be adapted

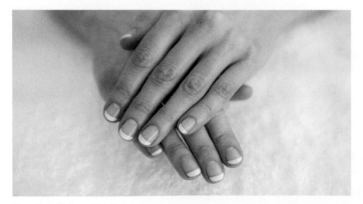

French polish application

by painting a narrow block of colour along the free edge, which is more complementary for a shorter nail. This technique can also provide product strength to a weaker nail.

◆ *Free lunula application* This style involves applying polish over the whole nail plate except the area of the lunula.

◆ *Painted lunula application* This style involves painting the lunula a contrasting colour.

◆ *Painted free edge application* This style involves painting the free edge a contrasting colour.

TOP TIP
Choosing colours
For short nails, select a pale, neutral colour. Darker, more dramatic colours suit healthy, long nails, especially on clients with darker skin tones. Remember, it is always the client's choice, but you will often be asked to recommend.

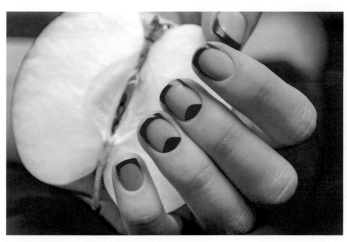
Painted free edge and Lunula application

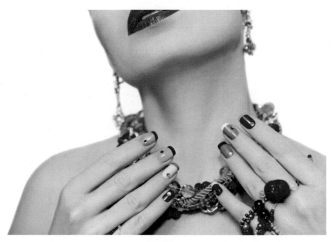
Nail art, contrasting free edge colour with rhinestone adornments

◆ *Application to give the appearance of longer nails* This style creates an optical illusion that the nails are longer than they really are. The whole nail plate is painted, leaving a slightly larger gap than usual (usually 1.5 mm) along the nail walls.

Tips for nail painting

◆ Ensure the surface of the nail plate is grease-free. If grease is present this will result in nail polish peeling or chipping.

◆ Select colours that suit the client's nail length, condition and skin colour.

◆ Dark colours will draw attention to the nails, and will make small/short nails appear smaller/shorter.

◆ If the nails are very broad leave a margin at the sides of the nail's wall free of polish, this will help them to appear slimmer.

◆ Avoid pearlised polish if the client's nail surface is uneven or ridged. The polish will emphasise the imperfection.

◆ Always apply a good quality base coat suited to the client's nail condition. This helps to prevent staining from pigment in the polish, and may strengthen the nail or smooth ridges depending on its formulation.

◆ When applying nail polish colour, apply two coats, allowing the nails to dry between each coat to prevent the appearance of brush marks.

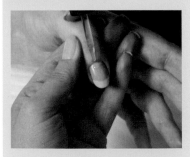

"Painting the nail is a skill in its own right. It takes practice! Polishes differ and colours within the same range can differ. Even the temperature will make a difference. The longevity of polish will depend on the condition of the nail, e.g. a peeling nail will not hold polish as well as a smooth nail."

Marian Newman

◆ Ensure your polish is a good quality. If it has become thickened use a specialised solvent to restore to the correct consistency. This should be done 20 minutes prior to use to ensure an even consistency.

◆ Ensure good colour coverage.

◆ Allow nail polish to dry before **top coat** application.

◆ Always follow manufacturer's recommendations for their nail polish application.

ALWAYS REMEMBER

Essential nail polish qualities

Nail polish should:

◆ if coloured polish, achieve the required colour shade in one to two coats
◆ adhere to the nail plate and be flexible to resist peeling and chipping
◆ have good durability on exposure to water, detergents and other chemicals it may come into contact with
◆ not stain the nail plate
◆ flow freely onto the nail plate and be easy to apply.

Reasons for peeling and chipping nail polish Chipping may be explained by any of the following:

◆ The nail polish was not thick enough because of over-thinning with solvent.

◆ No base coat was used.

◆ Grease was left on the nail plate prior to painting.

◆ The natural nail plate is flaking. Nail health can affect the durability of the polish.

◆ The polish was dried too quickly by artificial means.

◆ Non-compliance with manufacturer application instructions.

Peeling polish may have the following explanations:

◆ No top coat was used.

◆ Polish application at each coat was too thick. Thin coats of colour should be applied.

◆ Successive coats were not allowed to dry between applications.

◆ The nail polish was too thick, due to evaporation of the solvent.

◆ Grease was left on the nail plate prior to painting.

◆ Non-compliance with manufacturer application instructions.

Nail polish storage Nail polish should be stored in a cool, dark place, to avoid separation and fading. The caps and the rims of bottles **must** be kept clean, not only for appearance but also to ensure that the bottle is airtight to avoid exposure to chemical vapours. Always use stock rotation to ensure that the oldest product is used first, remember FILO – first in, last out.

Types of polish The following types of polish may be used:

◆ *Cream* This has a matt finish, and requires a top coat application to give a sheen.

◆ *Pearlised* This is also known as crystalline. It has a frosted, shimmery appearance due to the addition of natural fish scales or synthetic ingredients such as bismuth oxychloride.

◆ *Base coat* This protects the nail from staining from a strong-coloured nail polish; it also gives a good grip to polish, and smooths out minor surface irregularities. Many base coats are formulated using ingredients to treat different nail problems such as weak, brittle, peeling or ridged nails.

◆ *Top coat* This gives a sheen to cream polish, and adds longer wear as it helps to prevent chipping.

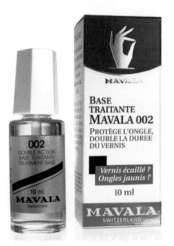

Base coat

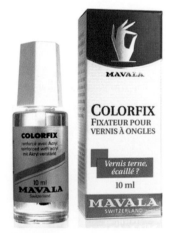

Top coat

REVISION AID

What are the different nail finishes that a client may choose to have?

ALWAYS REMEMBER

Nail polish Flooding

Take care to avoid touching the cuticle or the nail wall. If nail polish flooding occurs, remove the polish immediately with a disposable pointed cuticle stick and polish remover.

TOP TIP

Cleaning the nail plate before polish application

Use a lint-free pad as cotton wool may leave fibres, which may spoil the application of nail polish.

Contra-indications to nail polish Do not apply polish in these circumstances:

◆ if there are diseases and disorders of the nail plate and surrounding skin

◆ if the client is allergic to nail polish.

In addition, pearlised nail polish should not be applied to excessively ridged nails as it may appear to exaggerate the problem. Short or bitten nails are more suited to pale polishes, to avoid attracting attention.

HEALTH & SAFETY

Nail painting environment

Ensure the area is well ventilated to avoid inhalation of excessive fumes. Lighting should be good to enable you to avoid eyestrain. It is a good idea to use a table lamp when painting the nails.

STEP-BY-STEP: DARK POLISH APPLICATION

Confirm the client's choice of nail colour. A cream formulation is being demonstrated.

Ensure the free edge is smooth, the cuticles are neat and smooth and the nail plate is free from grease.

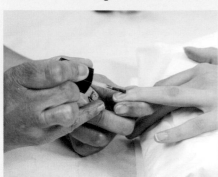

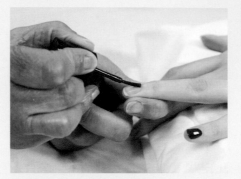

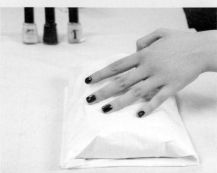

1 Starting with the thumb, apply three brush strokes down the length of each nail from the cuticle to the free edge, beginning in the centre, then down either side close to the nail wall. Apply one coat of base coat to each nail on one hand, followed by the other hand.

2 Starting with the thumb apply the coloured polish; apply one coat of polish to each nail of each hand followed by a second coat. Avoid applying the polish too thickly at each application. This is then, followed by one coat of top coat to each nail.

3 The completed dark polish application. Confirm with the client that the finished result is to their satisfaction. Complete details on the client's service record.

"Few clients can paint their own nails beautifully. The polished nails are what your client will take away with them and see every day. They will forget the relaxing hand massage but will remember how beautiful their nails looked and how much longer the polish lasted compared to when they do it."

Marian Newman

Manicure for a male client

A man's hands differ slightly from a woman's, usually with thicker skin, larger in size, and there may be coarse terminal hair on the fingers. Males tend to wear their nails shorter too. The hands may be drier and with areas of rough skin which often relate to hand care and occupation. The manicure service sequence does not differ greatly, the main difference usually being the selected finish. Confirm requirements at the consultation. Consider the following in your service plan:

◆ File the nails to a shorter length.

◆ Complete cuticle work as required to achieve a healthy, groomed appearance.

◆ Usually coloured nail polish is omitted. A nail treatment base coat may be included if advised or requested.

◆ Shape the nails square rather than oval.

◆ Buff the nails with paste, if a shine is required.

TOP TIP

Engaging male clients with manicure service

It may be preferable to use treatment description which explain to the client clearly what is involved with the service such as *hand care and condition*.

◆ include an exfoliant treatment product to target and smooth any rough areas of skin.

◆ Use massage mediums that are fragranced or non-fragranced according to the client's preference. Stimulating fragrances such as mint and menthol are popular.

◆ Use an oil or oil based cream for massage, to provide slip and avoid dragging body hair.

◆ Use firmer pressure during hand and arm massage as the skin is thicker and the arms often more muscular.

◆ Pressure points are a popular addition to include to induce relaxation. Pressure is applied at specific points on the skin to release muscular tension. Training is required before this technique can be incorporated into your massage routine.

◆ A treatment oil may be applied at the end of the service to condition the nail.

ACTIVITY

Comparing hands

Write down as many differences as you can between the appearance of male and female client nails, hands and lower arms.

From your observations, can you think of any further adaptations or recommendations that may be necessary when manicuring a man's hands?

STEP-BY-STEP: MALE MANICURE

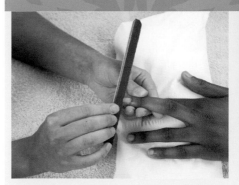

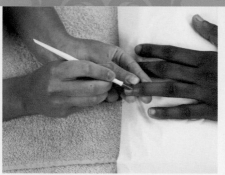

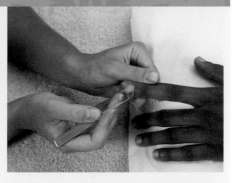

1 File the nails to a shorter length and bevel the free edge. The nails are usually filed to a square shape rather than oval.

2 Improve the appearance of the cuticles. Following the previous manicure procedure for preparation and application of cuticle nail products, push back the cuticles gently. Cuticle conditioner products may be recommended for home use and maintenance.

3 A cuticle knife is used to remove the excess eponychium from the cuticle area. Remember to keep the blade dampened and hold flat to the nail plate to avoid scratches to the nail plate.

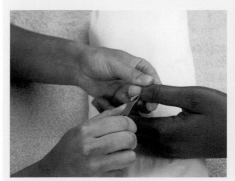

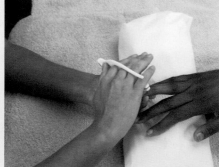

4 Remove excess cuticle using cuticle nippers.

5 Buff the nails to improve blood circulation to the nail bed, giving a healthy appearance to the nail. Buff the nails with a buffing paste if a shine is required. This may be included at this stage or at the end of the manicure as a nail plate finish. Apply a massage lotion to the hands if required.

Specialist hand and arm treatments may be included if required such as exfoliation service and paraffin wax treatment. A hand massage is shown in the next step-by-step, but you may wish to include massage to the lower arm also. This example may be suitable for an express hand massage service.

After massage, the nail plate is cleaned with acetone if buffing is required as a finish, or a specialist nail polish finish is applied.

STEP-BY-STEP: MALE HAND AND ARM MASSAGE

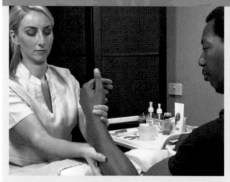

1 Select a massage medium compatible with the client's preference. Effleurage to the hand and forearm. This movement starts and concludes the hand and arm massage. Use long, sweeping strokes from the hand to the elbow, moving on both the outer and inner sides of the forearm.

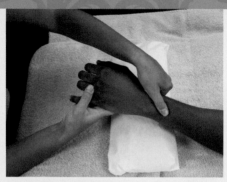

2 Petrissage to the lower arm, picking up the flexor and extensor muscles. Firmer pressure may be applied as the skin is thicker.

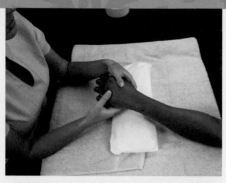

3 Perform frictions over the back of the hand working between each metacarpal bone.

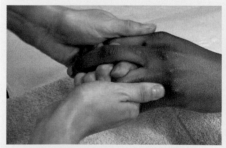

4 Perform small friction movements down the length of each finger (phalange).

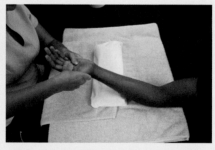

5 Thumbs kneading movement to the palm of the hand. Perform deep localised stroking to the palm of the hands using the thumbs. Repeat step 1 effleurage to conclude the massage. Remove excess massage medium following massage if preferred.

REVISION AID

How can you ensure the client gets the best possible result from their nail finish?

Advice and recommendations

It is important when carrying out a nail service that the client knows how to care for their nails and hands at home. It is your duty as a beauty therapist to ensure that the correct aftercare advice and recommendations are provided. If it isn't, the client may undo all the good work you have done during the service.

"A manicure is not just about sending a client away with lovely polished nails. It is also about improving the condition and appearance of the nails and surrounding skin. This usually takes some daily help. If you explain to your client what they need to do in an informative and interesting way you will automatically be retailing useful products without any hard sell techniques. They will also be impressed with your expert knowledge and care of them as your valued client."

Marian Newman

When giving aftercare advice you have a good opportunity to recommend additional nail treatments and retail products, such as polish personalised to their nail-treatment requirements, emery boards, cuticle-care products or hand cream, thereby enhancing retail sales and the business profit.

Aftercare advice will differ for each client, personalised according to their individual requirements, but there is some generic advice as follows:

◆ Wear protective gloves when washing up to avoid contact with water and detergents, which will dry the nails and skin.

◆ Wear protective gloves when gardening or carrying out domestic chores to avoid accidental damage and dirt entering the nail plate and hands.

◆ Just as when caring for the skin of the face, recommend a cuticle product and hand cream/lotion are applied daily. This is important when a client is improving their nails following general neglect, ill health or when breaking the habit of nail biting or picking skin around the nails.

◆ Mini retail versions of products are a good idea for clients to try. For example, trying a nail polish when matching to a dress. They are also ideal for travel.

◆ Always wear gloves in cold weather as this will help maintain healthy blood circulation in the area.

◆ Dry the hands thoroughly after washing, and apply hand cream. Some hand creams contain UV filters, which reduce hyperpigmentation (seen as darker areas of skin) to the backs of the hands occurring.

◆ Avoid harsh soaps when washing hands.

◆ Advise the client on how to file their nails, and the correct type of nail file to use. They should never use metal files.

◆ Do not use the fingernails as tools (for instance, to prise lids off tins).

◆ Advise on appropriate nail/skincare products to remedy the problems present, e.g. dry skin, weak nails.

◆ Advise the client that a healthy diet is related to the health and appearance of the nails and skin.

◆ Advise the client on what other professional services/treatments you could recommend.

◆ Advise the client on a service plan to improve the nail/skin condition; discuss time and costs and the time intervals recommended between each service. If working towards a special occasion such as a wedding, identify the date and schedule the appointments in advance with the bride.

ALWAYS REMEMBER

Provide advice and tips for your clients electronically

Use electronic and social media to communicate with your client.

◆ Inform them of new products you are excited about.

◆ Share nail finish looks that are eye-catching.

◆ Tips on how to care and maintain their nails.

◆ Advice on any promotions sent at times when they are most likely to be read.

◆ Use hashtag to pick up keywords.

◆ Consider and target all current and potential clients.

TOP TIP

Products for purchase

Present retail products for the client in the service area. This will mean that you will maximise sales, as the client will have already committed to purchase before they go to the payment point.

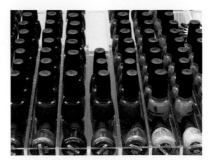

A range of nail polishes for retail

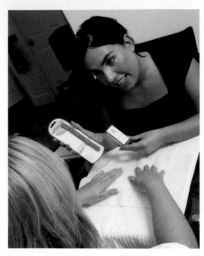

Recommending aftercare retail products to meet the client's needs

It is also necessary to tell the client what to do in the event of a contra-action.

It is a good idea to have available the nail polish colours that you have used. The client can then touch up any accidental chips themselves.

Recommend the use of top coat applied every three to four days to protect the nail polish, increase its durability and impart shine.

Finally, at the end of the nail service ensure the client's records are updated, accurate and signed by the client. Ensure that the finished result is to the client's satisfaction and meets the agreed service plan.

ACTIVITY

Designing an aftercare leaflet

Devise an aftercare leaflet for clients. It is good practice to provide the client with an aftercare leaflet outlining all recommendations following service, or make this available electronically.

Exercises for the hands

Hand exercises play an important role in the homecare advice given to clients, for the following reasons:

◆ They keep the joints supple, allowing greater mobility.

◆ Circulation is increased, encouraging healthy nail and skin growth.

◆ Good circulation helps to prevent cold hands.

◆ Exercises keep the client interested in their hands, and so more likely to keep regular salon appointments.

TOP TIP

Hand exercises

Remember recommended, hand exercises should be performed by the manicurist also to keep the hands supple, reducing the possibility of the effects of RSI in the hands.

Pedicure

The word **pedicure** is derived from the Latin word *pedis*, meaning 'foot' and *cura*, meaning 'care'. The service is very similar to manicure except that it is carried out on the feet instead of the hands. A pedicure cares for the feet and nails to achieve the following effects:

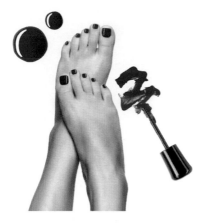

◆ to improve and maintain the appearance of the foot and nails

◆ to keep the skin and cuticles soft and supple

◆ to reduce the amount of hard skin present and prevent it building in localised areas

◆ to relax tired, aching feet

◆ to keep the nails smooth and healthy.

A pedicure therefore aims to improve and maintain your client's feet, nails and surrounding skin. The pedicure procedure includes filing the nails to shape, using specialised nail or cuticle products, tools and equipment and foot treatments, massaging the lower leg and foot and providing a complementary nail finish to suit the client and their service requirements.

Health and safety is an important feature of every service and delivery of the pedicure service must ensure cross-contamination and harmful chemical exposure are avoided.

Dealing with your clients in a polite, efficient manner, using good communication and questioning skills to find out exactly what they require from the pedicure service forms an important part of this technical service.

INDUSTRY ROLE MODEL

MARGARET DABBS Founder and Chief Executive of Margaret Dabbs (Footcare) London

What do you find rewarding about your job? It might sound like a cliché, but one of the most genuinely rewarding aspects of my job has to be seeing customers leave happy afterwards. It's always lovely to get positive feedback, and there's nothing better than having customers leave the salon feeling relaxed and pampered. It's also great establishing strong relationships with clients who then come back to the salon again and again.

What do you find challenging about your job? As a foot expert who sees so many clients, it's often a challenge to convince people that we can absolutely transform the way they look and feel – in just one appointment. However after one appointment, our clients are always converted, and never allow their feet to deteriorate to such an extent again.

What makes a good beauty therapist? A good beauty therapist is one who strikes up an instant rapport with their clients and puts them at ease so that they can truly relax and enjoy the spa environment. Another important skill to have is to be able to listen and

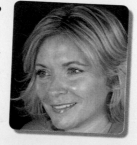

fully understand a client's needs and concerns. Beauty is such a fast paced industry, with new products and treatments constantly appearing on the market, you'll also need to keep on top of these developments. This will allow you to give your clients the best possible advice about what will work best for them.

The necessary anatomy and physiology knowledge for this unit is listed on the checklist in **CHAPTER 2**. There are also questions at the end of the chapter to check your knowledge and understanding.

ALWAYS REMEMBER

Transferable knowledge, understanding and skills

When providing foot and nail services it is important to use the skills you have learnt in the following chapters:

◆ The Business of Beauty Therapy (Chapter 1)

◆ The Science of Beauty Therapy (Chapter 2)

◆ Consultation Practice and Techniques (Chapter 3)

ALWAYS REMEMBER

Foot and nail treatments

Foot and nail services include different products and specialised treatments applied to improve and maintain the overall appearance and health of the nails and skin.

ALWAYS REMEMBER

Foot and nail service products

Foot and nail service products, that may be used within a pedicure include:

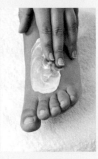

cuticle cream/oil; cuticle remover; foot cream/lotion; nail polish (**base coat**, **top coat** and different nail finishes, which may be coloured); range of specialist nail treatment products **nail polish drier**; nail polish remover.

Increasingly popular as a finish is gel polish as it is more durable.

ALWAYS REMEMBER

Anatomy and physiology

When performing foot nail services you are required to apply your knowledge of the structure and function of the skin including its appendages:

◆ identifying skin conditions

◆ the structure of the nail, thickness and nail shapes

◆ identifying nail conditions

◆ nail growth and factors affecting it

◆ the bones of the foot and lower leg

◆ the muscles of the foot and lower leg

◆ the blood circulation to the foot and lower leg.

Products, tools and equipment

Before beginning the pedicure, check that you have the necessary products, tools and equipment to hand and that they meet the legal hygiene and industry requirements for pedicure service.

The basic equipment required is the same as for manicure – refer to the manicure section earlier in this chapter for the full list of resources.

In addition, each pedicure work area should have the following equipment listed below. Further supplementary products, tools and equipment relevant to pedicure service are discussed below.

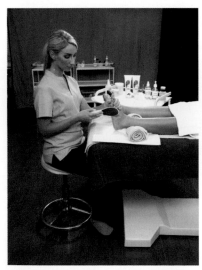

Pedicure service improves skin condition of the feet

Pedicure spa chair

Pedicure spa chairs provide comfort and luxury for the client. Some chairs can be independently plumbed, and electronically positioned and adjusted. The client immerses their feet in a tray, which may be equipped with hydrotherapy jets to massage the feet, while the chair may also feature a vibrating massage system.

Doing your research is important as this equipment can offer a variety of additional features:

◆ water temperature control
◆ hand sprayer, ideal for removing spa treatment products
◆ music system
◆ manicure tray facility in the arm rests.

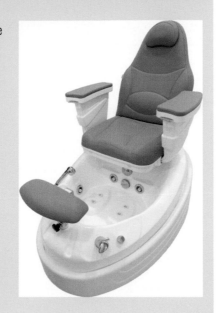

Products, tools and equipment

◆ **Scissors and toenail clippers** To shorten nail length.

◆ **Foot rasp or callus file** To remove areas of dead, dry skin from the plantar surface (sole) of the foot. For hygiene the foot rasp is available with water-resistant paper pads providing different grades of abrasive grit that adhere to the file. These are disposed of after each service.

◆ **Foot massage lotion or oil** To massage the skin of the foot and lower leg.

◆ **Disposable toe separators** Used to keep the toes separated during nail polish application. Alternatively, disposable items such as biodegradable cotton toe ropes, cotton wool or tissues may be used for this purpose.

◆ **Disposable footwear (optional)** Enabling the client to move immediately following polish application without smudging the nail polish.

◆ **Foot and nail treatment equipment** Including: paraffin wax heater, thermal boots, applicator brushes for masks and paraffin wax and brushes suitable for dry brushing exfoliation.

◆ **Foot and nail treatment products** Including: paraffin wax, exfoliator, foot mask.

◆ **Pedicure bowl or foot spa** To soak, soften and cleanse the foot. The foot spa also revitalises and refreshes the skin by stimulating the sensory nerve endings, and improving blood and lymph circulation.

◆ **Liquid soap or cleansing tablets** Specialised foot cleaning products added to the spa bath to cleanse, soften and deodorise the feet.

◆ **Towel steamer** To prepare towels to cleanse and remove product from the skin.

Products used in pedicure services
For full details of products used for both manicures and pedicures, their ingredients and uses, see the table earlier in the chapter. In addition to these, an exfoliating pedicure scrub and foot mask may also be used for the feet (see below).

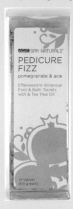

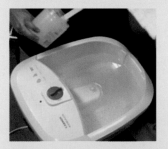

Adding revitalising spa agent to the foot spa water

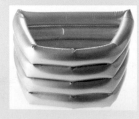

Product	Ingredients	Use
Exfoliating pedicure scrub	Abrasive ingredients such as pumice, sea salt, detergent, water and water-soluble ingredients, added moisturisers, refreshing agents, e.g. peppermint oil.	To remove dead skin cells, cleanse the skin, condition, soften and refresh the skin, improving blood and lymphatic circulation in the area.
Foot mask	Absorbent ingredients, such as clay, e.g. kaolin, and bentonite gel to cleanse and soften the skin. Mildly abrasive ingredients, such as pumice, may also be added. Antioxidant vitamins to brighten the skin and counteract the damaging action of free radicals and added moisturisers to hydrate the skin. Glycerine to transport the active ingredients on to the skin. Marine ingredients such as mineral rich sea kelp may be included and essential oils such as peppermint to cool and refresh or teatree for its anti-bacterial properties.	To cleanse, soften, hydrate and refresh the skin.

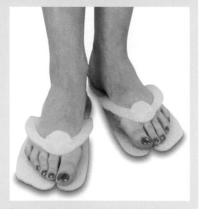

Disposable footwear

Safety and hygiene

Safety and hygiene must be maintained in a number of ways:

◆ Ensure that tools and equipment are clean, disinfected and, where required according to legal requirements, sterile before use.

◆ Sterilised or disinfected tools and equipment should be stored in a chemical disinfectant, UV cabinet or closed container until ready for use. Remember, they will remain clean but will not be sterile after 24 hours.

◆ Ensure sufficient breaks are timetabled to breathe fresh air if carrying out concurrent nail services.

◆ Dispense products from containers, e.g. creams and lotions, with a disinfected or disposable spatula.

◆ Dispose of waste as advised by the manufacturer and your workplace policy. Disposal containers used during service delivery should have tightly fitting lids, to avoid volatile vapours unnecessarily entering the air in the work environment.

◆ Disinfect all work surfaces after every client.

◆ Hygiene issues have been addressed by the design of many items of equipment with disposable accessories that can be replaced for each client.

◆ Use disposable tools, products and equipment wherever possible. When using disposable items ensure, wherever possible, that these are produced ethically from sustainable sources.

◆ Care must be taken when using products that could spill, such as oils and paraffin wax, and could result in an accidental fall. Work tidily and throughly clean the area after each service. The floor covering in the treatment area should be suitable for effective cleaning and hygiene.

Pedicure tools and equipment can be disposable or can be sterilised and disinfected by the methods shown earlier in this chapter.

Preparation of the service area for pedicure

Ensure that all pedicure products, tools and **equipment** are clean, sterilised and disinfected, as appropriate, and that all necessary resources are neatly organised on the nail workstation, which should be suitably positioned.

> "It is down to you to make the environment professional. Ensure the service area is kept spotless at all times. Have pride in what you are doing and how you are doing it."
>
> *Margaret Dabbs*

All metal tools should be sterilised in the autoclave prior to use. Non-metal instruments should be disinfected by immersing them in a suitable disinfecting fluid. Prepare equipment neatly on the nail workstation so that everything you need is to hand and the client need not be disturbed during service. Ensure adequate time is allowed to heat paraffin wax or oil used in specialised treatments.

The work area should remain in a condition suitable for further nail services during the working day.

Exactly how you arrange the work area will depend upon how your work area is equipped to deliver the service.

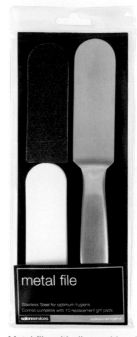

Metal file with disposable adhesive abrasive grit surface used for the removal of excess dead skin

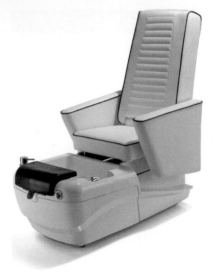

Pedicure chair

TOP TIP

Benefits of pedicure service

The beneficial effects of pedicure should be explained to a client at consultation and how regular treatments will help maintain healthy nails and skin.

REVISION AID

Why is it good practice to maintain the appearance of your nail workstation and keep it orderly?

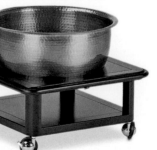

Non-fixed pedicure bowl, castors must be locked in position when stationary.

REVISION AID

How many bones are there in the foot? Can you name them?

If using a non-fixed pedicure bowl, place a towel on the floor between you and the client. A foot bowl or foot spa containing warm, soapy water should be placed on this towel. A non-fixed pedicure bowl is shown and also a fixed pedicure chair.

Towels should be placed on your lap: one is for protection, the other is for drying the client's feet. Keep the other towels close by for wrapping the client's feet during the pedicure sequence. If the pedicure is performed on a beauty couch or in a pedicure chair towels are only required for drying and wrapping up the feet.

When cutting the client's nails and removing hard skin, disposable tissue should be placed to collect nail and skin debris, then removed before continuing service.

Personal protective equipment, e.g. safety glasses and single use disposable non-latex (synthetic) powder-free gloves may be worn for protection from skin and nail debris at this stage. It is recommended that gloves are worn when checking for contra-indications to prevent cross contamination.

TOP TIP

Nail service hygiene guidance

Refer to the Habia Code of Practice for Nail Services for health and safety best practice guidance.

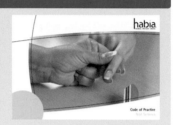

"Take an interest in your client list and always look at ways to maximise the treatment experience."

Margaret Dabbs

When the client is comfortably seated, clean your hands using an approved hand cleaning technique, preferably in view of the client, who will observe hygienic procedures being carried out. This will assure them that they are receiving a professional service.

Client care, consultation and communication skills

Treatment information to provide to the client at the initial point of interest

When a client makes an appointment for a pedicure service, the receptionist should advise the client how long the service will take. This will include sufficient time for the nail polish to dry before replacing footwear, if part of the service.

To allocate the appropriate length of time ask if they require a specialist foot service with their pedicure.

Allow 50 minutes for a pedicure.

Allow up to 1 hour for a specialist foot service including treatment.

All staff, especially the staff communicating with clients at reception, should be familiar with the different pricing structures for the range of pedicure services and products available for retail.

Ask the client whether they are currently receiving service from a chiropodist for any conditions such as verrucas or athlete's foot. These would contra-indicate service: the receptionist should advise the client it will be necessary to wait until the condition has cleared. However, a consultation would be recommended to provide the opportunity to discuss alternative or future services.

It is important that accurate records are kept and stored in compliance with the Data Protection Act for future reference.

Consultation

Before carrying out a pedicure service, it is necessary to assess the condition of the client's skin, nails and cuticles. This is done in order that the most appropriate **foot and nail treatments** and products may be chosen. Also, by correctly assessing and analysing the client's foot condition and writing this on their client record, you will be able to see over a period of time how the condition is progressing. Remember things can change between each treatment and must be checked for.

Assess the condition of the following:

◆ **The cuticles** Are they dry, tight, cracked or overgrown, or are they soft, intact and pliable?

◆ **The nails** Are they strong or weak, thickened, discoloured or stained? Sometimes this may indicate a nail disorder. The nails of the foot should be filed straight across into a square shape. Shaping the nails at the corners can cause ingrowing toenails.

◆ **The skin** Is the skin dry, rough or cracked, or is it soft and smooth? Is the colour even? Also check the skin between the toes.

It is important that accurate records are kept and stored in compliance with the Data Protection Act for future reference.

HEALTH & SAFETY

Disposing of waste

All waste should be disposed of as instructed by your local authority requirements and in compliance with the Environmental Protection Act 1990.

HEALTH & SAFETY

Lighting and ventilation

Ensure the area is well ventilated to remove atmospheric moisture and avoid inhalation of excessive fumes. Lighting should be good to enable you to avoid eyestrain and for reasons of health and safety when completing cuticle work, especially when painting the nails.

HEALTH & SAFETY

If the client is a minor, under 16 years of age, it is necessary to obtain parent, carer or guardian permission for service. They will also have to be present when the service is received.

TOP TIP

Recommended footwear when receiving a pedicure service

Advise the client booking a pedicure service that they will have to allow the nail polish to dry thoroughly before replacing footwear. It is a good idea to wear footwear such as flip flops, that will enable the toes to dry thoroughly to avoid spoiling the nail polish.

Service plan

After analysing the client's nails and adjacent skin, a **service plan** should be considered and agreed with the client. In order to correct any skin and nail problems the client should attend the salon weekly as part of a treatment package. They should also be advised of the appropriate retail products to use at home, so as to

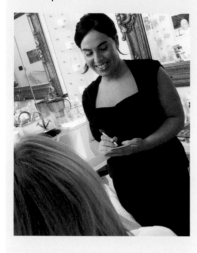

support the salon service and the objectives identified at consultation. Specialist foot treatments to use will depend upon the skin and nail condition; they include:

- **Revitalising foot spa agents** These may be in tablet form or as a foaming soak often containing ingredients with anti-bacterial properties. They are dissolved in warm water, in which the feet are then immersed, cleansing and softening the skin and nails.

- **Exfoliator** This product is used following immersion of the feet in the foot spa. It removes surface dead skin cells, preventing the formation of a callus (excess dead tissue).

- **Massage lotion or cream** This is a massage preparation that hydrates and nourishes the skin and often includes refreshing essential oils such as peppermint. It is recommended for the relief of tired, aching feet.

- **Foot mask** A **mask** may be applied to cool and to refresh the feet. Anti-ageing ingredients may be included such as anti-oxidants, vitamin A, C and E, to increase healthy cell function. Booties (unheated) may be worn while the mask penetrates the epidermis.

- **Foot gel or spray** This may be applied to create an immediate cooling, refreshing effect.

Provide the opportunity for your client to ask any questions relating to the pedicure service or service plan.

The service plan should be signed and dated by the client and pedicurist following the consultation to confirm the suitability and consent with the agreed pedicure service.

While assessing the client's feet, you should also be looking for any contra-indications to the pedicure service.

"The key to customer loyalty relies on communication with your client. It is important that you introduce yourself, but do not talk too much about yourself, explain what it is you are doing and why you are doing it. Promote the products you are using and show an interest in your client. Your pride and passion for what you are doing is what will shine through every time."

Margaret Dabbs

For more information on diseases affecting the skin see **CHAPTER 3** Consultation Practice and Techniques.

Skin and nail disorders of the feet

When a client attends for a pedicure service, as part of the consultation and assessment of the client's needs, the beauty therapist should always look at the client's skin and nails to check that no infection or disease is present that might contra-indicate service.

These include bacterial, fungal, parasitic and viral infections, which are described in more detail in Chapter 3, where **contra-indications** are illustrated and discussed.

If the client is wearing nail polish this must be removed before checking.

Contra-indications The following disorders contra-indicate pedicure services. If you suspect the client has any disorder from the chart below, do not attempt a diagnosis, but refer the client tactfully to their GP or a podiatrist without causing unnecessary concern.

Disorder	Description
Broken bones Cuts or abrasions on the feet **Diabetes** **Paronychia** Scabies or itch mites Severe **eczema of the nail** Severe eczema of the skin Blue nail Severe nail separation (**onycholysis**) Severe **psoriasis of the nail** Severe psoriasis of the skin **Tinea corporis (body ringworm)** **Tinea unguium**	*For full details, see earlier in this chapter.*
Phlebitis	Recognised by swelling and pain in the leg caused by inflammation of the vein wall (veins transport blood from the tissues back towards the heart). If a vein becomes inflamed a blood clot commonly forms inside the inflamed area (termed thrombophlebitis) Venous problems can also lead to skin ulceration. Massage to the lower leg may cause a blood clot to move through the bloodstream, causing a blockage elsewhere that could prove fatal.
Ingrowing toenail 	The side of the nail penetrates the nail wall: redness, inflammation and pus may be present, depending on the severity of the condition. The client should be referred to a chiropodist for appropriate service. To prevent ingrowing toenails clients should be advised to cut the toenails straight across, and not too short.
Tinea pedis (athlete's foot) 	Fungal infection of the foot occurring in the webs of the skin between the toes. Small blisters form, which later burst. The skin in the area can become dry, with a scaly appearance.
Verrucae or plantar warts on the feet 	A viral infection. Small epidermal skin growths. Warts occurring on the sole of the foot grow inwards, due to the pressure of body weight. Warts vary in size, shape, texture and colour. Usually they have a rough surface and are raised. Plantar wart – found on the sole of the foot.

TOP TIP

The role of the podiatrist

A podiatrist, which is the modern term for a chiropodist, is a healthcare professional who is trained and qualified to diagnose, treat and rehabilitate abnormalities of the foot and lower leg. Refer the treatment of non-cosmetic foot conditions to a podiatrist, e.g. conditions such as excessive callus (hard skin).

Below is a list of common disorders that may be seen on the feet. Not all of these contra-indicate service but may require service modification. See also 'bruised nails', earlier in this chapter.

Disorder	Cause	Appearance	Salon service	Homecare advice
Bunions 	Long-term wear of ill-fitting shoes, especially those with high heels or pointed toe areas force the foot into a position where pressure is placed on the joint and where the feet cannot spread. The ligaments and tendons tighten, altering the shape of the toes. A weakness in the arches of the feet. May also be hereditary or medically related, e.g. rheumatoid arthritis.	The large joint at the base of the big toe protrudes, forcing the big toe inwards towards the other toes. The joint grows larger over time.	None – refer the client to a podiatrist if the bunion is painful; gentle massage may help to ease any pain or discomfort.	Try to keep pressure off the affected area. Follow preventative measures.
Calluses 	Incorrect footwear.	Thick, yellowish, hardened patches of skin, usually found on prominent areas of the foot such as the heel and the ball of toe: may be painful.	Soak the feet in a foot bath containing cooling, soothing ingredients. Use a foot file or rasp when the skin is softened, to gently remove any build-up of hard skin: painful calluses should be treated by a podiatrist. Specialised foot treatments such as exfoliation and foot masks will be of benefit.	Ensure that shoes fit correctly. Avoid standing for long periods. Alternate style of footwear regularly. Keep the skin of the foot moisturised with a specialised skin conditioner for the feet. Use an exfoliant to remove excess dead skin.

Disorder	Cause	Appearance	Salon service	Homecare advice
Chilblains	Poor blood supply to the hands and feet, aggravated in cold weather.	Fingers and toes may swell and become red, blue or purple in colour; the client may complain of painful or itchy areas of skin. Severe cases of chilblains may result in blisters and broken skin.	Permission to treat to be received from the client's GP. Regular pedicures, with special attention paid to massage, which will help to improve the circulation.	Keep affected areas warm and dry. Avoid scratching the irritated area. Avoid tight footwear, which might restrict the circulation. If the condition is severe, seek medical advice.
Corns	Incorrect footwear (corns are often found on toes that have been squeezed together by tight shoes).	Similar to calluses except that the affected area is smaller and more compact; corns often look white, and may be extremely painful.	Small corns may be treated in the same way as a callus, but if the client has large or painful corns they should be treated by a podiatrist.	Ensure that shoes fit correctly. Avoid standing for long periods. Alternate style of footwear regularly.
Pitting	Eczema and/or psoriasis.	Pitting, resembling small, irregular pin pricks, appear on the nail plate.	Refer the client to their GP for permission to treat if required. Regular pedicure with gentle buffing.	General pedicure advice. Ridge-filling **base coat** polish.

Contra-actions Certain cosmetic ingredients are known to cause allergic reactions in some people.

The client – or the pedicurist – may at some time develop an allergy to a nail treatment product that has been successfully used previously. This could be for a number of reasons, including new medication being taken or illness. This is known as a contra-action. This may occur during or following a service.

The symptoms of an allergic reaction could be:

◆ redness of the skin (erythema)   ◆ skin irritation, e.g. itching

◆ swelling   ◆ raised blisters.

The symptoms do not necessarily appear on the feet. In the case of nail polish allergy, the symptoms often show up on the face.

HEALTH & SAFETY

Pedicure contra-indication

When initially preparing your client's feet during a pedicure procedure, check further for contra-indications. If you notice anything potentially contra-indicated or that could be aggravated by the service, it would need to be identified before you soak the feet.

HEALTH & SAFETY

Contact dermatitis

Contact dermatitis is a skin problem caused by intolerance of the skin to a particular substance or a group of substances. On exposure to the substance the skin quickly becomes irritated and an allergic reaction occurs. This may occur when a beauty therapist's skin is exposed to dust and chemicals on a regular basis. Follow all HSE guidelines to reduce the risk of developing this skin disorder, which could result in the need for a career change!

Always follow manufacturer's guidelines on the use of products.

In the case of an allergic reaction:

◆ Remove the offending product immediately, using water or, in the case of polish, **nail polish solvent**.

◆ Apply a cool compress and soothing agent to the skin to reduce redness and irritation.

If symptoms persist, seek medical advice. If the client receives medical advice, ask them to inform you of the advice and/or treatment received so you can include this in your records.

Always carry out a skin sensitivity patch test if a client has known sensitivity to product ingredients, identified at consultation. The patch test should be performed 24–48 hours before using any new or known ingredient within the pedicure service or treatment that may cause sensitisation. A negative patch test result is required.

Always record any allergies or contra-actions on the client's service plan, so that the offending product may be avoided in future.

Further contra-actions could occur as a result of incorrect use of pedicure tools and equipment, for example:

◆ sore, sensitised skin following excessive hard skin removal

◆ sore, reddened skin in the cuticle area due to excessive trimming of the cuticle

◆ tissue damage could result in blood loss, e.g. incorrect nipping removal technique when using cuticle nippers may result in pulling and tearing of the skin, potentially leading to infection

◆ incorrect positioning and use of the cuticle knife may lead to piercing the cuticle with the knife blade

◆ paraffin wax – heat intolerance to the temperature of the paraffin wax

◆ using sharp tools under the free edge, piercing the hyponychium, the skin's protective seal, exposing the nail bed to potential infection.

◆ cutting the nails too short as again this can result in possible damage to the hyponychium, the part of the epidermis under the free edge of the nail. This may affect its protective function, leading to possible infection.

REVISION AID

Which foot conditions should not be treated by a beauty therapist?

Preparing the client

Ensure that the client is seated at the correct height, so that you can work comfortably and healthily and the client can enjoy the service without strain to the muscles and joints of the leg.

Ensure that the client is warm and comfortable when preparing for the pedicure. Client privacy and modesty should also be considered. Not all clients would be happy to be on view while receiving the service. Ensure that lighting is good to avoid eyestrain and to enable the service to be performed competently. Avoid positioning the nail workstation in direct sunlight however, to prevent discomfort to the client and pedicurist. Heat and light can also damage the quality of the nail products.

Before service begins, ask the client to remove their tights or socks if worn and any clothing that might restrict access to their lower leg, such as tight jeans or trousers. Cover their upper legs with a clean towel or provide appropriate protective clothing, such as a robe. This will help them to be more comfortable and allow you to work without restriction.

Ask your client to remove any jewellery from the area to be treated, to prevent the jewellery being damaged by creams and to avoid obstructing massage movements. Place the jewellery where the client can see it. Alternatively, ask the client to take possession of it for safe keeping – following your workplace security policy.

When the client is comfortably seated, clean your hands using an approved hand cleaning technique – preferably in view of the client, who will observe hygienic procedures being carried out. This will assure them that they are receiving a professional service.

Explain each stage of the service and check client comfort and satisfaction throughout.

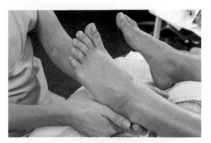

Ensure client is sitting at the correct height so they can enjoy the treatment without strain to the leg and that you can safely perform the service without risk of injury

HEALTH & SAFETY

Avoiding repetitive strain injury(RSI)

Remember to consider your posture and prevent any awkward movements during delivery of the pedicure service. Ensure the work station is at the correct height to avoid stretching and straining your upper body and limbs.

STEP-BY-STEP: PEDICURE PROCEDURE

This process briefly shows the stages in the pedicure. Each step is discussed in detail later in this section. The procedure may start with either the right or left foot.

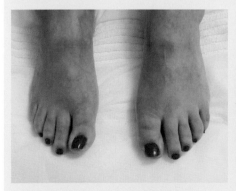

1 Nails and feet before pedicure procedure.

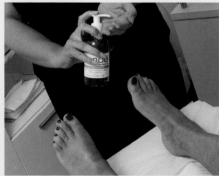

2 Clean your hands using an approved hand cleaning technique.

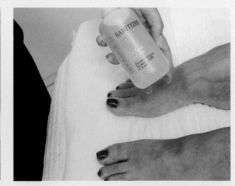

3 Wipe both feet including between the toes with cotton wool soaked in skin disinfectant (product example shown here) or a specialised hygiene spray for the feet. Use separate pieces of cotton wool for each foot.

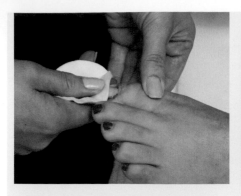

4 Remove any existing nail polish if worn. Check again for contra-indications below the nail plate. (If a nail contra-indication is present, service must not continue. Tactfully explain why and give appropriate referral advice.)

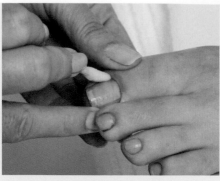

5 Remove any remaining polish around the cuticle with nail polish remover applied with a cuticle stick tipped with cotton wool.

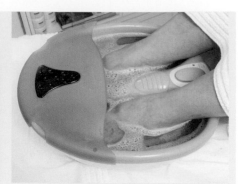

6 Soak both feet in warm water to which a liquid soap or similar professional foot soak product has been added. Take out left foot and towel dry.

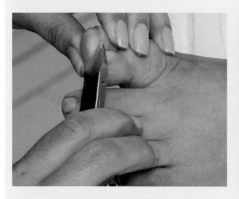

7 Cut the toenails straight across, using toenail clippers or scissors.

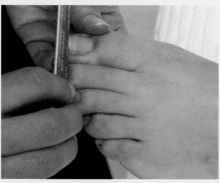

8 File the nails smooth with the coarse side of the emery board. Hold the emery board at a 45 degree angle to the free edge, and apply strokes in one direction. Do not shape the nails at the sides to avoid ingrowing nails. Ensure the free edge is smooth by bevelling.

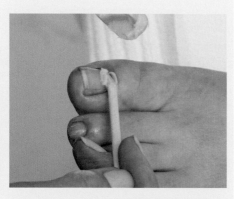

9 Apply cuticle massage cream or oil and massage into the cuticles. Place the foot back in the water. Remove the right foot and repeat steps 7–9.

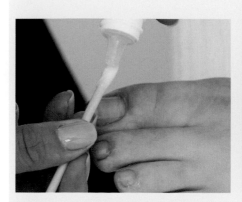

10 Dry the left foot and apply cuticle remover. To avoid excessive application and contaminating the applicator apply to a cotton wool-tipped **cuticle stick**.

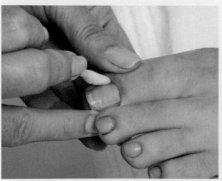

11 Push back the cuticles with a cotton wool-tipped cuticle stick, hoof stick or cuticle pusher.

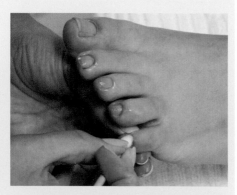

12 Clean under the free edge with a separate clean cotton-tipped cuticle stick.

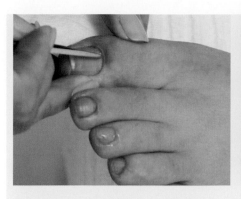

13 Use the **cuticle knife** where indicated to remove excess eponychium and perionychium. Collect excess skin in a tissue or a clean piece of cotton wool and dispose of immediately.

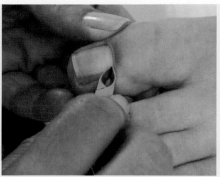

14 Use cuticle nippers where necessary to remove excess cuticle. Wipe off any remaining cuticle remover with damp cotton wool, and apply cuticle oil to the nails again if necessary.

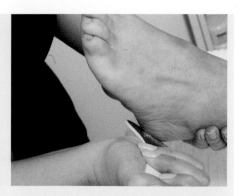

15 Remove any hard skin. This may be done with exfoliating cream, pedicure callus file or a foot rasp, This will depend on the severity of the condition, but remember you are not a chiropodist/podiatrist.

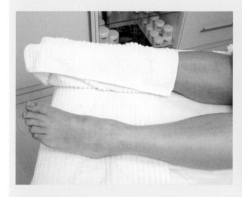

16 Wrap the foot in a dry towel to keep it warm.

Repeat steps **10–15** for the other foot.

Remove the pedicure foot bowl from the working area if non-fixed.

Perform a foot and lower leg massage. (See later in this chapter.)

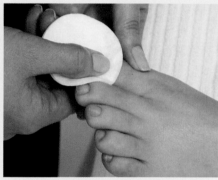

17 Remove any remaining grease from the nail plates with a cotton wool pad soaked in nail polish remover. Re-file the nails as necessary to ensure the free edge is smooth and even. Polish may be applied or, if left natural, the nail may be buffed and a conditioning oil applied. Natural polishes are available which can colour correct the nail plate achieving a healthy appearance.

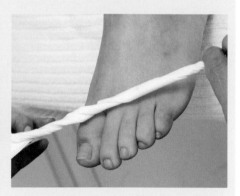

18 Place disposable toe separators or other hygienic equivalent to separate them and facilitate polish application.

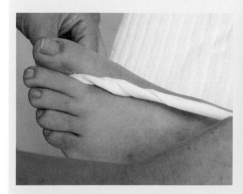

19 Continued

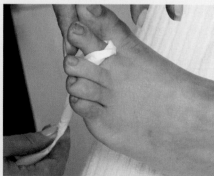

20 Continued

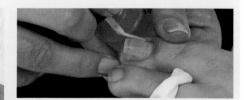

21 Apply the polish: base coat (once), cream polish (twice) and top coat (once). If a pearlised polish is used a top coat is not required and a third coat of polish may be applied.

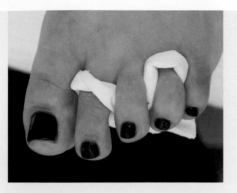

22 Apply one coat of nail polish to each nail plate, followed by a second coat to provide even coverage.

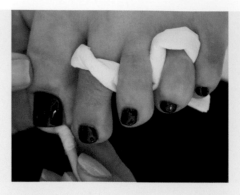

23 A cotton wool-tipped cuticle stick may be used to apply nail polish remover to remove any excess polish from the surrounding skin.

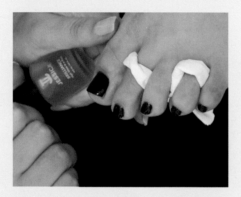

24 Application of top coat as the product is a cream polish, requiring a top coat.

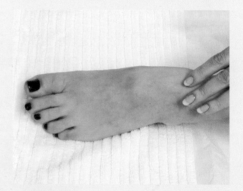

25 Completed nail pedicure service.

Cutting and filing toenails

Toenails should be cut straight across, using nail clippers or strong sharp scissors, then filed smooth at the free edge using the bevelling technique. Not shaping the nails at the corners helps to avoid ingrowing toenails. Do not cut the nails too short to ensure there is adequate protection at the free edge to avoid discomfort and infection of the nail bed.

Cuticle work Cuticle work is carried out to keep the cuticle area attractive and also to prevent excess eponychium skin from adhering to the nail plate, which could lead to splitting of the cuticle as the nail grows forward, and subsequently infection of the area, e.g. paronychia.

A cuticle remover product is used to prepare and soften the cuticle. The cuticle knife blade should be damp when using and is held flat to avoid scratching the nail plate. Clean the blade of the tool as necessary during each use to remove excess tissue.

The cuticle nipper points, used to remove excess dead cuticle, should face downwards and the skin should never be pulled during removal. Clean the points of the tool as necessary during each use to remove excess tissue.

Excess cuticle should be collected hygienically in a tissue and disposed of immediately following this stage of the pedicure service. Excess cuticle remover should be removed from the area with damp cotton wool to avoid drying or irritating the skin following its use.

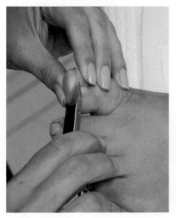

Cutting toenails

REVISION AID

How can an ingrowing toenail be avoided when filing?

HEALTH & SAFETY

Contaminated waste

If you accidentally cut the skin causing bleeding at the cuticle area, protect your hands with disposable non-latex (synthetic) powder-free gloves and wipe the skin with an antiseptic wipe. Any waste is classed as clinical waste or contaminated waste and should be disposed of in a yellow medical bin liner in accordance with the **Environmental Protection Act (1990)** and **Controlled Waste Regulations (2012)**.

The work is carried out after soaking the feet in warm soapy water, having previously applied a cuticle cream or oil. This step softens the skin in the cuticle area before cuticle work.

STEP-BY-STEP: CUTICLE WORK

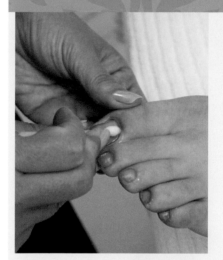

1 Pushing back the cuticles following application of cuticle remover using a cotton wool tipped cuticle stick.

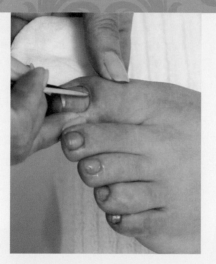

2 Using a cuticle knife to loosen excess eponychium skin from the nail plate. The blade must be kept damp.

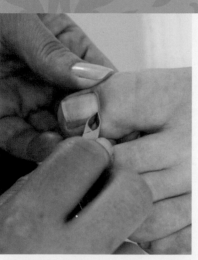

3 Using cuticle nippers to remove excess cuticle and dead skin.

Removing hard skin

Hard skin develops on the feet as a form of protection, either caused by friction from footwear or from standing for long periods of time. The skin in this area also becomes drier as part of the ageing process.

It is not advisable to remove *all* the hard skin from an area, as this would remove the protective function of the skin in this area. Hard skin should be removed only to improve the appearance and condition of the feet. Hard skin build-up that causes pain or discomfort should be referred to a podiatrist for treatment.

Excess hard skin may be removed from the feet in a number of ways, including exfoliators, foot rasp and callus files. Exfoliator is a product which should be applied using a deep circular massage movement that is comfortable for your client: it is ideal when only a very small build-up of hard skin is present. Files and foot rasps should be used with a swift

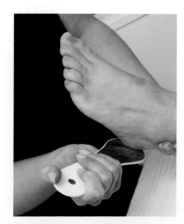

Removing hard skin with a pumice file. Pumice is a type of volcanic rock.

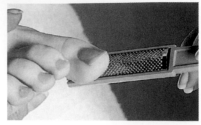
Removing hard skin with a foot rasp

stroking movement in one direction only (similar to buffing). Sawing back and forth would lead to friction and discomfort for the client.

Always finish off a hard skin removal procedure with the application of a specialised foot moisturiser or lotion, to soften the newly exposed skin.

Foot and nail treatments

In addition to the pedicure, further treatments may be added as appropriate. Here are some examples:

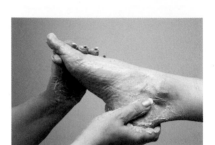
Exfoliating treatment

◆ **Exfoliating treatment** is usually carried out prior to massage or as part of the massage routine if an exfoliating massage medium is used. A cosmetic product containing an abrasive ingredient or beta hydroxy acid such as salicylic acid with exfoliating properties is massaged over the skin of the foot in circular movements, concentrating over the ball and heel of the foot. It may be extended to the lower limb in order to improve blood and lymphatic circulation. Exfoliation removes dead skin, increases blood and lymphatic circulation and improves the condition and appearance of the skin and the absorption of further treatment products.

◆ **Foot treatment mask** is applied according to the client's service plan. The mask is applied to the skin, then usually covered with a plastic protective cover. The feet can then be enclosed in thermal booties to assist in the absorption of the mask depending on the manufacturer's instructions and the aim of the chosen mask. Sometimes a cooling effect is required. The mask further softens the skin, aiding desquamation, improves blood and lymphatic circulation and improves generally the condition of the skin of the feet.

REVISION AID

What must you consider when designing the client's nail and foot treatment?

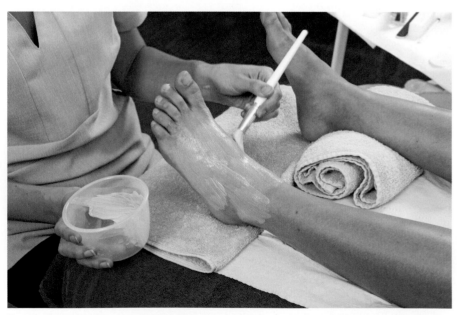
Foot treatment mask

◆ **Paraffin wax service** – this wax is heated in a special bath to a temperature of 50–55°C. The therapeutic heating effect stimulates the blood and lymphatic circulation, eases the discomfort of arthritic and rheumatic conditions, soothes sensory nerve endings and softens the skin, improving the appearance and condition of dry skin.

After checking the client's tolerance to the wax temperature, the client's whole foot and ankle is covered with paraffin wax. The liquid wax may be applied with a brush or gauze can be dipped into the wax a number of times and then wrapped around the feet, or alternatively a spray attached to a heated cartridge of paraffin wax. The initial wax application quickly sets, becoming solid and then further layers of paraffin wax are applied to provide a waterproof covering. Once applied the feet should then be placed in a plastic protective covering and covered for example with cotton booties to retain heat. The wax may be removed after 10–15 minutes. It is a good idea to remove the wax with the polythene covering, which is usually in one action. After use the wax is disposed of.

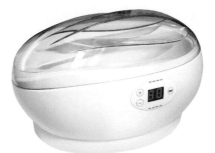

Paraffin wax heater

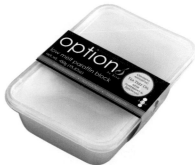

Paraffin wax

◆ **Thermal booties** are electrically heated booties. They are used to stimulate, rejuvenate and moisturise the skin of the feet. The feet are prepared with the application of a foot treatment mask, protected in a polythene covering and placed inside warm booties for 10 minutes to enable the mask to penetrate the skin of the epidermis and cuticles of the nail.

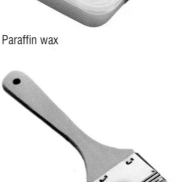

Brush for paraffin wax application

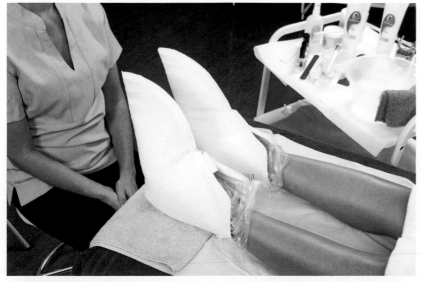

Thermal booties used to aid absorption of specialist foot treatments

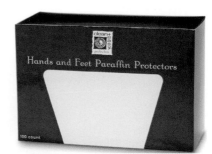

Polythene protectors

Always follow manufacturer's guidelines in the application procedure for feet and nail treatments.

STEP-BY-STEP: SPECIALIST FOOT AND LEG TREATMENTS

Specialist treatments should be offered to your client when there is a specific need or if they feel they would like to benefit from such a treatment for maintenance or relaxation purposes. Specialist training in these techniques is usually offered by the manufacturers of such products. They can also advise you of associated retail products.

The model for this specialist foot and leg is a client who regularly visits the gym and wishes to benefit from a well-being spa therapy revitalising foot and lower leg treatment following a workout.

The following foot and leg treatment will:

◆ stimulate the blood and lymphatic circulation locally

◆ aid with the localised removal of toxins and waste products

◆ have a skin-cleansing action through increased sweating and removal of skin debris

◆ remove dead skin cells (desquamation)

◆ improve the moisture content of the skin through absorption

◆ relax tense/stiff muscles in the foot and leg.

Your treatments should be adapted to meet the service plan objectives for the client. Allow 30 minutes for the specialist foot and leg treatment below.

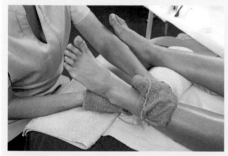

1 The skin of the feet, between the toes and lower legs is cleansed using warm towelling mitts infused with lime oil for its therapeutic refreshing and energising properties. Support of the client's limb is important, shown under the ankle and the knee.

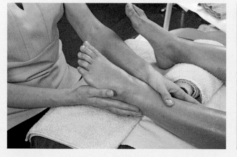

2 The feet and legs are exfoliated to remove all dead skin cells and brighten the skin. A sea salt-based preparation with emollient, skin softening ingredients is applied to each foot and leg. Gloves may be worn to protect the hands from the abrasive action of the exfoliation.

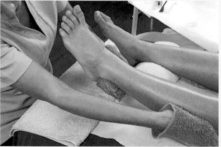

3 Towelling mitts are used to remove the exfoliating product. These have been steamed and are warm when used.

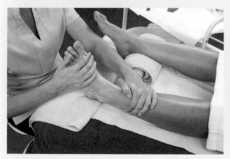

4 A skin-nourishing lotion is applied to each foot and leg. The lotion is particularly beneficial for dry skin. Massage movements are applied using **effleurage** and **petrissage** manipulations to introduce the massage medium into the skin.

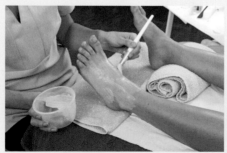

5 A skin treatment mask is applied and massaged into the skin. This will soften and condition the skin in the treatment area.

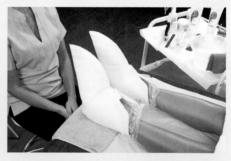

6 The feet are then placed in polythene bags before being placed in electrical thermally heated booties for 10–15 minutes. The heat will help the skin to absorb the therapeutic ingredients of the mask. Excess product can be removed with warm mitts or towels. Further pedicure service can follow following removal such as preparing the nails and providing a nail finish.

Foot and lower leg massage

As with a manicure massage, the pedicure massage is carried out near the end of the service, prior to nail polishing. However, if required it may be applied with other services such as during a facial whilst the treatment mask is on. The pedicure massage includes the foot and the lower leg, and offers the following benefits to the client:

◆ moisturises the skin with the massage medium, cream, lotion or oil, improving skin hydration

◆ increases blood circulation locally, transporting oxygen and nutrients to the lower leg and foot

◆ increases lymph circulation, transporting waste products in the lymph away from the lower leg and foot

◆ helps maintain joint mobility through the application of passive massage techniques

◆ eases discomfort from arthritis or rheumatism, although pressure and massage techniques that may cause discomfort must be considered where there is limited joint movement

◆ relaxes the client, soothes sensory nerve endings and relieves tension in muscles

◆ muscle tone is improved as the muscles receive an improved supply of oxygenated blood, essential for cell growth; massage techniques such as tapotement can provide a toning effect

◆ helps remove any dead skin cells (desquamation).

The massage incorporates classic massage movements, each with different effects:

◆ **Effleurage** – a stroking movement, used to begin the massage as a link manipulation, and to complete the massage sequence.

◆ **Petrissage** – movements, including **kneading**, where the tissues are lifted away from the underlying structures and compressed. Pressure is intermittent, and should be light yet firm.

◆ **Tapotement**, also known as **percussion**, may be included – **tapotement** movements are performed in a brisk, stimulating manner to increase blood supply and improve tone of the skin and muscles. Movements include clapping and tapping.

◆ **Joint manipulations** – ankle joints and toes are manipulated through their range of movement, dependent upon the type of joint. This helps to maintain good mobility within the range of movement but must be avoided if the client has any joint disorders.

◆ **Frictions** – small circular movements using the pads of the fingers or thumbs. The skin and muscle below is massaged against the underlying bone. This can be used to loosen any adhesions in the tissues.

You can adapt the massage application according to the needs of the client. A firmer massage is usually required when treating a male client. Either the *speed of application* or *depth of pressure* can be altered.

"Luxury manicure and pedicure treatments can be very important to the elderly client. The sensory nature of the treatment, the warmth in the oil and paraffin wax application, can promote a feeling of well-being."

Laura Dicken

REVISION AID

What are the massage techniques you may use during a foot and lower leg massage?

TOP TIP

Pressure point technique can be incorporated to aid relaxation if you are qualified to do so.

For detailed information on the different classifications of massage movement and their benefits refer to CHAPTER 4 Facials.

STEP-BY-STEP: FOOT AND LOWER LEG MASSAGE

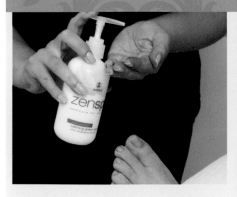

1 Select an appropriate massage medium for the service and for the client's skin type and condition. Dispense the massage medium into the hands. This should be sufficient to perform the massage, but dependent upon skin condition further product may be required to provide sufficient slip during massage.

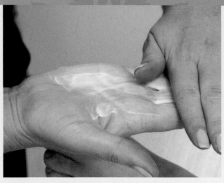

2 Distribute and warm the product over the palms and apply to the client's skin using effleurage technique.

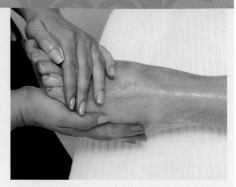

3 Effleurage from the foot to the knee. Use long sweeping strokes from the toes upwards to the knee, massaging on both the posterior (back) and the anterior (front) of the leg.

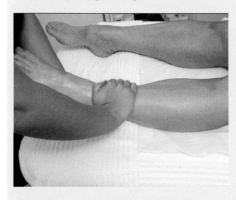

4 Effleurage from the foot to the knee. Effleurage can be interspersed throughout the massage to aid removal of excess tissue fluid and toxins.

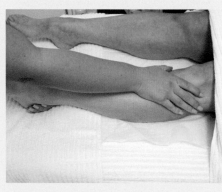

5 Effleurage from the foot to the knee.

Repeat steps 3-5 a further five times.

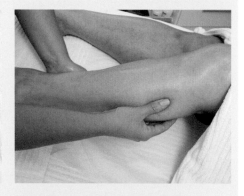

6 Flex the client's knee and using a petrissage movement knead the gastrocnemius muscle in an upwards direction, then pick up and gently squeeze the gastrocnemius muscle as shown.

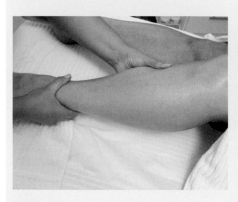

7 Repeat on the inner side of the leg.

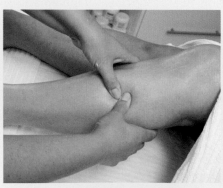

8 Slide the palms of your hands down to the ankle and using the thumbs knead gently upwards along the tibialis anterior muscles on the outer shin.

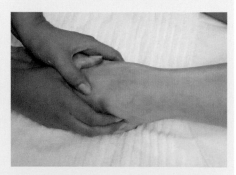

9 Using the pads of the fingers perform small circular kneading movements around the malleolus (ankle) bone. Massage both sides of the ankle bone at the same time.

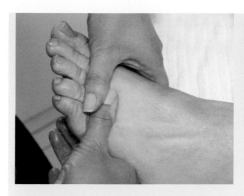

10 **Thumb frictions to the dorsal aspect of the foot.** Use the thumbs, one in front of the other, and move backwards and forwards in a gentle sawing action. Move from the toes to the ankle, then slide back down to the toes.

Repeat step 10 a further two times.

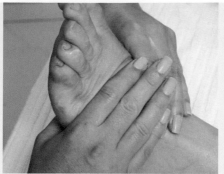

11 **Thumb frictions to the plantar aspect of the foot.** Use the same movement as in step 10, but on the sole of the foot, moving from the toes to the heel.

Repeat step 11 a further two times.

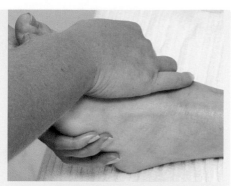

12 **Palm kneading to the plantar surface of the foot.** Place the heel of the hand into the arch of the foot and massage with deep circular movements.

Repeat step 12 a further five times.

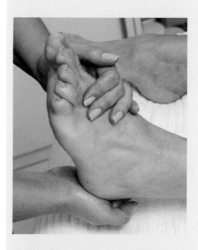

13 Support the foot with one hand, and using the palm, cup the heel and perform a circular kneading movement.

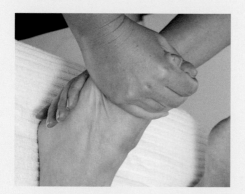

14 Place the hand either side of the toes; gently press together and rotate all the toes three times clockwise and three times anticlockwise.

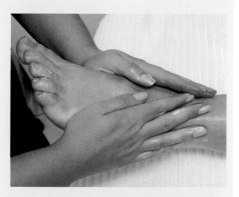

15 Effleurage from the foot to the knee, using the same movements as in step 3.

Repeat step 15 a further five times.

Repeat massage on the other foot and lower leg.

Nail polish application

Confirm the client's choice of nail polish colour finish. Whatever the finish, ensure the nail plate is clean and free from grease, which would affect adherence of the polish. Also make sure the free edge is smooth and the cuticles are neat and smooth. Before nail polish is applied, any jewellery worn in the area should be replaced to avoid smudging the polish afterwards.

When choosing nail polish discuss the reasons for choice of colour. If exposed, the client may wish it to complement the nails of the hands, but it does not necessarily need to do so.

Consider the skin colour of the client in order to advise which colour would suit their skin. Alternatively, matt colour corrector polishes are available to create a natural healthy nail finish.

> Nail finishes including polish, types, use and application techniques are discussed earlier in the chapter.

REVISION AID

When providing a nail polish finish, what do you consider a professionally applied nail polish would look like?

STEP-BY-STEP: FRENCH POLISH APPLICATION

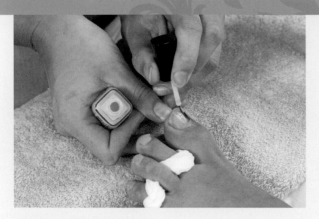

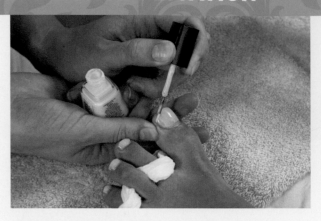

1 After ensuring the nail plate is free from oil and the nails are neat, start polish application with the big toe. Using a base coat, apply three to four brush strokes down the length of the nail from the cuticle to the free edge, beginning in the centre, then down either side close to the nail wall. Follow this with a pink colour, cream formulation polish, applied in the same way as the base coat. A second coat may be required as necessary.

2 Using a white cream polish take the polish horizontally across the free edge, enhancing and creating the appearance of a white free edge. A second coat may be required as necessary.

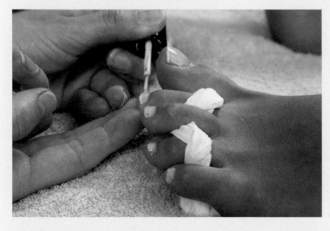

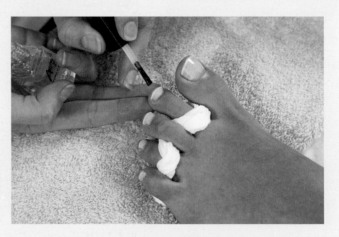

3 When all nails have been painted, apply a top coat to add gloss and durability to the finished nails.

4 Advise the client how long the nail will take to dry; a quick drying spray or oil may be applied to accelerate this.

Client advice and recommendations

Offering advice and recommendations on-going from the consultation, throughout the service and at the end of a pedicure service will raise the client's understanding of how to look after their feet between salon visits, and is also an ideal opportunity to recommend retail products to support this.

Advice will differ for each client according to their personal requirements but there is some generic advice as follows:

◆ Provide relevant advice to the service/treatment received. For example, avoid immediate UV exposure where certain ingredients could cause photo sensitivity, such as lemon oil and skin brightening ingredients.

◆ Advise the client that a healthy diet is related to the health and appearance of the nails and skin.

REVISION AID

What information should be recorded on the client's service plan during and following treatment?

- Lifestyle activities that may affect care of the feet should be considered, such as running, swimming, etc.

- Change socks or tights daily.

- Gently scrubbing the feet daily is recommended to avoid skin conditions such as athlete's foot.

- Apply moisturising lotion daily to the feet, preferably after bathing when the skin is softened.

- Ensure that the feet are thoroughly dry after washing, especially between the toes.

- Apply a special foot powder between the toes to help absorb moisture.

- Foot sprays containing peppermint or citrus oil to cleanse and refresh are useful to refresh the feet during the day.

- Go barefoot wherever it is safe and practical to do so.

- Ensure that footwear fits properly. Foot problems such as bunions can be aggravated by incorrect footwear.

- Avoid wearing high heels for long periods of time. They can cause postural problems and increase hard skin callus formation.

- Advise on appropriate nail/skincare products to remedy the problems present, e.g. dry skin, nails, stained nails.

- Advise the client of any other professional services you could recommend.

- Advise the client on a service plan to improve the nail/skin condition and the time intervals recommended between each service.

- When filing the nails, always file straight across in one direction.

- If any pain is felt in the feet visit a podiatrist.

- It is also necessary to advise the client what to do in the event of a contra-action.

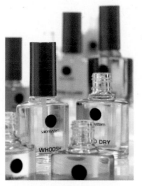

Specialised nail polishes to treat nail condition identified

ALWAYS REMEMBER

Advise on further professional services

Professionally advise the client on further services that would benefit them. For example, if a client has dry skin on their heels, take the opportunity to recommend an **exfoliant** treatment.

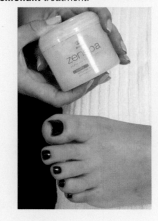

"If you are passionate about what you do and work hard, you will inevitably do well. Learn from your colleagues and always try to do that bit more for your client. When you are ready, ask to take on more responsibility. If you have an interest in one area, develop your skills further with training courses. As you progress, share your expertise with others and think about where you would like to be in the future."

Margaret Dabbs

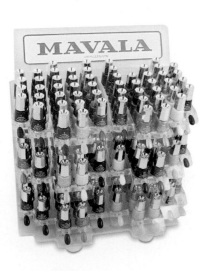

Have retail products available for the client to purchase. These include nail files, coloured nail polishes, nail polish remover and nail/skin service products.

It is a good idea to have available the nail polish colours that you have used. The client can then touch up any accidental chips themselves.

Recommend the use of top coat applied every three to four days to protect the nail polish, increase its durability and impart shine.

"Consider the three Rs:

Recognise the issue being presented.

Recommend the proper pedicure service, products and home maintenance.

Refer the client to a medical professional when necessary."

Laura Dicken

More information on anatomical terminology can be found in **CHAPTER 2**.

Finally, at the end of the pedicure service ensure the client's records are updated, accurate and signed by the client and beauty therapist. Ensure the finished result is to the client's satisfaction and meets the agreed treatment plan.

Exercises for the feet and ankles

As part of the advice given to a pedicure client **foot exercises** may be mentioned – these can play a very important role in keeping the client's feet healthy. They help:

◆ to stimulate blood and lymphatic circulation

◆ to keep joints mobilised, allowing a greater range of movement in the toes and ankles

◆ to keep muscles strong, reducing the chance of fallen arches (flat feet).

Here are some examples of exercises:

1 Sit on a chair with the feet flat on the floor, raise the toes upwards and then relax.

2 Stand on tiptoes, and relax down again.

3 Sit on a chair with the feet flat on the floor, lift one leg slightly and draw a circle with the toes so that the ankle moves through its full range of movement.

4 **Dorsiflexion**: bend the foot backwards towards the body.

5 **Plantar flexion**: point the foot down towards the ground.

6 Move the foot inwards towards the middle of the body – this is termed inversion.

7 Move the foot out towards the side of the body – this is termed eversion.

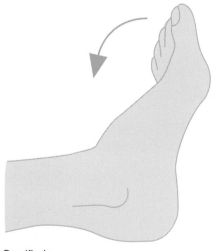

Dorsiflexion

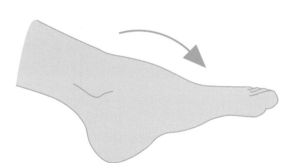

Plantarflexion

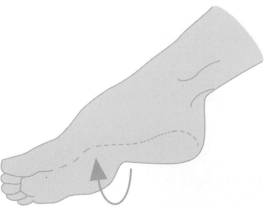

Inversion

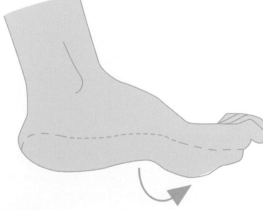

Eversion

Nail Art

This section is about how to provide **nail art**. Nail art provides a decorative nail finish where nail polish and other mediums are used. It includes paints, **glitters** and transfers to achieve different textures and nail looks for both the hands and feet. In addition to the skills required, creativity and imagination are just as important for the nail artist. It can be as simple as a single stripe across the nail or as intricate as a tiny repeated pattern embellished by flat stones.

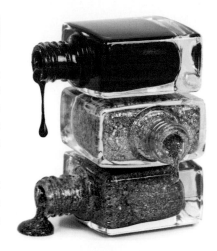

Consultation is important to ensure that you fully understand the expectations of the client according to their nail art requirement. To assist this, it is a good idea to have a portfolio of images. These may be in an electronic format or samples of pre-prepared nail art to show your client.

The anatomy and physiology knowledge and understanding required is found in the checklist in Chapter 2, and is also discussed within this chapter.

Nail art is a skill that takes practice and requires a very good eye for detail and a steady hand.

ALWAYS REMEMBER

Anatomy and physiology

When performing hand and foot nail services, including nail art services, you are required to apply your knowledge of the structure and function of the skin including:

◆ identifying skin conditions

◆ the structure of the nail and nail shapes

◆ identifying nail conditions

◆ nail growth.

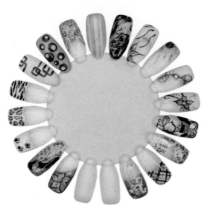

Nail art wheel: these are great to share at consultation when deciding upon the nail art look to be achieved

INDUSTRY ROLE MODEL

NATALIYA, N-Style, Edinburgh

"My passion and interest in the nail and beauty industry led me to pursue my dream and change direction in life. I attended Mary Reid International School of Beauty and graduated in 2006 with ITEC qualifications in beauty and body therapy. I then worked as a senior therapist in PURE Spa in Edinburgh. As the only nail professional in the team, I realised that nail design is what I wanted to do for life. Shortly after leaving the spa and opening my first beauty salon, I attended various nail courses in the brand Creative Nail Design (CND). I became a CND Shellac education Ambassador in 2011 and have taken nail art to a new level. In May 2013 I attended CND's Education Boot Camp in San Diego and qualified as a full systems CND Education Ambassador, bringing home two awards. I regularly contribute to the industry with my Nail Trail article in *Scratch* Magazine. I work full time in my own salon N-Style in Edinburgh, with responsibility for hygiene, marketing and business development."

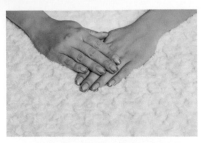

French manicure style with light blue free edge and gold lines

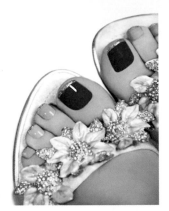

Free edge painted gold on toes

The nail art skill starts when a 'French manicure finish' is applied, demonstrated earlier in this chapter as this is actually two colours that need to be painted accurately, resembling the distinction between the free edge and the nail plate. The shape of the free edge can be changed and enhanced depending upon the effect required. Nail art technique becomes more advanced when other colours and designs are included. You do not need to be a great artist in order to create quite stunning and commercially acceptable designs. There are many easy commercial **nail art techniques** and products that allow even the most 'artistically challenged' to produce some stunning designs!

There is an extensive range of nail art products or mediums available on the market today that, with a few guidelines and hints, can create stunning 'masterpieces' at minimal cost and effort. The real effort is practising! Nail art is visual and there are a relatively small number of basic **painting techniques** that, using readily available products, can be demonstrated in a few step-by-step pictures. Every newcomer to nail art will find that, with the attainment of the basic traditional techniques and access to the necessary equipment and range of products, a few initial ideas will lead on to many, many more.

Although some more unusual designs are included, the aim of this section is to provide the underpinning knowledge and practical skills of the various techniques of nail art that may be performed commercially in a beauty salon or freelance situation.

How to convince clients to try nail art

"Wear it yourself, usually clients will ask for what you are wearing on your nails. Encourage your clients with a complementary simple design on their ring finger to introduce them to artistic designs. Take into consideration clients' profession, lifestyle and fashion preferences. Ask clients about preferred shape and length, colours they love and dislike, and keep a note of them for future appointments."

Nataliya

Preparing for nail art

Preparing the work area

Prepare the nail work station to meet the requirements for all related health and safety legislation. The work surface must be stable to avoid products being knocked over or spilt. The area must be free of any other previously used materials and debris. Dust created from services such as artificial nail enhancements can spoil the effect of a client's newly painted nails. Lighting must be good to enable you to avoid eyestrain, especially when performing intricate artwork. It is a good idea to use a magnifying lamp when necessary.

All the health and safety rules and legislation that you learnt in Chapter 1 The Business of Beauty Therapy and this chapter must be followed. With increasing availability of online resources it is important that products are purchased from a reputable supplier and meet all legal hygiene and industry safety requirements for nail services.

Ensure all products, tools and equipment are available, clean and disinfected as appropriate and are neatly organised on the nail workstation.

TOP TIP

Looking for inspiration

Nail trade magazines and websites are extremely useful to keep you updated on the latest colours, nail products and designs, as these are the forums for many nails artists to display their designs. Also, many nail technicians share their 'blog' of latests nail products, techniques and looks.

Products, tools and equipment

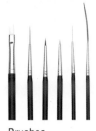

Brushes

◆ **Brushes** A variety of shapes and sizes of brushes for freehand painting including detail brush, striping brush, flat brush and fan brush.

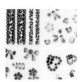

Foils/transfers/
tapes/stencils

◆ **Foils/transfers/tapes/stencils** A variety of materials for creating designs.

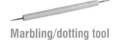

Marbling/dotting tool

◆ **Marbling/dotting tool** For creating 'marbling' or 'dotting' designs with the paint.

Nail piercing tool

◆ **Nail piercing tool** For making small holes in the nail for jewellery attachments. Also known as a jewellery tool.

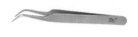

◆ **Nail art tweezers** To pick up nail art materials; to enable its secure placement on the nail plate.

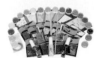

Nail art paints

◆ **Nail art paints** Specialised water-based acrylic paints for nail art.

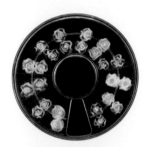

◆ **Embellishments** Small stones including rhinestones, flat stones and any pre-made shapes for attaching to the nail as part of the design.

Glitter polishes/dusts

◆ **Glitter polishes/dusts** Can be used to create or enhance nail art designs

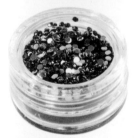

Embellishment

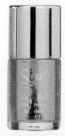

Specialised nail
art sealer/top coat

◆ **Specialised nail art sealer/top coat** For sealing the design once the paint is dry.

Dappen dishes

◆ **Dappen dishes** For keeping polish secures or glitter in.

YOU WILL ALSO NEED:

◆ **Palette** For placing nail art paints on for use or mixing.

◆ **Nail scissors** For trimming nail length and also cutting nail art media such as striping foil.

◆ **Disinfectant solution** To store small stainless steel sterilised tools.

◆ **Nail work station** On which to place everything. You will require manicure tools and equipment to prepare the nails for nail art. A light is useful when carrying out detailed techniques.

◆ **Nail polish remover** To remove nail polish/products as required.

◆ **Nail polishes** Including base coat and a range of coloured polishes.

◆ **Medium sized towels (3)** To dry the skin, nails, etc. and protect the client's clothing.

◆ **Water spray** For re-wetting the nail art paints when they start to dry out.

◆ **Cuticle stick** for application and removal of nail art.

◆ **Skin disinfectant** To cleanse and disinfect the client's skin and nails.

◆ **Waste container** This should be a lined metal bin with a lid to contain vapours from solvents.

◆ **Tissues or disposal towels** To cover the work area when using paints and protect the client's clothing.

◆ **Cotton buds** A damp cotton bud can be used to remove mistakes made with nail art paint.

◆ **Cotton wool or lint free nail pads** For preparing the nail plate and removing previous nail art.

◆ **Client service record** To record the client's personal details, products used and details of the service.

TOP TIP

Product range

As the range of nail art services and products develops, it is important to keep up-to-date with all those products that are available to improve efficiency and have been designed to keep the nails healthy. For example, glitter polish is hard to remove and formulations of nail polish remover are available to make this a less arduous process. This may be a great retail product for clients too.

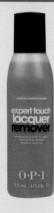

TOP TIP

Spoilt polish

It is a good idea for the client to pay before their service to prevent spoiling the nail art. Gel polish nail art is a popular alternative as the finish dries immediately.

ALWAYS REMEMBER

Be realistic

Although designs look effective displayed on quite large plastic tips, remember that the design will look very different on a much smaller nail and on a finger or toe and some designs are much easier to apply on a tip than a real nail as the surrounding skin can get in the way!

Safety and hygiene

Hygiene must be maintained in a number of ways:

◆ Ensure that your nail workstation is positioned and prepared to avoid unhealthy working positions and posture which could lead to strain and injury of the body and limbs.

◆ Ensure that tools and equipment are clean and, where applicable, disinfected before use.

◆ Having sterilised or disinfected tools and equipment, store them in a chemical disinfectant, UV cabinet or closed container until ready for use. Remember, they will remain clean but will not be sterile after 24 hours.

◆ Disinfect work surfaces after each client.

◆ Clear discarded waste and debris after each client.

◆ Refer to your workplace policy, manufacturers' guidelines and related legislative guidelines to ensure safe usage, prevention of cross-infection/contamination and the health and welfare of yourself, clients and others.

HEALTH & SAFETY

Legislation

It is important that you comply with all relevant health and safety legislation while performing nail art.

Examples include:

◆ Control of Substances Hazardous to Health Regulations (COSHH) (2002)
◆ Personal Protective Equipment (PPE) at Work Regulations (1992).

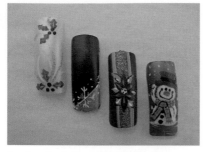

Freehand painting with a festive theme

Sitting properly is important. Ideally sit on a properly designed manicure stool or chair that offers adequate back support. When completing nail art it is important to sit upright with both feet flat on the floor.

Protection of the skin on the hands and wrists is important to avoid contact with any skin irritants. There should be no exposure to any harmful chemicals. Decant only small amounts of products, such as brush cleaner, and always replace the tops on products after using them. Ensure lighting is adequate in the service area. Position the client to avoid unnecessary strain or discomfort.

Treatment information to provide to the client at the initial point of interest

Nail art should be priced as a stand alone service, not just included in the cost of a manicure or pedicure with finish. When a client makes an appointment and requests nail art, discuss the requirements of the service and associated cost. Prices will vary depending on the products and materials used, or the time involved to create the design. If a client is booking a manicure or pedicure ask them if they would like nail art too.

If there are promotional events it is important that clients have the opportunity to consider these as part of their nail service. Nail art is popular for seasonal events such as Halloween and Christmas. Also, following winter, complimentary nail art finishes may be provided to encourage the promotion of pedicure services.

Allocate sufficient time. Some designs are very quick and use little product, for example a flick of paint with a nail art brush or a simple **marbling** technique using a **dotting tool**. Other designs are very quick but use more costly products, for example, **polish secures** that are fast to apply, but cost much more than a flick of nail art paint or a couple of blobs of **nail polish**. When booking their appointment, ask the client whether they have had the service before, and what nail art look they are considering.

Nail art can be time consuming but must be cost effective. If it costs too much this may be a barrier as it will only last a short time. Longevity is why gel and hybrid gel polishes are becoming increasingly popular. You must always be realistic in your pricing, ensuring that the most popular designs are quick to apply but will equally look stunning. The simplest designs are often the most effective and may appeal to a wider client base.

A website or social media are good places to share nail tips, comments about products, designs and any promotions.

If the client's natural nails are in poor condition it will be necessary to allow extra time to perform a simple nail treatment, to improve the nails' appearance, and facilitate application. Care must be taken if buffing is required to avoid thinning the nail plates. The client must be aware that it may take time for the nail products to harden.

ALWAYS REMEMBER

Consider how best to promote your nail art.

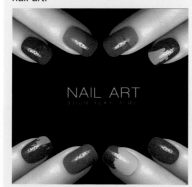

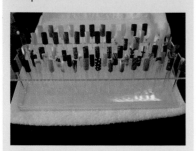
"Don't forget to display your creations at your nail station, so that your clients will see them. If clients don't know what you can do, they will never ask for it. Display artistic designs on colour wheels or colour pops. It is advisable to change your designs according to the seasonal colour schemes and latest colour arrivals by your brand.

Remember that nail art is an artistic skill and requires a little extra time for the appointment, hence it should be charged accordingly. It is normal practice to add at least 20 per cent extra to the total cost of the appointment."

Nataliya

ALWAYS REMEMBER

Minors

If the client is a minor under the age of 16, it is necessary to obtain parent, carer or guardian permission for the service. They will also have to be present when the service is received.

It is popular for salons to offer 'princess' pamper parties to minors where nail art is often applied in the form of glitter polish to the hands and feet. It is important to check the requirements of your insurance when treating minors. There is often a requirement to be checked by the Disclosure and Barring Service (DBS) when working with young children and vulnerable adults. In the UK many local authorities issue treatment licenses, supported by a code of practice for treating minors.

Commercial timing

Allow 30 minutes for nail art application.

Consultation

If a client expresses an interest in nail art, the next step is careful questioning. Find out at the consultation the client's likes and dislikes and how adventurous they are; do they have a specific idea for a design or are they prepared to allow you to choose and create the design? Make sure you understand what your client is saying and that you are clear about the degree of 'statement' they are interested in making with their nails. For example, a client usually known for their conservative taste in clothes and natural nails with sheer or delicate colours, who is interested in nail art for a special occasion, is only likely to be interested in a very subtle design. Alternatively, a client who likes to try out new ideas, such as the latest fashion trends, may be open to a more interesting suggestion such as embellishments or an unusual nail polish application technique.

Share prepared designs with the client. These may be applied to false nail tips or they may be images of nail art designs that you have created and photographed. On your display have designs in two or three colours to demonstrate that a design can be customised to suit the client and show how different colour combinations can change design appearance dramatically. Start the display with the simpler and less expensive designs and progress to the more elaborate and more involved designs.

Assess the condition of the client's nails and cuticles before the service. If the client's expectations are unsuitable because of the client's natural nail shape or size or condition of the nail, offer a suitable alternative. For example, if the client's nails are too short, if qualified, you could apply nail enhancement tips to the natural nail, blend and paint these. Decide upon the nail shape and length. It is important that the nail shape and length selected suits the client's hands and fingers. Refer to earlier in this chapter for further guidance on finger nail shapes and filing the nails of the hands and feet.

Contra-indications Whilst assessing the client's hands/feet you should be looking for any contra-indications to nail art. Contra-indications are the same as for any other nail service (see earlier in this chapter). If the client has a disease or disorder of the skin or nail it is in the interest of the client and beauty therapist not to proceed with the nail art service. Treating a client with a contra-indication may lead to cross-infection or a worsening of the client's condition. It is important to advise the client to seek medical advice to ensure a correct diagnosis and treatment for their condition. Some conditions will require restriction and adaption of the nail art service.

Contra-actions Certain cosmetic ingredients are known to cause allergic reactions in some people. These substances are known as allergens and may cause irritation, excessive erythema, inflammation and swelling. This is known as a contra-action and may occur during or following service.

The client may at any time develop an allergy to a nail art product that has been successfully used previously. This could be for a number of reasons, such as new medication being taken or illness. If an allergic reaction occurs, remove the product immediately and a soothing substance may be applied. This product should not be used again. See earlier in this chapter for more information on contra-actions.

As with all treatments/services, accurate client records must be kept. If the client has received nail art services before, consult their records and review the success and satisfaction of this with the client. Details of the products used should be recorded on the client service record. This is useful if the client returns for this service, also it is important in the event of a contra-action such as an allergic reaction.

> **HEALTH & SAFETY**
>
> **Avoiding a contra-action**
>
> Always check at the consultation for any known allergies to substances or ingredients. Always follow the manufacturer's instructions to ensure that products are used correctly and safely.

Preparation of the client

Ensure that the client is warm and comfortable when preparing them for their nail art service.

- Confirm the client's choice of nail art.
- File the nails to achieve the desired shape and length.
- The cuticles should be neat and trimmed and excess eponychium removed from the nail plate.

> **REVISION AID**
>
> How would you decide upon the recommended nail art for a client?

> **REVISION AID**
>
> What are the different nail shapes?

> **HEALTH & SAFETY**
>
> **Dealing with a contra-indication**
>
> Remember, never advise the client as to what the contra-indication may be; you are not qualified to do so. Always refer the client to their GP if you are at all unsure. Do not treat the client.

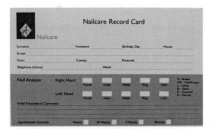

Nail service record

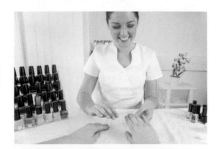

Following consultation confirm the client's choice of nail art finish that will suit their nails

> **TOP TIP**
>
> **Costing**
>
> When allowing for time in costing a design, use an average time that the design would take. Initially, when inexperienced, it will take you longer to achieve the finished nail art but you shouldn't be charging the client extra for that time.

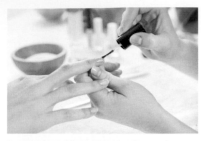

Application of base coat to ensure adhesion of the nail colour and prevent nail staining

◆ Ensure the surface of the nail plate and under the free edge are clean and grease-free.

◆ Wipe with polish remover or an alcohol such as isopropyl alcohol to prepare the nail. Use a lint-free pad as cotton wool may leave fibres, which may spoil the application of the nail polish/paint.

◆ Apply the required nail art base (usually a good quality base coat and the chosen base colour).

Basic nail art techniques

The basic techniques are easy! All that is required are ideas, a bit of imagination and the right products, tools and equipment. You also need to have an understanding of colour to mix colors, to select harmonious colours in a scheme and to suit skin tone.

Paints, if used, are different from nail polishes. They are usually water-based acrylic artist's paint, as this gives a very dense colour, can be mixed and is easier to use for fine detail. There are lots of effects that can be achieved with paints, a selection of nail art brushes and a marbling/dotting tool.

Nails need to be painted with a base colour that will be part of or enhance the finished design. This is usually a nail polish.

TOP TIP

Nail polish storage

Store nail polish stock in a cool, dark place to avoid separation and fading. Use good stock control, FIFO – First In, First Out, to ensure optimum quality of resources.

If exposed to light, most hybrid gel polishes will thicken. Carefully consider where to display and store your products for retail to avoid spoilage.

"Nail Art is all about colour. It is very important to learn and understand colour theory prior to offering nail art to your clients. Understanding colour will help you to identify the client's skin tone correctly and choose a method that would complement, neutralise or accessorise the client's skin tone. Learning colour theory is so much fun, in fact this is my favourite subject to teach. Nail artists must have a colour wheel in their kit; this will be your ultimate partner in choosing the colour schemes for your designs."

Nataliya

Decide if the skin colour is light, medium or dark. Then decide if is it warm or cool in tone. Skin can be neutral where it is hard to distinguish between the two, and has equal amounts of warm and cool.

Cool tones have blue and pink undertones, suiting cool toned shades.

Warm tones have yellow/orange or olive undertones, suiting warmer toned shades.

Neutral tones suit most colours.

If you divide the colour wheel, cool and warm colour shades can be seen.

The colour wheel shows the various colour combinations that can be created from the initial three primary colours, resulting in 12 main divisions.

When carrying out nail art you can select complementary colours which work well visually when placed together. These are the opposite colour on the wheel such as green and red.

There are three **primary** colours, these do not have any other colours mixed with them and are the colours blue, red and yellow.

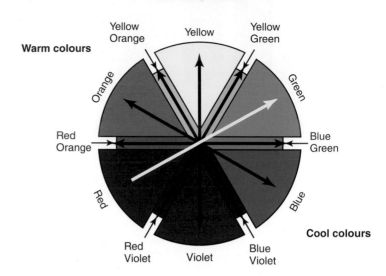

Primary and secondary colours

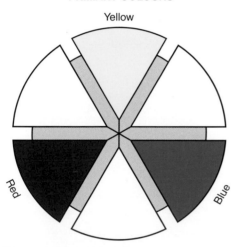

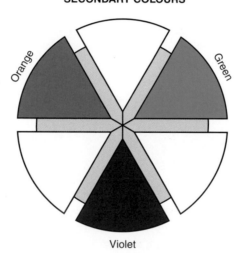

When two primary colours are mixed they form **secondary** colours, these are:

◆ green: a mix of blue and yellow

◆ orange: a mix of red and yellow

◆ violet: a mix of blue and red.

Primary colours can be mixed with secondary colours and form **tertiary** colours; these include:

◆ blue-green

◆ red-violet

◆ yellow-orange

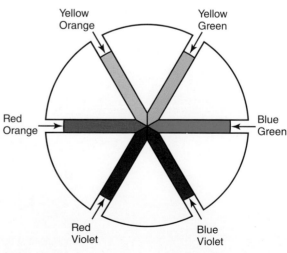

Tertiary colours

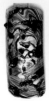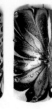

Designs using dotting and marbling techniques

Dotting and marbling technique Very simple but effective designs can be achieved by placing dots of colour. Use either a very small round brush or a 'marbling or dotting tool' to apply the dots. Care needs to be taken on the size and regularity of the dots as this can spoil a good design.

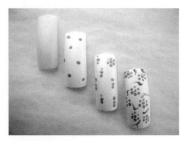
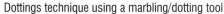

Dottings technique using a marbling/dotting tool

Steps: White base colour applied, yellow flower centres and blue flower petals applied with a dotting tool, finish design with green stems added with a short detailing brush.
Seal the finish with a top coat.

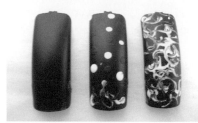

Marbling technique: Apply aubergine base colour, add two or more different coloured dots, red and white shown, with a dotting tool, swirl together to achieve a marbling effect

Striping technique A very long, thin brush referred to as a **striping** brush dipped in paint can achieve fine stripes and create quite sophisticated designs.

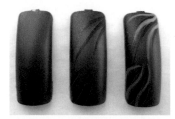

Striping technique
Steps: Purple base colour applied and stripes placed first in black, the brush is cleaned and then alternate pink stripes are applied using a striping brush.
Seal the finish with a top coat.

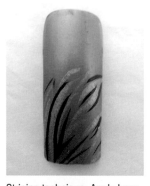

Striping technique: Apply base colour; using different diameter striping brushes, apply alternate colours to create the design

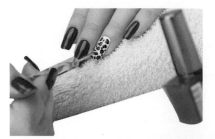

Abstract patterns or marbling can look stunning with a good choice of colour combinations. Flicking the colour from side to side with a fine brush or placing spots of colour on the nail and mixing them together with the marbling or dotting tool achieves this effect.

Application of dots of colour using a dotting tool to achieve a leopard-print effect. Following the application of a base colour, applied to the whole nail plate, a dotting tool is used to apply non-uniform colours of brown polish. The tool is then cleaned and irregular dots of red polish are placed with the brown polish, breaking its shape to achieve a leopard-print look.

Stencils Those who are not so good at hand painting designs can use stencils. The types that are readily available have a sticky back to keep them in place. These are applied to a dry nail and painted over. When the nail paint is completely dry they are removed, leaving the chosen design behind.

An easy example is to apply a sticky shape of the lunula to the nail and paint. When this stencil is removed this area is left free from polish. This can be left or filled in using an alternative colour as shown, with polish applied with a detail brush.

Freehand designs Pictures and designs of all sorts can be recreated and painted on the nail freehand with a steady hand, a good imagination or an easy picture to copy. (Most nail artists keep large numbers of pictures to copy onto a nail or just to give them inspiration to create an original design.)

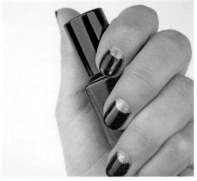

Lunula painted gold in contrast to rest of nail

"Arm yourself with plenty of ideas for artistic designs. Where to get ideas? Simply look around, you can see colour everywhere. We are surrounded by colour. I love getting my ideas from the shops – fruit and vegetable arrangements at the supermarket, fashion departments, fabric shops, fashion programmes on TV and the Internet are full of ideas, you just need to learn to see them. Choose colours that are enjoyable to wear and look at, so your designs are very well thought through and are pleasurable to look at."

Nataliya

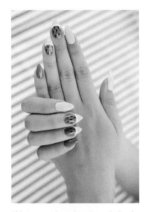

Water melon freehand design

A palette is required for this, it can be any plastic surface that can be easily cleaned. This can be used to place nail art paints on for use or mixing. Have a small water spray to hand then, if your paints start drying out, give a small spray of distilled water to keep them workable. Nail art paint is water-based and any mistakes can be easily removed with a wet nail wipe, or a cotton bud will remove a small part.

In all nail art, sealing the design is very important and, when the paint is dry, a sealer or top coat must be applied to fix the paint and also bring out the colour. The manufacturer's recommended sealer should be used, as some top coats may react to the paints. Clients should be advised to reseal the nails every couple of days to keep them fresh-looking and avoid any chips. This also provides a link selling opportunity.

Nail art brushes

There are many brushes specifically sold for nail art purposes but also remember that art shops sell many shapes and sizes too. A small collection of brushes is necessary for the nail artist in order to create a wide range of styles and these can be purchased relatively cheaply from suppliers and, with care, may last a long time.

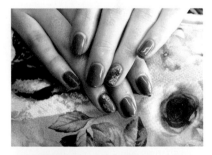

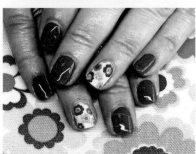

Hand painted flower designs

◆ *Detail brush*. This is the smallest brush and is used for hand painting details or placing dots.

◆ *Striping brushes*. These are available in different sizes. Their length and the number of hairs are relevant. A shorter brush with several hairs will produce lines that are thick. The longer and thinner the brush, the finer and longer the line they produce. It is worth having at least two of these: a medium one for lines and flicks and a very long one for fine stripes.

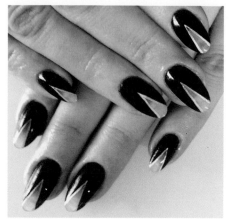
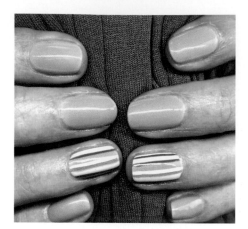

Designs using striping technique

"Nail Art requires tools; invest in good quality tools that will last a long time and become your partner in success. Research what is available. It is great to ask for advice from experienced nail artists. Take good care of your tools, clean them after every use and store them properly when not in use."

Nataliya

◆ *Flat brush*. This is a brush with a small flat head that can create several effects and is used to fill in colours. It can shade and smudge and create swirls.

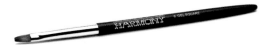

◆ *Fan brush*. This brush can create texture and blend colours together. It is probably not as versatile as the others but worth having.

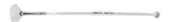

Foiling

Foiling is another very easy technique that uses various application techniques of specialised foil. This is almost instant nail art, as some foils have designs on them and just need applying to a painted nail.

◆ Nails should be painted before using foils. They can be painted with a base coat, but it is worth spending the extra time to paint a colour, as this will enhance the effect.

◆ Foils are supplied with a special adhesive that should be painted onto the nail in a very thin coat. The adhesive is usually white and needs to turn clear before the foil is applied; this takes a very short time. The foil is then applied to the tacky adhesive, pattern side uppermost, gently pressed onto the nail with either a finger or a cotton bud and the backing pulled off leaving the foil behind. It is not necessary to cut any foil from the roll, as it will only stick to where the adhesive is.

◆ This is an amazingly quick process that can have spectacular results. As the foil only sticks to where the adhesive has been applied, patterns or pictures can be drawn with the adhesive. The foil needs a special sealer, as most top coats will destroy the delicate layer. Several layers of sealer are also needed, as with all nail art, to keep it intact.

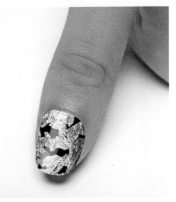

Foiled nail

Embellishments

Embellishment technique requires polish to secure the embellishment and design. They are often therefore referred to as polish secures. Many different products are available for this easy technique. Embellishment is the term for small stones or shapes with a flat back that are placed into the wet nail varnish and held secure when it dries. The products that fall into this category sometimes have different brand names. Most of them are available in different sizes and, although it depends on the design, the smaller versions are usually the most effective for durability.

ACTIVITY

Nail conditions

Identify the cause of the **nail conditions** below and what salon service and homecare/action you would recommend for a client who wished to receive nail art and to improve the appearance/condition of the nail.

◆ Pterygium.
◆ Onychopagy.
◆ Weak, dry, brittle and split nails.
◆ Hangnails.
◆ Longitudinal or horizontal ridges.
◆ Allergies to products.

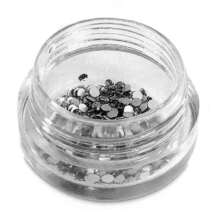

Square rhinestones

◆ *Rhinestones (or diamantes or crystals)*. These are clear or coloured stones that look like precious or semi-precious stones. They are usually made of glass or crystal and cut with facets to reflect light. They can be used to encrust a design or a throughfully placed single stone can bring a simple design to life. In relative terms they are more expensive and the designs using them should reflect this cost. Good quality rhinestones will not dull or lose their sparkle if sealed with a top coat and this will ensure they stay on the nail for the maximum time, especially if the client re-applies a top coat. Although stunning, even the smallest rhinestone stands quite proud from the nail.

◆ *Flat backed beads*. These, like rhinestones are usually coloured glass but they are rounded rather than cut with facets. Applied in the same way to wet polish, they look like beads on the nails.

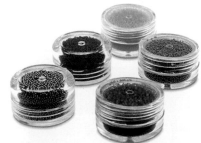

Flat back beads

◆ *Flat stones*. These are a less expensive version of rhinestones. As the name suggests, they are quite flat and usually very small, but they sparkle well. They can, however, lose their sparkle under a top coat. If this is the case, then apply a thicker layer of top coat than usual and push the stones into the wet polish. This should hold them in place without the need to seal them.

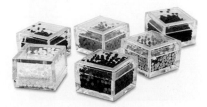

Flat stones

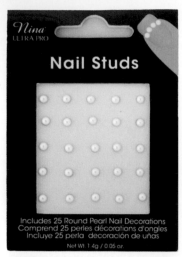

Pearls

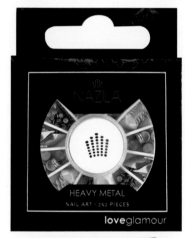

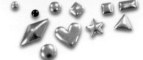

Stone shapes

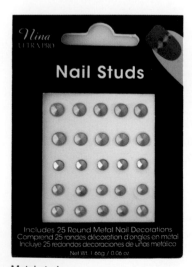

Metal studs

◆ *Pearls*. These are flat backed plastic shapes coloured to look like pearls. Although white is the obvious colour, they can be obtained in pastel colours, such as pink or lilac. They can look very pretty, especially in a design for a bride. Again, take account of their size.

◆ *Stone shapes*. Interesting shapes are available, such as a flower made of coloured glass.

◆ *Foil shapes*. These are tiny pieces of shiny or holographic plastic cut into different shapes that can look very effective incorporated into a design. The shapes may be circular, stars, moons, hexagons, even tiny hands and dolphins! These are applied in the same way, but care must be taken with the top coat. They need to be sealed, as edges that are not covered by top coat can catch and be pulled off, although some top coats have a solvent that is too strong. This will cause the colour to be affected and it will often streak.

◆ *Metal studs*. A very effective and less 'glitzy' polish secure are metal studs. These are available in gold or silver colours and different sizes.

◆ *Fimo canes*. These can be bought in ready cut or in long 'canes'. There is a vast variety of designs that can be laid on the nail once a very thin 'slice' has been cut. Some of these can be partially transparent.

◆ *Crushed shells*. These are available in many colours and can be applied as a base for other decorations to go on top or can be used alone or with colour variations. They have an opalescence that can look spectacular.

◆ *Dried flowers*. Various tiny dried real flowers and leaves are available and applied in the same way.

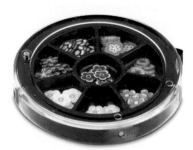

Fimo canes

Embellishment placement tool

After the base colour has been applied (or other design) a top coat or sealer must be painted onto the nail. While this is still wet, the 'embellishment' can be placed on it. The easiest way to pick up 'the embellishment' is with a wet cuticle stick, nail art tweezers or nail art tool such as a sticky pick, which makes picking up the tiny shapes easier.

When all the shapes have been placed, the whole nail needs to be sealed with a thick coat of sealer or top coat. Make sure your top coat does not affect the colour of the foil shapes.

Recommend to your client that they re-apply a top coat every two to three days to keep the design fresh and avoid damage to or loss of stones.

Nail art enhanced by embellishment

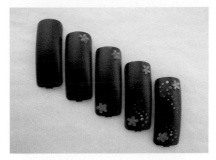

Dotting and flat stone embellishment

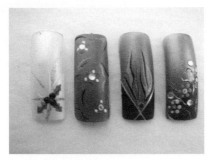

A range of nail art techniques enhanced with embellishment

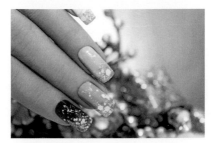

Glitter dust applied to the free edge with flat-shaped embellishments to create a snowflake effect

Embellishment design incorporating studs

REVISION AID

What is the purpose of a marbling tool?

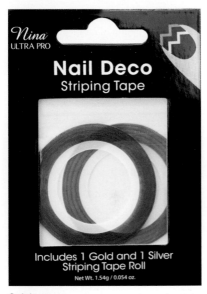

Striping tape

Glitter dusts

Glitter polishes and **glitter dusts** are a very versatile range of products to create or enhance nail art. Obviously, glitter can be applied to the whole nail, but it can also be used to make patterns or designs; a well-placed highlight on a painted or airbrushed design can make a simple piece of nail art spectacular. Make sure your loose glitter is of a cosmetic quality and the colour will not run with the top coat. Cosmetic glitter is plastic rather than metal.

◆ Glitter polishes can be painted straight from the bottle with either the brush supplied or a fine nail art brush. Glitter dusts can be used to create more specific designs by picking up the dust with a brush dipped in sealer, as this will give an effect that is denser than glitter polish. The dust will also stick to wet sealer, so the tip of a nail dipped into the pot will collect the dust on the tip only or where the sealer is wet.

◆ Like all nail art, glitter dusts need sealing. The sealer must be painted on thickly and gently to avoid moving the dust.

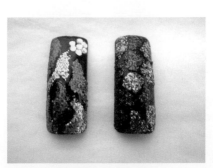

Designs using glitter dusts

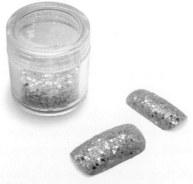

Glitter dust finish applied to nail tips

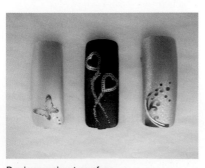

Designs using transfers

TOP TIP

Striping tape as a template

Use striping tape as a guide when placing products or embellishments where a straight line is required. Its sticky back can be easily removed when your design is dry.

"Photograph finished designs and use those to promote your business on your website or Facebook. The best advertisement is word of mouth, make your clients' nails stand out with beauty and fashion. Always give your clients a couple of extra business cards so they can recommend your services to their friends."

Nataliya

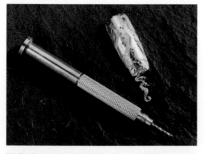

Nail piercing tool and nail pendant attached

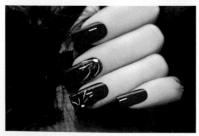

Nail art incorporating feather medium

Transfers and tapes

There are many **transfers** available to apply to nails. These are ready-made nail art and can be very effective. Some need to be soaked off their backing with water (place a few drops onto the backing paper to soak through and then the transfer slides off) or they peel off their backing and stick straight on to the nail.

Tapes are also available in many plain colours and patterns. They have a sticky back and must be placed on the nail and then trimmed with a small pair of very sharp scissors.

The nails are prepared with a base colour. The chosen transfer is applied following the manufacturer's instructions and then sealed.

Wraps

Wraps are available in many designs and textures. Wraps can be heat released material or self adhesive. The wrap is cut to the shape of the nail plate. On removal the chosen design transfers to the nail.

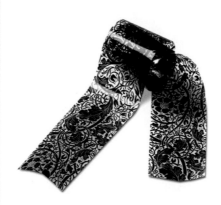

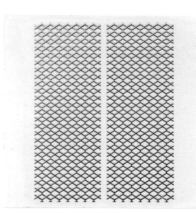

Foil sticker meche

Nail jewellery

Many different types of nail jewellery are available.

◆ Some of the designs are applied to the nail as an embellishment that is stuck to wet varnish or nail adhesive. These can only be very light and small. Larger designs can be applied to the nail with nail adhesive . Both of these are reusable, as they can be removed with nail varnish remover.

◆ Other types of nail jewellery involve making a small hole in the free edge of the nail. This can be done with ease using a specially made tool that has a very sharp but tiny drill. There is no problem at all when piercing an artificial nail, but care must be taken when piercing a natural nail:

◆ a natural nail should be strengthened with a coating of resin as used in a fibre system.

◆ the free edge must be long enough to provide a space for the hole without being too close to the hyponychium. If the hole is made on a nail that is too short the seal at the hyponychium could be damaged.

If a pendant has been applied, advise the client to remove it while dressing, doing housework, washing hair, etc., as it is possible to catch it and split the nail.

Having learnt the fundamental techniques of nail art, all the various techniques can often be incorporated into your design. Foil can be mixed with embellishments and paint mixed with glitter. The possibilities are endless and the only limit is imagination.

Water Marbling (Technique and images courtesy of Natash Lee, Divine by Design)

The water **marbling** technique is a quick and fun way to create very impressive designs. It produces an effect that would be very time-consuming if painted by hand and would not be as sharp. It can be a messy process but this method is quick and clean.

There is very little special equipment required:

Products, tools and equipment

◆ A variety of contrasting colours (avoid mixing creams, metallics and shimmers) including a very pale cream colour, e.g. white

◆ A dotting tool (or other sharp object, e.g. a cuticle stick)

◆ Cotton buds

◆ Cotton pads (plastic backed pads are more effective)

◆ Polish remover

◆ A small dish with a wide surface (e.g. a ramekin dish)

◆ Top coat

◆ A small stiff brush with square shape (optional)

STEP-BY-STEP: WATER MARBLING

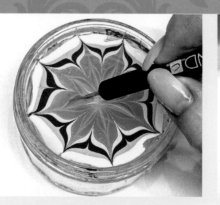
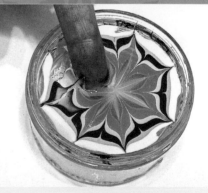

1 Prepare all your equipment. Fill the dish with room temperature water.

Paint the nails with a very pale colour (e.g. the white). Have the caps of all the bottles unscrewed.

2 Drop the white from the brush into the water. Follow with each of the colours, dropping each one into the middle until you are happy with the number of colours.

With a fine dotting tool, place it into the middle and draw it out so the polish touches the side of the dish. Repeat a few times around the circle.

Place your dotting tool between each line drawn into the colour next to the white (not the whole as that will break the pattern) and draw into the middle. This will give you a flower-like pattern.

3 Choose an area of the pattern you like and place the finger, nail side down, into the pattern, tip first and hold the finger there.

With a cotton bud, sweep around the water to pick up all the remaining pattern. When all the polish is cleared away lift out the finger.

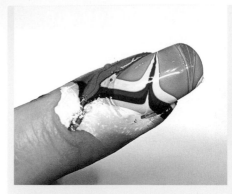

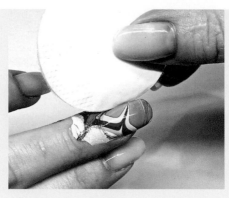

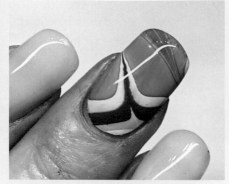

4 The nail (and some of the skin) will have the pattern on it.

With your dotting tool, run the tip around the base of the nail to break the polish seal, leaving the polish on the nail separate from that on the skin.

5 Soak your plastic backed cotton pad with polish remover.

With the plastic side against the nail, carefully remove the polish by the nail and the skin.

With your brush dipped in remover, carefully run it around the edges of the nail to tidy up the design. Repeat with the other fingers.

6 The finished design. Apply a top coat to give it shine.

Client advice and recommendations

Confirm with the client that the finished result is to their satisfaction. Complete details of the nail art service on the client record. Clear instructions should be provided on how to care for their nails and also what action to take in the event of a contra-action.

Aftercare advice will differ for each client according to their individual needs, but generally it will be as manicure/pedicure aftercare advice: see earlier in this chapter.

When giving aftercare advice, it is a good opportunity to recommend retail products, such as nail polish, hand cream or cuticle oil, thereby enhancing retail sales and the salon profits. It is a good idea to have the nail polish colours that you have used available for sale. The client can then touch up any accidental chips. Recommend the use of a top coat applied every three to four days to protect the nail art, increase its durability and impart shine if traditional nail polish has been used.

Nail art will last approximately five to 10 days with traditional polish, so recommend the client books their next appointment after this. Ideally, the client should return to the salon to have their nail art removed. However, nail art with traditional polish can usually be removed with nail polish remover. Care should be taken when removing embellishments and nail jewellery to avoid damage to the natural nail.

Contra-actions A contra-action is an unwanted reaction to the service and might include an allergic reaction. It is possible to become allergic to a product after having been in contact with it for years. The reaction would be recognised if the skin becomes red, itchy and inflamed.

Advise the client that if an allergic reaction occurs, all nail products should be removed and a cool compress and soothing agent applied to the skin to reduce redness and irritation.

A further contra-action is loss of a nail embellishment; follow your salon workplace policy on replacement.

Gel polish services

A further popular nail finish is gel polish, requiring curing through exposure to UV light. This creates a chemical reaction where the gel hardens, achieving a high gloss durable finish.

Key terms

◆ capping

◆ catalyst

◆ curing

◆ exothermic reaction

◆ inhibition layer

◆ monomers

◆ photo-initiators

◆ polymerisation

UV cured gel polish application as a nail finish saw a 35% growth rate between 2013 and 2015, according to new research by analysts at Mintel. Reasons for this increase in popularity varies, with women stating that gel polish outlasts regular polish (30% more durable), is worth the additional cost (18% more expensive), and makes the nails look thicker (16%).

ALWAYS REMEMBER

The development of non-UV cured gel polishes – long-lasting polishes

Innovation in the development of polish finish has seen a gel polish that provides durability (lasting up to 10 days), gloss and depth of colour without the need for UV curing. It already has gel polymers (chains of molecules) in the gel.

These are becoming a popular and convenient alternative choice for the consumer.

It is important that the client recognises the difference when a gel polish is applied and removed professionally and is willing to pay for this service.

The application technique differs according to the non-UV gel polish manufacturer, but may include the following stages and the requirement for exposure to natural light:

◆ Buff the nail plate gently to remove surface irregularities; this will enhance gel adherence. The hands are then cleansed to remove any surface debris.

◆ Apply the recommended preparatory base coat gel polish, which will enable the colour to adhere to the nail plate. Ensure that the free edge is sealed, or capped.

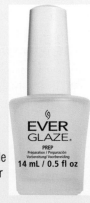

◆ Apply chosen gel polish, ensuring that the nail plate free edge is capped.

◆ Apply gel polish topcoat, often containing acrylic and shellac, which will seal the finish and prevent cosmetic damage such as chipping.

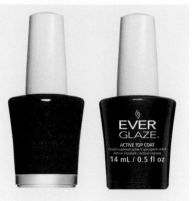

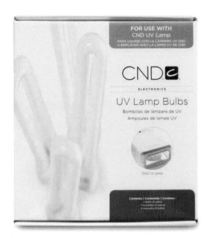

UV lamp bulbs

Traditional gel polish finish hardens when exposed to ultraviolet (UVA) light. Intensity of this UV light is affected by the wattage of the bulbs used in the lamp and is increased by the number of bulbs used in its design.

Chemicals in the gel called **photo-initiators** create a chemical reaction in the product on exposure to UV light. **Polymerisation** occurs, a chemical reaction that creates polymer chains (joined molecules) from **monomers** (smaller molecules). This results in **curing** or hardening of the product. This reaction occurs when exposed to UV light of a specific wavelength and intensity, which acts as a **catalyst** for polymerisation. Heat is produced during this process, called an **exothermic reaction**. Following curing, most gels have a sticky layer called the **inhibition layer** on the surface. This is uncured monomer, as a result of atmospheric oxygen and requires removal.

Each manufacturer designs its lamp to be compatible with their gel product. The wavelengths of UV lamps differ. LED lamps cure the product faster than traditional UV due to the intensity of its UVA wavelength exposure so this can be a benefit. It is important, however, that you comply with the manufacturer's curing instructions and recommendations at all times.

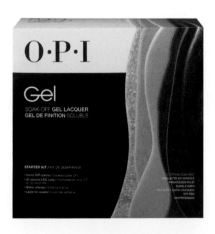

HEALTH & SAFETY

Curing

Always cure the gel polish for the correct length of time.

Check client comfort at all times and ask them to inform you if they can feel any heat or discomfort on the nail plate.

Benefits of gel polish

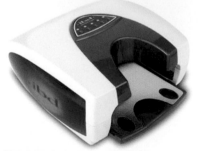

This light source is supplied by either a UV or Light Emitting Diode (LED) lamp

◆ Durability – it lasts up to 14 days therefore ideal for special events, e.g. holidays, weddings.

◆ Polish instantly sets through a process called curing, therefore more time efficient and convenient for the client.

◆ Nail designs are easily created with curing between each stage of the design.

◆ Clients don't smudge their nails following polish application!

◆ It can benefit fragile nails, as the gel provides strength and protection.

Disadvantages

◆ Removal soak-off technique takes longer than the removal of regular polish.

◆ Changing nail polish colour for the client is not as straightforward as regular polish.

◆ Maintenance is a necessity or nail damage may occur.

Anatomy and physiology

When performing gel polish services you are required to apply your knowledge as required for hand and foot services. This is found in the checklist in Chapter 2.

Products, tools and equipment

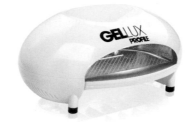
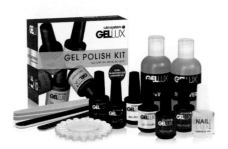

Safety and hygiene

◆ Maintain good ventilation to remove chemicals from the air. Poor ventilation may lead to eye, skin and respiratory irritation.

◆ Never treat clients with nails that are too fragile and may be harmed further through the process of gel application and removal. Offer manicures initially and nail-strengthening preparations.

◆ Gloves may be worn by the beauty therapist to avoid sensitisation and irritation from contact with the gel.

◆ Store gels in a cool, dark environment – exposure to light will cause product hardening. COSHH guidelines should be followed.

◆ Always secure caps on bottles/containers when not in use.

◆ Regularly clean the inside of the lamp with a dry cloth when switched off to ensure the bulbs are clean and will effectively and evenly emit UV light.

◆ Dispose of chemical solvents and remover pads in a sealed bag after each service.

Preparation of the area

Prepare the area as for nail services.

Position the nail workstation away from natural light that may spoil the product. An electrical supply will be required for the lamp. Ensure that there are no trailing wires, which could be a trip hazard.

Ventilation should be adequate.

Treatment information to provide to client at the initial point of interest

Allow approximately 35 minutes for application.

Allow approximately 20 minutes for removal.

Allow 55 minutes for removal and reapplication.

Inform the client that maintenance is a requirement and it is necessary for them to return to the salon in two to three weeks. This will depend upon the growth rate of the natural nail.

When a client makes an appointment for the service part of the consultation, check the nails and skin in the service area. Check the health of the nails and skin ensuring there is no infection or disease, which might present a contra-indication to treatment.

Contra-indications

Examples of contra-indications that **prevent** gel polish application include:

◆ bacterial infections termed pseudomonas (green between nail plate and gel overlay)

◆ paronychia

◆ fungal infections, e.g. onychomycosis, tinea pedis

◆ viral infections, e.g. verruca (feet), warts (hands)

◆ parasitic infection, e.g. scabies

◆ allergy to ingredients or subsequent allergic reactions – red, itchy, inflamed tissue

◆ broken skin in area

◆ onychia

◆ onycholysis

◆ onchocryptosis

◆ severe eczema, dermatitis, psoriasis.

Examples of contra-indications that **restrict** gel polish application include:

◆ minor eczema, dermatitis, psoriasis

◆ onychopagy (severely bitten nails); gel polish can be applied if there is sufficient nail plate and a manicure has been received in advance of the service application

◆ dry, overgrown cuticles; gel polish can be applied if a manicure has been received in advance of the service application and there is no sign of redness or inflammation following this

◆ broken bones; gel polish can be applied if the area can be avoided during service application

◆ cuts and abrasions; gel polish can be applied if the area can be avoided during service application.

Inform the client and be aware of contra-actions that may occur during or following gel polish application. These include the following:

Contra-actions

Allergic reaction Allergy can occur at any time for both the beauty therapist and the client. As there should be no contact with the skin, allergic reactions are less probable so care must be taken when applying the gel to avoid the skin. Allergy is recognised by redness, irritation, swelling, blisters and inflammation. Remove the product immediately in a professional manner. The client's record should be updated to record the reaction and the action taken. An alternative product may be trialled.

It is important to have a period where the nails are free from product. Discuss this with your client as part of the maintenance advice and then this can be planned for.

Shrinkage The polymerisation process results in some shrinkage. This can occur also if the product is too thick or the environment is too warm.

Lifting This may relate to poor preparation of the nail plate. The nail condition is too moist and requires dehydration; uneven application of the base coat, which should evenly cover the nail plate; curing is incomplete.

Cracking Poor preparation of the nail; trauma; product consistency is too thick, which may be associated with incorrect storage of products.

Peeling Ineffective preparation of the nail plate; incorrect product consistency if too thin or too thick; free edge not capped, enabling moisture to enter the finish; incorrect curing of product; contact of product with the skin at the borders.

Pitting Indentations appearing on the nail plate, often caused by poor preparation and removal technique where layers of the natural nail are removed also.

Heat sensitisation Exothermic chemical reaction occurs too quickly; this may happen when using incompatible products, or through incorrect application technique, affecting the curing rate. If the nails are thin, there is less resistance and the heat will be felt more quickly.

Trauma to the nail plate Poor nail preparation and removal technique, removing layers of the natural nail, resulting in areas of leuconychia (white spots), peeling, nail thinning and scratching of the nail plate; poor aftercare advice or client non-compliance with instructions.

Dullness of colour Ineffective preparation of the nail plate, which will affect curing; incomplete curing of each gel polish layer – allow the nails to cool slightly following final cure before removal of the inhibition layer; poor protection and care of the hands post service.

TOP TIP

Hand placement

Positioning of the hands/feet in the lamp is important to ensure that curing is adequate. Some lamps will have a position indicated in the lamp for each digit and thumb.

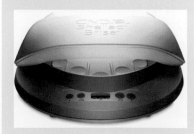

REVISION AID

What are the different nail shapes a client may have?

HEALTH & SAFETY

Record the condition of the client's nails

The condition of the nails will influence the application but is also important for reference when comes to removal. It is important that the client understands the importance of their care for the nails between services too.

Service modification – weak nails

Gel may be applied as a basecoat to provide strength for the nail, with the colour being applied later as the nail regains strength.

ALWAYS REMEMBER

Avoid immersing the hands and nails in water as this will hydrate the nails, which will affect adhesion as the nail later dries.

HEALTH & SAFETY

Use of cuticle tools

Care should be taken when using tools on the nail plate when preparing the nail for gel polish service, to avoid causing skin sensitivity and scratching the nail surface.

Preparation of the beauty therapist

PPE may be worn to protect the skin from contact with products.

Consultation and assessment techniques including post service

Assessment of the skin and nails should take into consideration:

◆ skin condition – dry, sensitive, allergic

◆ nail condition, e.g. bitten, dry, damaged from previous nail services and moist nail plates

◆ cuticle condition, e.g. dry, normal, overgrown, split, hangnails present

◆ nail shape and length; this will influence preparation requirements and choice of colour.

Explain the service outcomes, products and equipment used, and their effects and the expected sensations they might experience. If the client is unable to commit to homecare requirements then a regular manicure may be a preferred option using a hybrid gel style polish.

Preparation of the client

Position the client at the nail station and ensure that they are comfortable and their arm and wrist are supported.

The client's clothing should be protected against accidental contact with the products when applying or removing gel polish.

Clients should cleanse their hands thoroughly with an anti-bacterial skin preparation, including the nail plates. Surface oils, moisture and skin debris on the nails will affect gel polish adhesion and create lifting of the gel finish.

The nails are prepared by pushing back the cuticle with a cuticle pusher, removing excess cuticle and excess dry skin from around the nail plate, using cuticle nippers as required. Always follow the manufacturer's product guidance. The nails are then filed and shaped as agreed at the consultation. All debris should be removed from the nail plate, including the free edge, using the appropriate cleansing, dehydrating product. Drying the nail plates is essential; if the plates are moist this will affect the curing process.

Service application

Always follow the manufacturer's instructions when applying gel products.

Most UV gels are self-levelling, so time must be allowed for this to take place after the application.

A layer of gel base coat is applied using a traditional polish application technique, ensuring the layer provides a thin application of the gel. If the gel is too thick the UV will not effectively cure the polish. It will also be more difficult to remove. The polish should be placed close to the border of the nail plate without touching the skin – approximately 1mm.

A layer of gel is applied horizontally along the free edge, termed **capping**. This seals the gel and prevents moisture and debris getting between the gel and nail plate. This process is repeated to the nail plates of one hand.

The nails of the fingers are placed flat within the UV lamp and are exposed to the UV light for the required time as stated by the manufacturer. This is called curing. Most lamps will have a timer and the lamp will switch off after the allocated time. Some lamps accommodate all five fingers; others may require the thumb to be cured independently. Whilst curing is taking place you can repeat the process of base coat application to the other hand and cure as previously.

If using a block colour, a thin layer of the chosen colour is applied to each nail on the first hand. Again, cover the nail plate and cap the free edge. The colour may appear patchy, but avoid trying to correct this with a thicker application. A second colour application will address coverage issues. Cure for the required time, whilst applying colour to the second hand. Apply the second layer to both hands and cure as before.

Apply a gel top coat to the first hand, evenly covering the coloured polish. Cure for the required time and repeat for the second hand.

When the top coat is cured, saturate a cotton pad with gel cleanser, which removes the sticky surface referred to as the inhibition layer from each nail plate. Stroke the cotton pad over the nail plate of each finger and thumb from the base of the nail to the tip, avoiding getting the product on the skin.

Apply oil to the skin surrounding each nail plate and massage in. This will moisturise the skin and avoid the appearance of hang nails.

Toenails

The process is the same if treating the feet.

Clients should cleanse their feet thoroughly with an anti-bacterial skin preparation, including the nail plates. Surface oils and skin debris on the nails will affect gel polish adhesion and create lifting of the gel finish.

The free edge is shortened, neatly shaped straight across to prevent the formation of ingrowing toenails.

The cuticles are prepared and treated as per the hands following the manufacturer's product guidance.

Surface debris is removed from the nail plate.

Apply gel polish as per nails of the hands.

Colours

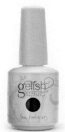

Dark colours

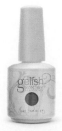

Light colours

ALWAYS REMEMBER

Avoid thick gel application

If the gel is too thick, curing may not be complete throughout, even when following manufacturers' curing timings. The client may also feel compelled to pick the thicker border of gel.

ALWAYS REMEMBER

Gel product consistency

Ensure the pigment in the gel product colour is evenly suspended through the product, shaking it gently before use.

ALWAYS REMEMBER

Colour removal

If colour comes off when removing the inhibition layer, the product is not cured sufficiently.

TOP TIP

Purchase of UV/LED lamp

When purchasing your lamp, consider how it is to be used. It is more time efficient to be able to place all the fingers and the thumb of one hand in the lamp.

Also, if performing pedicures, choose a lamp that will accommodate gel polish service to the toes.

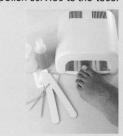

French

1   Apply base coat to the nail plate, cap the free edge and cure.

2   Apply a sheer colour in pink or light caramel to the nail plate and cap the free edge, then cure.

3   Apply a thin layer of white gel polish to the free edge, in depth and shape to suit the natural nail shape, length and size. To define the shape a detail gel brush may be used. Cure.

4   Apply top coat to the nail plate, cap the free edge and cure.

5   Remove the inhibition layer.

6   Condition the cuticle and surrounding skin.

Design

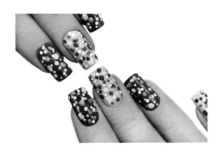

Gel polish can be used to create long-lasting, striking looks, personalised for your client. It may be applied to one or all nails.

A simple design is to apply Contrasting dots of colour applied using dotting tools of different diameters on a base colour and cured.

At the end of the service, update the service plan recording details of the service.

Removal

The client should wash their hands in an anti-bacterial agent before gel polish removal.

A professional hand disinfectant can then be applied.

The nail polish should be removed according to manufacturer's instructions. Some gels require that the surface is gently buffed to remove shine using a medium grit file to break the gel surface and enable penetration of the solvent.

Allow approximately 20 minutes for this service.

Removal using a bowl

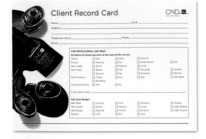

Update the client record following service

Prepare the nail surface by buffing if required. Place the client's fingers in bowls containing acetone or gel remover and allow to soak. There should only be sufficient liquid to cover the nail plate. A towel may be placed over the bowl to retain heat in the area, which will accelerate removal. Check the nails after the recommended time to see if the gel is breaking down.

After the required time the polish should have lifted ready for removal; remaining polish is gently lifted from the plate using the appropriate tool, such as a pointed cuticle stick, without damaging the nail plate, which is softened at this stage. It may be necessary to apply further gel polish remover or acetone for stubborn areas of polish still adhering to the nail.

Following removal, replenish moisture in the nail plate with the application of cuticle oil.

Removal using a foil wrap

Saturate a cotton wool pad with the gel polish remover (or pure acetone) and place on the nail, ensuring it extends over the free edge. Wrap with foil, folding the end over the finger, and leave for the recommended period, between 8 and 15 minutes.

The cotton pad enclosed in the foil is then squeezed against the nail plate, side to side, to soften the gel polish, and then the wrap is removed. The polish will have lifted ready for removal; remaining polish is removed as described previously.

Client advice and recommendations

◆ Clients must never pick at the nails. Inform them of the damage this will cause, which may prevent future application until the nail has improved.

◆ Avoid contact with extreme temperatures.

◆ The skin around the nails should be nourished regularly, e.g. daily with cuticle nail oil.

◆ Any damage that occurs should be fixed by the beauty therapist immediately, to avoid infection.

◆ It is important to have a period where the nails are free from product to enable nail hydration and avoid nail thinning through maintenance/removal technique. Discuss this with your client as part of the maintenance advice to plan for this.

◆ Up-sell other services in a package such as a 'holiday ready' package, which may include an exfoliation, leg wax or spray tan and gel polish to the hands and feet.

◆ Identify suitable retail products and their use, e.g. restorative nail products that help improve the condition of the natural nail plate.

◆ Every two to three weeks a maintenance service should be scheduled, where the gel polish product is removed and, if required, reapplied.

At this appointment any damage to the nail should be repaired, such as cracks or lifting.

The client's hands are cleaned and the health of the nails should be checked.

◆ At the time the client comes in for the gel nail polish to be removed, another short service may be offered and provided.

TOP TIP

Heat

Heat may be applied with some systems, which will increase the rate of removal.

The design of some prepared foil remover wraps ensures acetone remains in contact with the nail plate and heat is retained, speeding the action of gel breakdown.

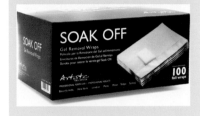

ASSESSMENT OF KNOWLEDGE AND UNDERSTANDING

Having covered the learning objectives for this chapter test what you need to know and understand by answering the following short questions below.

The information covers:

◆ Organisational and legal requirements

◆ How to work safely and effectively when performing manicure services

◆ Consult, plan and prepare for treatments with clients

◆ Contra-indications and contra-actions

◆ Anatomy and physiology

◆ Manicure services

◆ Pedicure services

◆ Nail finish

◆ advice and recommendations for clients

Organisational and legal requirements

For full legislation details, see Chapter 1.

1. What actions must be taken before a client under 16 years of age receives a nail service?

2. Taking into account health and safety hygiene requirements, provide five examples of how cross-infection can be avoided when carrying out nail services?

3. How should all client records be stored to comply with the Data Protection Act (1998)?

4. How long would you allow to complete a basic manicure treatment and a specialised manicure including a hand and nail treatment?

5. What is the commercially acceptable service time for a basic pedicure and a specialised pedicure including a foot and nail treatment?

6. Why is it important for staff to be familiar with the different nail service pricing structures?

7. What details should be recorded on the client's nail service record and why is it important to maintain up-to-date accurate records?

8. What is the cause of repetitive strain injury and how can this be avoided when performing nail services?

How to work safely and effectively when performing nail services

1. What personal protective equipment may be used when performing hand and feet nail services? Explain their purpose.

2. What are the symptoms of the skin disorder contact dermatitis and how can it be caused when performing nail services? What steps could you take to minimise the risk of developing contact dermatitis?

3. Why is it important that the client is warm and comfortable when receiving a nail service?

4. Why is good lighting important when carrying out nail services ?

5. Give **three** examples of tools and equipment that are sterilised and disinfected. What are the methods of disinfecting and sterilising used for the tools and equipment you have identified?

6. Personal presentation and hygiene are important to create a good impression. Give **three** examples of good personal presentation and hygiene practice which may be observed by the client.

7. Why is it important to complete your nail service in the allocated time?

8. How would you dispose of general and contaminated waste in connection with a manicure and pedicure service considering environmental best practice?

Consult, plan and prepare for treatments with clients

1. Communication is important. Give three examples of good communication techniques.

2. Why should the beauty therapist consult the client's record prior to each service?

3. How would you recognise each of the following, and what would you recommend to improve the appearance and condition of each:

   a. weak nails
   b. dry nails
   c. brittle nails
   d. ridged nails
   e. dry cuticles
   f. overgrown cuticles
   g. dry skin
   h. hard skin?

4. Why is it important to discuss and agree the service plan and outcomes with your client at the consultation?

5. Why should you record your client's responses to questions asked at consultation on the client's service plan?

6. Following the consultation what should be considered in the design of your service plan for a manicure/pedicure and nail art service?

Contra-indications and contra-actions

1. Name **three** contra-indications observed at consultation that would prevent a nail service being carried out.

2. What types of hand, feet and nail disorders would restrict treatment application?

3. Name three contra-actions that could occur during or following a manicure and pedicure service.

4. If you suspected a client had a contagious contra-indication what actions would you take for the welfare of the client, yourself and others?

5. Contra-indications are not always visible. How can you ensure the client's suitability for a nail service?

Anatomy and physiology

For full anatomy and physiology details, see Chapter 2.

1. How many bones form the hand? Name them.

2. Name the bones of the forearm.

3. Name the main arteries of the arm and hand.

4. Name two muscles of the hand.

5. What are the group of muscles called that bend the wrist, drawing it towards the forearm?

6. How many bones form the foot? Can you name them?

7. Name the bones of the lower leg.

8. Name the main arteries of the lower leg.

9. Name two muscles of the foot.

10. Name two muscles of the lower leg.

Hand, foot and nail treatments and services

1. Why would you choose to include the following hand, foot and nail treatments in your treatment plan:

   a. paraffin wax therapy
   b. hand/foot mask
   c. warm oil
   d. thermal mitts/booties
   e. exfoliators?

2. How can buffing improve the appearance of the natural nails? What product may be used with buffing to enhance its effectiveness?

3. Which tools are used to improve the appearance of the cuticles?

4. Describe how a cuticle knife should be used in order to avoid damage to the surface of the nail plate and cuticle.

5. If used incorrectly, cuticle remover can cause drying of the cuticle. Explain how this can occur and how this can be avoided.

6. What products applied to the cuticles help to prevent them from drying and splitting?

7. When filing the nail how is the shape of the client's free edge determined?

8. Why should the toenail be cut and filed straight across and not shaped at the corners?

9. Why are several treatments often necessary to improve the condition of the nails and skin to their full potential?

10. What are the differences in formulation and treatment benefits of the following massage mediums:

   a. cream
   b. oil?

11. How may you adapt your manicure service when treating a male client?

12. What are the terms used for the different types of massage techniques used in a nail service massage?

13. State **four** benefits of massage service.

Nail finish

1. How would you remove excess moisture and general debris created during the nail service/treatment from the natural nails before nail finish application?

2. What is the difference between a base coat and a top coat in terms of purpose and application technique?

3. What is the application technique to achieve a 'French Manicure' nail polish finish?

4. What nail finishes are available to the client? What would you consider when recommending the type of nail finish for a client?

5. If a client had very short nails, what nail shape and colour and type of polish would you suggest they chose and why?

6. Which nail polish product helps to reduce the appearance of ridges on the natural nail plate?

7. How is the natural nail prepared before a gel polish finish?

8. What is the equipment required to cure the gel polish and what happens to the gel product during the curing process?

9. If a client has their nails polished professionally, what would be the recommended time interval between

each service if using a UV cured gel polish and a regular nail polish?

10. Why is it a good idea to retail the nail polish colours used with the treatment?

11. What is the correct procedure for removing regular nail polish and UV cured gel polish?

12. Considering the nail art brushes and tools available select three and describe the techniques they may be used for.

Pedicure services

1. What is the purpose of the soaking medium usually added to the warm water to soak the client's feet?

2. Describe the methods available for removing hard skin from the feet.

3. How should the skin be left following hard skin removal?

4. Name **three** service products used in pedicure and their effect on the nail, cuticle or skin of the foot as applicable.

5. What modifications can you make when treating a male client for a pedicure?

6. How is the quantity and type of massage medium selected for each client?

7. How and why should massage be adapted for each client?

8. State **four** benefits of foot and leg massage.

Client advice and recommendations

1. What general advice should be given to a client on maintaining the condition and appearance and health of their natural nails following a manicure service?

2. When shaping the nails of the hands which side of the emery board should be used when filing the

natural nail shape? Why is it important to advise the client to avoid a sawing action when filing their nails?

3. List **three** retail products that you could recommend to a manicure and pedicure client.

4. For each of the clients below suggest a treatment routine. Detail the treatment plan to include: cause of the condition, aims of the treatment, products used, treatments recommended, relevant retail sales and aftercare advice.

   a. A hairdresser with very soft, weak, stained nails.

   b. An engineer with a bruised nail, overgrown cuticles and cracked skin on the fingers.

   c. A teenager who has badly bitten nails.

   d. An elderly client with strong, ridged nails and dry skin on the hands.

   e. A middle-aged retail worker who has very hard cracked skin on the soles of her feet around both heels.

   f. An elderly male client who has little movement in his ankle joints and slightly distorted joints in his toes.

   g. A pregnant woman who has tired, aching feet and swollen ankles.

8 Wax Depilation

LEARNING OBJECTIVES

This chapter covers how to provide wax depilation services. It covers the different wax depilation products and hair removal techniques that are used to remove unwanted hair growth to achieve an agreed result. You will learn more about:

◆ Wax depilation services to remove unwanted hair.

◆ The different techniques of wax depilation application and removal using hot and warm wax types.

◆ How to maintain safe effective methods when working, for both yourself and the client.

◆ The information that must be obtained at the consultation. This includes an assessment of the skin to be treated to check suitability and will incorporate skin sensitivity patch and thermal tests. The assessment results may mean the service needs to be modified to ensure it is suitable for the client and their welfare.

◆ How to prepare the client and body area for hair removal to ensure an effective final result with minimal discomfort.

◆ How to select the tools required, waxing products and methods of wax application and, hair

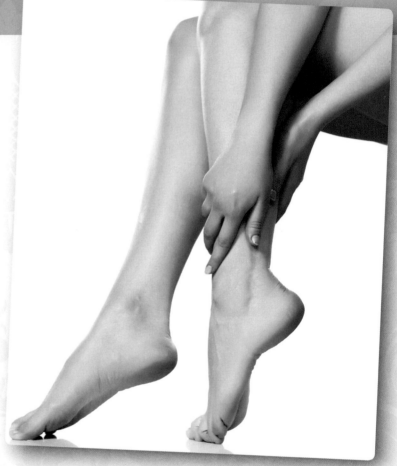

removal techniques that will best suit the client's skin and hair type to meet the service objectives.

◆ How to provide advice to the client and recommendations following service on any additional waxing products or services that will enhance the results achieved and maintain a healthy skin condition, or further products or services that you consider will be of benefit to them.

KEY TERMS

after-wax lotions

allergic reaction

bruising

cold wax

congenital hair growth

consultation

contra-action

contra-indication

disposable applicator

erythema

hair follicle

hair growth cycle
   (anagen, catagen and
   telogen)

hair removal techniques

histamine reaction

hot wax

ingrowing (hair growth)

pre-wax lotion

service areas

skin removal

skin sensitivity patch test

superfluous (hair)

systemic hair growth

terminal hair

thermal patch test

topical hair growth

vellus hair

warm wax

wax depilation

waxing products

WHEN PROVIDING WAXING SERVICES YOU WILL BE REQUIRED TO

◆ apply environmental and sustainable working practices

◆ follow relevant laws and manufacturers' instructions

◆ use different consultation and assessment techniques to correctly identify your client's needs

◆ use products, tools and equipment that will achieve the required results

◆ adapt and modify the service to meet the client's service and physiological requirements

◆ carry out the necessary on-going checks during the service to ensure client welfare

◆ take the necessary actions where a contra-action, contra-indication or service modification is required

◆ provide relevant advice and recommendations to support your client's service objectives.

INTRODUCTION

Hair removal is a popular service in the beauty salon for males and females, where both temporary and permanent methods of removal are often available. Wax depilation is a service used to temporarily remove facial and body hair. Areas for hair removal include the eyebrows, face (usually the upper lip and chin), forearms, underarms, legs (divided into the part being treated, such as a half or full leg) and for female clients the bikini line area (which involves removing hair growth that extends beyond a high-leg brief, around and underneath the upper thigh).

As wax depilation is a temporary hair removal method it must be repeated regularly, as hair re-grows. Temporary hair removal can be of benefit on areas such as the eyebrows where the shape and extent of hair growth can be influenced by fashion, and you will require the hair to regrow. Another benefit is that temporary hair removal is quick and instant!

Aftercare advice and recommendations form an important part of this service to promote skin healing and maintain healthy skin appearance and hair regrowth with the optimum period of hair-free skin. Health and safety are an important consideration when carrying out waxing services and guidance is available from your Local Authority, professional bodies, waxing manufacturers and Habia, which developed a best practice Waxing Code. Dealing with clients in a polite, efficient manner and using good communication and questioning skills to find out exactly what they require from the waxing service form an important part of this technical service.

INDUSTRY ROLE MODEL

ANNETTE CLOSE General Manager, Australian Bodycare UK Ltd

I trained in all aspects of beauty therapy and hairdressing, worked in salons for a couple of years then moved abroad and worked in spa therapy. When I returned to the UK, I opened my own salon, went back to college to do my teaching certificates, and worked as an examiner. Subsequently, I sold the salon and taught beauty therapy full-time in various colleges throughout Kent, working for adult education and implementing fully accredited beauty therapy and alternative therapy courses to adult learners.

From here I decided to change direction and applied to an international company as a UK development manager where I stayed for eight years and became the UK sales and marketing manager.

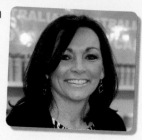

I was then approached by Australian Bodycare, and now, after ten years, have established a solid foundation for our brand throughout the UK, Ireland and Europe. As General Manager I am actively involved in new product development and research along with all the sales and marketing aspects, PR, and brand awareness. The job is challenging and rewarding and allows me to be creative, stay in touch with therapists at student and salon level and exercise management skills all in one role.

INDUSTRY ROLE MODEL

ANDY ROUILLARD Owner of Axiom Bodyworks (male grooming salon) and Axiom Wax Academy (training school)

I became involved in the beauty world almost by accident: while working as a massage therapist, an increasing number of my male clients started asking for hair removal treatments. At the time there were very few places in the UK offering grooming treatments for men so I took up the mantle and trained in waxing before going on to complete my full beauty therapy NVQ. I joined forces with a local barbershop to open a one-stop male grooming centre in Hampshire, providing skincare, massage and holistic treatments for guys alongside traditional hairdressing services.

Hair removal is still our most popular treatment. Some clients travel over an hour just to get their monthly defuzzing. I also

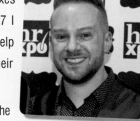

work with a leading international wax brand, developing new waxes and skincare products. In 2007 I opened a training school to help fellow therapists advance their hair removal skills.

My work takes me all over the UK and further afield, speaking at industry events, writing for magazines and demonstrating the art of waxing across the globe. It is tremendously rewarding to work in an industry that is all about helping customers to look and feel their best.

TOP TIP

Importance of client waxing recommendations

Waxing service offers a high profit margin. It is also a service where it is important to get it right. Clients will wish to receive this service all year round and industry expert Annette Close, general manager for waxing brand Australian Bodycare, says, "most salons tell us waxing makes up between 30–40% of their business".

It has also been found that a waxing service is most likely to be recommended by word of mouth. BABTAC surveyed more than 2000 beauty treatment clients and found that 68% would recommend a beauty therapist following a good waxing treatment.

Development of your waxing skills

Areas requiring hair removal such as 'intimate waxing' are advanced techniques and can be studied when you are skilled and competent with the delivery of Level 2 waxing services. It is important only to carry out hair removal in your area of competence; your insurance is likely to be invalid if this is not complied with.

Keep up-to-date with all the industry developments that take place with wax depilation hair removal products and systems. Courses for professional updating of skills are often advertised through professional bodies and Habia.

Wax removal products

Wax products differ as they are formulated to suit the treatment requirements for different skin and hair types. Some wax types set, contracting around the hair as they harden, being especially suited for the removal of strong terminal hair the coarse hair type found when treating the underarm and bikini areas. Others stay pliable whilst contracting and remain as a sticky residue on the skin, usually requiring a strip to remove the wax from the skin and embedded hair from the hair follicle.

Non-setting warm wax heated in and dispensed from a cartridge

Hot wax pellets melt, becoming liquid when heated and then harden on cooling

Transferable knowledge, understanding and skills

When providing wax depilation services it is important to use the skills you have learnt in the following chapters:

◆ The Business of Beauty Therapy (Chapter 1)

◆ The Science of Beauty Therapy (Chapter 2)

◆ Consultation Practice and Techniques (Chapter 3)

◆ Eyelash and Eyebrow Treatments (Chapter 5)

Anatomy and physiology

When performing wax depilation you need to apply your knowledge of the structure and function of the skin, including:

◆ identifying skin characteristics

◆ the structure and function of the hair

◆ the different types of hair growth

◆ the basic principles of the hair growth cycle.

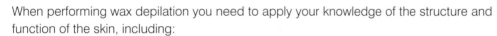

Hair removal methods

Hair removal services carried out are either temporary or permanent. With temporary methods of hair removal the service is repeated where as permanent methods aim to destroy the parts of the hair follicle that produce the hair. Different methods of temporary and permanent hair removal methods are discussed.

Temporary methods of hair removal

Depilatory waxing Wax depilation, using a warm or hot wax, involves applying wax to the service area and embedding the unwanted hairs in it. When the wax is removed from the skin in the area, all the visible hairs in the area, both vellus and terminal, are removed at their roots from the hair follicle, so the regrowth is of completely new hairs with soft, fine-tapered tips. They grow again in approximately four weeks, depending upon the stage of the client's hair growth cycle, hair type and area treated.

The necessary anatomy and physiology knowledge for this unit is listed on the checklist in CHAPTER 2. There are also questions at the end of the chapter to check your knowledge and understanding.

REVISION AID

What are the three stages of the hair growth cycle?

ALWAYS REMEMBER

Vellus and terminal hair type

When waxing the area it is usually the terminal hair the client wishes to be removed, waxing will remove the vellus hair type also.

Vellus: fine, downy hair found on the face and body, often unpigmented.

Terminal: longer, coarser hair, usually pigmented.

Please see CHAPTER 5 Eyelash and Eyebrow Treatments for more information on temporary eyebrow hair removal method using tweezers.

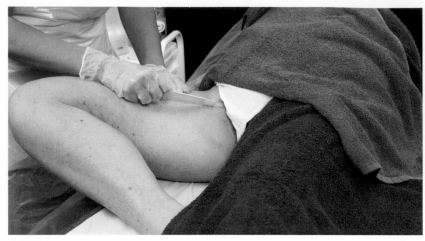

Bikini line wax service using warm wax, spatula method

Tweezing Tweezing or plucking uses a pair of tweezers to remove the hair from the hair follicle. Tweezers grasp the hair near the surface of the skin, and the hair is then removed or plucked in the direction of growth, again removing it at its root from the hair follicle. The hair grows again in approximately four weeks, depending on hair type, growth and area treated.

Due to the sensitive nature of the skin in the eye area, tweezing is often considered a suitable choice for temporary hair removal from the eyebrows.

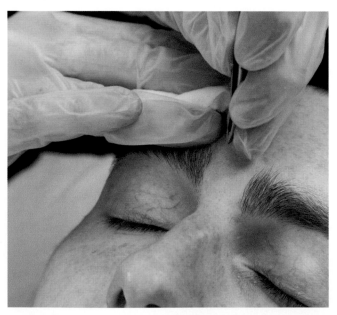

Tweezing hair following eyebrow wax hair removal

Tweezing may be used after waxing to remove hairs that are too short for the wax to remove or to remove specific hairs, e.g. to define the final brow shape following eyebrow wax removal.

Threading Threading involves the use of a thread of twisted cotton, which is rolled over the area from which the hair is to be removed: the hairs catch in the cotton, and are pulled out from the hair follicle. See Chapter 5 for more information on this hair removal method. Hair regrowth can appear again in four weeks depending on hair type, growth and area treated.

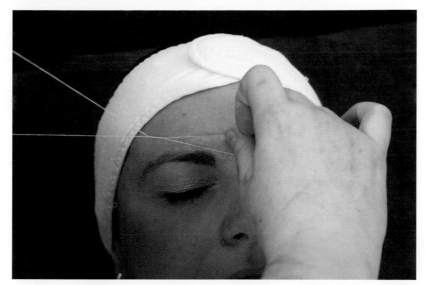

Threading method eyebrow hair removal, defining the shape above the brows

Waxing, tweezing and threading remove the entire hair, including the visible hair above the skin's surface (the hair shaft) and the part that cannot be seen below in the hair follicle.

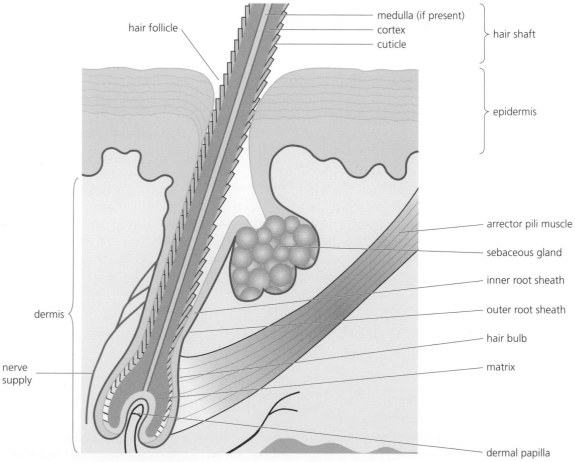

Skin cross section of the hair in its follicle

ALWAYS REMEMBER

Eyebrow shaping (choice of shape)

When carrying out eyebrow hair removal using the wax depilation method refer to Chapter 5 to inform you of eyebrow-shaping procedures to consider to ensure that the finished brow shape will be to the client's satisfaction.

Please see **CHAPTER 5** for more information on threading hair removal technique to shape the brows. Facial threading hair removal is discussed later in this chapter.

Other temporary methods of hair removal

There are also other methods of temporary hair removal that the client may have previously used.

At the **consultation** it is important to find out which method of hair removal the client has previously used and discuss the suitability of each. If the client chooses to replace these with wax depilation, the temporary methods discussed below should stop being used unless recommended by the beauty therapist.

◆ *Cutting the hairs with scissors* Scissors are used to trim the hair close to the skin's surface. This does not affect hair growth as only the dead hair above the skin's surface, the hair shaft, is removed. The hair, however, is left with a blunt end and feels stubbly. This leaves the skin hair free for a very short time, usually only one to two days, dependent upon the client's hair growth.

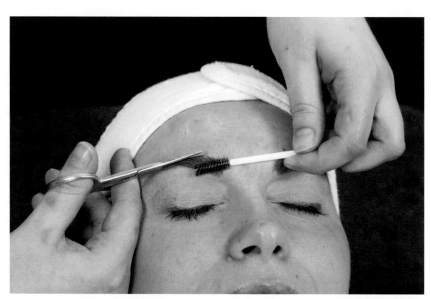

Cutting eyebrow hair with scissors

◆ *Shaving* A razor blade is stroked over the skin, against the natural hair growth after the skin has been prepared with a suitable skin lubricant such as shaving foam or oil. This removes the hair at the skin's surface. This leaves the skin hair free for a very short time, usually only one to two days, depending upon the client's hair growth rate. The hair feels sharp as it grows because the hair is left with a blunt end. Shaving is unsuitable for sensitive, thinner areas of skin such as the eyebrow area. Accidental damage to the skin can result in skin scarring.

◆ *Depilatory cream* A chemical reaction occurs between ingredients contained in the cream, such as potassium thioglycollate and calcium hydroxide.

This breaks down the protein bonds that give hair its structure. The cream is applied to the hair and then removed following manufacturers' instructions, usually after five to ten minutes. The hair will have been dissolved at the skin's surface.

As the chemical is strong enough to dissolve the hair protein keratin, it can sometimes cause skin irritation because the skin also contains keratin. Hair can reappear in two to four days depending on the hair growth rate.

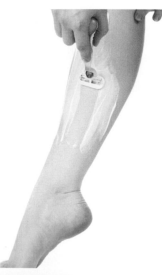

Shaving leg hair

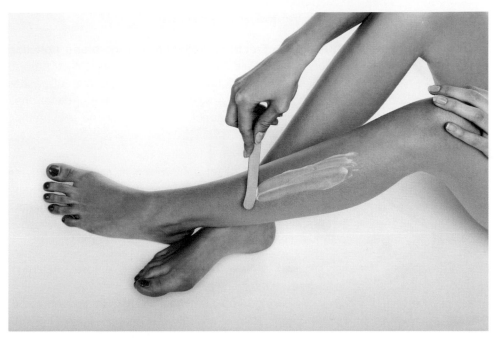

Depilatory cream application to leg hair

◆ **Abrasive mitt** An abrasive glove is rubbed against the skin and the hair is broken off at the skin's surface. The result and its effectiveness are similar to shaving and is unsuitable for a sensitive skin as the skin can become reddened quickly and becomes further sensitised. Hair can reappear in one to three days depending on hair growth rate.

◆ **Electrical depilatory** An electrical hand-held device performs the action of mass tweezing. As the device is moved over the skin's surface, hairs are grasped and removed. This method does not take into account direction of hair growth and can be problematic when the hair regrows. It may lead to distortion of the hair follicle, which affects how the hair is positioned when it grows back. Hair breakage and **ingrowing hairs** may also occur. Hair can appear again in three to four weeks depending on hair growth rate.

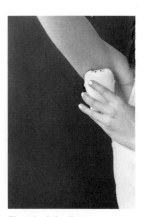

Electrical depilatory

ACTIVITY

Methods of temporary hair removal

As well as the professional use of depilatory waxing, threading and tweezing, other methods of temporary hair removal include the home use of tweezing, **cold wax** using ready-waxed strips, electrical depilatory devices, chemical depilatory creams, shaving and pumice powder. Find out the effect of each on the actual hair in its follicle. Are there any risks associated with each method?

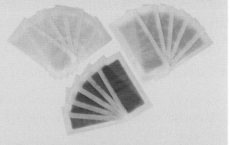

Cold depilatory wax strips popular for client home use

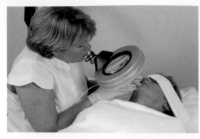

Electrical epilation

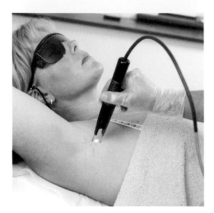

Laser hair removal

Permanent methods of hair removal

Electrical current methods Electrical epilation and the **blend epilation technique** are techniques that use an electrical current. The current is passed to the hair root via a fine needle inserted into the **hair follicle**. The current causes destruction of the hair follicle, affecting hair regrowth and resulting in permanent hair removal. Depending on hair growth, several treatments may be required until the hair is permanently removed.

Light-based hair reduction The use of light, which is absorbed into the melanin in the skin and hair, is converted to heat. This damages the target area, stopping the activity of the hair follicle. Generally this type of hair removal is most effective for dark hair as the more melanin that is present, the more destruction occurs. It is less effective on blonde or white hair. Hair removal is permanent.

Several treatments are often required to achieve permanent hair removal. Treatment timing will depend on the coarseness of the hair type and the size of the hair follicle. It is most effective when the hair is in the **anagen** (growth) stage of the **hair growth cycle**. Subsequent treatments therefore target different hairs in their anagen stage of growth until all hairs cease to grow.

The client needs to understand that the hair will never grow back if effectively treated with any of the above permanent methods. This is an important consideration, especially when treating an area such as the brow hair, as the desired shape and thickness of the brows change frequently under the influence of fashion.

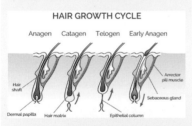
Hair regrowth following temporary methods of hair removal

Because of the cyclical nature of hair growth and the fact that follicles will be at different stages of their growth cycle when the hair is removed, the hair will not all grow back at the same time. Waxing, along with threading and tweezing, can therefore appear to reduce the *quantity of* hair growth. This is not so, however, and the hair will all grow back eventually: this is why waxing is termed as a temporary form of hair removal. Occasionally hair regrowth will increase, which is not a normal reaction and may be related to medication being taken or the medical health of the client. That is why it is important to carry out a thorough consultation before waxing service is provided. Waxing may be considered unsuitable as a hair removal method in this instance.

Nevertheless, certain bodily changes (such as ageing), when *combined* with waxing, can result in permanent hair removal. This effect is so erratic and unpredictable, though, that waxing cannot reliably be sold as a permanent method of hair removal.

Products, tools and equipment

Before beginning the waxing service, check that you have the necessary products, tools and equipment to hand and that they meet legal hygiene and industry requirements for waxing services.

Basic equipment

Each wax depilation work area should have the following basic equipment listed on next page.

Products, tools and equipment

◆ **Couch** With sit-up and lie-down positions and an easy-to-clean impermeable surface.

◆ **Trolley** To hold all the necessary products, tools and equipment.

◆ **Cotton wool** For cleaning equipment and applying various skin soothing/cleansing preparations.

◆ **Disposable paper tissues** (white) For blotting skin dry and protecting the client's clothing in the area.

◆ **Protective plastic couch cover** A durable covering that can be cleaned with a disinfectant agent before each client service. It is then covered with disposable tissue roll.

◆ **Disposable paper tissue couch roll** Placed over the couch cover prior to each service to prevent the client sticking to the couch cover and for reasons of hygiene.

◆ **Towels** (medium-sized) For draping over the client and providing modesty.

◆ **Disposable briefs** These may be provided for the client when carrying out bikini line waxing.

◆ **Head band** To protect the hair when carrying out waxing service to the face.

◆ **Disposable wooden spatulas** (a selection of differing sizes) For use on different body areas.

◆ **Tweezers** Sterilised, for removing stray hairs following wax depilation or defining the brow shape following a brow waxing service.

◆ **Small scissors** For trimming over-long hairs, and in the event that hairs in different growth patterns become stuck.

◆ **Disinfecting solution** In which to immerse all sterile small metal tools following sterilisation in the autoclave. This must be changed regularly as stated in manufacturer's instructions.

◆ **Wax solvent commercial cleaner** Designed for cleaning waxing equipment to remove waxy residue.

◆ **Hand disinfectant gel** To clean hands before each waxing service.

◆ **Single-use disposable non-latex (synthetic) powder-free gloves** To comply with Personal Protective Equipment (PPE) at Work regulations and ensure a high standard of hygiene and to reduce the possibility of contamination.

◆ **Disposable apron** To comply with Personal Protective Equipment (PPE) at Work regulations, protect work wear from spillages and for hygiene.

◆ **Waste container** This should be a lined metal bin with a lid. Specific disposable bags may be required for contaminated waste.

◆ **Mirror** (clean) For facial waxing treatments.

◆ **Magnifying lamp** To provide additional assistance when observing the area of hair removal.

◆ **Wax-removal strips** Thick enough that the wax does not soak through, but flexible enough for ease of work. These strips should be cut to size and placed ready in a container. Alternatively they may be purchased in different sizes, according to the size of area being treated. These may be paper or muslin.

◆ **Skin thermal test applicators** To hold both hot and cold water.

◆ **Anti-bacterial skin cleanser** (Also known as **pre-wax lotion**) or professional antiseptic wipes.

◆ **Wax heater** With a thermostatic control. Wax heaters are referred to with further waxing systems.

◆ **Pre-depilation powder** Or alternative talc-free powder formulation to avoid allergic responses in some clients. To absorb body perspiration and oil on the skin's surface, and to facilitate hair removal.

◆ **Pre-depilation oil** Conditions the skin before wax application, helps the wax to adhere to the area, facilitating hair removal. The use of such an oil will be advised by the wax manufacturer.

◆ **Wax depilation products** A choice of warm and hot wax with ingredients to suit different skin types and conditions and hair types.

◆ **Petroleum jelly** This may be applied to hair that is not to be removed, as it will prevent wax adherence.

◆ **After-wax lotion** With soothing, healing and antiseptic qualities.

◆ **Mirror** To consult with the client before, during and after their service when performing eyebrow and facial waxing.

◆ **Wax cleaner** For removing accidental spillages of wax, and wax from the work area, equipment and tools such as tweezers. Manufacturer's instructions must be followed for safe use and storage.

◆ **Client record** Confidential card recording details of each client registered at the salon to record the client's personal details, products used and details of the service.

◆ **List of contra-indications** To discuss with client prior to treatment.

◆ **Aftercare leaflets** Recommended information and advice for the client to refer to following service.

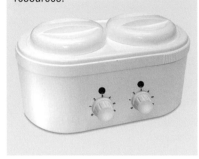

Types of wax

There is a broad range of waxes available. This means you can select a wax for the client, so personalising their treatment.

When choosing a hair removal waxing product, select one with the following qualities:

◆ It should be easy to remove from work surfaces and equipment.

◆ It should be able to efficiently remove short, strong hairs (2.5 mm).

◆ It should have a pleasant fragrance or no smell.

◆ It should not stick to the skin, but only to the hair.

◆ A low melting temperature is beneficial as it reduces post-treatment redness.

Wherever possible, it should be suitable for all skin types, including sensitive skin, and all facial and body areas; however, it is common to have different **waxing products** to suit the removal of different hair strengths.

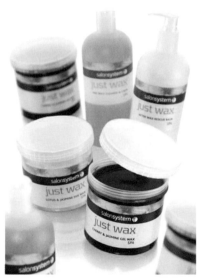

Warm wax

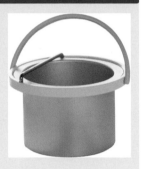

Warm wax This first became available in 1975 and is now the market leader for hair removal. It is clean and easy to use.

Warm wax is used at a low temperature, around 43°C, so there is little risk of skin burning, and in less sensitive areas the wax can be reapplied once or even twice if necessary.

Warm wax does not set but remains soft at body temperature. It adheres efficiently to hairs and is quick to use; service is relatively pain-free. It can remove even very short hairs (2.5 mm) from legs, arms, underarms, the bikini line, the torso, the face and the neck.

Warm waxes are frequently made of mixtures of glucose syrup, resin to help the wax stick, oil to help removal (e.g. almond oil), water and fragrances. Honey (fructose syrup) can be used instead of glucose syrup and this formulation is often called honey wax. Zinc oxide is added to cream wax to provide an opaque colour. This type of warm wax is capable of providing a thin, liquid consistency at lower temperatures making it less sensitising to the skin. Gel waxes contain synthetic hydrocarbon resin such as polycyclopentadiene, which leaves the skin less sticky. These are easy to colour and a great choice of waxes from mint chocolate to pina colada colour and fragrance have been developed.

Hot wax This takes longer to heat than warm wax, and is relatively slow to use, taking approximately double the time of a warm waxing. This time reduces when skill is attained.

As **hot wax** is used at quite a high temperature, 50°C, extra care must be taken to avoid accidental **burns**. Because of this risk, hot wax cannot be reapplied to already treated areas.

Hot wax cools on contact with the skin. It contracts around the hair shaft, gripping it firmly. This makes it ideal for use on stronger, short hairs.

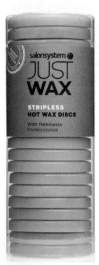

Hot wax discs

Hot waxes for hair removal need to be a blend of waxes and resins so that they stay reasonably flexible when cool. **Beeswax** is a desirable ingredient, and often comprises 25–60 per cent of the finished product.

Cetiol, azulene and vitamin E are often added to wax preparations to soothe the skin and minimise possible skin reactions.

In addition to wax, new generation peelable waxes are increasingly used which have a lower melting point due to the use of microcrystalline, a fine grained crystal structure which increases their flexibility and reduces skin irritation, whilst being effective when removing terminal hair.

HEALTH & SAFETY

Sensitive skin

Increasingly products are being formulated which contain only natural ingredients which can reduce skin irritation. Ingredients include sugar and plant extracts such as chamomile and lavender to soothe the skin.

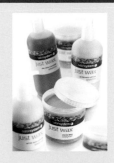

ACTIVITY

Wax heaters

Research using current beauty trade magazines, online manufacturer suppliers, visiting wholesale suppliers or tradeshows for at least five different types of wax heater and applicators. Where possible see demonstrations of them working. Discuss their suitability, considering size, cleaning practicalities, safety, hygiene and any other points that you think are important. Which heater would you choose out of preference, and why?

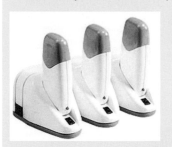
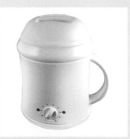
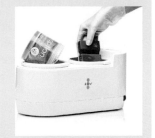

REVISION AID

What is the difference between removing hair with wax depilation and threading method?

TOP TIP

After-wax lotion

After-wax lotions reduce redness and promote skin healing. They contain ingredients such as tea tree oil, aloe vera, azulene and witch hazel to soothe, calm and reduce the possibility of secondary infection. These are an ideal retail product to recommend to your client to ensure effective skin healing and to reduce the possibility of the formation of pustules and folliculitis.

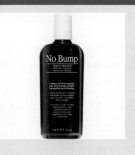

HEALTH & SAFETY

Personal Protective Equipment Act (PPE) at Work Regulations (2002)

Waxing is a service where there is a risk of contamination and cross-infection, therefore protective equipment such as gloves and an apron should be available and worn.

TOP TIP

Wax collars

Disposable collars may be applied at the neck of the wax heater to prevent spillages, and to provide a professional appearance in the work area.

ACTIVITY

Safe storage of related products

List and state how should products used in the waxing service be stored?

ACTIVITY

Electrical testing

How can you ensure that your wax heater is safe to use? What checks should you make before use?

How can you ensure you comply with the Electricity at Work Regulations (1989)?

Safety and hygiene

Ensure all relevant **skin sensitivity patch tests** are completed in advance to avoid allergic reactions. The plastic-covered couch should be clean, having previously been washed with hot water and detergent and wiped thoroughly with a disinfectant that is bactericidal, fungicidal and virucidal. The use of an additional heavy-duty plastic sheet is recommended: this is easier to wipe than the couch, and can be replaced if damaged.

All surfaces must be disinfected after thorough cleaning between services.

The couch should then be covered and protected with a disposable paper tissue couch roll. Place a towel(s) neatly on the couch, ready to protect the client's clothing and to cover them when they have undressed. These tend to be of a medium size as large towels can make the client too warm. The tissue should be disposed of after use, and the towel freshly laundered for each client.

Check all electrical safety precautions have been followed; examples include ensuring water is not placed next to electrical equipment and avoiding trailing wires.

Heat the wax to its optimum temperature as guided by the manufacturer's instructions. Test wax temperature before use on yourself and client to avoid thermal burns and to check consistency of wax.

Use the correct wax and technique for the body area to avoid potential **contra-actions**.

Disposable waste from waxing may have body fluids on it: potentially it is a health risk. It must be handled, collected and disposed of according to the local environmental health regulations. It is a requirement to wear disposable gloves while carrying out bikini line and underarm wax services, to protect yourself from body fluids and the client from contamination. These too should be disposed of after each waxing service.

ALWAYS REMEMBER

Waxing service legal requirements

Habia have provided a best practice Code of Practice for Waxing. This should be referred to ensuring that you are complying with your responsibilities under relevant health and safety related to the service. Also refer to manufacturers' instructions and local council guidelines. If you are a member of a professional organisation they too will keep you up-to-date with best practice guidelines. Website: www.habia.org

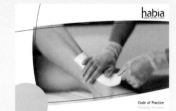

Habia Code of Practice for Waxing

Wash your hands regularly with antibacterial soap, before and after preparing the work area and before application of the disposable gloves. This shows the client that you have a high standard of hygiene.

HEALTH & SAFETY

Avoiding cross-infection

Never filter hot wax after use: it cannot be used again as it will be contaminated with skin cells, tissue fluid and perhaps even blood.

HEALTH & SAFETY

Contaminated waste

Any wax waste that contains bodily fluids should be bagged separately from other regular waste and special arrangements made for its disposal by a registered waste carrier in an approved incinerator in accordance with the Local Authority Waste Regulations legislation.

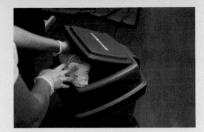

Disposal of waxing waste

This may include spatulas, wax strips and wax waste, consumables such as tissues and cotton wool, disposable underwear, aprons and tissue couch roll.

An apron should be worn to protect work wear from wax spillage.

All metal tools should be sterilised in the autoclave before use, this includes tweezers and scissors. After the waxing service they must be replaced and re-sterilised.

Increasingly systems that minimise the risk of cross-infection are being adopted. These include single use pots, cartridges and **disposable applicator** heads.

Environmental and sustainable working practice

◆ Select waxing products with a low melting point and in pellet form as they require less energy to heat to the optimum working temperature.

◆ Manufacturers' packaging may be made from recycled paper and be recyclable, making it a preferable choice.

◆ Post Consumer Resin (PCR – a recycled product) may be used in plastic container packaging.

◆ Organic waxes are available and becoming increasingly popular.

◆ The adhesive rosin, an ingredient in wax sourced from resins of pine trees, may be sustainably sourced. Synthetic resins are becoming increasingly popular.

◆ Bamboo is an alternative material to wood for spatulas for wax application; it grows faster than wood.

◆ Source locally manufactured wax wherever possible.

◆ Provide online client aftercare information, reducing paper.

Preparing the work area for wax depilation

Check the suitability of the environmental conditions in the work area.

To enable the hairs to be removed effectively the service area should be well lit; a magnifying lamp may be available to assist observation of the area. It must also be warm, (but not hot) as the client must be made as comfortable as possible when performing the service. If the client is cold the follicles will constrict, making hair removal more difficult.

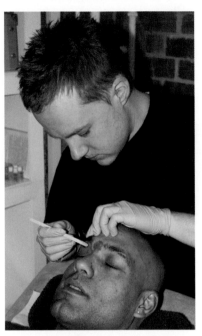

Wear disposable gloves when carrying out waxing services

Ensure ventilation is adequate to remove odours and humid air, providing sufficient air movement to keep the air fresh.

Before the client is shown through, the work area and its contents should be checked to ensure that they are clean and tidy. The bins should have been emptied since the previous client.

The couch should be in the sit-up position, unless the client is only having their bikini line or underarm areas waxed, in which case it should be positioned at a lower angle for the comfort of the client and accessibility to the treatment area.

Check the trolley to ensure that you have all that you need for carrying out the service and that it is suitably positioned to prevent unnecessary stretching or walking, which will affect commercial timing and could cause RSI. The wax should be of a suitable consistency, i.e. ready for application.

Client care, consultation and communication

Treatment information to provide to the client at the initial point of interest

When the client is booking their service they should be asked whether they have had a waxing service before in the salon. If they have not, a small area of waxing should be carried out as a skin sensitivity patch test, to ensure that the client is not sensitive to the technique or allergic to any of the products used. If the **sensitivity test** patch causes an unwanted reaction within 48 hours, then the service must not be undertaken. Unwanted reactions include excessive redness, irritation and swelling, referred to as contra-actions.

Ideally the hair should be of two to three weeks' growth.

Advise the client not to apply any lotions or oils to the area on the day of the service – these could prevent the adhesion of the wax to the hairs being removed. Ask them also to allow at least one week, and preferably two, between any home shaving or other depilatory service and a salon waxing service. This is to let the hairs grow to a length sufficient for effective removal when waxing.

No UV tanning should be received 24-48 hours before service. This includes self tanning service.

Exfoliation before service is beneficial to remove dead skin cells from the treatment area, facilitating hair removal.

Loose clothing is preferable, to avoid irritation of the treated area.

When a client makes an appointment for a wax depilation service, the receptionist should advise the client how long the service will take.

The first consultation for a waxing service will take longer as you assess the client's suitability for service and agree their service needs. This information will be reviewed at each service to check for changes to their service record since the last service.

It is important to complete the service in the time allowed in order to be efficient in service application and to ensure the appointment schedule runs smoothly and clients are not kept waiting.

Inform the client briefly what the waxing service will entail so that they have an understanding of what will be required from them. This will help clients who have not received the more intimate wax removal services, e.g. to the underarms and bikini line area, to be prepared and to relax.

Allow a four- to six-week interval between successive wax depilation appointments. Following set intervals between waxing services will improve the effectiveness of the service as this will follow the hair growth cycle. Suggested timings that consider Habia maximum service times are tabled below. Times will always vary according to the skill of the beauty therapist and quantity of hair to be removed. However, repeat bookings vary according to the natural hair regrowth and client requirements.

All staff, especially the staff communicating with clients at reception, should be familiar with the different pricing structures for the range of waxing services and products available for retail.

Clients under 16 years of age (minors) must be accompanied by a parent/guardian who will be required to sign a consent form in order for service to proceed and they should remain present during the service.

REVISION AID

Why would you use a visual aid at consultation when explaining the hair growth cycle, and how might this affect the hair-free period?

Service	Warm waxing (minutes)	Hot waxing (minutes)
Half leg	30	30
Half leg and bikini line	45	45
Full leg	45	60
Full leg and bikini line	70	75–80
Bikini line	15	15–20
Underarm	15	15–20
Half arm	10–15	15–20
Full arm	20–30	20–30
Top lip	10	10
Top lip and chin	15	15–20
Eyebrows	15	15

Preparation of the beauty therapist

Consultation

A consultation must be performed for all clients who have not received the service before or are new clients to you. However, every time the client receives the service you should review their personal details to ensure their continued suitability and service requirements. For example their medical history may have changed. Discuss what methods of hair removal have been used before and when they were last used. Discuss the known sensitivity of the client's skin. If the client is taking any medication that causes skin thinning, such as tetracycline, or has received facial chemical peels or retin-A, skin lifting may occur because the wax is designed to stick to the skin before removal. This will result in skin damage so waxing must not be performed. If necessary a skin sensitivity patch test should

ALWAYS REMEMBER

Client service record

Accurately record your client's responses to mandatory questions at consultation on the service record. This is necessary for future reference.

TOP TIP

Sporting requirements for wax depilation

Some clients will require waxing to improve their sporting performance. Removal of the hair makes them more aerodynamic and therefore faster! Associated sports include swimming, cycling and athletics.

TOP TIP

Examples of waxing service modification include:

◆ hair removal around contra-indications that restrict service (such as hairy moles and skin tags)

◆ altering the choice of wax to suit skin condition and hair type

◆ care when treating older skin, which is drier, thinner and has reduced elasticity, meaning that it could easily bruise or suffer from skin removal.

TOP TIP

Hair growth cycle

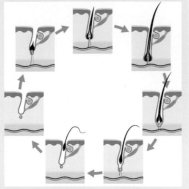

Using a visual aid will assist the clients in understanding why some hairs may appear soon after the waxing service.

be provided to assess tolerance. A positive reaction where there is redness, irritation or swelling means that the service cannot proceed. A negative reaction means that it can. Maintain client privacy at all times during the consultation. Explain what is involved with the method of hair removal technique to be used, the expected costs, sensations, service reactions and aftercare requirements. It is important that the client can see that you provide a professional waxing service and that each service is personalised – matched to meet the client's needs, including the choice of wax.

It is a good idea to discuss the hair growth cycle with the client using a visual aid. This will help the client to understand that hairs that grow through following hair removal were at a different stage of the hair growth cycle and were below the skin's surface at the time of the service and therefore could not be removed. It also helps to show the need for regular intervals between waxing appointments as hairs will be at a similar hair growth pattern. Some waxes are designed to remove shorter hairs. This is useful if regular wax appointments are not maintained and in this circumstance is a preferable choice.

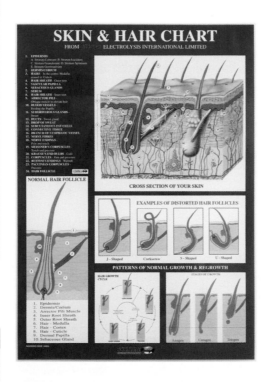

TOP TIP

Describing the sensation

Here are some useful explanatory phrases: 'It's a bit like quickly ripping a plaster off and taking the hairs with it. It isn't so bad, or so many people wouldn't have it done time and time again!'

The skin looks and feels great after hair removal, making any possible discomfort experienced worthwhile!

Immediately following hair removal, the skin becomes slightly red around the hair follicle from where the hair has been removed. There may also be slight swelling of the skin in the area. This will soon disappear following service but this will vary according to skin sensitivity and hair strength and the quantity of hair that has been removed. Occasionally spot bleeding may occur where a particularly strong terminal hair type hair has been removed, usually when in the anagen stage where it is receiving blood from the dermal papilla, resulting in capillary damage. This too may be explained at consultation.

Inform the client that it may be necessary to trim hairs, which will help reduce discomfort.

Invite the client to ask questions. It is important that they understand fully what the service includes.

Following the consultation and completion of the service record, advise the client of the most appropriate method of hair removal having considered the type of hair (vellus/terminal) and quantity, sensitivity of the skin and any other related factors such as treatment area, skin age and condition.

When a client attends a wax depilation service, you should always check that there are no **contra-indications** that might prevent or restrict service.

Contra-indications

Certain medical conditions or medications and hormonal changes in the body, such as those that occur in females at pregnancy, puberty and menopause can affect hair growth, causing an increase, so it is important to discuss the hair growth observed in the area to be removed with the client. This will confirm client suitability for treatment. Types of hair growth and factors affecting hair growth are discussed in Chapter 2, The Science of Beauty Therapy.

If the client has any of the following, wax depilation must not be carried out:

◆ *failure of skin sensitivity thermal test patch* – the client will be unable to tell you if the wax is too hot

◆ *positive reaction to skin sensitivity patch test* – a lack of tolerance to product ingredients

◆ *skin conditions* such as thin and fragile skin

◆ *skin disorders* such as severe eczema or psoriasis

◆ *contagious skin disease* – medical referral required

◆ *eye disorders* such as conjunctivitis when treating the face

◆ *swellings* – the cause may be medical

◆ *diabetes* – a client with this condition is vulnerable to infection as they have slow skin healing

◆ *defective circulation* – poor skin healing may occur. This may be a symptom of conditions such as diabetes, heart disease and multiple sclerosis

◆ *recent scar tissue (under 6 months old)* – the skin lacks elasticity

◆ *broken bones*

◆ *fractures or sprains* – discomfort may occur

◆ *phlebitis* – an inflammatory condition of the vein

◆ *retin-A, tetracycline medication* as the skin is more sensitive, weaker and prone to skin irritation and tearing

◆ *loss of skin sensation* – the client would be unable to identify if the wax was too hot

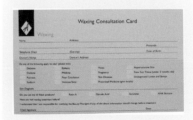

◆ *allergies to products* – such as the ingredient rosin, an ingredient found in sticking plasters and wax

◆ *clients under 16 years of age.*

HEALTH & SAFETY

Diabetes

Clients who have the medical condition diabetes should be treated with care. This is because diabetics generally have poor blood circulation and are slower to heal. As there is some tissue damage to the skin during wax depilation when the hair is removed from the follicle, secondary infection could occur. Approval to treat should be obtained by the client from their GP before temporary hair removal service.

Further contra-indications that prevent waxing service

(Continued)

REVISION AID

How often should a client have a waxing service?

Name	Description
Excessive bruising	Injury to an area causes blood to leak from damaged blood vessels. Bruises may swell, appearing dark purple or blue at first and then turn, brown, green or yellow as they fade. Use your professional judgment if the bruise is old or can be avoided it may be possible to carry out the service.
Folliculitis	A bacterial infection where the skin becomes inflamed around the hair follicles and pustules develop in the skin tissue around the hair follicle. Antibiotics may be required to clear the infection. Effective post-service aftercare is essential to avoid the possibility of folliculitis.
Severe varicose veins	Veins are vessels that carry blood away from the body tissues and back to the heart. Veins have valves to prevent backflow as they carry blood under low blood pressure back towards the heart. If valves become weak and their elasticity is lost, it becomes a *varicose vein*. The area appears knotted, swollen and bluish-purple in colour.

Name	Description
Heat rash	A reaction to heat exposure where the sweat ducts become blocked and sweat escapes into the epidermis. Red pimples occur and the skin becomes itchy.

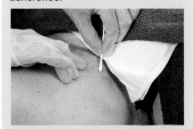
Certain contra-indications *restrict* service application. This may mean that the service has to be adapted or modified for the client. For example, in the case of a small, localised bruise the area could be avoided.

Other contra-indications that restrict service include the following:

◆ *Cuts* – secondary infection could occur.

◆ *Mild skin disorders* such as psoriasis or eczema and skin tags.

◆ *Abrasions* – secondary infection could occur.

◆ *Self-tan* – waxing will remove the surface skin cells and the chemically tanned skin.

◆ *Bruises* – client discomfort may be caused and the condition made worse.

◆ *Sunburn* – the skin is damaged due to acute overexposure to the sun.

◆ *Varicose veins* (non-severe) – avoid the area.

◆ *Moles* – avoid wax application to the areas.

◆ *Ingrowing hairs* – the area should be avoided as the hair will not be removed. Also, infection commonly occurs at the site of an ingrowing hair, leading to folliculitis.

Further contra-indications that restrict waxing service

Name	Description
Warts	Small epidermal skin growths. Warts may be raised or flat, depending upon their position. Usually they have a rough surface and are raised.

(Continued)

Name	Description
Hairy moles	Moles exhibiting coarse terminal hairs on their surface. Hair growing from a mole should be cut, not plucked: if plucked, the hairs will become coarser and the growth of the hairs further stimulated.
Skin tags	Skin-coloured threads of skin 3–6 mm long, projecting from the skin's surface. Skin tags often occur under the arms and can be found on the groin when treating the bikini area.

Contra-actions

Inform the client at consultation of any contra-actions that may occur during or after service and the action to take.

A contra-action is an unwanted reaction to a waxing service which may occur during or following the service.

Contra-actions which may occur with waxing include:

◆ ingrowing hairs

◆ folliculitis

◆ burns – caused by both excessive wax temperature and friction burns from repeated removal of wax

◆ removal of skin

◆ **erythema** – increased blood flow to the skin, causing an extreme redness.

Ingrowing hairs Ingrowing hairs can arise in three ways:

◆ *Over-reaction to damage* An excessive reaction by the skin and the follicle to the 'damage' produced by depilation may cause extra cornified cells to be made. These may block the surface of the follicle, causing the newly growing hair to turn around and grow inwards.

◆ *Overtight clothing* If after the service the client wears clothing that is too tight, this too can block the follicle.

◆ *Dry skin* Likewise dry skin can cause blockage of the follicle.

Ingrowing hairs can usually be recognised to be one or other of three types:

◆ *A hair growing along beneath the surface of the skin* Identify the tip (the pointed end); then pierce the tissues over the root end with a sterile needle. Free the tip, trim the hair if required and leave it in place so that the follicle can heal around it.

HEALTH & SAFETY

Contra-actions

If a contra-action occurs during the waxing service occurs, discontinue the service and provide appropriate advice.

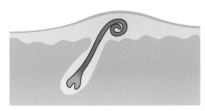

Coiled ingrowing hair

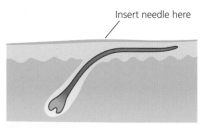

Insert needle here

Hair growing beneath the surface of the skin

◆ *A coiled ingrowing hair* This looks like a small black spot or dome on the skin. If this is gently squeezed and rolled between the fingertips, using a tissue, it will release the coiled ingrowing hair and some hardened sebum. If the hair does not fall out, it should be left in place (as above).

◆ *An infected ingrowth* If the trapped sebum or hair starts to decay, either of the two preceding forms can become infected or begin to display an immune response. The area first becomes red (irritation); then an infected white dome-shaped pustule develops. Release the trapped tissue (as above), and cover the affected area – which may bleed, or leak tissue fluid – with a sterile non-allergenic dressing.

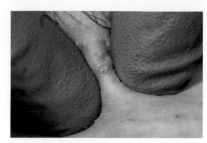
Infected ingrowth

Skin removal If the granular layer of the epidermis is exposed – the skin should be treated as if it has been burnt. This is often a result of poor removal techniques such as not holding the skin sufficiently taut or lifting the wax too high rather than parallel to the skin. This can also occur as a result of the client having used exfoliating skin medications, cortisone steroid medications and recent exfoliating beauty therapy services such as micro-dermabrasion. Cool the area immediately by applying cold-water compresses for 10 minutes. Dry it carefully; then apply a dry, non-fluffy dressing to protect the area from infection. The dressing should be worn for three to four days, and the area then left open to the air. (Antiseptic cream by itself should be used only when the injury is very minor.) Medical attention should be sought if necessary.

REVISION AID

What must be performed if a client has a sensitive or allergic skin type?

HEALTH & SAFETY

Ingrowing hairs

Training should be received before treating ingrowing hairs.

When handling ingrowing hairs the surface of the skin to be treated should be disinfected.

PPE gloves should be worn.

All hazardous clinical waste should be disposed of in line with waste legislation.

An antiseptic should be applied to the area to promote skin healing.

No further contact with the area should be made at the service.

Contra-action advice should be provided. An antiseptic may be applied by the client for 48 hours. If any redness remains continue to apply the antiseptic. Signs of infection should be reported to the beauty therapist for further advice e.g. swelling, inflammation and pus present.

Reinforce post-treatment advice to those clients prone to infection.

Burns A burn should be treated as **skin removal**. If blisters form, they should not be broken – they help prevent the entry of infection into the wound. Medical attention should be sought.

Always remember the importance of testing the wax temperature on yourself and the client before service commences and make ongoing checks throughout the service.

Excessive erythema Erythema is a visible redness, which is a normal reaction to skin-waxing treatment. If excessive, it will be accompanied by an increase in warmth on the surface of the skin. This is created by an increased blood flow through the capillaries near the surface of the skin, caused by the **histamine reaction** after waxing. Ask the client to follow the recommended aftercare advice and recommendations.

Certain waxing ingredients such as rosin, a resin, may cause an **allergic reaction** in some people.

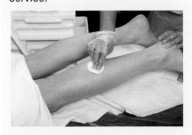

The symptoms of an allergic reaction could be:

- redness of the skin (erythema)
- swelling
- itching
- blisters.

Poor hygiene practice such as inadequate skin cleansing, application of aftercare lotion infecting the area of treatment and non-compliance by the client with aftercare instructions, may result in bacterial infection seen as erythema and pustules in the area.

In the case of an allergic reaction, if it occurs during waxing application stop service and remove any remaining product. Apply a cool compress and soothing agent to the area to reduce redness and irritation. Identify the possible cause of the allergic reaction. If symptoms persist, seek medical advice.

Always record any allergies on the client's service record so that the offending product may be avoided in the future. Try an alternative **waxing product** to assess skin tolerance. In some cases the skin is too sensitive and intolerant to waxing service.

Always date and record any contra-actions on the client service record with actions taken/ recommendations provided and the outcome.

After the service plan has been completed, the client should be asked to read the list of contra-indications and sign to state that they are not suffering from any of the contra-indications stated.

The beauty therapist must not carry out a wax service immediately after a heat service, such as a sauna, or steam or UV services, as the heat-sensitised tissues may be irritated by the wax service.

If you are unsure if service may commence, tactfully refer the client to their GP for permission to treat. A copy of the GP's letter on receipt should be kept with the client's record card. If the service cannot be carried out for any reason, always explain why, without naming a contra-indication, as you are not qualified to do so. Clients will respect your professional advice.

Following the consultation an appropriate service plan will be confirmed with the client. Their understanding of the service is important to ensure that their needs are met and that they will not be disappointed.

Preparing the client

The client should be shown through to the service area and asked to remove specific items of clothing as necessary so that the service may be carried out. Disposable briefs may be provided if a bikini line wax service is to be received.

If it is the first time the client has had the service, explain to them that the service can be uncomfortable, but reassure them that it is quick and any discomfort experienced is tolerable.

Be efficient and quick, so that the client does not have to wait. Try to get the client talking about something pleasant, such as a holiday, to take their mind off the service. Throughout the service, reassure them, praising them in order to motivate them to continue with the services. Do try to be sympathetic to your client's feelings, and provide support and encouragement when necessary. Waxing, although a necessity for many people, is not a particularly pleasant or relaxing service.

Preparation of the client

After the initial consultation, the correct choice of wax formulation and technique for the client's hair removal requirements are identified and agreed with the client.

1   Use a towel to protect the client's remaining clothing. Even if performing an eyebrow wax, protect the scalp hair and chest area in case of wax spillage.

2   Wipe the area to be waxed with a professional antiseptic pre-wax cleansing lotion on clean cotton wool. This is usually dispensed from a pump or spray bottle. Blot the area dry with tissues before applying the wax. While wiping the skin, look for contra-indications that restrict the service, e.g. varicose veins.

   Record any minor abrasions, scars or **bruising** on the service record to avoid potential problems later.

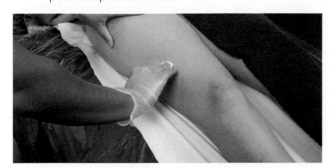

Cleansing the skin of the leg with pre-wax lotion

3   If the client's skin is very oily or they may for example have applied oil before coming to the salon, cleanse it using a suitable pre-wax lotion. Professional tissue wipes are available that both cleanse and exfoliate the skin. These are ideal for preparation of the skin. Powder may be applied lightly to the area to absorb moisture and facilitate hair removal depending on wax system used.

4   Immediately before starting the service, wash your hands. Apply PPE as required according to the body part being treated.

5   Perform a **thermal sensitivity patch test**: before applying the wax, check its temperature. Test the wax on yourself first, to ensure that it's not too warm; then try a little on the client on the area to be treated (to check tolerance to the heat) before spreading it on other areas.

HEALTH & SAFETY

Avoiding cross-contamination

It is unhygienic to return a spatula to the wax after it has been in contact with the body part (double dipping). It is therefore *recommended* that a new spatula be used for each entry to the wax. Another method is to use one spatula for dipping in the wax pot and then transferring the wax onto a second spatula that is applied to the client. Therefore cutting out the risk of cross-infection or contamination, by this transfer technique method.

Please refer to Habia's code of practice for more information. This applies to warm and hot wax methods.

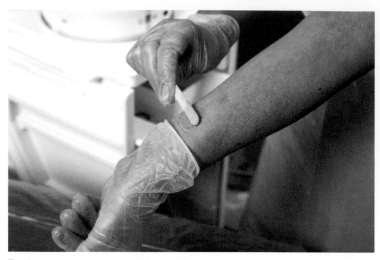

Testing wax temperature on inner wrist

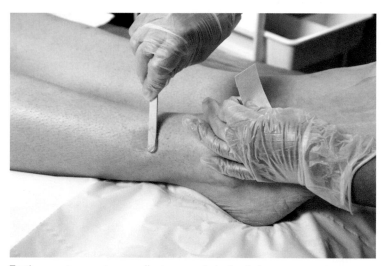

Testing wax temperature on client on area to be treated

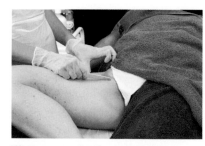

Warm wax application to the bikini line area; the wax is applied in sections considering direction of hair growth

Warm wax techniques

Warm waxing has a few basic rules, which must be followed to ensure a good result.

If the manufacturer's instructions say that oil is to be used with the warm wax, apply this now.

Observe the direction of hair growth. Warm wax must always be *applied with* the direction of hair growth, and *removed against* the direction of growth. This ensures both maximum adhesion between the hair, the strip and the wax, and that the hair will be pulled back on itself in the follicle and thus removed complete with its bulb.

Spatula application technique

1   Dip the spatula into the wax. Remove the excess on the sides and tip by wiping the spatula against the metal bar or the sides of the tub. Place the strip under the spatula while transferring it to the client: this will control dripping and improve your technique.

2　Place the spatula onto the skin at a 90° angle, and push the wax along in the direction of the hair growth. Do not allow the spatula to fall forward past 45°. The objective is to coat the area with a very thin film of wax. Quite a large area can be spread with each sweep of the spatula, as warm wax does not set. Do not attempt to smooth out or go over areas on which wax has already been spread, however, as the wax will have become cooler and will not move again, but will drag painfully on the client's skin.

3　Fold back 20 mm at the end of a strip and grip the flap with the thumb widthways across the strip. The flap should provide a wax-free handle throughout the service.

4　Place the strip at the bottom end of the wax-covered area, and make a firm bond between the wax and the strip by pressing firmly along the strip's length and width, following the direction of hair growth. If the strip is placed anywhere but at the bottom of a waxed area, the hairs at the *bottom* of the strip will become tangled together and held in the wax on the area below the strip: the removal of the strip will then be far more painful for the client.

5　Using the non-working hand, stretch the skin to minimise discomfort. Gripping the flap tightly, use the working hand to remove the strip against the direction of hair growth. Use a firm, steady pull. Make sure that the strip is pulled back on itself, close to the skin. (To obtain the correct angle of pull, stand at the side of the client, facing them.) Maintain this same horizontal angle of pull until the last bit of the strip has left the skin: *do not pull the strip upwards at the end of the pull* as this would break the hairs at the end of the strip and be very painful.

6　The strip may be used many times; in fact it works best when some wax builds up on its surface. When there is too much wax on the surface it will stop picking up more: throw it away and start with a new one.

7　Do not repeatedly spread and remove wax over one area. In particular, wax should not be spread and removed more than twice on sensitive areas such as the bikini line, the face and the underarms. Any remaining stray hairs must instead be removed using sterilised tweezers.

Alternatively, warm wax may be applied using a disposable cartridge/tube applicator system. This system is discussed later in this chapter.

Different temperatures
Summer heat and winter cold can each give rise to problems with the wax service. In summer, the wax can remain too warm on the body, becoming sticky and difficult to work with, and tending to leave a sticky residue on the treated areas. In winter, the client's legs may be cold, causing the wax to set too quickly as you spread it, so that it becomes too thick. This prevents the efficient removal of both the wax and the hair growth.

To some extent these problems can be overcome by using thicker waxes with higher melting points in the summer, and thinner waxes with lower melting points in the winter.

TOP TIP

Thin wax application

The thinner the wax, the easier the service is to carry out when using the strip removal technique and the better the result. Also, less wax and fewer strips are used. Gel and cream waxes both provide a thin consistency for application.

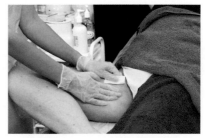
Hair removal from the bikini line area using a disposable strip

REVISION AID

Why is it necessary to consider hair growth direction for hair removal?

TOP TIP

Soothing the skin

To take the sting out of the removal, immediately place a hand or finger over the depilated area and apply gentle pressure.

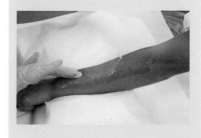

STEP-BY-STEP: HALF-LEG WAX SERVICE

The areas of the body where warm-wax hair removal is most frequently used are the lower legs. This is often referred to simply as a **half-leg service**. A 'pair of half legs' should take 20–30 minutes to treat, and use no more than two or three strips.

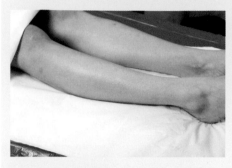 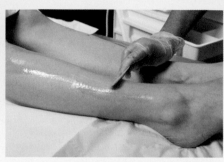 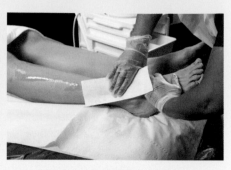

1 Before the service, the area to be waxed should be cleansed as previously described.

2 Sit the client on the upraised couch, with both legs straight out in front of them.

3 Spread the wax on the *front* of the leg furthest away from you. Use three sweeps of the spatula: each sweep should go from just below the knee to the end of hair growth at the ankle.

Repeat this pattern of spreading on the leg nearest to you. (By spreading the leg furthest away first, you will not have to lean over an already waxed area.)

4 Starting with the leg nearest to you, remove the wax using the strip. Start at the ankle and work upwards towards the knees. Stretch the skin with the other hand, near where you are removing the wax from.

Repeat for the other leg.

5 Ask the client to bend her legs to one side. Beginning again with the leg furthest away, spread wax on one *side* of the leg, from the knee to the ankle, using two sweeps of the spatula.

Repeat for the leg nearest to you.

6 Starting with the leg nearest to you, remove the wax from the bottom upwards.

Repeat for the other leg.

7 Repeat steps **5** and **6** for the other side of the legs.

8 Bend one knee. Spread the wax from just above the knee, downwards to cover the knee.

9 Remove this wax from the bottom upwards, remembering that strips cannot pull around corners effectively. To keep the angle of the pull horizontal, remove wax below the knee first, then that above the knee.

10 Repeat steps **8** and **9** for the other knee.

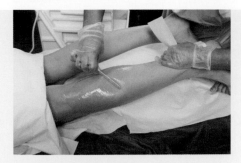
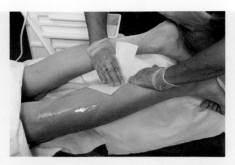

11 Lower the backrest and ask the client to turn over. To ensure efficient application and removal of wax in the ankle area, ask the client if possible to support their foot on their toes which will keep the skin at the ankle taut.

12 On the *back* of the legs, the direction of hair growth is not from the top to the bottom but usually sweeping at an angle, from the outside to the inside of the calf muscle.

Starting with the leg furthest away, spread wax following the direction of the natural hair growth.

Repeat for the leg nearest to you.

13 Starting with the leg nearest to you, remove the wax against the direction of the natural hair growth.

Repeat for the other leg.

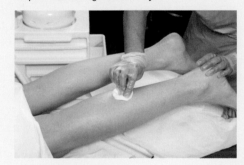
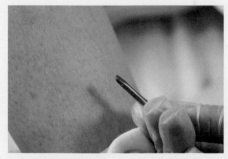

Tweezer hair removal, to remove the odd short or stray hair

14 Finally, apply after-wax lotion to clean cotton wool and apply this to the back of the client's legs, followed by the front of the legs to complete. As you apply the lotion, check for hairs left behind: if there are any, remove them using tweezers.

Remove any excess lotion using a tissue.

TOP TIP

Troubleshooting

The faults most commonly seen in warm-wax depilation are these:

◆ spreading the wax too thickly

◆ placing the strip in the middle of a wax-spread area, instead of starting at the bottom and working up

◆ pulling the strip upwards instead of backwards, away from the body part, causing breakage of the hair

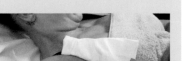

Wax application too thick

◆ wax left on the skin after strip removal – this may be because of poor skin preparation; the skin was damp before wax application; the skin was not held sufficiently taut on removal; insufficient pressure applied when rubbing the wax strip before removal.

TOP TIP

Seasonal problems

Thick lumps of wax stuck to the legs (a winter problem) after warm wax strip removal can be removed by pulling more slowly than normal, or by reversing the direction of pull on the strip. A sticky residue on the legs (a summer problem) must be removed using post-wax lotion.

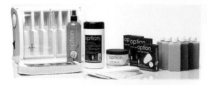

Cartridge wax system

Disposable warm wax application to the leg Wax is heated in its container and applied through the disposable applicator head directly to the skin area. A wax strip is used to remove the hairs from the area removing the wax strip against hair growth.

Toes Clients frequently request that their toes be waxed in conjunction with a half-leg or full-leg service. When doing this, follow the normal guidelines for waxing, but be aware that hair may grow in many directions. Apply wax with a small spatula and cut strips into small pieces to effectively remove hair.

HEALTH & SAFETY

Wax spills

If you spill wax on the couch cover, immediately place a quarter-width facial-sized piece of strip on top of the spill. This prevents the wax from damaging the client's clothing when they move.

TOP TIP

Intimate waxing

Intimate waxing is a range of waxing techniques that remove pubic and/or anal body hair. This is an advanced waxing service covered in Level 3 and differs from the requirements of a bikini line waxing service.

ALWAYS REMEMBER

Common faults

The most common fault seen in half-leg waxing is trying to remove too big an area at once over the calf muscle and not supporting the surrounding tissues adequately. This will result in a painful service for the client and possible skin bruising.

Providing a full-leg wax service

A full-leg wax should take 40–50 minutes and four to six strips should be sufficient.

When carrying out a full-leg wax, follow the same sequence of working as with the half leg. On the thighs, observe the direction of hair growth carefully, as the hair grows in different directions. It is best not to spread wax on too large an area at once, or you may forget the direction of growth. Each direction of hair growth should be treated as a separate area. It is of prime importance that you support the skin on the thighs as you remove the strip – the tissues in this area can bruise very easily. The two essential factors in preventing bruising, pain and hair breakage are:

◆ the correct angle for wax removal

◆ adequate support for the tissues.

STEP-BY-STEP: PROVIDING A BIKINI LINE SERVICE

A **bikini line service** takes 10–15 minutes, and requires a new strip for each section to ensure effective hair removal from this delicate area.

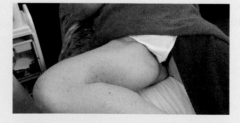

1 Treat one side at a time. It is best if the client lies flat, as the skin's tissues are then pulled tighter, but the service can be carried out in a semi-reclining position if the client prefers. Bend the client's knee out to the side, and put her foot flat against the knee of the other leg. This is sometimes referred to as the **figure-four position**.

2 Request and instruct the client how to place a protective tissue along and under the lower edge of their briefs. Raise this edge and agree with the client where she wants the final line to be. Hold the briefs slightly beyond this line, and ask the client to place her hand on top of the protective tissue to hold everything in place. This leaves you with both hands free, one to pull the strip and one to support the skin.

3 Cleanse and dry the areas to be waxed.

4 Using sterilised scissors, if necessary trim both the hair to be waxed and the adjacent hairs down to about 5–12 mm in length. This is essential to avoid tangling, pulling and pain, and to prevent wax going onto hair that you do not want to remove.

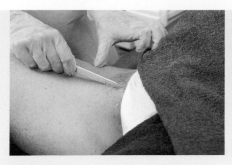

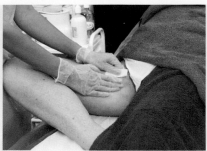

5 Spread and remove the wax in two or three separate and distinct areas, the number depending on the directions of hair growth.

6 Use half of the strip length to remove the wax. Do not cover the whole area and tear it off at once! Treat the top plane of the thigh (Plane 1) and then the plane underneath this (Plane 2).

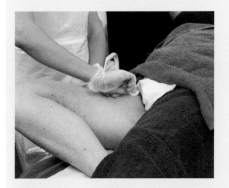

8 With both legs straight out in front on the couch, request and instruct the client how to place a protective tissue along the top edge of the client's briefs, against the abdomen. Lower the briefs as necessary to expose just the hair to be removed – check this with your client. Usually the direction of hair growth here sweeps in from the sides and then up to the navel.

9 Trim the hair as before.

10 Apply and remove the wax in small sections, carefully observing hair growth. On completion, apply after-wax lotion.

7 Repeat to the other side and check each side is symmetrical, confirm satisfaction with the client. As soon as an area is completed, apply after-wax lotion. If necessary, hygienically remove any stray hairs with sterilised tweezers. If necessary, use a clean tissue to remove excess lotion.

TOP TIP

Trimming hair

Trim long hair before waxing to avoid unnecessary client discomfort and to enable the hair growth direction to be more easily viewed. Skin disorders such as skin tags can be hidden if the hair is too long.

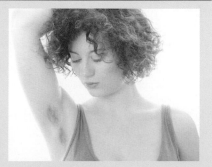

Long terminal underarm hair

REVISION AID

What contra-action may occur during the waxing service?

ALWAYS REMEMBER

Bruising

Bruising is neither normal nor acceptable, but a sign of faulty technique.

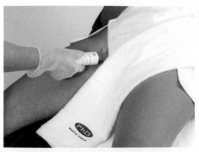

Bikini line wax using disposable applicator warm wax technique

Disposable warm wax application to bikini line area Wax is applied in small sections through the applicator head to the skin area. A wax strip is used to remove the hairs from the area, removing the wax strip against hair growth.

STEP-BY-STEP: UNDERARM SERVICE

An underarm service should take 5–15 minutes and two strips, one for each underarm.

1 If a client is wearing a bra this remains worn, ask your client to lie flat on her back with their hands behind her head, elbows flat on the couch.

2 Cleanse both underarms with pre-wax lotion on clean cotton wool; blot with a tissue.

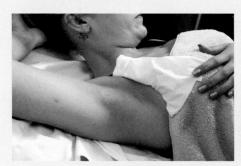

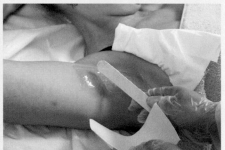

3 Place a protective tissue under the edge of the bra cup on the side away from you. Ask the client to bring her opposite arm down and over, and to pull the breast area away from the underarm being waxed and across towards the middle of her chest. This pulls the tissues tight, making the service a lot more comfortable for them; it also leaves you with both hands free, one to pull and one to support.

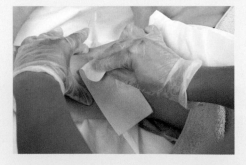

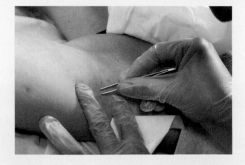

4 Underarm hair usually grows in two main directions. Observe the directions of hair growth, then apply and remove the wax separately for each small area.

5 Apply after-wax lotion to the treated area. Check for stray hairs; remove these hygienically with sterile tweezers. Repeat on the other underarm area.

6 Blot any excess lotion with a clean tissue.

HEALTH & SAFETY

Contaminated waste

Both bikini line and underarm waxing can be uncomfortable, especially if the hair growth is thick – always bear this in mind when carrying out the service. Some slight bleeding can be expected as the hairs in this area are very strong and have deep roots. Any waste contaminated by blood must be disposed of hygienically in a sealed bag.

Disposable warm wax application to the underarm Wax is applied in small sections following the direction of the hair growth through the applicator head to the skin area. A wax strip is used to remove the hair from the area, removing the wax strip against hair growth.

STEP-BY-STEP: FOREARM SERVICE

Depilation in this area should take 10–15 minutes for a **half-arm service** and 20–30 minutes for a **full-arm service**. Half the length of the strip should be used. Avoid harsh lines between waxed areas which are hair free and non-waxed areas. Subtly, soften this line by removing some hair in this area.

The roundness of the arm means that in order to effect a horizontal pull the work must be done in short lengths. Other than this, follow the general rules for waxing.

Arms are usually waxed with the client in the sitting position, with their general clothing protected with a towel. Sleeve edges can be protected with tucked-in tissues although, ideally, upper outer clothing should be removed.

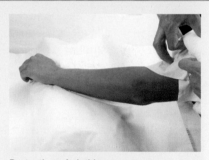

Protection of clothing

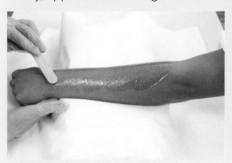

1 Following cleansing of both forearms with pre-wax lotion wax applied in sections following the direction of hair growth.

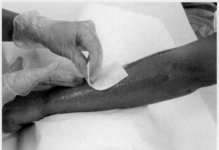

2 Wax is removed against hair growth, commencing at the wrist area ensuring that the skin is held taut to minimise discomfort and ensure effective hair removal, continue until the area is hair free. Move the arm supporting at the wrist, to enable access to all areas of hair growth.

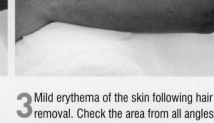

3 Mild erythema of the skin following hair removal. Check the area from all angles to ensure all hairs have been removed.

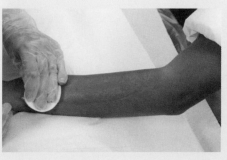

4 Sterilised tweezers may be used to hygienically remove any stray hairs. A soothing afterwax lotion is applied with clean cotton wool to reduce erythema and any discomfort and to prevent secondary infection.

Repeat wax application and removal sequence on the other arm.

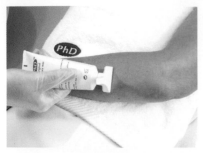

Forearm wax using disposable application warm wax technique

Disposable warm wax application to the forearm Wax is applied in sections following the direction of the hair growth through the applicator head to the skin area. A wax strip is used to remove the hair from the area, removing the wax strip against hair growth.

> **TOP TIP**
>
> **Dark superfluous facial hair**
>
> Avoid obvious lines when removing facial hair. Ensure the outer border of the area treated blends into the adjacent area of skin.

STEP-BY-STEP: FACIAL WAXING SERVICE

The **service** must always be approached with extra care as facial skin is more sensitive than skin elsewhere on the body. Faulty technique can result in the top layer of skin being removed. (If this happens, a scab will form after about a day and the mark will take days to heal and fade completely.) In darker skins this may result in hyper pigmentation.

The client should be in a semi-reclining position, with their head supported and a clean towel draped across their shoulders to protect clothing. A clean headband can be used to keep the hair away from the face.

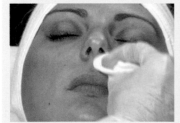

Cotton wool applied to cleanse the skin

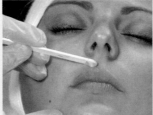

Wax application to outer upper lip area

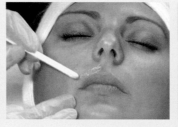

Wax application to under the nose area

1 Cleanse and wipe over the area thoroughly until the cotton wool used to apply the pre-wax lotion or pre-wax cleansing wipe shows clean. Blot area dry with a tissue.

2 Application of warm wax to the upper lip using a disposable small spatula, paying close attention to the direction of natural hair growth. Spread one-half of the top lip with wax; remove this in two or three narrow strips; repeat the process on the other half of the lip.

3 Apply wax to the upper lip area immediately below the nose. The client is requested to pull the skin taut, moving the skin over the upper teeth. This position will assist hair removal.

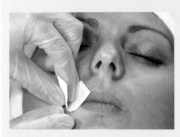

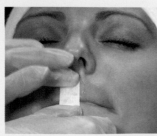

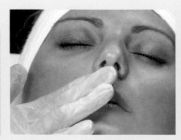

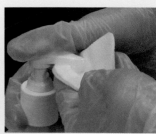

4 Removal of wax against hair growth. The area is held taut to minimise discomfort and ensure effective hair removal.

5 Strip removal under the nose in an upwards direction. The client continues to hold the skin taut in this area.

6 Pressure is applied to the area to minimise discomfort.

7 Application of after-wax lotion to the hair free area.

A **top-lip wax** should take approximately five minutes, and a **lip and chin wax** approximately 15 minutes. A removal strip of no more than one-eighth normal size should be used on the face. Do not allow wax to build up on the facial wax strips – such a build-up could lead to skin removal. Use a new strip for each area.

If the chin is to be treated this area is less sensitive than the upper lip so if treating both areas complete the chin area last. Apply the wax according to the type of wax used. You may find that when treating a female client there may be small groupings of hairs and the wax may be applied to these areas only. If the client has dark **superfluous** facial hair it may be necessary to treat the sides of the face also.

A disposable warm wax application to facial area Wax is applied in small sections through the applicator head to the skin area. A wax strip is used to remove the hair from the area removing the wax strip against growth.

> ### TOP TIP
>
> **Neck and face applications**
>
> Other areas of the neck and face can be treated by wax depilation – for example, to tidy up a haircut at the neckline, or to remove sideburns – provided that you follow the general guidelines for facial services.

> ### HEALTH & SAFETY
>
> **The lips**
>
> The lips are extremely sensitive. To avoid possible irritation, do not allow the wax to come into contact with them.

REVISION AID

How can a client reduce the possibility of developing ingrowing hairs following waxing service?

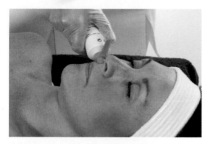

Facial wax application using disposable applicator warm wax technique

ALWAYS REMEMBER

Bleached hair

Previously bleached hair tends to break off at skin level when waxed. Clients should be told not to bleach facial hair if it is to be waxed.

STEP-BY-STEP: EYEBROW WAXING SERVICE

Eyebrows, as a part of the face, are treated accordingly (see above). An **eyebrow wax** should take approximately 10–15 minutes.

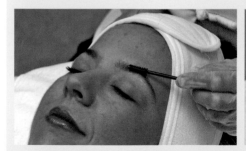

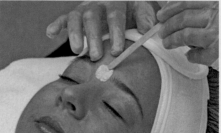

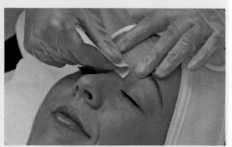

1 Study the eyebrows and confirm with the client the final shape to be achieved. Use a mirror to discuss the shape and hairs requiring removal. Brow length, arch position and thickness of the shape are all factors to consider. Male eyebrows usually require a natural shape where stray hairs and hairs between the brows are removed.

2 Brush the eyebrows and separate the unwanted (superfluous) hair from the line of the other hairs.

3 Commence wax application between the brows, the skin is firmer in this area and allows the client to become accustomed to the sensation, especially if this treatment is new to them.

Using a small spatula, apply a thin film of wax in an upwards direction to the unwanted hairs between the brows, above the nose.

4 Remove the wax and hair against the growth using a clean wax strip.

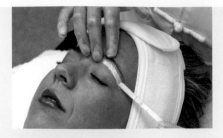
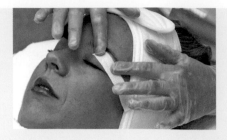

5 Repeat application and removal in different areas. It is important to support the skin when removing wax to avoid stretching delicate skin in the area. Apply wax in the direction of hair growth and remove until all the unwanted hairs have been removed. Change the strip as required. Ensure you avoid excessive wax build-up on the strip (the strip should make good contact with the waxed area). For each eye use a new strip. When applying the wax strip to the area, ensure you can see the hairs below to avoid accidental removal of those not requiring removal.

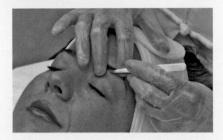
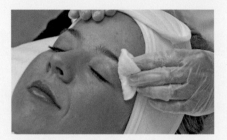

6 Apply an after-wax lotion suitable for the eye area and use sterile tweezers to remove any remaining stray hairs, this should be minimal as this is the benefit of waxing service it provides mass tweezing.

7 The finished look. Ensure the client is satisfied with the brow shape achieved

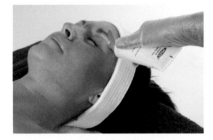

Eyebrow wax application: disposable applicator technique

A disposable warm wax application to the eyebrow area Wax is applied in small sections through the applicator head to the skin area. A wax strip is used to remove the hair from the area, removing the wax strip against growth.

HEALTH & SAFETY

Protect against spillage

When performing an eyebrow wax, eyebrow hair that does not need to be removed may be protected with petroleum jelly. This is a useful tip when first performing eyebrow waxing to prevent mistakes.

Cotton wool pads may be placed over the eyes to protect the eye and eyelashes from accidental wax spillage.

TOP TIP

Hot wax

When selecting a hot wax, choose one that does not go brittle when cool. Wax sold as small blocks or pellets is preferable as this melts quickly, or choose a wax with a low melting point. Also available are peelable waxes which have a lower melting point and remain pliable when cool and are a popular alternative to traditional hot wax type.

Hot waxing

In **hot waxing**, the wax is applied at a higher temperature than warm wax. The hairs embed in the wax and are gripped tightly as the wax cools and contracts. When the wax is pulled away, it removes the hair from the base of the follicle.

Equipment and materials

The equipment and materials required for hot waxing are the same as for warm waxing (covered earlier in this chapter), except that:

◆ *a wax heater* suitable for hot wax should be selected

◆ *wax-removal* strips are not necessary

◆ *pre-wax oil* may be applied to the skin according to manufacturer's instructions before wax application to make wax removal easier.

Remember double dipping should be avoided. Some therapists prefer to apply the hot wax with disposable brushes rather than spatulas, but either can be used.

STEP-BY-STEP: PROVIDING HOT WAX SERVICE

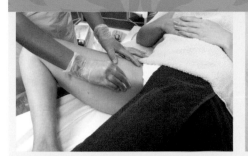

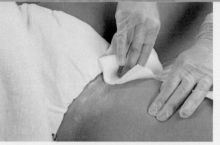

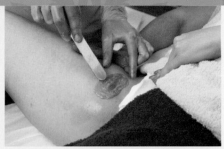

1 Prepare the client as for warm waxing. Ensure that the area to be waxed is clean and grease-free.

2 Apply a small amount of pre-depilation talc against the direction of hair growth. This will make the hairs stand away from the skin and embed more firmly into the wax. Alternatively apply oil if compatible with your wax type.

3 Carefully observe the direction of hair growth and the size of the area to be waxed. Trimming the hair in this area will facilitate this.

4 Test the heat of the wax on the inside of your wrist and on the client on the service area.

5 The client can hold their skin taut next to the area being waxed but their hands must not be in the way. Using either a disposable spatula or a brush, for legs apply a layer of wax about 5 cm × 10 cm *against* the direction of hair growth. The skin must be taut surrounding the area of application. Apply a second layer *with* the direction of growth; and a third layer against the direction of growth. (If two or three strips are applied at the same time, you can work faster. Removing one as the other strips harden.) Always follow the manufacturer's instructions as some hot wax products may be applied with growth. Keep the edges of the wax thicker than the middle, to make it easier to remove. Overlap the lower edge by about 2 cm onto a hair-free area: this makes it less painful later, when you lift the edge to make a lip to pull.

8 Check the area for any remaining wax and any stray hairs. Remove hairs hygienically using tweezers. Second applications are not advisable when using hot wax, because of the risk of burning. However, some manufacturers allow a repeat waxing where necessary as the wax contracts and grips the hair not the skin, minimising skin reaction. This will also depend on skin sensitivity and reaction to the waxing service.

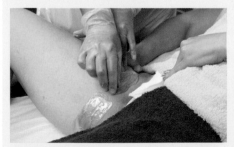

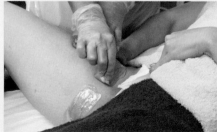

6 The wax can be removed when it has cooled sufficiently to grip the hairs, but whilst still pliable so that the wax does not become brittle and break on removal. As it sets, it starts to lose its gloss: it should be removed when this happens and while it is still pliable.

Curl up the lower end of the wax to make a lip, and press and mould the wax firmly onto the skin.

Further wax may be applied, working in sections.

7 Support the area below the wax, grasp the lip, and remove swiftly the wax off the skin *against* the direction of hair growth in one movement (as with warm-wax removal). Immediately apply pressure to the area with your hand: this takes away some of the discomfort.

TOP TIP

Wax temperature

If the wax becomes too cool and brittle for removal, fresh hot wax may be applied with care over the area to soften it.

ALWAYS REMEMBER

Hot wax temperature

If the wax is *not hot enough* when it is applied, it will not contract effectively around the hair and will therefore not grip it properly. This may result in poor depilation and possible hair breakage.

If on the other hand the wax is allowed to *overheat*, it may cause burns. Also, the quality of the wax will deteriorate and the wax will become brittle as it cools.

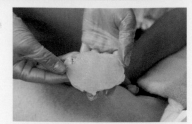

Hot wax should be removed when set but whilst still pliable

REVISION AID

What bacterial infection causes pustules to develop in the skin tissue around the hair follicle?

If this general application technique is followed, any area of the body can be depilated – use the same order of work as for warm waxing: observe the direction of hair growth and take into account the body area; use smaller strips in smaller areas; support the skin; and use the correct angle of pull for removal.

Apply a soothing antiseptic cream and use sterile tweezers to remove any stray hairs. Follow with appropriate aftercare advice.

Disposable applicator head waxing systems

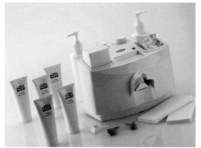

Disposable application starter kit

Roller head and flat applicator techniques wax systems are hygienic methods of removing hair as they use disposable applicators that are new for each client. A disposable applicator head screws onto the wax applicator tube/cartridge in place of a cap for each client. This reduces the possible risk of contamination through cross-infection. The tubes/cartridges of wax vary in size, as does the applicator head, to treat the different body areas. The method is less messy, as the wax is contained in the tube or cartridge and is not exposed until application.

Each tube/cartridge of wax as needed is heated to working temperature, which minimises the risk of burning. A thin film of wax is applied in the direction of hair growth. A wax removal strip is used to remove the wax from the skin against hair growth.

STEP-BY-STEP: WAXING THE LEGS USING A DISPOSABLE APPLICATOR

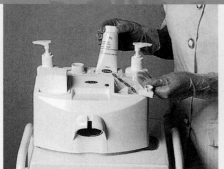

1 Remove the disposable applicator from the right-hand heating and storage compartment.

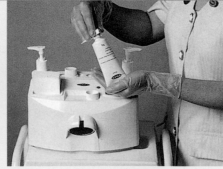

2 Remove the cap from the tube of wax. Attach the applicator head to the tube.

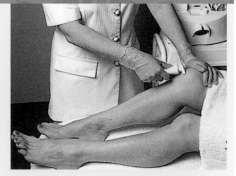

3 Release the applicator by lifting the lever upwards. Squeeze until a small amount of wax appears on the front of the applicator, then apply the wax. Hold the applicator at a 45° angle to the leg, and glide it smoothly down the leg.

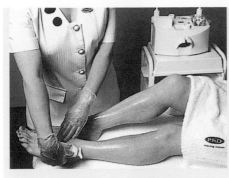

4 Apply a thin film of wax to the front of both legs, then press down the closing device on the applicator to stop wax flow.

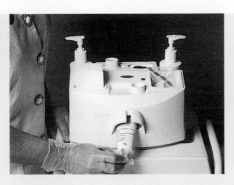

5 Wipe any wax residue from the front of the applicator and return the tube to heat.

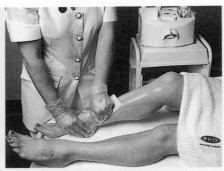

6 Remove wax from the leg, starting at the ankle and working towards the knee. Support the skin with one hand, and firmly stretch it against the removal of the wax.

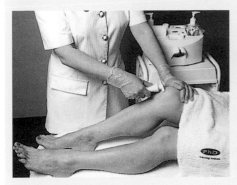

7 Continue application and removal to the sides and back of the legs.

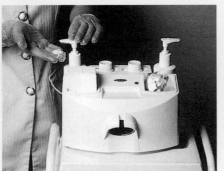

8 When service is complete, apply antiseptic soothing lotion (shown). Record details of the service on the client's record card.

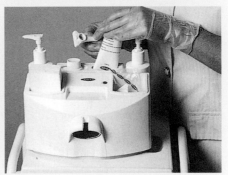

9 Remove the applicator from the tube, replace the cap and return the tube to the heater. Dispose of the applicator head.

Client advice and recommendations

The following aftercare advice and recommendations should be provided after each waxing service is completed to reconfirm the client's understanding of these important procedures.

A post-wax antiseptic lotion with soothing properties should be applied, using clean cotton wool, at the end of the service. This breaks down any wax residue, reduces skin reddening, helps to guard against secondary infection and irritation, and takes away any feelings of discomfort. Encourage your client to continue with the use of such a lotion at home for up to three days: it will protect against dryness, discomfort, infection and ingrowing hairs.

Products have been formulated to apply to the skin following wax depilation to slow hair regrowth. The product when entering the empty hair follicle aims to weaken the cell's matrix, slowing cell division in this area, which is responsible for creating the new hair. An additional benefit is that it also keeps the skin moisturised. These are available for your client to purchase as a retail product.

Advise the client against wearing any tight clothing (such as tights or hosiery) over the waxed areas for 24 hours following a service. Such clothing could lead to irritation and ingrowing hairs.

If the client suffers from ingrowing hairs, they should **exfoliate** their skin every four to seven days, starting two or three days after the service. It is also advisable to recommend the client carry out exfoliation before a waxing service. Exfoliation prevents the build-up of dead skin cells on the surface of the skin; these would otherwise block the exit from the follicle and cause

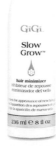

After-wax product to slow hair growth

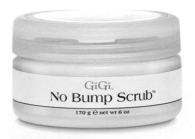

Exfoliating scrub

a growing hair to turn back on itself and grow inwards. Ingrowing hairs should be freed and, if possible, left in place so that the follicle exit will reform around the hair's shaft. Demonstrate to the client the correct use and benefits of the exfoliant product. Circular movements when using cosmetic products will ensure hairs growing in different directions are treated.

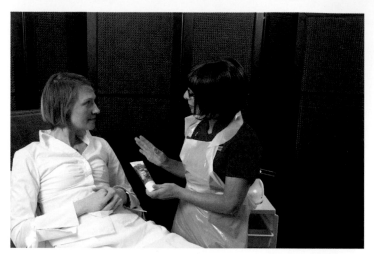

Recommending retail a post-wax products

Advise the client that for 24 hours following their service they should not apply any talcum powders, deodorants, antiperspirants, perfumes, self-tanning products or make-up over the treated areas. Any of these products could enter the hair follicles causing irritation or allergic reactions on the temporarily sensitised area. During this time they must use only plain, unperfumed soap and water to cleanse the treated area.

For the same 24-hour period they should preferably avoid exercise, especially swimming, and not apply heat or UV – hot baths, for example, or the use of a sun bed or sauna – as these would add to the heat generated in the skin following the service and would probably cause discomfort or irritation. They must also refrain from touching or scratching the area; explain to the client that this is to avoid infecting the open follicles.

Aftercare advice and recommendations should contain this information: as best practice these can be given to the client at the end of the service to remind them what to do at home or direct them to an electronic format if available. Images may be incorporated to visually demonstrate the text.

HEALTH & SAFETY

Sensitisation

Under no circumstances should wax be applied to facial hair, underarm hair or bikini line hair more than twice during any one service. If any hairs remain after two applications, they must be removed with tweezers. The delicate skin in these areas readily becomes sensitised.

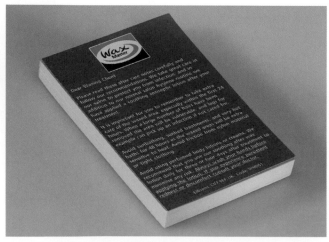

Aftercare leaflet

If there is a contra-action following service such as excessive redness and irritation, advise the client to apply a cool compress with soothing antiseptic lotion. If the redness does not disappear she must contact the salon. Advise the client to receive the service as follows: facial waxing three to four weeks; body waxing four to six weeks. Repeat bookings vary according to the natural hair regrowth and client requirements.

Remind the client that the hair grows in a three-stage cycle and not all hairs are in the same cycle at the same time. Some hairs will not be visible on the skin's surface at the time of waxing and some in **telogen** will be replaced by a new hair in the anagen growth cycle. This will explain why some hairs may appear following the waxing sevice.

Many salons incentivise their clients, offering complementary treatments following waxing service. An example is to include a foot massage.

Ensure that the client's records are up-to-date, accurate and complete following the waxing service and provide written instructions in an aftercare leaflet or direct them to an electronic format if available.

HEALTH & SAFETY

Post-wax lotion

Before post-wax lotion is applied, ensure that the area treated is free of waxing product and hair and check that the finished result is to the client's satisfaction.

The client expects all hairs to be removed.

Any residue left will cause dirt and materials in the area to stick, which could lead to secondary infection.

ACTIVITY

Aftercare advice and recommendations

Discuss why aftercare information should be provided to clients, as well as giving them the advice and recommendations verbally.

What could happen if aftercare advice is not given?

Design a suitable aftercare guidance sheet suitable for paper-based or digital production that you could provide for your clients following waxing service.

Threading

Threading, as a temporary method of hair removal, was discussed in Chapter 5 Eyelash and Eyebrow Treatments. Threading may also be used to remove hair from other body areas, but typically it is used to temporarily remove facial hair as described in the following pages.

It may be an option for clients who wish to have facial hair removed but who have an allergy to waxing service.

The advantages and disadvantages of this service are listed as follows.

TOP TIP

Minimising discomfort

Thread in small sections on the upper lip and brow area to minimise discomfort as the hairs are removed.

Advantages	Disadvantages
◆ Only removes hair not skin	◆ Some clients may experience side-effects following the treatment; these include excessive skin reddening (erythema) and short-term puffiness of the skin tissue treated
◆ Good for removal of short hairs	◆ The area may be uncomfortable for a short while
◆ Can isolate one hair at a time	◆ Itching may occur following hair removal
◆ Can go over an area more than once without causing skin irritation	◆ Ingrowing hair may occur when the hair regrows or as a result of poor technique
◆ Sharp, defined shape can be achieved	◆ Infections may occur (e.g. folliculitis), if homecare advice is not followed as the follicle will remain open for up to 24 hours following the treatment
◆ Inexpensive to perform as minimal resources required	
◆ Fast results	
◆ Ideal for eyebrows and facial hair	
◆ Minimal skin irritation – good for delicate, sensitive skin types	

Facial hair threading

The client's skin is prepared as for facial waxing service. Agree the hair to be removed. It is important to protect the scalp hair to avoid accidentally catching the hair in the thread. For the upper lip the client is asked to keep the skin of the upper lip taut, keeping the skin firmly stretched. Ask your client to place their tongue into the area of treatment or to stretch their upper lip over their upper teeth. This will facilitate hair removal. Hair is removed in small sections, using the preferred threading technique from the side of the lip working towards the centre of the face.

When removing hair from the chin position the neck so that it is taut. Position the client's hands so that they are holding the skin taut adjacent to the area of threading. Work from one side of the face to the other.

Threading client advice and recommendations is provided in chapter 5.

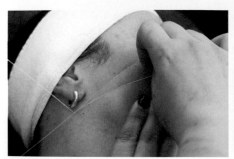
Removing facial hair from the sides of the face

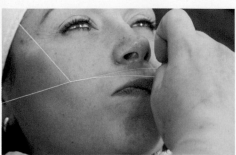
Removing facial hair from the upper lip

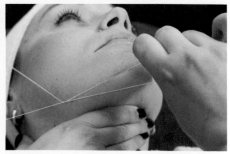
Removing facial hair from the chin and jawline

ASSESSMENT OF KNOWLEDGE AND UNDERSTANDING

Having covered the learning objectives for this chapter, test what you need to know and understand by answering the following short questions below.

The information covers:

◆ Organisational and legal requirements
◆ How to work safely and effectively when providing waxing services
◆ Client consultation and preparation
◆ Anatomy and physiology
◆ Contra-indications and contra-actions
◆ Products, tools and equipment
◆ Waxing service application
◆ Client advice and recommendations

Organisational and legal requirements

For full legislation details, see Chapter 1.

1. What are your responsibilities under the relevant local and national health and safety legislation when carrying out waxing services? Give **three** examples.

2. What actions must be taken before a client under 16 years of age receives a waxing service?

3. Give an example of how you may need to modify your service to treat a client with a particular disability, e.g. mobility, visual or hearing impairment.

4. Why must a client's signature be obtained before commencing waxing service?

5. How would you prepare yourself for waxing service to comply with personal protective equipment (PPE) legislation requirements?

6. How should all clients' records be stored to comply with the Data Protection Act (1998)?

7. How long would you allow to complete a full leg and bikini line waxing service when using warm wax technique?

8. Why is it important for staff to be familiar with the waxing pricing structures?

9. What details should have been recorded on the client's record by the end of the service?

10. What is contaminated waste and when might it be generated during a waxing service and how should this be disposed of following waxing service?

How to work safely and effectively when providing waxing services

1. Why is it important to wear PPE?

2. How can you minimise the risk of acquiring the skin condition contact dermatitis when performing waxing services?

3. Give **three** examples of when both sterilisation and disinfection methods are used to comply with hygiene regulations when performing a waxing service.

4. What is the recommended temperature of wax when using:

   a. hot wax
   b. warm wax spatula method?

5. Why is it important to disinfect your hands before each service even though disposable gloves are to be worn?

6. What are the necessary environmental conditions required for waxing? Consider lighting, heating and ventilation in your answer.

7. How can cross-infection be prevented when carrying out waxing service? Provide **three** examples.

8. Why is your posture and position of the client an important consideration when carrying out the waxing service?

Client consultation and preparation

1. To reassure the client, how would you explain the waxing service sensation and expected post-service skin reaction to them?

2. It is necessary to check the hair growth before hair removal. How long should hair growth be for successful wax depilation to be carried out?

3. A client complains that on their previous service (which was their first), stubbly hairs appeared the following week. What could have been the cause?

4. How would you position the client for wax depilation for:

    a. a bikini line wax
    b. an underarm wax
    c. a chin wax?

5. Why would you refer to the menstrual cycle when performing a waxing service on a female client?

6. What skin tests should be carried out before a waxing service? When and why would you perform each?

7. How should the area to be treated be prepared for wax depilation, to ensure effective hair removal?

8. Why is it necessary to explain contra-actions that may occur with the client at the consultation?

9. It is necessary to consider the direction of hair growth for the hair removal technique chosen. Why is this?

10. Why is it important to consider the client's privacy and modesty?

Anatomy and physiology

For full anatomy and physiology details, see Chapter 2.

1. How many layers form the epidermis of the skin? From which layer are cells removed when carrying out a waxing service?

2. What is the name of the structure that the hair grows from in the skin?

3. What is the difference between a sebaceous and sudoriferous gland?

4. What are the three stages of the hair growth cycle? Briefly explain what happens to the hair at each stage. When is this knowledge shared with the client?

5. If the client was too cold or too warm when receiving waxing service how would this affect the wax and hair and surrounding skin being treated?

6. What are the main functions of the skin?

7. What is the normal reaction to the skin following waxing service and what is its cause?

8. What are the three main parts if you looked at a cross-section of the hair?

9. What is the name given to coarse pigmented hair and where is it mainly found on the body?

Contra-indications and contra-actions

1. What would be **three** undesirable post-service skin reactions? How would these be avoided?

2. Which contra-indications restrict service, meaning that the service may proceed, but the area contra-indicated must be avoided?

3. When observing the area for hair removal you identify what you think to be a contra-indication requiring referral. What action would you take?

4. Why is diabetes normally regarded initially as a contra-indication to waxing service?

Products, tools and equipment

1. Certain ingredients may cause an allergic reaction; therefore it is important that you know what the product contains. What are the main ingredients in:

    a. warm wax
    b. hot wax?

2. What is the purpose of pre-wax lotion when used in a waxing service?

3. What should be applied to the skin following wax depilation? What action does this product have on the treated area?

4. When might you apply talc or oil to the skin in a waxing service?

Waxing service

1. It is important to select the most suitable method to remove the hair type. From the following temporary hair removal methods – warm wax and hot wax – identify which you would select for:

    a. the face
    b. the underarm
    c. the bikini line.

2. How do hot wax and warm wax usually differ in relation to:

    a. application
    b. removal?

3. Give an example of the precautions you would need to take when performing waxing service around an area where there is a contra-indication that restricts service. State what your contra-indication is.

4. Explain **three** other temporary methods of hair removal and **three** permanent methods of hair removal. If a client had received these services previously how would this affect the service plan for waxing?

5. Why should the skin be supported during the waxing service by the beauty therapist and the client?

6. What is the normal skin reaction to waxing service that should be explained to the client at the consultation?

7. What additional precautions should be taken to ensure that the wax is used at a comfortable temperature for the client?

Client advice and recommendations

1. What activities should be avoided immediately following the waxing service and for how long should they be avoided?

2. In what forms should aftercare instructions be provided to the client following waxing service to ensure compliance with insurance requirements?

3. If your client suffers from ingrowing hairs, what advice would you give them that could possibly prevent them recurring?

4. When would you book a client to return for the following repeat waxing services, and how long would you allow for treatment of the:

   a. eyebrow
   b. full leg
   c. bikini line
   d. underarm
   e. lip and chin?

5. What contra-actions could occur following waxing service? What advice should you provide regarding actions to take?

6. Which other services should not be performed on the treatment area at the same service as waxing?

7. What opportunities for retail sales may be linked to this service?

Glossary

Acid mantle the combination of sweat and sebum on the skin's surface, which creates an acid film. The acid mantle is protective and discourages the growth of bacteria and fungi.

Accident an unfortunate, non-deliberate event that may result in harm or loss. In the workplace, a written record of an accident must be made in an accident book, if need be, and reviewed to see where improvements to working practice can be made.

Adhesive specialised glue used to attach artificial lashes to the natural lashes. This glue differs in formulation according to the lash type.

Adipose tissue body tissue layer that stores fat.

Advice and recommendations information provided to clients about the treatment, including how they can prolong the treatment benefits, home care routines, recommended time intervals, additional products and services, and how these will benefit them.

After-wax lotion a product applied to the skin following hair removal to reduce redness and promote skin healing.

Age group different classifications of age groups that are generally grouped as follows: 16–30, 31–50 and over 50 years.

Allergen a substance that the skin is sensitive to and which causes an allergic reaction.

Allergic reaction response by the body to a substance or ingredients in a product, producing symptoms including erythema, swelling, itching and bruising.

Alternating current (AC) an interrupted electrical current that reverses the direction of flow of electrons.

Anagen the active growth stage of the hair-growth cycle.

Antioxidant properties of some foods that maintain the health of the skin, reducing the damaging effects of free radicals (unstable molecules that can cause skin cells to break down) in the body. Antioxidant ingredients are increasingly included in skincare preparations to keep products stable and to reduce the harmful effects of free radicals.

Appointment arrangement made for a client to receive a service or treatment on a particular date and time.

Apprenticeships training model, where you work towards your qualification developing the necessary workplace skills and experience to perform the job role, combining 'on-the-job' training in a real workplace with classroom or e-based learning and assessment at a college or other training provider. You will work towards your technical qualification alongside additional transferable skills and qualifications, including English, Maths, and employment rights and responsibilities.

Astringent toning lotion containing alcohol, formulated to remove sebum and tighten the skin's surface.

Atoms the smallest parts of an element that can exist by themselves and possess the element's characteristics. An atom is the basic unit of all matter.

Bacteria minute, single-celled organisms of various shapes which inhabit the body. These may be harmless, referred to as non-pathogenic bacteria; others are harmful and can cause disease, referred to as pathogenic bacteria.

Base coat a nail polish product applied to improve the health and appearance of the nail, provide protection, prevent staining from coloured nail polish, and give an even surface to improve nail polish application and adherence.

Behaviours these relate to your conduct and underpin the delivery of all beauty therapy treatments, which ensure that the client receives a positive impression of the workplace and its employees.

Bevelling a nail filing technique used at the free edge of the nail to ensure it is smooth and to prevent splitting.

Blending nail art paints applied and blended together without definite lines, creating a marbling or iridescent effect dependent upon products and brushes used.

Blood liquid circulating through the blood vessels. It transports essential nutrients to the cells and other important substances such as oxygen and hormones as well as removing carbon dioxide and waste products.

Blood vessel part of the circulatory system that carries blood around the body. The main types of blood vessel are arteries, veins and capillaries, which differ in their structure and role in blood transportation.

Body language communication involving the body, rather than speech. It includes facial expressions and hand gestures.

Bruising nail condition where the skin appears blue/black in colour due to bleeding which has occurred on the nail bed, beneath the nail plate, following injury.

Buffer a tool that can be used for manicure and pedicure services. It is used on the nail plate to remove surface cells, provide a sheen, increase blood supply to the nail bed and, if used with an abrasive paste, help smooth out nail surface irregularities.

Catagen a brief, transitional stage in the cycle of hair growth in which the hair moves up the hair follicle.

Cell the smallest and simplest unit capable of life.

Central nervous system (CNS) composed of the brain and the spinal cord, which coordinate the activities of the whole body.

Cheque an alternative form of payment to that of using cash or a credit/debit card.

Circulatory system transports materials around the body. It supplies cells with oxygen and nutrients and then carries away waste products.

Cleanser a skincare preparation that removes dead skin cells, excess sweat and sebum, make-up and dirt from the skin's surface to maintain a healthy skin condition. These are formulated to treat different skin types, conditions and facial areas.

Client care standards on how clients should be treated to ensure their treatment meets expectations and without harm.

Client records confidential information recording the personal details of each client registered at the salon.

Code of practice the expected standards and behaviour for the professional beauty therapist to follow, which will uphold the reputation of the industry and ensure best working practice as well as protect members of the public. Beauty therapy professional bodies produce codes of practice for their members. A business may have its own code of practice.

Cold wax pre-prepared wax strip used for removal of unwanted hair. It is ready for use without the need for heating.

Comedone extraction facial technique used to extract (remove) comedones (blackheads) from the skin. A small tool called a comedone extractor is used for this purpose.

Communication the exchange of information and the establishment of understanding between people. It can be verbal and non-verbal.

Complaints procedure a formal, standardised approach adopted by an organisation to handle any complaints.

Congenital (hair growth) inherited predisposition (tendency) to grow excessive hair all over the body.

Connective tissue sheath surrounds both the hair follicle and sebaceous gland, providing a sensory supply and a blood supply. The connective tissue sheath includes, and is a continuation of, the papilla.

Consultation assessment of the client's needs using different techniques, including questioning and natural observation.

Continuing professional development (CPD) activities undertaken to develop technical skill and expertise and to ensure current, professional experience in the industry is maintained.

Contra-action an unwanted reaction occurring during or after treatment application.

Contract of employment an agreement between an employer and employee identifying the terms and conditions of employment.

Contra-indication a problematic symptom which indicates that treatment may not proceed.

Credit card an alternative form of payment to that of using cash. These cards are held by those who have a credit account, where there is a pre-arranged borrowing limit. These can only be used if your business has an arrangement to deal with the relevant credit card company.

Curing equipment devices used in the process of polymerisation, such as UV and LED.

Cuticle cream a cosmetic preparation used to condition and rehydrate the nail and skin of the cuticle.

Cuticle nippers a metal tool used to remove excess cuticle and neaten dead skin around the cuticle area.

Cuticle oil a cosmetic preparation used to condition the skin of the cuticle.

Cuticle remover a cosmetic preparation used to soften and loosen the skin cells and cuticle from the nail plate.

Debit card alternative method of payment, where the card authorises immediate debit of the cash amount from the client's bank account.

Demonstration an activity that allows you to show clients a product or treatment to enhance their awareness and understanding of it.

Dermal papilla a structure that provides the hair follicle with blood, necessary for hair growth.

Dermis the inner portion of the skin, situated underneath the epidermis composed of dense connective tissue containing other structures such as the lymphatic system, blood vessels and nerves. It is much thicker than the epidermis.

Diagnostic assessment tools and techniques used for gaining information about the client at consultation which will inform the treatment plan objectives.

Direct current (DC) an electrical current using the effects of polarity. The electrons flow constantly, uninterrupted, in one direction.

Disciplinary if expected workplace procedures and standards of behaviour are broken, it may lead to appropriate measures being applied as identified in the workplace disciplinary procedure.

Discrepancy a disagreement, for example, over amounts of money, etc. This is referred to in instances where clients disagree with what they are being asked to pay or the amount of change received.

Disposable applicator a tool used to apply products hygienically to an area of the body without the risk of client contamination. The applicator is disposed of after each service.

Dotting technique placement of dots of nail paint or polish using a nail art tool referred to as a dotting/marbling tool. The dots may create a design or be blended together to create a marbling nail art technique.

Dotting tool also known as a marbling tool, it is a nail art tool that can have different sized balls on each end which are used for applying dots of colour to the nail plate and for marbling techniques.

Effleurage a massage movement which has a sedating and relaxing effect; applied with the whole palm it can be made superficially or deeply.

Elastin a protein fibre giving the skin elasticity, produced by specialised cells called fibroblasts.

Electric current the flow of electrons along an electric circuit between the electrical supply and the appliance.

Elements the basic unit of all matter, it is the simplest form of matter that cannot be broken down further.

Embellishment a nail art decorative addition including rhinestones, flat stones or any pre-made art products such as bows and flowers.

Endocrine system coordinates and regulates processes in the body by means of chemicals (hormones), released by endocrine glands into the bloodstream. Hormones control activities such as growth or the development of the secondary sexual characteristics.

Enquiries questions presented by clients or business contacts to find out more information.

Epidermis the outer layer of the skin located directly above the skin dermis. Composed of five layers, with the surface layer forming the outer skin, which has a protective function.

Erythema reddening of the skin.

Ethics behaviour and standards which are morally correct, and consider the outcomes of all professional decisions made.

Exfoliation to remove excess dead skin cells from the surface of the skin, which has a cleansing action. This process can be achieved using a specialised cosmetic, or mechanically, using facial equipment applied over the skin's surface.

Express facial a quick facial treatment that usually lasts 30 minutes. Applied for a variety of reasons, this allows the customer to experience the benefits of the products or service.

Extraction the manual removal of minor impurities from the skin including comedones (blackheads) and milia (whiteheads).

Eyebrow artistry a combination of techniques of hair removal and colour products applied to define and emphasise the shape of the brow.

Eyebrow pencil a cosmetic product applied to eyebrows to provide colour, emphasise or alter their shape, and which can make sparse eyebrows look thicker.

Eyebrow powder a cosmetic product applied to eyebrows to provide colour, emphasise or alter their shape, and which can make sparse eyebrows look thicker.

Eye make-up remover a product that cleanses the eye area, gently emulsifying the make-up and conditioning the delicate skin in this area.

Eyebrow shaping the removal of eyebrow hair to create a new shape (reshape) or to remove stray hairs to maintain the existing brow shape (maintenance). Shaping treatments can be performed with tweezers, threading or waxing, or a combination of techniques.

Eyebrow template a shaped stencil-like template which can be filled with colour to create and define the eyebrow shape.

Eyebrow threading a method of hair removal using specialist thread.

Eyelash and eyebrow tinting the permanent colouring of the eyelash or eyebrow hairs to enhance and define their appearance by applying specialised dye formulated for use around the delicate eye area.

Eyelash attachment made from small threads of nylon fibre or real hair, they are attached to the client's natural lash to provide additional length and thickness.

Eyelash extension adhesive a specialised glue used to attach artificial eyelashes to the natural eyelashes. Formulations differ according to the artificial eyelash chosen, including flare, strip and single lash systems.

Eyelash extension solvent a specialised solvent used to dissolve lash adhesive for flare and single lash extension systems when removal is required.

Eyelash extensions made from small threads of nylon fibre or real hair, they are attached to the client's natural lash to provide additional length, thickness and to achieve a balanced look.

Facial products skincare used within a facial treatment or for home use, with specific benefits to care for and improve the function, health and appearance of the skin.

Facial treatment the application of different techniques using the hands, tools and equipment, and scientifically formulated skincare products with key ingredients to maintain and improve the function, health and appearance of the skin.

Fibres these are found in the dermis and give the skin its strength and elasticity. Yellow elastin gives the skin its elasticity, white collagen gives skin its strength.

Fitzpatrick Classification this is a skin classification system on a scale of 1 to 6 based on photosensitivity reaction to UV light. It was devised in 1975 at Harvard University.

Flare lashes a collection of individual false eyelash hairs of differing colours and lengths attached to a non-adhesive bulb.

Fluid retention accumulation of tissue fluid creating swelling; termed oedema.

Foiling a technique used in nail art that uses a specialised foil attached to decorate the nails.

Folliculitis a bacterial infection where pustules develop in the skin tissue around the hair follicle.

Foot and nail treatments specialised products and equipment designed to improve the condition and appearance of different nail and skin conditions.

Foot rasp a pedicure tool used to remove excess dead skin from the foot.

Foot spa a foot bath incorporating massage and water aeration, creating a bubbling effect to cleanse and relax the feet.

Freehand techniques freehand drawing using nail art medium on the nail plate.

Frictions a massage manipulation which causes the skin and superficial structures to move together over the deeper, underlying structures. The movements help to break down fibrous thickening and fat deposits, and aid the removal of any non-medical oedemas (areas of fluid retention).

Fungal infection caused by different parasitic fungi which are dependent upon a host for their existence.

Gel polish a polish system of base, top coats and colours that are cured (set) under a UV or LED lamp.

Gift voucher a pre-payment method for beauty therapy services or retail sales.

Glitters sparkly powders or foil material applied to add shimmer to create or enhance a nail art design.

Hair a long slender structure that grows out of, and is part of, the skin. Each hair is made up of dead skin cells, which contain the protein called keratin.

Hair analysis to learn more about the appearance, hair type and growth.

Hair colour characteristics natural hair colouring, including fair, red, dark and white. It should be considered and may influence treatment application such as compatibility of colour and development time when eyelash tinting.

Hair cuticle the protective outer layer of the hair, composed of unpigmented, flat, scale-like cells. These cells contain hard keratin and overlap each other from the base to the tip of the hair.

Hair follicle a structure in the skin formed from epidermal tissue. Cells move up the hair follicle from the bottom (the hair bulb), changing in structure, to form the hair.

Hair growth cycle the cyclical pattern of hair growth, which can be divided into three stages: anagen, catagen and telogen.

Hair removal techniques the use of temporary and permanent methods to remove unwanted (superfluous) hair.

Hand and nail treatments specialised products and equipment designed to improve the condition and appearance of different nail and skin conditions.

Hazard something with potential to cause harm.

Health and Safety Executive (HSE) the UK government organisation responsible for setting legislation for health and safety and overseeing its regulation and enforcement.

Health and safety policy each employer of more than five employees must have a written health and safety policy issued to their employees outlining their health and safety responsibilities.

Hirsutism hair growth pattern considered to be abnormal for the person's gender, e.g. female hair growth following a male hair growth pattern. The hair growth is usually terminal when it should be a vellus type.

Histamine a chemical released when the skin comes into contact with a substance to which it is allergic. This causes a reaction referred to as a histamine reaction. Cells called mast cells burst, releasing histamine into the tissues. This causes the blood capillaries to dilate, which increases blood flow to limit skin damage and begin repair.

Homeostasis regulation of internal chemical balance within the body.

Hormones chemical messengers transported in the blood. They control the activity of many organs in the body, including the cells and glands in the skin.

Hot wax a system of wax depilation used to remove hair from the skin. Hot wax, also known as hard wax, traditionally cools and sets on contact with the skin. Hot wax products are made from a blend of waxes and resins which keep the wax flexible as well as soothing ingredients to avoid skin irritation.

Human resources (HR) employees that make up the workforce in the business.

Hydrogen peroxide (H_2O_2) an oxidant, a chemical that contains available oxygen atoms and encourages certain chemical reactions.

Hygiene the recommended standard of cleanliness necessary in the salon to prevent cross-infection and secondary infection as laid down by law, and industry codes of practice or written procedures specified by the organisation.

Hyper-pigmentation increased pigment production.

Hypertrichosis excessive hair growth for a person's gender, age and race. It is usually due to abnormal conditions in the body caused by disease or injury.

Hypo-pigmentation loss of pigmentation.

Ingrowing hair a hair that has not grown above the surface of the epidermis and grows abnormally into the surrounding tissue.

Inner root sheath grows from the bottom of the hair follicle at the papilla, both the hair and inner root sheath grow upwards together until level with the sebaceous gland when it ceases to grow.

Integumentary system the largest organ of the body, comprising the skin and its associated components such as hair, nails and glands.

Insulators poor conductors of electricity often used to prevent the flow of electrons. Insulators include rubber, plastic and wood.

Jewellery tool a nail piercing tool that has a sharp, tiny drill used to make a small hole in the free edge of the nail. The hole is used to accommodate jewellery with a post, secured by a tiny nut or ring attached through the hole.

Job description written details of a person's specific job role, duties and responsibilities.

Joint area where two points of the skeleton meet.

Keratin a protein produced by cells in the epidermis called keratinocytes. Keratin makes the skin tough and reduces the passage of substances into our bodies. Hair and nails contain keratin.

Lanugo hair a type of hair found on the unborn foetus; usually shed at the eighth month of pregnancy.

Legal requirements mandatory rules and regulations that affect workplace practice and procedures.

Liability insurance protects employers and employees against the consequences of death or injury to a third party while on the premises, also known as public liability insurance.

Lifestyle factors a set of personal considerations for each client that may have an impact on their health and skin condition. Examples include smoking, drinking alcohol, diet and stress levels.

Limbic system is involved in emotions and memory. It consists of a group of structures that encircle the brain stem.

Lipids these are fats or oils.

Lymph a clear straw-coloured liquid circulating in the lymph vessels and lymphatic system of the body, filtered out of the blood plasma.

Lymphatic system closely connected to the blood system. Its primary function is defensive: to remove bacteria and foreign materials in order to prevent infection. The lymphatic system consists of the fluid lymph, the lymph vessels and the lymph nodes (or glands).

Magnifying light used to direct light onto the area of the body with some magnification, providing a useful tool for skin and hair analysis.

Make-up products different cosmetics available to suit skin type, colour and condition. Make-up products include primers, tinted moisturisers, concealing and contour cosmetics, foundations, powders, eyeshadows, eyeliners, eyebrow cosmetics, mascara, lip cosmetics and setting sprays.

Make-up style the client's preference and the context in which the make-up is to be viewed and that will influence application. This includes natural light, evening and special occasions such as parties or weddings.

Make-up techniques choice and application of make-up products to enhance and minimise the skin and facial features and achieve a make-up look or style.

Make-up tools a range of different shapes and sizes of tools including sponges, brushes and disposable items to create different make-up looks and application considerations.

Manicure a service to care for and improve the condition and appearance of the hands and nails.

Marbling a technique used in nail art that mixes two or more colours together to create a design.

Marbling tool also known as a dotting tool, this is a nail art tool available with different sized balls on each end used for applying dots of colour to the nail plate. These are then combined to create a marble effect.

Marketing methods used to raise publicity for the business, its brand image, products and treatments, in order to support sales and growth.

Mask a setting or non-setting skin treatment preparation containing different ingredients applied to the skin. It can have a deep cleansing, toning, nourishing or refreshing effect. It may be applied to the face, hands and feet or targeted areas such as the eyes.

Massage manipulation of the body's soft tissues, using a series of movements or manipulations selected according to their effects which may be stimulating, relaxing and toning. Their effects produce localised heat, relaxation and stimulation affecting the circulatory, muscular and nervous systems.

Massage medium a product used to suit skin types, e.g. oil, balm and cream, to facilitate massage manipulation of soft tissues and, dependent upon formulation, to benefit and improve skin condition.

Massage techniques movements that are selected and applied according to the required effect, which may be stimulating, relaxing or toning. Massage manipulations include effleurage, petrissage, percussion (also known as tapotement), vibrations and frictions.

Matter anything that takes up space. It exists in three physical forms – solid, liquid and gas – and is made up of chemical elements.

Medical history a client's past and present health record that may include current medication, recent operations, allergies to products, etc.

Melanin a pigment in the skin that contributes to skin and hair colour.

Melanocytes the cells that produce the skin pigment melanin, which contributes to skin and hair colour.

Message taking communication of information to another person in written, electronic or verbal form.

Method of payment different forms of payment that may be accepted to pay for a product or service including cash, cash equivalents, cheque and payment cards.

Moisturiser a skincare preparation often with a formulation of oil and water that helps maintain the skin's natural moisture, offering protection and hydration.

Motor nerves these are nerves situated in a muscle tissue and act on information from the brain, causing a particular response, typically muscle movement.

Motor point a location on the muscles where the motor nerve can be most easily stimulated.

Muscle tone the normal degree of tension in healthy muscle.

Muscular system responsible for movement of the body, when muscular tissue contracts and shortens.

Nail the structure on the end of each finger and toe formed from hard, keratinised, epidermal cells that protect the living nail bed of the fingers and toes.

Nail analysis to learn more about the shape, condition and cause of the nails' appearance.

Nail art nail decoration using a variety of techniques and materials.

Nail art techniques application methods used to create different visual effects including dotting, striping, marbling, freehand painting, foiling and blending.

Nail conditions the nail appearance is assessed at the consultation, called nail analysis. This will identify the nail condition. Nail condition examples include brittle, discoloured, pitted, ridged, split, dry, dehydrated and bitten.

Nail finish the product finally applied to the natural nail to enhance its appearance; for example, buffed nail or nail polish colour application and style.

Nail growth cells divide in the matrix and the nails grow forward over the nail bed until they reach the end of the finger. The nail cells harden as they grow through a process called keratinisation.

Nail plate a tough hard covering on top of the nail bed, composed of keratinised skin cells.

Nail polish a clear or coloured nail product that adds colour/protection to the nail. Cream polish has a finish that benefits from a top coat application to increase durability. Pearlised polish produces a frosted, shimmery appearance and top coat is not required.

Nail polish drier an aerosol or oil preparation applied following nail polish application to increase the speed at which the polish hardens.

Nail polish remover a solvent (often acetone) used to remove nail polish and grease from the nails prior to applying polish.

Nail polish solvent used to thin nail polish and to restore its quality and consistency.

Nail shapes if there is sufficient length at the nail's free edge, this can be shaped by filing. There are several popular shapes, selected according to the client's natural nail shape, condition and length, finger length and hand size, fashion and client preference. Nail shapes include oval, square, squoval, pointed and round.

Nail strengthener a nail polish product that strengthens the nail plate, which has a tendency to split.

Nail structure composed for protection, the nail is made up of the following parts: nail plate, nail bed, matrix, cuticle, lunula, hyponychium, eponychium, perionychium nail wall, free edge and lateral nail fold.

Natural nail shapes these include fan, hook, spoon, oval and square.

Nerve a collection of single neurones surrounded by a protective sheath through which impulses are transmitted between the brain or spinal cord and other parts of the body.

Neurones nerve cells which makes up nervous tissue.

Node (lymphatic) small, oval shaped glands of the lymphatic system responsible for storage and filtration of lymph.

Non-pathogenic harmless microorganisms that can provide a positive benefit to the health of the body.

Nutrition the nourishment derived from food, required for the body's growth, energy and repair.

Oedema the retention of fluid in the tissues, causing swelling.

Olfactory system located high inside the nose and responsible for the sense of smell. When we breathe in aromas, nerve endings in the olfactory system are stimulated and relay messages to the brain, which cause the body to respond.

Open questions a questioning technique that requires more than a one word response.

Outer root sheath forms the hair follicle wall. This does not grow up with the hair but is stationary, a continuation of the growing layer of the epidermis.

Oxidisation the addition of oxygen to a compound resulting in a chemical reaction where one or more substances are changed into others.

Papillae projections near the surface of the dermis, which contain nerve endings and blood capillaries. They supply the upper epidermis with nutrition.

Paraffin wax a substance that is heated and applied to the skin of the hands and feet to provide a warming effect. This improves skin functioning, aids the absorption of products and is beneficial to ease the discomfort of arthritic and rheumatic conditions.

Parasite organisms that require a host to live on or in, and gain their nutrients from to survive.

Patch test a pre-treatment test applied to the skin, which checks for sensitivity to an ingredient or nerve stimuli responses to heat or touch.

Pathogenic harmful microorganisms that can cause disease or infection in the body.

Pedicure a service to care for and improve the condition and appearance of the skin and nails of the feet.

Personal protective equipment (PPE) all of the items, clothing and tools that are required for specific activities to ensure the health and safety of the employee and the client.

Petrissage massage manipulations which apply intermittent pressure to the tissues of the skin, lifting them from the underlying structures. Often known as compression movements.

Pigmentation the colouring of the skin or hair. The amount of pigment varies for each client, resulting in different skin/hair colour.

Pilosebaceous unit hair follicles together with the sebaceous gland form the skin structure: the pilosebaceous unit.

Polish secures embellishments in nail art that stick to the nail using nail polish such as rhinestones and flat stones.

Posture the position of the body, which varies from person to person. Good posture is when the body is in alignment.

Pre-wax lotion an antibacterial skin cleanser applied to clean the skin before wax depilation hair removal.

Primer provides a base for make-up and acts as a barrier preventing absorption of the make-up products into the skin.

Promotion an event that aims to benefit the business and meet specified objectives.

Promotional activities actions carried out to benefit the business to meet specified objectives.

Receptionist person responsible for maintaining the reception area, scheduling appointments and handling payments.

Repetitive strain injury (RSI) injury incurred through repetition of movement of a particular part of the body.

Risk the likelihood of potential harm happening from a hazard.

Salon services a general term, covering all of the treatments and services offered in a salon or workplace.

Scissors (nail) tools used to shorten the length of the nail before filing.

Sebaceous gland a minute sac-like structure usually associated with the hair follicle. The cells of the gland decompose and produce the skin's natural oil, sebum. Found all over the body except the soles of the feet and the palms of the hands. It is usually associated with the hair follicle, which together form the pilosebaceous unit.

Sebum the skin's natural oil which keeps the skin supple.

Self-management taking responsibility to manage oneself to improve productivity and the achievement of business outcomes.

Sensory nerves these nerves receive information and relay it to the brain. They are found near to the skin's surface and respond to touch, pressure, temperature and pain.

Service areas the areas of the body that will be treated.

Single (or individual) lashes single artificial lashes which are attached to a single natural lash by a specialised adhesive.

Skeletal system supports the softer tissues of the body and maintains the shape of the body.

Skills the ability to perform tasks competently that underpin workplace activities.

Skin allergy if the skin is sensitive to a particular substance an allergic skin reaction will occur. This is recognised by irritation, swelling and inflammation.

Skin analysis assessment of the client's skin type and condition.

Skin appendages structures within the skin including sweat glands (excrete sweat), hair follicles (produce hair), sebaceous glands (produce the skin's natural oil, sebum) and nails (a horny substance that protects the ends of fingers and toes).

Skin colour the colour of the client's skin tone. This should be considered when selecting colours to suit the skin colour.

Skin conditions (sensitive, dehydrated, mature, young) additional characteristics observed when identifying skin type as part of the analysis that indicates the condition of the skin.

Skin disease abnormal condition that affects the skin's health and its normal functioning.

Skin disorder abnormal condition that affects normal functioning and may affect the skin's health.

Skin removal accidental removal of the upper, dead, protective cornified layer of the skin, leaving the granular layer exposed.

Skin sensitivity patch test this is performed to determine if the client is allergic to a product being applied or to assess skin response.

Skin structure the largest organ and the external protective covering of the body. The skin is made up of two main divisions: the epidermis and dermis.

Skin tone the strength and elasticity of the skin.

Skin type the different physiological functioning of each person's skin provides their skin type. Skin types include dry (lacking in oil), oily (excessive oil) and combination (a mixture of two skin types, i.e. dry and oily).

Skin warming device a piece of equipment or other resource that can be used to warm the client's skin. A facial steamer is one example, which heats water to boiling point so that the steam can be directed safely at the client's skin. Another example is a hot towel cabinet which heats towels.

Specialised skin products additional skincare preparations available to target improvement. These products include eye gels, neck creams, serums and lip balms.

Strip lashes a length of artificial lashes attached to a non-adhesive strip which are attached to the natural lash line using a specialised adhesive.

Striping a nail art technique, creating lines or stripes of different lengths, thickness and definition using a nail art striping brush. These are available in different sizes, lengths and the number of hairs is relevant for the look to be achieved.

Subcutaneous layer a layer of fatty tissue situated below the dermis layer of the skin.

Superfluous hair considered to be in excess of the amount of normal downy hair for the person's age and gender, but is considered unwanted.

Sweat glands (or sudoriferous glands) are small tubes in the skin of the dermis and epidermis which excrete sweat. Their function is to regulate body temperature through the evaporation of sweat from the skin's surface. There are two types of gland: eccrine gland and apocrine gland.

Systemic (hair growth) a type of hair growth that can be normal (as caused by hormones at puberty, pregnancy and menopause) or abnormal (caused by hormonal imbalance due to disease, tumour, surgery, medication or emotional stress).

Tapotement also known as percussion. A massage manipulation that is used for its general toning and stimulating effect.

Telogen the resting stage of the hair growth cycle where the hair is finally shed.

Terminal hair deep-rooted, thick, coarse, pigmented hair found on the scalp, underarms, pubic region, eyelash and brow areas.

Thermal test patch used to test the skin's ability to detect differences in temperature and comfort with the heat of a product such as wax when applied to the skin during wax depilation.

Threading hair removal using a length of specialised thread that is moved over the skin's surface, gripping hairs and removing them from the skin against hair growth.

Threading technique (hand, mouth and neck) hair removal techniques using a length of thread that is held in the hands, mouth or around the neck.

Tissues groups of cells sharing function, shape and size that specialise in carrying out particular functions. These include: epithelial, connective, muscular and nervous.

Toe-nail clippers used to shorten nail length before filing.

Toluenediamine small molecules of permanent dye used in the eyelash/brow tinting service.

Toning lotion a skincare preparation formulated to treat the different skin types and facial characteristics. It is applied to remove all traces of cleanser from the skin. It produces a cooling effect on the skin and has a skin-tightening effect.

Top coat a nail polish product applied over another nail polish to provide shine, additional strength and durability to the finish by reducing peeling and chipping.

Topical hair growth localised hair growth in an area caused by irritation of the skin, such as friction, e.g. a plaster cast on a broken arm can result in increased hair growth, which is soon shed upon cast removal.

Towel steaming an alternative to facial steaming using an electrical facial steamer. Small, clean facial towels are heated in a bowl of warm water or specialised hot towel heater before application to the face to warm, cleanse and stimulate the skin.

Transfers ready-made nail art designs, secured to the nail plate. Transfers are available in water release and self-adhesive for application.

Treatment plan following the client consultation, appropriate treatment objectives are identified, agreed and scheduled to treat the conditions and needs of the client. It includes the areas to be treated, type of treatment, product and equipment to be used, treatment advice and recommendations, client signature and client feedback.

Tweezers small metal tools used to remove body hair by pulling it from the bottom of the hair follicle (small opening in the skin from where the hair grows). There are two main types: one is designed to remove the bulk of the hair – automatic – and the other is designed to remove stray hairs – manual tweezers which are available with various shaped ends.

Values importance of personal beliefs reflected in attitude and standards of behaviour that underpin service delivery.

Vellus hair fine, downy and soft hair; found on the face and body.

Vibrations massage manipulation used to relieve pain and fatigue, stimulate the nerves and produce a sedative effect. The movements are firm and trembling, performed with one or both hands.

Virus the smallest living organisms, too small to be seen under an ordinary microscope. They are considered to be parasites, as they require living tissue to survive. Viruses invade healthy body cells and multiply within the cell. Eventually, the cell walls break down and the virus particles are freed to attack further cells.

Vouchers alternative payment method where pre-payment has already taken place.

Warm wax a system of wax depilation applied by spatula or other mechanical method. Warm wax remains soft at body temperature. It is frequently made of mixtures of glucose syrup and zinc oxide. Honey can be used instead of glucose syrup; this is referred to as honey wax. Additives such as lavender and tea tree oil are popular.

Warm-oil service involves gently heating a small amount of oil and soaking the nails and cuticles in it to nourish the nails and soften the cuticles and surrounding skin.

Wax depilation the temporary removal of excess hair from a body part using wax.

Waxing products cosmetic preparations used with a waxing service that have specific benefits to cleanse the skin, assist in hair removal care, and improve the appearance and healing properties of the skin following hair removal.

Glossary of legislation for beauty therapy

Consumer Protection (Distance Selling) Regulations (2000) these Regulations are derived from a European Directive and cover the supply of goods/services made between suppliers acting in a commercial capacity and consumers. They are concerned with purchases made by telephone, fax, Internet, digital, television and mail order.

Consumer Protection Act (1987) protects consumers from unsafe, defective services and products that do not reach safety standards. It also covers misleading price indications.

Consumer Safety Act (1978) outlines the minimum safety standard to be met for products and reduce the risk to consumers.

Control of Noise at Work Regulations (2005) as an employer a safe working environment should be provided, therefore noise levels should be kept within safe levels. There is a duty to assess any risks in the workplace in this.

Control of Substances Hazardous to Health (COSHH) (2002) these Regulations require employers to identify all hazardous substances used in the workplace and state how they should be stored and handled.

Controlled Waste Regulations (1993) categorises waste types. The Local Authority provides advice on how to dispose of waste types in compliance with the law.

Cosmetic Products (Safety) Regulations (2004) part of consumer legislation that requires that cosmetics and toiletries are safe in their formulation and are safe for use for their intended purpose as a cosmetic and comply with labelling requirements.

Cosmetic Products Enforcement Regulations (2013) requires that cosmetics and toiletries are safe in their formulation and for use for their intended purpose.

Data Protection Act (1998) legislation designed to protect client privacy and confidentiality.

Electricity at Work Regulations (1989) these Regulations state that every piece of equipment in the workplace should be tested every 12 months by a qualified electrician. It covers the installation, maintenance and use of electrical equipment. It is the responsibility of the employer to keep records of the equipment tested and the date it was checked in order to keep it in a safe condition.

Employers Liability (Compulsory Insurance) Act (1969) this provides financial compensation to an employee should they be injured as a result of an accident in the workplace.

Environmental Protection Act (1990) pollution control measures for the disposal of waste to land, water and air.

Equality Act (2010) protects people from being discriminated against in the workplace and in society. This single Act replaced a number of different laws such as the Sex Discrimination Act, Race Relations Act and Disability Discrimination Act.

Hazardous Waste Regulations (2005) these ensure that hazardous waste produced or handled by a business causes no harm or damage, and stipulate that the business has a duty of care.

Health and Safety (Display Screen Equipment) Regulations (1992) these regulations cover the use of visual display units (VDUs) and computer screens. They specify acceptable levels of radiation emissions from the screen and identify correct posture, seating position, permitted working heights and rest periods.

Health and Safety (First Aid) Regulations (1981) legislation which states that workplaces must have first aid provision.

Health and Safety (Information for Employees) Regulations (1989) these regulations require the employer to make health and safety information via notices, posters and leaflets published by the Health and Safety Executive (HSE) available to all employees.

Health and Safety at Work Act (1974) legislation which lays down the minimum standards of health, safety and welfare requirements in each area of the workplace.

Local Government Miscellaneous Provisions Act (1982) legislation that requires that salons offering any form of skin piercing be registered with the local health authority. This registration includes both the beauty therapists who will be carrying out the treatment and the salon premises where it will be carried out.

Management of Health and Safety at Work Regulations (1999) this legislation requires the employer to make formal arrangements for maintaining a safe, secure working environment under the Health and Safety at Work Act. This includes staff training for competently monitoring risk in the workplace, known as a risk assessment.

Manual Handling Operations Regulations (1992) legislation which requires the employer to carry out a risk assessment of all activities undertaken which involve manual handling (lifting and moving objects) the aim being to prevent injury due to poor working practice.

Pensions Act (2008) every employer in the UK must enrol certain employees into a pension scheme and contribute towards it.

Personal Protective Equipment (PPE) Regulations (2002) this legislation requires employers to identify, through a risk assessment, those activities which require special protective equipment to be worn or used. Instruction should be provided on how the personal protective equipment should be used/worn to be effective.

Prices Act (1974) states that prices of goods and services must be displayed to prevent the buyer being misled.

Provision and Use of Work Equipment Regulations (PUWER) (1998) this Regulation lays down important health and safety controls on the provision and use of equipment to prevent risk. They state the duties required by employers and for users.

REACH 2007 is a European Union Regulation concerning the Registration, Evaluation, Authorization and Restriction of CHemicals. It operates alongside COSHH and is designed to improve the information provided by chemical manufacturers through the provision of adequate safety data sheets.

Regulatory Reform (Fire Safety) Order (2005) this legislation requires that the employer or designated 'responsible person' must carry out a risk assessment for the premises in relation to fire evacuation practice and procedures.

Reporting of Injuries, Diseases and Dangerous Occurrences Regulations (RIDDOR) (2013) RIDDOR requires the salon/business to notify the HSE incident contact centre (ICC) in any case of personal injury, disease or dangerous occurrence in the workplace.

Resale Prices Acts (1964 and 1976) the manufacturer can supply a recommended retail price but the seller is not obliged to sell at this price.

Sales and Supply of Goods Act (1994) goods must be as described and of satisfactory quality.

Supply of Goods and Services Act (1982) provides protection when a contract is agreed for the supply of goods or services.

Trade Descriptions Act (1968 and 1972) prohibits the use of false descriptions of goods and services.

Waste Electronic and Electrical Equipment Regulations (2013) place responsibilities on manufacturers, importers, retailers and salons to ensure the safe disposal of electrical products.

Working Time Regulations (1998) these regulations implement the European Work Time Directive into British law and aim to ensure that employees are protected against adverse conditions as a result of working excessively long hours with inadequate rest or disrupted work patterns.

Workplace (Health, Safety and Welfare) Regulations (1992) these Regulations ensure the workplace is a safe, healthy and secure working environment meeting the needs of all employees.

Index